Concise Text of

HISTOLOGY

SECOND EDITION

Concise Text of

HISTOLOGY

SECOND EDITION

WILLIAM J. KRAUSE, Ph.D.
J. HARRY CUTTS, Ph.D.

Department of Anatomy
University of Missouri
School of Medicine
Columbia, Missouri

WILLIAMS & WILKINS
Baltimore • London • Los Angeles • Sydney

Editor: John N. Gardner
Associate Editor: Victoria M. Vaughn
Copy Editor: Stephen C. Siegforth
Design: JoAnne Janowiak
Illustration Planning: Lorraine Wrzosek
Production: Raymond E. Reter

Printed in the United States of America

First Edition, 1981

Library of Congress Cataloging in Publication Data

Krause, William J.
Concise text of histology.

Bibliography: p.
Includes index.
1. Histology. I. Cutts, J. Harry, 1926– . II. Title
QM551.K89 1986 611′.018 85-9325
ISBN 0-683-04785-X

Composed and printed at the
Waverly Press, Inc.

86 87 88 89 90
10 9 8 7 6 5 4 3 2 1

Preface to the Second Edition

In this second edition, as in the first, our aim has been to present a concise coverage of Histology without sacrificing any of the detail that is essential to an understanding of the subject. *Concise Text of Histology* was not conceived of as a "basic" or "introductory" level text; generally, it contains the same kind of information that can be found in the larger "comprehensive" volumes. Thus, while useful for introductory or elementary courses, it also can serve for more advanced presentations of Histology, since we have eliminated only the historical considerations, the more speculative aspects of recent histological research, and the "chatty" garrulities of many of the larger (and smaller) texts.

We have maintained the format of the first edition—the division of the subject matter into learning units preceded by key words, the functional summaries and the arrangement of photographic material into self-standing atlases at the end of each chapter. However, in addition to a complete revision of Chapter 1, the remaining 18 chapters have been updated and a short segment on histogenesis/organogenesis has been added to each chapter. Of the nearly 100 new photographic illustrations, most are devoted to features of development.

We have been gratified by the reception that the text has received, and appreciate the number of positive comments that have been made. We particularly value those of the students for whom this text was especially prepared, and are pleased that so many have found it useful not only in their initial introduction to the discipline of Histology, but in reviewing for National Board and Flex examinations. If we have eased the burden of studying in any way, then we have accomplished our goals.

Acknowledgments

We gratefully acknowledge the permission of S.T.E.M. Laboratories, Inc. for the use of several illustrations in the text, developed previously by W. J. Krause as 2 × 2 color projection slides in conjunction with S.T.E.M. Laboratories, Inc., Kansas City, Missouri.

We also thank the following individual contributors for the illustrative materials they provided:

Allison, O. L., S.T.E.M. Laboratories, Inc., Kansas City, Missouri
Figures 4-12, 4-15, 5-2, 5-3, 5-5, 5-7, 5-11, 12-9, 15-5, 18-22, 18-23, 18-24

Andrews, P., Georgetown University, Washington, D.C.
Figures 16-5 (*American Journal of Anatomy*, vol. 140, 1974, with permission of Wistar Press), 16-7, 16-9, 16-10, 16-21 (*Laboratory Investigation*, vol. 32, 1975, with permission of Williams & Wilkins)

Breipohl, W., Universitätsklinikum des Gesamthochschule, Essen, West Germany
Figure 14-5 (*Cell Tissue Research*, vol. 183, 1977, with permission of Springer-Verlag)

Brink, P. R., State University of New York, Stony Brook, New York
Figures 2-25, 2-26 (*American Journal of Anatomy*, vol. 154, 1979, with permission of Wistar Press)

Campbell, G. T., University of Nebraska, Omaha, Nebraska
Figures 19-6, 19-7, 19-8, 19-9, 19-10

Chan, B. S. T., University of Hong Kong, Shatin, Hong Kong
Figure 5-15 (*Acta Haematologica*, vol. 42, 1969, with permission of S. Karger AG)

Decker, J. D., University of Missouri, Columbia, Missouri
Figures 8-33, 17-30, 17-31, 17-32, 19-27, 19-28, 19-29

Dow, P., University of British Columbia, Vancouver, Canada
Figure 7-15

Dunkerly, G. B., University of Missouri, Columbia, Missouri
Figure 10-7

Engstrom, H. H., Uppsala Universitet, Uppsala, Sweden
Figures 10-13, 10-14, 10-18, 10-19
Feeney-Burns, L., University of Missouri, Columbia, Missouri
Figures 9-11, 9-13, 9-14, 9-20, 9-23
Fujita, T., Niigata University, School of Medicine, Asahi-Machi, Niigata, Japan
Figures 12-20, 12-21, 16-16, (*Archivum Histologicum Japonicum*, vol. 37, 1974, with permission of the Japan Society of Histological Documentation)
Haggis, G. H., Canada Department of Agriculture, Ottawa, Canada
Figures 15-56 (*Laboratory Investigation*, vol. 29, 1973, with permission of Williams & Wilkins)
Hirakow, R., Saitama Medical School, Iruma-Gun, Saitama, Japan
Figures 7-18, 7-19, 7-20, 7-21 (*Electron Microscopic Technique*, with permission of Ishiyaku Publishers, Inc.)
Huxley, H. E., University Medical School, Cambridge, England
Figures 7-12, 7-13 (*Scientific American*, vol. 199, 1958, with permission of Scientific American, Inc.)
King, J. S., Ohio State University, Columbus Ohio
Figures 8-9, 8-18
Kuwabara, T., National Eye Institute, National Institutes of Health, Bethesda, Maryland
Figures 9-21, 9-22 (Greep and Weiss: *Histology*, with permission of McGraw-Hill Book Company)
Murakami, T., Okayama University, Medical School, Okayama, Japan
Figure 16-6 (*Archivum Histologicum Japonicum*, vol. 34, 1972, with permission of the Japan Society of Histological Documentation)
Sherman, D. M., University of Missouri, Columbia, Missouri
Figures 2-19, 19-11, 19-26
Stachura, J., Institute of Pathology, Copernicus Medical Academy, Krakow, Poland
Figures 5-16, 11-9
Stranock, S. D., Merchiston Castle School, Edinburgh, Scotland
Figure 1-20 (*Journal of Anatomy*, vol. 129, 1979, with permission of Cambridge University Press)
Tyson, G. E., Mississippi State University, Mississippi State, Mississippi
Figure 16-8 (*Virchow Arch B. Cell Pathology*, vol. 25, 1977, with permission of Springer-Verlag)
Weisbrode, S. E., Ohio State University, Columbus, Ohio
Figure 4-25 (*Calcified Tissue Research*, vol. 25, 1978, with permission of Springer-Verlag)
American Society of Biological Chemists, Inc.
Figure 5-14 (*Journal of Biological Chemistry*, vol. 179, 1949)

We also acknowledge the following publishers for permission to use illustrative materials that we have previously published:
Archivum Histologicum Japonicum
Figure 15-75 (vol. 43, 1980)
British Medical Association
Figure 15-27 (*British Medical Journal*, vol. 2, 1972)
Cambridge University Press
Figures (all from the *Journal of Anatomy*) 1-23 (vol. 123, 1977), 2-23 (vol. 104, 1969), 2-24 (vol. 125, 1978), 2-36 and 2-37 (vol. 122, 1976), 15-59 (vol. 120, 1975), 16-15, 16-18, 16-22 (vol. 129 1979), 15-77, 15-78, 15-79, 15-80, 15-82 (vol. 122, 1976), 15-86

(vol. 123, 1977), 16-29, 16-30, 16-31, 16-32, 16-33, 16-34, 16-35, 16-36, 16-37, 16-38, 16-39 (vol. 129, 1979)

S. Karger AG

Figures 2-14, 5-14 (*Acta Anatomica*, vol. 92, 1975), 15-90, 15-96, 15-97 (*Acta Anatomica*, vol. 101, 1978), 8-31 (*Acta Anatomica*, vol. 120, 1984)

Wistar Institute Press

Figures 1-12 (*American Journal of Anatomy*, vol. 132, 1971), 2-38 and 6-23 (*Journal of Morphology*, vol. 140, 1973)

Use of the Text

To understand Histology, it is essential to learn a specialized vocabulary and to assimilate a rather large body of facts. Learning, as distinct from rote memorization, depends to a great degree on repetition and reinforcement and is made easier if the material to be learned can be presented in discrete, manageable segments. The format of *Concise Text of Histology* has been designed specifically to meet these requirements and if used properly, will enable the student to master the discipline quickly and efficiently. From our experience, the text can be used most effectively by adopting a study plan similar to that suggested below.

1. Read the key words carefully: they introduce the main features of the subject to be discussed and provide the basic vocabulary for that unit. As each segment is read, again note the key words (identified by **boldface** print) and how they contribute to the discussion.

2. After completing the text segment, return to the key words, using them as "prompts" to recall the details of the material just read.

3. As each chapter is completed, use the key word segments for rapid review of all the material covered. If a key word fails to prompt a response, it and its associated text can be found quickly from the **boldface** type in the appropriate segment.

4. The functional summaries briefly outline the structural/functional relationships and serve to draw the information together and to provide an additional review of the topic.

5. The developmental summaries describe how the adult tissues "got to be the way they are" and provide another means of reinforcement for an understanding of organ and tissue structure.

6. When study of the descriptive material has been completed, the atlases at the end of each chapter provide a final pictorial review of structure. Each is introduced by a table in which the key points for identification of an organ/tissue are presented, offering the briefest possible summary. The atlases also are useful as laboratory guides and can be used when examining histological preparations with the microscope.

7. As a final short review, an appendix has been added in which are presented a few short tables that outline the basic differences of several structures that frequently present difficulties in recognition. They, too, can be used, in conjunction with the atlas portions, as laboratory guides for the identification of tissues.

Contents

1

The Cell

Multicellular organisms are composed of two distinct structural elements: cells and those products of cells that form the intercellular substances. Cells are the fundamental units of living material and show a variety of functional specializations that are necessary for the survival of the organism. Each cell is a distinct entity, contains all the machinery for independent existence, and is separated from its external environment by a limiting membrane.

PROTOPLASM

KEY WORDS: protein, carbohydrate, lipid, nucleic acids, inorganic materials, water

The living substance of a cell, protoplasm, consists of protein, carbohydrate, lipid, nucleic acids, and inorganic materials, dispersed in water to form a complex, semifluid gel. The consistency of protoplasm varies in different cells and within a cell may change from a viscous to a more fluid state.

Protein, alone or in combination with lipid or carbohydrate, forms the major structural component of the cell and the intercellular substances. Enzymes and many hormones are proteins. The major **carbohydrates** are glucose, which provides the chief source of energy in mammalian cells, and glycogen, the storage form of glucose. Complexes of carbohydrates and proteins form the main constituents of the intercellular substances that bind cells together. Other carbohydrate-protein complexes form some enzymes and antibodies. **Lipids** not only serve as an energy source but also have important structural functions and are major components of the membrane systems of cells.

Two classes of **nucleic acids** can be distinguished. Deoxyribonucleic acid (DNA) is found mainly in the nucleus, where it forms the genetic material, whereas ribonucleic acid (RNA) is present in both the nucleus and the cytoplasm. Ribonucleic acid carries information from the nucleus to the cytoplasm and serves as a template for synthesis of proteins by the cell.

The **inorganic materials** are as much an integral component of protoplasm as are proteins, carbohydrates and lipids; without them physiological processes are impossible. Among the inorganic constituents are: calcium, potassium, sodium and magnesium as carbonates, chlorides, phosphates and sulfates; small quantities of iron, copper and iodine; and trace elements such as cobalt, manganese, zinc and other metals. The inorganic constituents have many diverse functions. Maintenance of intercellular and extracellular osmotic pressures, transmission of nerve impulses, contraction of muscle, adhesiveness of cells, activation of enzymes, transport of oxygen and the rigidity of tissues such as bone all depend on the presence of inorganic materials.

Water makes up about 75% of protoplasm. Part of the water content is free and available as a solvent for various metabolic processes and part is bound to protein.

Properties of Protoplasm

KEY WORDS: irritability, conductivity, contractility, absorption, metabolism, secretion and excretion, growth and reproduction

Protoplasm is characterized by several physiological properties that distinguish it from inanimate material. All living cells show these properties, but in some a particular property may be emphasized.

Irritability is a fundamental property of all living cells and refers to their ability to respond to a stimulus.

Conductivity refers to the ability of a cell to transmit a stimulus from the point of origin to another point on the cell surface, or to other cells. Conductivity also is a property of all cells but, like irritability, shows its greatest development in nerve tissue.

Contractility is the ability of a cell to change its shape in response to a stimulus and generally is manifested by a shortening of the cell in some direction. This property is especially prominent in muscle.

Absorption involves the transfer of materials across the cell membrane into the interior of the cell, where it might be used in some manner. All cells show the ability to absorb materials, some very selectively.

Metabolism refers to the ability of the cell to break down absorbed materials and produce energy.

Secretion is the process by which the cell elaborates and releases materials for use elsewhere. **Excretion**, on the other hand, is the elimination from the cell of the waste products of metabolism.

Growth and Reproduction

Growth of an organism can occur by increasing the amount of protoplasm in existing cells or by increasing the number of cells. There are limits to the size a cell can attain without sacrificing the efficiency with which nutrients and oxygen reach the interior of the cell. Beyond the maximum size, an increase in protoplasm is brought about by cell division.

ORGANIZATION OF CELLS

KEY WORDS: nucleus, nuclear envelope, cytoplasm, plasmalemma (cell membrane), organelles, inclusions, cytoplasmic matrix (hyaloplasm), karyolymph

Although cells differ in size, shape and function, the protoplasm of each cell consists of two major components, nucleus and cytoplasm. The **nucleus** contains the hereditary or genetic material and is completely surrounded by cytoplasm, from which it is separated by a **nuclear envelope**. The **cytoplasm** is limited by the **plasmalemma (cell membrane)**, which separates the cell from the external environment. Contained within the cytoplasm are several structures that may be classified as organelles or as inclusions. **Organelles** are highly organized, living structural units of the cytoplasm which perform specific functions in the cell. In contrast, **inclusions** generally represent cell products or metabolites that often are transitory in nature. The majority, but not all, of the organelles are membranous structures whose size and concentration vary with the type and activity of the cell. The different organelles tend to be localized within discrete areas of the cytoplasm so that they and the metabolic processes associated with them remain separated from other components of the cell.

The organelles and inclusions are suspended in an amorphous medium called the **cytoplasmic matrix (hyaloplasm).** The nuclear material also is suspended in a structureless ground material that has been called **karyolymph**, but other than the difference in their locations, karyolymph and hyaloplasm appear to be equivalent.

Cytoplasmic Organelles

Organelles are specialized units of the cell that perform specific functions and constitute part of the living substance of a cell. Included as organelles are cytoplasmic structures such as the plasmalemma, granular and agranular forms of endoplasmic reticulum, ribosomes, Golgi complex, mitochondria, lysosomes, peroxisomes, filaments, microtubules and centrioles. Many organelles are limited by membranes similar in structure to those which form the boundary of the cell itself. These membranes, including the cell membrane, are metabolically active sheets that are essential to the life of the cell. In electron micrographs the membranes show a trilaminar structure consisting of inner and outer dense lines separated by a light zone. Because the trilaminar structure is representative of all biological membranes of a cell, it has been called a unit membrane. The thickness of the unit membrane varies from organelle to organelle and generally is greatest where it forms the plasmalemma. While the membranes appear to show only minor variations among different organelles, they vary considerably in chemical composition, enzymatic properties and functions.

Plasmalemma (Cell Membrane)

KEY WORDS: unit membrane, phospholipid bilayer, intrinsic protein, glycocalyx, P-Face, E-Face, phagocytosis, endocytosis, pinocytosis, micropinocytosis, fluid-phase micropinocytosis, adsorptive micropinocytosis, coated pits, coated vesicles, clathrin, exocytosis

Each cell is enclosed by a plasmalemma which measures about 8 to 10 nm in thickness and shows the typical trilaminar appearance of the **unit membrane**. It appears as two dense lines, each 3 nm wide, separated by a 2- to 4-nm clear zone. The cell membrane is composed of proteins, lipids and carbohydrates; the lipids are mainly phospholipid with some neutral fat and cholesterol-like substances. Structurally, the cell membrane is thought to consist of a **phospholipid bilayer** in which the hydrocarbon chains are directed inward and the polar groups are directed outward. **Intrinsic proteins** within the phospholipid bilayer may extend through the full thickness of the membrane and serve as sites for transmembrane transport, or may lie only partially within the bilipid layer. Other proteins are thought to be present on the external surface, which also may be coated by a polysaccharide material that forms the **glycocalyx.** This coat varies in thickness, depending on the type of cell with which it is associated.

Freeze-fracture splits the cell membrane between the hydrocarbon chains of the phospholipid bilayers, permitting observation of the interior of the plasmalemma (Fig. 1-1); the outwardly directed, inner half membrane closest to the cytoplasm is the **P-face**, which generally shows numerous globular particles, 6 to 9 nm in diameter. The **E-face**, closest to the external environment, is relatively smooth. Only occasional particles are present which are thought to be proteins that reside within the cell membrane.

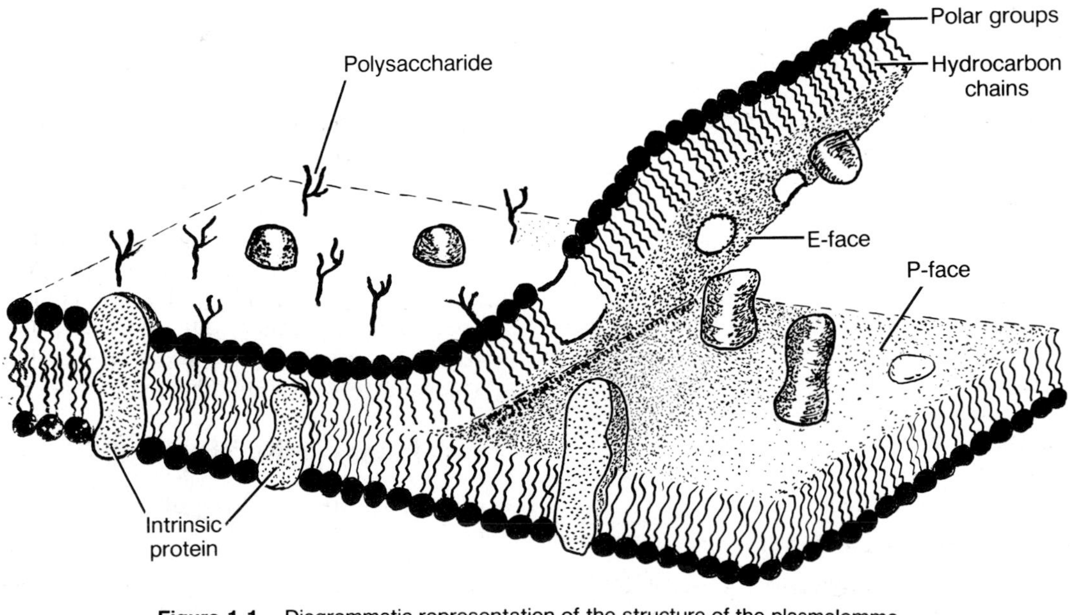

Figure 1-1. Diagrammatic representation of the structure of the plasmalemma.

The cell membrane is selectively permeable and plays an active role in bringing material into, or discharging it from, the cell. **Phagocytosis** is a form of endocytosis in which particulate matter is taken into a cell. During the **attachment phase**, particles bind to receptors on the cell surface, while in the **ingestion phase** the cytoplasm forms pseudopods which flow around the particles to engulf them and take them into the cell in membrane-bound vacuoles. In a similar fashion, fluid may be incorporated into the cell in small cytoplasmic vesicles, in a process called **pinocytosis.** Both phagocytosis and pinocytosis can be seen by light microscopy. Some materials may enter the cell in even smaller vesicles that are formed by minute invaginations of the cell surface. This process, called **micropinocytosis**, is visible only with the electron microscope. A nonselective fluid phase and a selective adsorptive type of micropinocytosis have been recognized. In most cells, **fluid-phase micropinocytosis** occurs with the formation of small vesicles from the plasmalemma. The vesicles, which contain fluid and anything dispersed in the fluid, traverse the cytoplasm to the opposite side of the cell, where they discharge their contents (Fig. 1-2*A*).

Adsorptive micropinocytosis is the selective uptake of specific macromolecules at certain receptor binding sites in the cell membrane. This receptor-mediated micropinocytosis is important in the ingestion of regulatory and nutritional proteins. Short, bristle-like projections may occur on the cytoplasmic surface at these sites, forming **coated pits**, from which **coated vesicles** arise (Fig. 1-2*B*). The cytoplasmic surfaces of the vesicles are covered by **clathrin**, a protein that appears as radiating spikes giving a fuzzy appearance to the vesicles. Clathrin is thought to prevent fusion of coated vesicles with membranous organelles; when the protein coat is lost, the vesicles fuse with lysosomes, Golgi complexes, other vesicles or cell membranes.

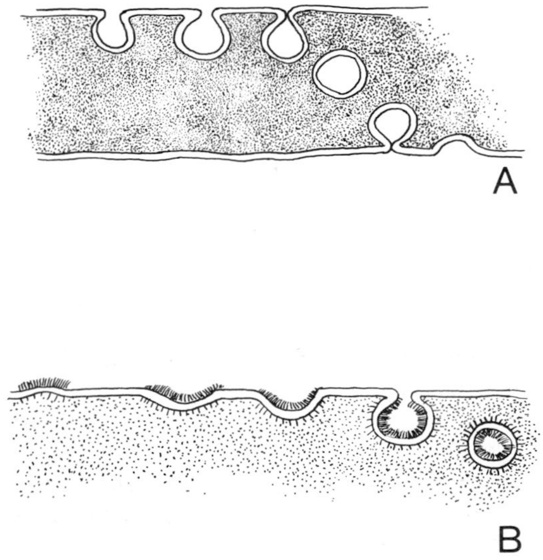

Figure 1-2. *A*, Diagrammatic representation of fluid-phase micropinocytosis. *B*, Diagrammatic representation of adsorptive micropinocytosis via coated vesicles.

Secretory granules are released from the cell by **exocytosis**, a process in which the limiting membranes of the secretory granules fuse with the plasmalemma before discharging the secretory material.

Endoplasmic Reticulum

KEY WORDS: tubules, cisternae, granular endoplasmic reticulum, ribosomes, smooth endoplasmic reticulum

The cytoplasm of nearly all cells contains a continuous, irregular network of membrane-bound channels called the endoplasmic reticulum. Typically, this organelle appears as anastomosing **tubules** but the membranes also form parallel, flattened saccules known as **cisternae**. Small vesicles, not attached to tubules or cisternae, may be present also and are considered to be part of the endoplasmic reticulum. Smooth and rough (granular) forms of endoplasmic reticulum can be distinguished.

Granular (rough) endoplasmic reticulum (GER; Fig. 1-3) usually consists of an array of flattened cisternae bounded by a membrane. The outer surface is studded with numerous particles of ribonucleoprotein, the **ribosomes**, which synthesize those proteins that, for the most part, are to be secreted by the cell. Synthesized on the external surface of the rough endoplasmic reticulum, the proteins then enter the lumen of the reticulum, where they are isolated from the surrounding cytoplasm.

Smooth endoplasmic reticulum (SER; Fig. 1-4) lacks ribosomes. It consists primarily of a system of interconnecting tubules without cisternae.

In most cells, one form of endoplasmic reticulum usually predominates. Protein-se-

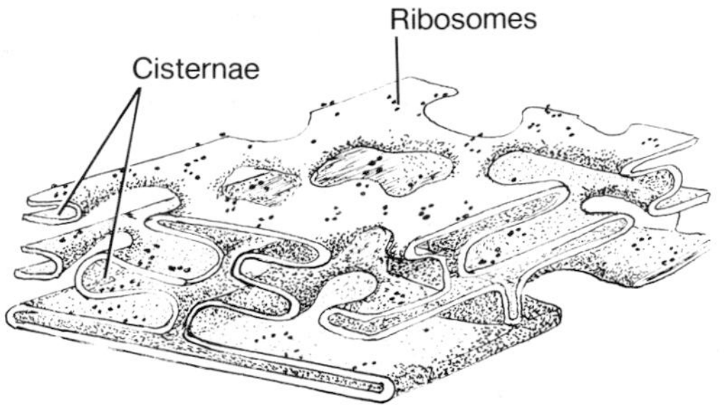

Figure 1-3. Diagrammatic representation of rough endoplasmic reticulum.

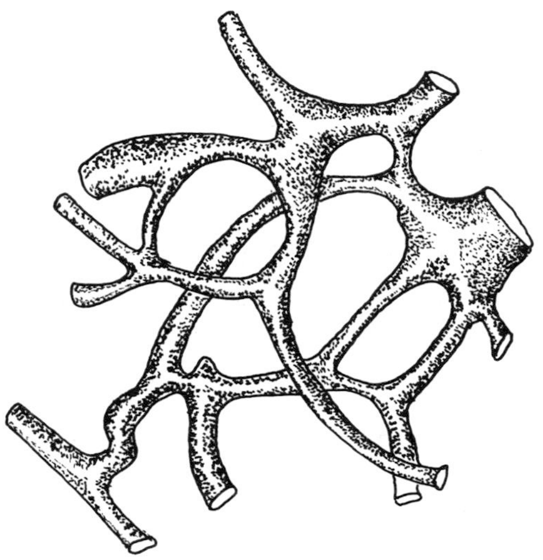

Figure 1-4. Diagrammatic representation of smooth endoplasmic reticulum.

creting cells such as pancreatic acinar cells or plasma cells, are characterized by an abundance of granular endoplasmic reticulum, whereas in cells that secrete steroid hormones, the smooth type predominates. In still other cells, such as liver cells, both types of endoplasmic reticulum are present in nearly equal amounts and may be continuous. Although the granular form of endoplasmic reticulum is known to be involved in the synthesis of protein, the exact function or functions of the smooth endoplasmic reticulum remain obscure. It has been implicated in different functions in different cells: synthesis of steroid hormones in certain endocrine cells, detoxification of drugs by liver cells, metabolism of lipid and cholesterol. It also is implicated in the release and recapture of calcium ions during the contraction and relaxation of striated muscle.

Ribosomes

KEY WORDS: ribonucleoprotein, free ribosomes, polyribosomes (polysomes), messenger RNA, protein synthesis, transfer RNA

Ribosomes are small, uniformly sized particles of **ribonucleoprotein**, 12 to 15 nm in diameter, composed of large and small subunits. They may be attached to the membranes of the endoplasmic reticulum or be present as **free ribosomes** suspended in the cytoplasm with no association with membranes. Free ribosomes often occur in clusters to form **polyribosomes (polysomes)**, in which the individual ribosomes are united by a thread of ribonucleic acid called **messenger RNA**.

Free ribosomes also are sites of **protein synthesis**, the protein formed being used by the cell itself rather than secreted. Individual free ribosomes are not active; it is only when they are attached to messenger RNA to form polysomes that ribosomes become active in protein synthesis. Similarly, ribosomes on the endoplasmic reticulum must be associated with messenger RNA before they engage in the synthesis of proteins.

Messenger RNA (mRNA) is formed in the nucleus on a template of uncoiled deoxyribonucleic acid. It contains a coded message that specifies the sequence in which amino acids are to be incorporated into the newly forming protein. During protein synthesis, mRNA enters the cytoplasm where it attaches to ribosomes which move along the messenger RNA, translating the code and assembling the amino acids in the proper order. On reaching the end of the mRNA, ribosomes detach and simultaneously release the newly synthesized protein molecule. Amino acids are brought to the ribosomes for incorporation into the protein by yet another form of ribonucleic acid, the **transfer RNA** (tRNA). There is a specific tRNA for each amino acid. Ribosomal and transfer RNA are thought to originate in the nucleolar region of the nucleus.

Golgi Complex

KEY WORDS: negative image, saccules, forming face, maturing face, transport vesicles, condensing vacuoles, secretory granules

The Golgi complex (Golgi apparatus; Fig. 1-5) does not stain in ordinary histological preparations, nor is it visible in living cells. However, it sometimes appears as a **negative image**—a nonstaining area of the cytoplasm usually located close to the nucleus. The size and appearance of the Golgi complex varies with the type and activity of the cell: it may be small and compact or large and net-like. In some cells, multiple Golgi complexes may be present.

In electron micrographs the Golgi complex is seen to consist of several flattened **saccules** or cisternae, each of which is limited by a smooth membrane. The saccules are disc-shaped, slightly curved and often appear to be compressed near the center and dilated at the edges. The saccules are arranged in stacks and because of their curvatures, the Golgi complex has convex and concave faces. The convex surface usually is directed toward the nucleus and is called the **forming face**; the concave or **maturing face** is oriented toward the cell membrane.

The saccules within the Golgi stack are separated by spaces 20 to 30 nm in width, but their cavities communicate by slender channels that extend between adjacent saccules. The convex surface of the Golgi apparatus is associated with numerous small vesicles and at this face the outer saccule is perforated by many small fenestrations. The saccules at the convex surface tend to be more dilated than those at the concave surface (Fig. 1-5).

Secretory products are concentrated in the Golgi complex, whose size varies with the activity of the cell. In protein-secreting cells, peptides first accumulate within the lumen of the rough endoplasmic reticulum (RER) and then are transported to the Golgi complex in small **transport vesicles**. Formed from ribosome free areas of the rough endoplasmic reticulum adjacent to the Golgi, the vesicles carry small quantities of protein to the Golgi complex, where they coalesce with and contribute membrane to the developing outer saccule at the forming face. Proteins accumulate within the cisternae of the Golgi membranes and are concentrated as they pass through the Golgi complex. At the maturing face, the saccules expand and bud off to form the limiting membranes that enclose the protein in structures known as **condensing vacuoles**. Addition of new membrane to the forming face balances the loss of membrane from the maturing face. Secre-

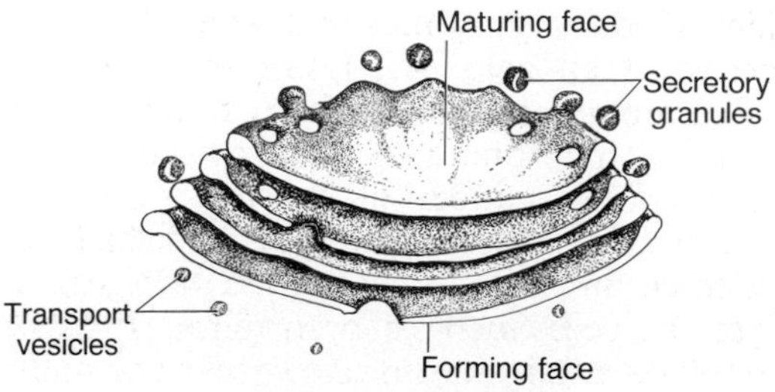

Figure 1-5. Diagrammatic representation of the Golgi complex.

tory materials within the vacuoles become more concentrated and the condensing vacuoles eventually mature into **secretory granules**. Golgi membranes are capable of synthesizing carbohydrate and depending on the cell type, protein may be complexed to newly synthesized carbohydrate to form a glycoprotein. Proteins synthesized by the RER may be complexed to lipids that enter the Golgi cisternae from the SER: the resulting lipoproteins are released by the Golgi as membrane-bound granules.

During release of secretory products, the membranes of the secretory granules fuse with the plasmalemma and become incorporated into the cell membrane. The membrane of secretory granules must have some special properties since they fuse specifically with the plasmalemma and not with the membranes of other organelles. From synthesis to exocytosis, secretory material is enclosed by membranes and thus is isolated from the cytoplasmic matrix.

There appears to be a continuous movement of membrane throughout the cell, from endoplasmic reticulum to transport vesicles to Golgi complex to secretory granules and then to the plasmalemma. Internalization of plasmalemma occurs during phagocytosis, pinocytosis and micropinocytosis.

Lysosomes

KEY WORDS: acid hydrolases, autolysis, primary lysosomes, secondary lysosomes, phagocytosis, phagosome, heterophagic vacuole, residual body, heterophagy, autophagy, autophagic vacuole, cytolysosome, multivesicular body

Lysosomes are small, membrane-bound, dense bodies measuring 0.2 to 0.5 μm in diameter. More than 50 enzymes have been identified in lysosomes and, since they are active at an acid pH, lysosomal enzymes often are referred to as **acid hydrolases**. The limiting membrane of the lysosomes protects the remainder of the cell from the effects of the contained enzymes which, if released into the cytoplasm, would digest or lyse the cell. Such an occurrence is called **autolysis** and is presumed to occur normally during resorption of tadpole tails at metamorphosis and in regression of the mesonephros in kidney development or of mammary tissue after the cessation of lactation. Increased lysosomal activity occurs during the regression of some tumors.

Lysosomes are one of the few organelles that cannot be identified with confidence solely on their morphology. Their appearance varies according to the state in which they occur and their association with cell structures or material brought into the cell. **Primary lysosomes** are those that have been newly released at the Golgi complex and have not engaged in digestive activities. The enzymes of the primary lysosomes are synthesized in the granular endoplasmic reticulum, transported to the Golgi complex and released from the maturing face as membrane-bound, electron-dense granules. Primary lysosomes are formed in a manner similar to that of secretory granules, but lysosomes usually are not secreted and remain within the cell. Some evidence suggests that primary lysosomes may form directly from smooth areas of the RER in the region of the Golgi complex.

Secondary lysosomes are vacuolar structures that represent the sites of past or current lysosomal activity and include heterophagic vacuoles, autophagic vacuoles and residual bodies. The relationships of these structures is best understood from a description of the processes involved in **phagocytosis** (Fig. 1-6).

Some cells, such as macrophages and some granular leukocytes of the blood, have a special capacity to engulf extracellular materials (such as bacteria) and destroy them. The process involves invagination of the cell membrane and containment of the material in a membrane-bound vacuole. Thus, the extracellular material taken into the cell is

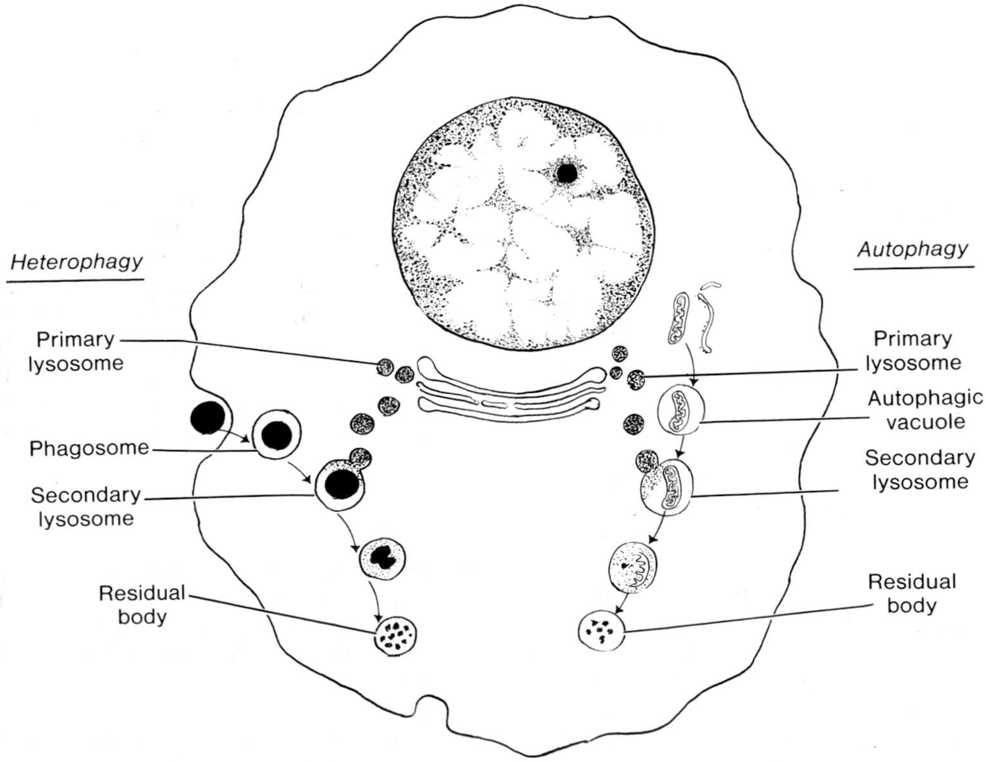

Figure 1-6. Schematic representation of autophagy and heterophagy.

sequestered in a vacuole called a **phagosome** and remains isolated from the cytoplasm. As the phagosome moves through the cytoplasm of the cell, it encounters a primary lysosome. The membranes of the two structures fuse and the enzymes of the lysosome are discharged into the phagosome. The combined primary lysosome and phagosome is now called a **heterophagic vacuole**, a type of secondary lysosome. The material within the heterophagic vacuole is digested by the lysosomal enzymes and any useful materials are transferred into the cytoplasm for use by the cell. Nondegradable materials, such as some dye particles, asbestos fibers, silica, carbon or other nondigestible substances, may remain within the vacuole, now called a **residual body**. Residual bodies are another form of secondary lysosomes which are thought by some to be eliminated from the cell by exocytosis. However, in many cells the residual bodies accumulate and persist for long periods of time. The process by which substances are taken into the cell from the external environment and broken down by lysosomal activity is referred to as **heterophagy**.

In contrast, **autophagy** refers to the lysosomal breakdown of cytoplasmic organelles in normal, viable cells (Fig. 1-6). The lysosomal system is involved in the destruction of worn or damaged organelles and the remodeling of the cytoplasm. During the process a portion of the cytoplasm containing aged or damaged organelles becomes surrounded by a membrane thought to be derived from the smooth endoplasmic reticulum. The membranous vacuole fuses with a primary lysosome to form still another type of secondary lysosome called an **autophagic vacuole** or **cytolysosome**. The fate of the materials within the autophagic vacuoles (which may be the cell's own mitochondria, ribosomes, endoplasmic reticulum, etc.) is the same as that in heterophagic vacuoles and again results in the formation of residual bodies. In many cells the indigestible components within autophagic vacuoles form a brownish material called lipofuscin pigment, the amount of which increases with age.

Another form of lysosome is the **multivesicular body**. It is a membrane-bound vacuolar structure, 0.5 to 0.8 μm in diameter, that contains several small, clear vesicles. The origin, function and exact relationship to other lysosomes is not known.

Peroxisomes

KEY WORDS: microbodies, hydrogen peroxide, glyconeogenesis

Peroxisomes or microbodies are yet another class of membrane-bound organelles. Usually larger than lysosomes, they vary in internal structure, which might be crystalline or dense. Peroxisomes contain enzymes such as urate oxidase and D-amino acid oxidase that produce **hydrogen peroxide** which, although essential for many cellular functions and capable of destroying micro-organisms, in excess is lethal to cells. Peroxisomes contain the enzyme catalase which degrades hydrogen peroxide to water. Peroxisomes have been implicated in glyconeogenesis and also are abundant in cells involved in steroid synthesis and cholesterol metabolism: their role in these activities is not understood.

Formation of peroxisomes does not appear to involve the Golgi complex. Inactive precursors of the peroxisomal enzymes are thought to be formed on free ribosomes and their limiting membrane is believed to be derived by a budding-off of vesicles from smooth regions of the rough endoplasmic reticulum.

Mitochondria

KEY WORDS: outer mitochondrial membrane, inner mitochondrial membrane, cristae, membrane space, intracristal space, intercristal space, mitochondrial matrix, Krebs cycle, elementary particle, electron transfer, deoxyribonucleic acid, ribonucleoprotein, matrix granule

Mitochondria are membranous structures that play a vital role in the production of the energy required by cells. They are visible in living cells examined by phase contrast microscopy and can be stained in fixed tissues where they appear as rods or thin filaments. They are not usually seen in routine tissue sections because of the lipid solvents used during tissue preparation.

Ultrastructurally, mitochondria show a variety of shapes and sizes, but all are enclosed by two membranes, each of which has the typical trilaminar substructure (Fig. 1-7). The **outer mitochondrial membrane** is a continuous, smooth structure that com-

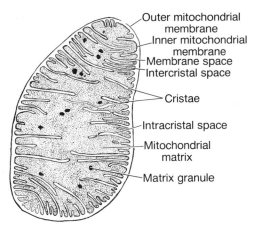

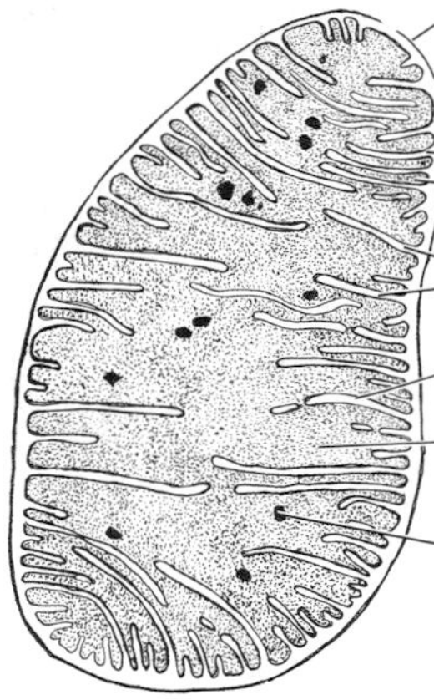

Figure 1-7. Structure of a mitochondrion.

pletely envelopes the organelle. An **inner mitochondrial membrane** runs parallel to the outer membrane but is thrown into numerous folds, the **cristae**, that extend into the interior of the mitochondrion. The narrow space between the inner and outer mitochondrial membranes, the **membrane space**, is continuous with the small **intracristal space** within each crista. The inner mitochondrial membrane surrounds the larger **intercristal space** that contains a slightly more electron dense material known as the **mitochondrial matrix**. Enzymes of the **Krebs cycle**, responsible for the final breakdown of fatty acids, monosugars and some amino acids, reside within the mitochondrial matrix.

The cristae greatly increase the surface area of the inner mitochondrial membrane and may be shelf-like or tubular in shape; the tubular form is seen most often in cells that are involved in steroid synthesis. The inner mitochondrial membrane is the site of many enzymatic reactions and is studded with club-shaped structures called **elementary particles**. These consist of a spherical head, 9 to 10 nm in diameter, attached to the inner mitochondrial membrane by a narrow stalk 5 nm in length. Phosphorylating enzymes and enzymes of the **electron transfer system** are located either on the elementary particles or within the inner mitochondrial membranes that form the cristae. Energy released by the enzymes operating in Krebs cycle is accepted by the electron transfer system of cytochromes and then incorporated into high energy phosphate compounds such as adenosine triphosphate (ATP), the primary source of energy for the activities carried out by the cell. Thus, a primary function of mitochondria is to synthesize ATP which is thought to diffuse into the adjacent cytoplasm.

Mitochondria are unique among organelles since they contain their own complement of **deoxyribonucleic acid** (DNA) and are capable of self-replication. Mitochondrial DNA differs from nuclear DNA in its lower molecular weight and is unusual in that it consists of branched filaments of variable thickness, arranged in a circular manner.

The mitochondrial matrix also contains small particles of **ribonucleoprotein**, 12 nm in diameter, that are similar in structure and function to cytoplasmic ribosomes. Scattered throughout the mitochondrial matrix are the more conspicuous **matrix granules**, which measure 30 to 50 nm in diameter. These granules are thought to regulate the internal ionic environment of the mitochondrion. In addition to the enzymes of Krebs cycle, enzymes involved in protein and lipid synthesis are present in the mitochondrial matrix of some cell types. Mitochondria also contain several enzymes associated with the synthesis of steroid hormones and at several steps in the synthetic pathway, substrate enters the mitochondrion for processing, then returns to the cytoplasm for the completion of additional steps. More than 50 enzymes have been localized to mitochondria.

Annulate Lamellae

This membranous organelle consists of cisternae arranged in parallel to form stacks. At regular intervals along their lengths, the cisternae show numerous small pores that appear to be closed by thin, electron dense diaphragms. The cisternae are spaced uniformly throughout the stack and frequently, the pores is successive cisternae are aligned. Annulate lamellae often occupy a perinucler position and might be continuous with elements of rough endoplasmic reticulum. They have been seen in germ cells, in various somatic cells and in tumor cells but their origin and function is unknown.

Cytoplasmic Filaments

KEY WORDS: actin, myosin, microfilaments, intermediate filaments, tonofilaments

Cytoplasmic filaments are responsible for contractility, a property shown to some degree by almost all cells. Filaments are best developed in muscle cells, where the proteins **actin** and **myosin** form two different types of filaments. These interact with one another, chemically and mechanically, to produce a shortening of the muscle cell.

Two types of intracellular filaments are present in nonmuscle cells also. One, the **microfilament**, has about the same diameter (7 nm) as actin, and in most cell types is located immediately beneath the plasmalemma. Actin has been identified in microfilaments by chemical means. Microfilaments may be organized into parallel bundles or may be randomly distributed to form an extensive, interwoven network. They function in cell locomotion and in the invagination of the plasmalemma during endocytosis, and form the contraction ring of dividing cells. A thin layer of microfilaments (actin) may occur along the cytoplasmic surface of the cell membrane and confer mobility to the plasmalemma, as in ruffling of the cell membrane.

The second type of filament, **tonofilaments** or **immediate filaments** are thicker, measuring 9 to 12 nm in diameter. They form a more diverse population of filaments and may be present as individual strands or loose bundles. Tonofilaments often are attached to the internal surface of the plasmalemma at cell junctions and are thought to contribute to the cytoskeleton of the cell and to provide support. Their chemical nature is unknown. Microfilaments and tonofilaments may both occur in the same cell.

Microtubules

KEY WORDS: tubulin, centrioles, cilia, flagella

Microtubules are straight or slightly curved, nonbranching tubules measuring 21 to 25 nm in diameter and several micrometers in length. Their walls, about 6 nm thick, are made up of 13 globular units, each 4 to 5 nm in diameter, arranged in a helix. The central zone is electron lucent and thus, the tubule appears to be hollow. Microtubules are composed primarily of the protein **tubulin** which occurs in *a* and *b* forms. Small quantities of high molecular weight proteins (microtubule-associated proteins, or MAPs) also have been isolated.

Microtubules usually are scarce in nondividing cells but are present in large numbers in dividing cells, where they make up the mitotic spindle. After the cell has divided, most of the microtubules disappear. In interphase cells, microtubules form prominent components of **centrioles**, **cilia** and **flagella**, contribute to the cytoskeleton of some cells and, as in platelets and nucleated red cells of nonmammalian species, form stiffening elements that help maintain the cell shape. In some cells, such as nerve cells, microtubules are believed to be important for transport of material from one region of the cytoplasm to another. A transient increase in the number of microtubules is seen in nondividing cells during changes in shape associated with cell movement and during differentiation. Thus, microtubules are important cytoplasmic structures that appear to be involved in cell division, cell movement and differentiation, intracellular transport of material and contribute to the cytoskeleton. Exactly how they serve these functions is unknown.

Centrioles

KEY WORDS: centrosome, diplosome, microtubules, triplet, procentriole, basal body, ciliogenesis

Under the light microscope, centrioles appear as minute rods or granules usually located near the nucleus in a specialized region of the cytoplasm called the **centrosome**. In some cells the centrioles might be located between the nucleus and the free surface of the cell at some distance from the nucleus. Two centrioles usually are present in the nondividing cell and together form the **diplosome**. Multinucleated cells contain several centrioles.

As seen in electron micrographs, the two centrioles that make up the diplosome are oriented perpendicularly to each other. The wall of each centriole consists of nine subunits, each of which is made up of three fused **microtubules**; the subunits are referred to as **triplets**. The nine sets of triplets are so arranged in the centriolar wall that they resemble a pinwheel when seen in cross section. The microtubules within each triplet are called the A, B and C microtubules, the innermost being the A microtubule, the central tubule the B, and the most peripheral tubule the C microtubule (Fig. 1-8). The clear center of the centriole contains a thin filament that passes in a helix immediately adjacent to the inner surface of the centriolar wall.

Centrioles are self-replicating organelles that duplicate just before cell division. A new centriole, called a **procentriole**, forms at right angles to each of the parent centrioles. Initially, the wall of the procentriole consists of a ring of amorphous material, with no microtubules. As the procentriole elongates by addition of material at its distal end, microtubules appear in the wall and the new structure assumes the configuration of the parent centriole. Immediately after duplication each parent centriole, together with a newly formed daughter centriole, migrates to the opposite poles of the cell, where they function in the development of the mitotic spindle.

A centriole can migrate close to the surface of the cell to form the **basal body**, from which may arise a cilium or flagellum: these also are microtubular structures. During the process of **ciliogenesis**, centrioles might arise de novo from fibrogranular material, in the absence of a parent centriole. Preceisely how the centriole initiates and directs the formation of microtubules in the mitotic apparatus, cilia and flagella is unknown.

Cytoplasmic Inclusions

Inclusions are nonliving elements found in the cytoplasm and include many diverse materials such as pigment granules, glycogen, lipid droplets, crystals and secretory granules. They are not essential to the life or functioning of the cell and represent metabolic products, storage materials or foreign substances taken into the cell from the environment.

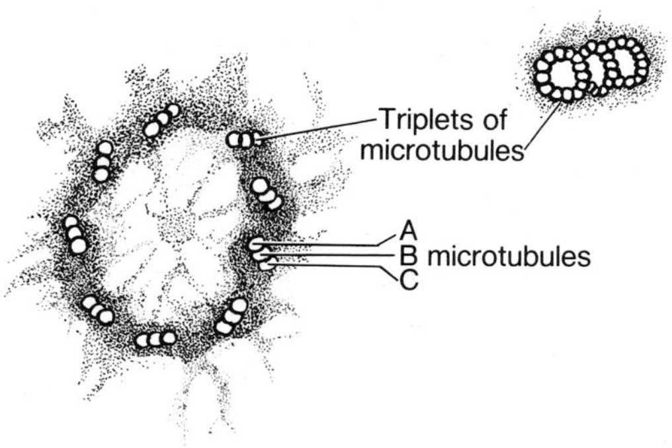

Figure 1-8. Diagrammatic representation of a centriole seen in cross section.

Pigment Granules

KEY WORDS: melanin, melanosomes, hemosiderin, lipofuscin

Naturally occurring pigments in man include melanin, hemosiderin and lipofuscin, in which the color is inherent in the inclusions and is not the result of staining methods. **Melanin** is contained within **melanosomes**, membrane-bound granules found in melanocytes. In man, this particular cell type chiefly occurs in the deep layers of the epidermis, where it contributes to the color of the skin. The pigment epithelium of the retina and iris and certain cells of the brain also contain melanin.

Hemosiderin is a golden brown pigment derived from the breakdown of hemoglobin present in red blood cells. Phagocytic cells of the liver, bone marrow and spleen normally contain this type of pigment.

Lipofuscin is found in many cells throughout the body, particularly in older persons. Sometimes called the "wear and tear" pigment, lipofuscin is light brown in color, increases with age and represents the end product of lysosomal activity.

Glycogen

KEY WORDS: glucose polymer, beta particles, alpha particles

Glycogen is a large **polymer of glucose** and is the storage form of carbohydrate. It is not visible in the usual light microscope preparations unless selectively stained with periodic acid-Schiff reagent or Best's carmine. Ultrastructurally, glycogen appears in two forms: **beta particles**, which are irregular, small, dense particles 15 to 45 nm in diameter, and **alpha particles**, which measure 90 to 95 nm in diameter and represent several smaller particles of glycogen clumped together to form rosettes.

Fat

KEY WORDS: fat cells, lipid droplets

Fat cells are the chief storage sites for lipid, but many other cell types store fat as **lipid droplets** of various sizes. Lipid synthesized by a cell accumulates in the cytoplasm as droplets that lack a limiting membrane. Intracellular lipid serves both as an energy source and as a supply of short-chain carbons for the synthesis of membranes by the cell. During preparation of routine histological sections, lipid usually is extracted and the sites of lipid storage appear as clear vacuoles. In electron micrographs, preserved lipid droplets are seen as homogeneous spheres of different densities.

Crystals

Crystalline inclusions are normal constituents in several cell types and might be free in the cytoplasm or contained in secretory granules, mitochondria, endoplasmic reticulum, the Golgi complex and even the nucleus. The chemical nature, significance or function of most crystalline inclusions is unknown.

Secretory Granules

These inclusions are limited by a membrane and represent cell products that are to be secreted by the cell. They are somewhat transitory, some granules being formed as others are released. Depending on the type of cell producing them, secretory granules contain different products that serve different functions.

Nucleus

The nucleus is an essential organelle present in all cells. The only cytoplasmic structures in which nuclei are absent are mature mammalian erythrocytes and blood platelets; these probably should not be regarded as cells. Generally, each cell has a single nucleus but some, such as the parietal cells of the stomach, cardiac muscle cells and some liver cells, may possess two nuclei. Giant cells, such as the osteoclasts of bone, megakaryocytes of marrow, and skeletal muscle cells, may have several nuclei.

The shape of the nucleus varies and may be spherical, ovoid or elongated, corresponding to the cell shape, or it might be lobulated, as in the granular leukocytes of the blood.

The nucleus contains all the information necessary to initiate and control the differentiation, maturation and metabolic activities of each cell. The nondividing nucleus is enclosed in a nuclear envelope and contains the chromatin material and one or two nucleoli. These are suspended in a nuclear ground substance called the karyolymph or nuclear matrix.

Chromatin and Chromosomes

KEY WORDS: karyosomes, heterochromatin, histones, euchromatin

Genetic information is stored in molecules of DNA which reside in the chromosomes. In nondividing nuclei, chromosomes are largely uncoiled and dispersed but some regions of the chromosomes remain condensed, stain deeply and are visible by the light microscope as chromatin. Individual masses of chromatin are called **karyosomes** and, although not entirely constant, the chromatin masses do tend to be characteristic in size, pattern and quantity for any given cell type. Collectively, the karyosomes form the **heterochromatin** of the nucleus, and represent the coiled portions of the chromosomes. Heterochromatin is believed to be complexed to **histones** and is considered to be nonactive. Histones are simple proteins that contain a high proportion of basic amino acids. The dispersed regions of the chromosomes stain lightly and form the **euchromatin**, which is thought to actively control the metabolic processes of the cell (Fig. 1-9). The distinction between heterochromatin and euchromatin disappears during cell division when all the chromatin condenses and becomes metabolically inert.

Nuclear Envelope

KEY WORDS: unit membranes, perinuclear space, nuclear pores, diaphragm, fibrous lamina

The nuclear envelope consists of two concentric **unit membranes**, each 7.5 nm thick, separated by a **perinuclear space** which measures 40 to 70 nm wide. The inner membrane appears smooth, whereas the outermost membrane often contains numerous ribosomes on its cytoplasmic surface and is

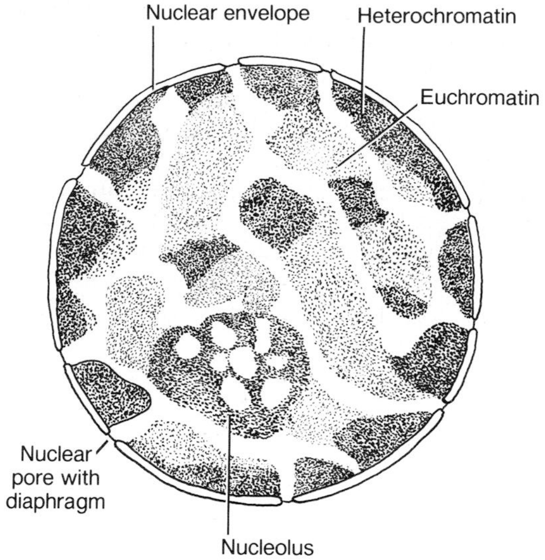

Figure 1-9. Diagrammatic representation of nuclear structures.

continuous with the surrounding endoplasmic reticulum. At irregular intervals around the nucleus, the inner and outer membranes of the nuclear envelope become continuous with one another to form small octagonal openings called **nuclear pores**. The pores measure about 50 nm in diameter and are closed by **diaphgrams** that are somewhat thinner than the usual unit membrane. The pores may be sites where materials are exchanged between the nucleus and cytoplasm.

In some types of cells a thin band of fine filaments lies along the inner surface of the nuclear membrane and forms the **fibrous lamina**. The significance of this structure is unknown, but it may provide support for the nuclear envelope.

Nucleolus

KEY WORDS: ribosomal RNA, transfer RNA, nucleolus-organizing region, pars granulosa, pars fibrosa, nucleolus-associated chromatin

A nucleolus appears as a dense, well-defined body 1 to 3 μm in diameter, contained within a nucleus. Nucleoli are the sites where **ribosomal RNA** (rRNA) and **transfer RNA** (tRNA) are synthesized. Since these sites (the **nucleolus organizing regions**) are located on five different chromosomes, any one cell may contain several nucleoli. Usually only one or two large nucleoli are found, since the nucleolus-organizing regions tend to associate and the RNA produced at these regions aggregates into larger masses.

As seen in electron micrographs, nucleoli lie free in the nucleus, not limited by a membrane. They show two regions each associated with a particular form of ribonucleoprotein. The dominant region, the **pars granulosa**, consists of dense granules of RNA about 13 to 15 nm in diameter. The second region tends to be centrally placed and consists of dense masses of filaments 5 nm in diameter; this portion is the **pars fibrosa**.

Deoxyribonucleoprotein also is associated with the nucleolus and is present as filaments of chromatin that surround or extend into the nucleolus. This chromatin forms the **nucleolus-associated chromatin**. Nucleoli are found only in interphase nuclei and are particularly prominent in cells that are actively synthesizing proteins. They are dispersed during cell division but reform at the nucleolus-organizing regions during reconstruction of the daughter nuclei after cell division.

FUNCTIONAL SUMMARY

Cells are the fundamental units of structure of all tissues and organs and perform all of the activities necessary for the survival, growth and reproduction of an organism. They carry out energy transformations, biosynthetic activities and are able to replicate themselves. The functional activities of a cell are carried out by specialized structures, the organelles, many of which consist of or are bounded by biological membranes. These membranes are essential to the organization of the cell. Besides forming the interface between the cell and its external environments, they are

important in transportation of materials, organization of various energy transfer systems, transmission of stimuli and provision of selectively permeable barriers and they serve to separate various intracellular spaces.

All materials that pass into or out of a cell must cross the plasmalemma, and this structure is instrumental in selecting what enters or leaves the cell. Large molecules are taken in by pinocytosis; particulate matter can be incorporated into the cell by phagocytosis while small molecules enter the cell by diffusion. The rate at which material diffuses into the cell depends upon whether it is soluble in lipid or water. Lipid-soluble materials readily dissolve in the lipid matrix of the plasmalemma and pass through the cell membrane relatively unhindered. The intrinsic proteins of the plasmalemma may act a sites for passage of water-soluble substances and as carrier proteins for materials such as glucose.

Although simple in microscopic appearance, the plasmalemma is very complex and variable in its molecular organization and function. Significant physiological and biochemical differences may occur at specific regions of the cell membrane according to the function of the cell. The cell membrane contains special receptor sites that can react with agents such as hormones or neurotransmitters to transfer information to the cell and elicit a specific response. The structure and composition of the cell membrane are important in determining the immunological properties of the cell and its relationships and interactions with other cells. The membrane may contain enzyme systems that act as ion pumps or that can initiate and control cellular activities by generating secondary messenger molecules. Membrane specializations also are involved in cell-to-cell attachments and communication.

The endoplasmic reticulum is associated with many synthetic activities of the cell. It is believed that the smooth endoplasmic reticulum in liver cells functions in lipid and cholesterol metabolism, in glycogen synthesis and storage, and in the detoxification of drugs. In endocrine cells, the smooth endoplasmic reticulum has been implicated in the synthesis of steroid hormones. It plays an important role in muscle contraction, being responsible for the release and recapture of calcium ions. The rough endoplasmic reticulum is involved in synthesizing proteins and provides the membranes for the transport vesicles that carry newly formed protein to the Golgi complex, where it is concentrated and packed into secretory granules. Golgi membranes are able to synthesize carbohydrate, complex it to protein and form glycoproteins. The Golgi also functions in the synthesis of lipoproteins, being responsible for complexing lipid to proteins produced by the rough endoplasmic reticulum. Synthesis of protein occurs on ribosomes. Protein formed by ribosomes attached to rough endoplasmic reticulum usually is secreted by the cell, whereas that formed on free polysomes is used by the cell itself.

Mitochondria perform a number of functions, chief of which is the production of energy for the cell. Pyruvate, produced by the degradation of glucose in the cytoplasm, enters the mitochondrion where, along with amino acids and fatty acids, it is processed by the enzymes of Krebs cycle located in the mitochondrial matrix. Transfer of electrons and hydrogen atoms to oxygen is mediated by enzymes of the electron transport system, which are located on the elementary particles or within the mitochondrial membranes that form the cristae. Energy released by the oxidations is incorporated into the high energy bonds of ATP, which then diffuses into the cytoplasm, where is is available for use by the cell. Mitochondria also play a role in the synthesis of proteins, lipids and steroids.

Lysosomes mainly function in intracellular digestion. The process takes place in membrane-enclosed digestion vacuoles which isolate the lysosomal enzymes from the remainder of the cytoplasm. Materials may be taken into the cell during phagocytosis or portions of cytoplasm containing aged or damaged organelles may be sequestered and digested by lysosomal activity. Any usable end products diffuse into the cytoplasm and the undigested residue remains within the vacuoles to form the residual bodies. Lysosomes might have other functions in normal cells: they have been implicated in the degradation of glycogen, in the removal from cells of excess substances such as unsecreted products, and in the release of thyroid hormone by splitting off the globulin to which the hormone is conjugated during its synthesis. Rupture of lysosomes in some cells may initiate mitosis.

Peroxisomes are similar in morphology to lysosomes but contain a population of enzymes capable of producing and degrading hydrogen peroxide. They play a role in the conversion of noncarbohydrate precursors to glucose and are instrumental in preventing the accumulation of lethal levels of hydrogen peroxide.

Microtubules and microfilaments perform a number of functions in the cell. Generally, microfilaments make up part of the cytoskeleton and serve as supporting elements. Microtubules contribute to the structure of cilia, flagella and centrioles, provide supporting structures (stiffening rods) in some cells, have been implicated in intracellular transport of materials and are essential for cell division and motility.

All of the information needed to initiate and regulate the activities of a cell is encoded in the nucleus. This structure controls the growth, differentiation, maturation and metabolic activities of the cell. The nucleus also is equipped to duplicate and pass on the DNA to its daughter cells. The nucleolus, which is the site of production of rRNA and tRNA, plays a central role in the control of protein synthesis by the cell.

MITOSIS

Nearly all multicellular organisms grow by an increase in the number of their cells. The zygote, which is formed at conception, divides repeatedly and gives rise to all the cells of the body. Every cell in the resulting individual contains a nucleus and each nucleus possesses identical genetic information. In the adult organism, most cells have a finite life-span and must be replaced continuously. Proliferation of somatic cells results from mitosis, which can be defined as the production of two daughter cells with exactly the same number of chromosomes and DNA content as the original parent cell.

Mitosis generally lasts from 30 to 60 minutes and involves division of the nucleus (karyokinesis) and the cytoplasm (cytokinesis). Both events usually take place during mitosis, but karyokinesis may occur without division of the cytoplasm, resulting in the formation of multinucleated cells such as megakaryocytes. Although a continuous process, for descriptive purposes it is convenient to divide mitosis into four stages: prophase, metaphase, anaphase and telophase. The time between successive mitotic divisions constitutes interphase and is the period during which the cell performs its usual functions, contributes to the total economy of the body and makes preparations for the next division.

Interphase

KEY WORDS: DNA replication, centromere

Replication of DNA takes place during interphase, before the cell visibly enters into mitosis. The double helix of the chromosome unwinds and each strand serves as a template for the development of a complementary strand of DNA. Thus a new double helix is formed that contains a new strand and a parent strand of DNA. By this means, an exact copy of the sequence of molecules in the DNA is produced.

Replication begins at the ends of the chromosomes and progresses towards the center, where a small area of the chromosome, the **centromere**, remains unduplicated. After a short time, the chromosomes begin to coil, shorten and become visible within the nucleus. The cell then enters into the prophase of mitotic division.

Prophase

KEY WORDS: chromatids, centriole replication

In this stage the cell assumes a more spherical shape and appears more refractile. Within the nucleus, the chromosomes become visible and appear as thread-like structures. At prophase each chromosome consists of two coiled subunits called **chromatids** which are closely associated along their entire lengths. The chromatids are the functional units of chromosomes and each contains a double strand of DNA. As prophase progresses, the chromatids continue to coil, thicken and shorten, reaching about 1/25th of their length by the end of prophase. The chromosomes then appear to approach the nuclear envelope.

As these events occur, the nucleoli become smaller and finally disappear, and the nuclear envelope breaks down. When this occurs, the center of the cell becomes more fluid and the chromosomes more freely, making their way to the equator of the cell. Simultaneous with the nuclear events, the **centrioles replicate** and the resulting pairs migrate to the opposite poles of the cell.

Metaphase

KEY WORDS: mitotic spindle, equatorial plate, continuous fibers, centromere (kinetochore), chromosomal fibers, splitting of centromeres

The breakdown and disappearance of the nuclear envelope marks the end of prophase and the beginning of metaphase. This stage is characterized by formation of the **mitotic spindle** and the alignment of chromosomes along the equator to form the **equatorial plate**. The mitotic spindle is a somewhat diffuse body that consists mainly of microtubules: those that pass from pole to pole of the spindle are called the **continuous fibers**. Other microtubules extend from the poles of the spindle to attach to the **centromere (kinetochore)** of each chromosome and are called the **chromosomal fibers**. The centromere is a special region of nonduplicated DNA and protein that serves both to hold together the chromatids of each chromosome and as the site of attachment of chromosomal fibers.

The final act of metaphase is duplication of the DNA at the centromeres, after which the **centromeres split**. The two chromatids of each chromosome separate and begin to migrate toward the centrioles at the opposite poles of the cell. Duplication of the centromeres and migration of the chromatids occur simultaneously in all chromosomes of a given cell.

Anaphase

KEY WORDS: telomeres, daughter chromosomes

The initial separation of chromatids marks the beginning of anaphase. As the chromatids move toward opposite poles, the centromeres proceed in advance of the arms or **telomeres** of the chromosomes, which trail behind. The movement of the chromatids, which now are **daughter chromosomes**, is an active and dynamic process but the mechanisms by which the movement is affected is not known.

Telophase

KEY WORDS: reforming nuclear envelope, nucleolus-organizing region, karyokinesis

As the daughter chromosomes reach their respective poles, discontinuous portions of granular endoplasmic reticulum form about each group of chromosomes and begin to **reform the nuclear envelopes**. This event initiates telophase. With complete reconstruction of the nuclear envelope, the chromosomes uncoil, become indistinct and the two nuclei reassume the interphase configuration. The normal complement of nucleoli also reappears at this time. Their development is associated with specific sites, the **nucleolus-organizing regions**, that are present on certain chromosomes. With this event, **karyokinesis** is complete.

Cytokinesis

KEY WORDS: interzonal fibers, midbody

During telophase the mitotic spindle begins to disappear. The fibers between the two forming nuclei appear to be stretched and often are called the **interzonal fibers**. Midway between the two nuclei, in the region formerly occupied by the equatorial plate, the plasmalemma constricts to form a furrow extending around the equator of the cell. The constriction extends more deeply into the cytoplasm, separating the daughter cells until they are united only by a thin protoplasmic bridge, the **midbody**, that contains interzonal fibers. Eventually, the two daughter cells pull away from each other by ameboid movement, thus completing the separation of the cells and ending cytokinesis.

The cell organelles are evenly distributed between the two daughter cells. Immediately after division, the daughter cells enter a phase of active RNA and protein synthesis, resulting in an increase in volume of the nucleus and cytoplasm. The endoplasmic reticulum and the Golgi complex are restored to concentrations originally present in the parent cell; mitochondia reproduce by fission; and the centrioles replicate in the daughter cell just before the next division (Fig. 1-10).

Chromosomes

KEY WORDS: diploid, haploid, homologous chromosomes, sex chromosomes, autosomes, karyotype, meta-

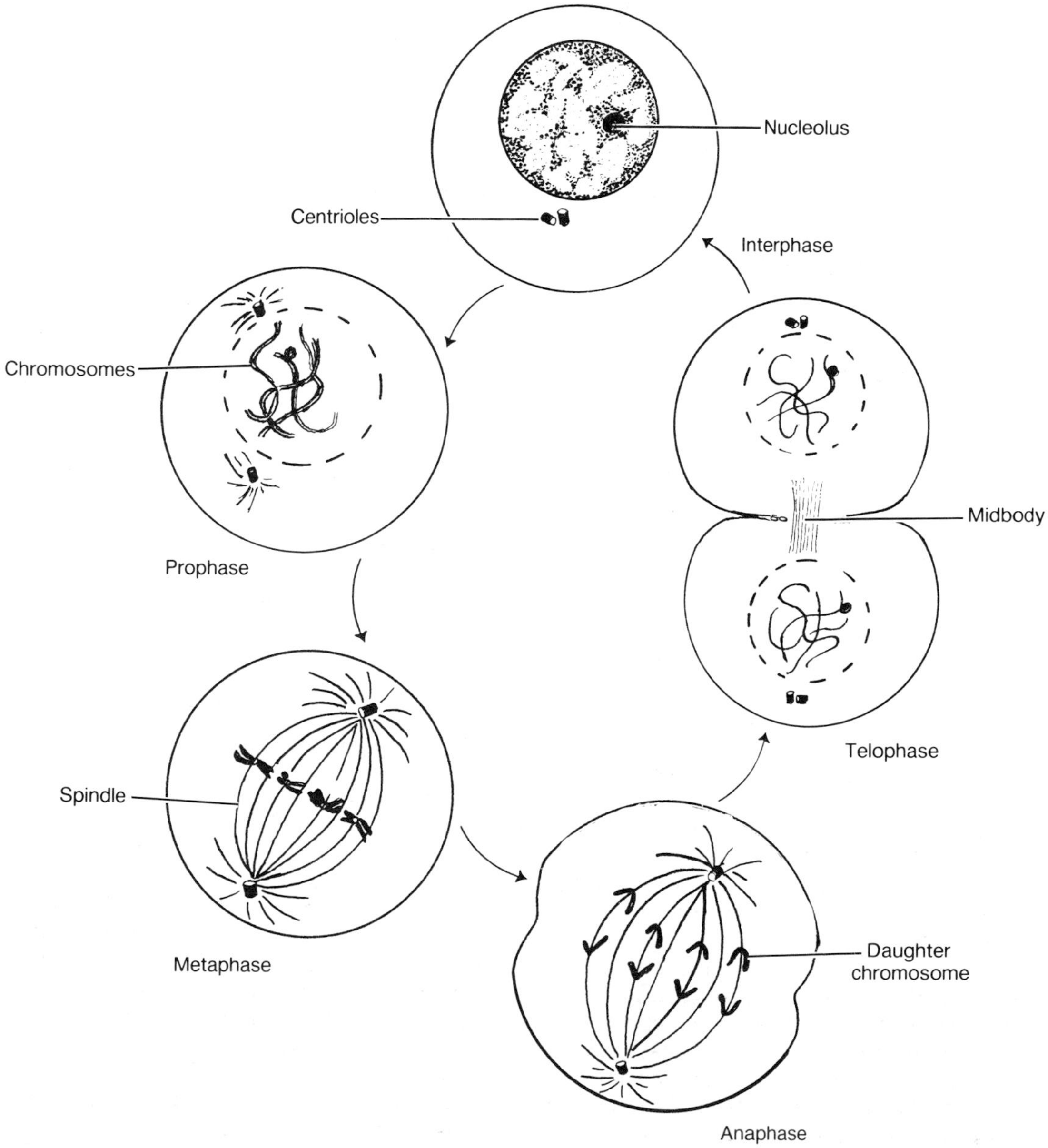

Figure 1-10. Changes occurring during mitotic division of a cell.

centric, acrocentric, submetacentric, polyploidy, aneuploid

Chromosomes are permanent entities of the cell and are present at every stage of the cell cycle, but their appearances depend on the physiological state of the cell. At interphase the chromosomes form delicate, tortuous threads and it is only during metaphase and anaphase that they assume the appearance of discrete, solid, rod-like structures. Analysis and study of chromosomes can be carried out most conveniently in dividing cells that have been arrested in metaphase. Alkaloids such as the vinca drugs and colchicine interfere with spindle formation and permit accumulation of metaphase chromosomes for study.

The number of chromosomes is constant for each species but varies considerably between species. In man the chromosome number is 46 compared with 22 in the North American opossum, 32 in the alligator and 78 in the dog. The figures given are for the **diploid** number in somatic cells. Germ cells (ova and sperm) contain half this number and are said to be **haploid**.The chromosomes present in somatic cells represent the inheritance of two sets of chromosomes, one from each of the male and female parents. Chromosomes in the male and female set that are similar are called **homologous chromosomes**. In most diploid organisms a pair of **sex chromosomes** have been specialized for the determination of sex; all other chromosomes are called **autosomes**. In the human there are 44 autosomes and a pair of sex chromosomes that are homologous (XX) in the female and heterologous (XY) in the male.

Homologous chromosomes can be recognized at metaphase and arranged in groups representing the **karyotype** of a species. Individual chromosomes can be identified by the length of their arms and the location of the centromere. If the centromere is in the middle of the chromosome and the arms (telomeres) are of equal length, the chromosome is said to be **metacentric**. If the centromere is close to one end, the chromosome is **acrocentric** and, if the centromere is between the midpoint and the end the chromosome is **submetacentric**.

Chromosomes may show abnormalities in number or configuration. An excess of chromosomes, usually some multiple of the haploid number, is called **polyploidy**; if the increase is less than an even number, the cell is said to be **aneuploid**. In rare instances the centromere may split transversely rather than longitudinally to yield chromosomes in which both arms are identical. Breaks may occur to give a fragment without a centromere; such a fragment will not move to the pole at anaphase and it and the genetic information it carries will be deleted.

FUNCTIONAL SUMMARY

Mitosis produces daughter cells that have the identical genetic constitution of the parent cell. What determines if and when a cell divides is not known but there are certain requirements that must be met before a cell can enter mitosis. Some relationship exists between cell mass and cell division. In *Amoeba proteus*, for example, mitosis can be prevented by periodic amputation of the cytoplasm. The cell then merely regenerates the lost cytoplasm without entering division. In general, each daughter cell achieves the mass of the parent cell before it undergoes division, but the relationship between cell growth and mitosis is not a causal one. The two events can be separated in time, as in cleavage of ova, where growth of the cell may occur long before division takes place.

Duplication of the entire DNA complement is essential for cell division. Depriving cells of thymidine blocks DNA synthesis and prevents cells from entering mitosis. Provision of thymidine to such cells results in a wave of DNA synthesis followed by a wave of cell divisions. Again, however, DNA replication may be completed long before division occurs. The existence and maintenance of polyploid cells argues against DNA synthesis being the trigger for mitosis.

The intense coiling and contraction of chromosomes at metaphase results in small, compact units that can be transported more easily to the poles of the cell. The destination of the chromosomes, their orderly arrangement at metaphase and the plane of cell cleavage are determined by the mitotic spindle. It would seem reasonable that one of the preparations for mitosis must be the synthesis of protein specifically concerned with formation of the spindle. Certain amino acid analogs result in the synthesis of faulty spindle proteins, and cells cultured in the presence of these analogs fail to divide. Upon removal to a normal medium, the cells enter mitosis but only after a delay during which the faulty protein is replaced by newly synthesized normal protein.

Centrioles are responsible for polarization of the mitotic spindle and may play a role in assembling the spindle, but how this is achieved is unknown. The centriole completes its duplication before mitosis begins and cell division can be headed off by suppressing the replication of centrioles.

Although mitosis would seem to be an energy-consuming process, cell division is not a period of intense respiratory activity. Restriction of energy sources and inhibition of respiration and oxidative phosphorylation does not stop mitosis once it has begun. Thus, it can be assumed that the energy requirements are met during the preparations for cell division.

Cell division often occurs in waves with patches of cells or whole tissues undergoing synchronous division, implying some kind of cellular or tissue control. Substances that promote or initiate mitosis have been isolated from epidermis and salivary glands in several species but other substances, called chalones, that *inhibit* mitosis also have been identified in a number of different tissues. Chalones are tissue specific, their action is reversible and they are not cytotoxic. Chalones appear to be produced by the mature cells of the tissue upon which they act. The mode of action is speculative, but in normal tissues the rate of mitosis might be inversely proportional to the concentration of chalone. Thus, when cells are damaged or removed from a tissue, a local decrease in chalone would result, allowing mitosis-promoting substances to become active and initiate a wave of cell division. As the cell population is restored, the balance between inhibitor (chalone) and promoter would be regained and mitosis would cease. Thus, autoregulatory tissue-specific systems may exist that normally control the rate of entry into mitosis and the rate of cell proliferation.

Atlas for Chapter 1

Organelles and Inclusions

1-11

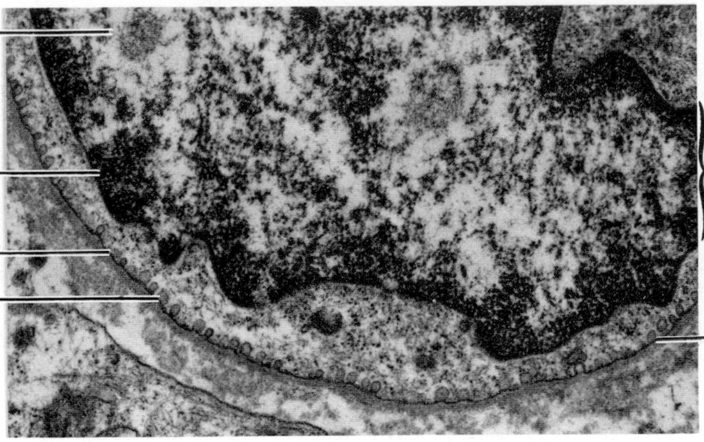

1-12

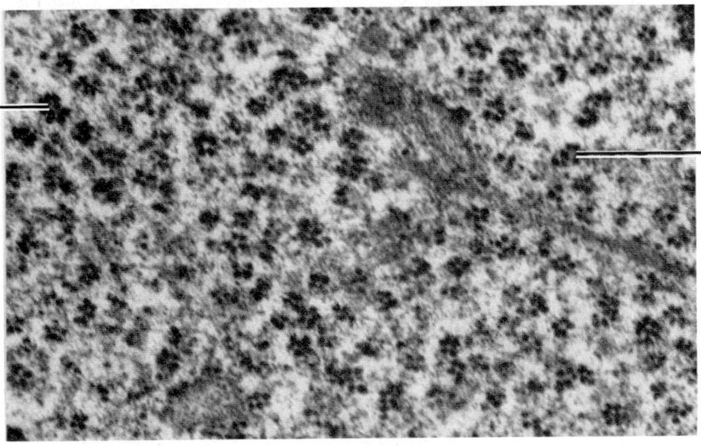

1-13

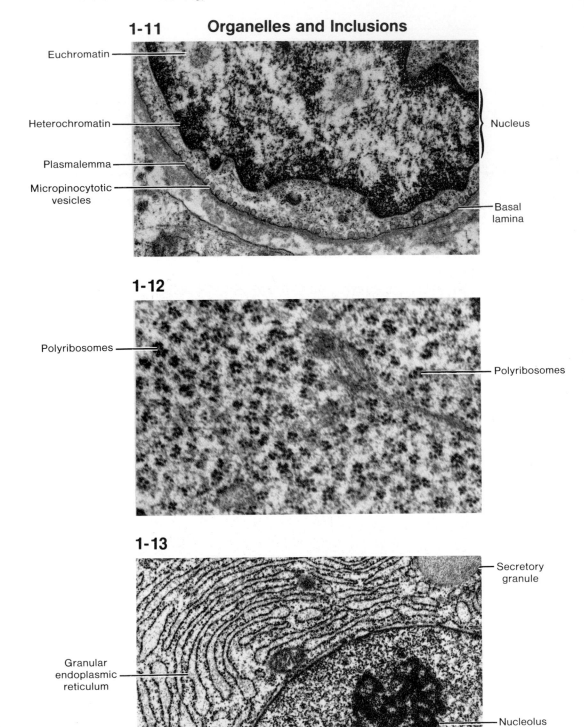

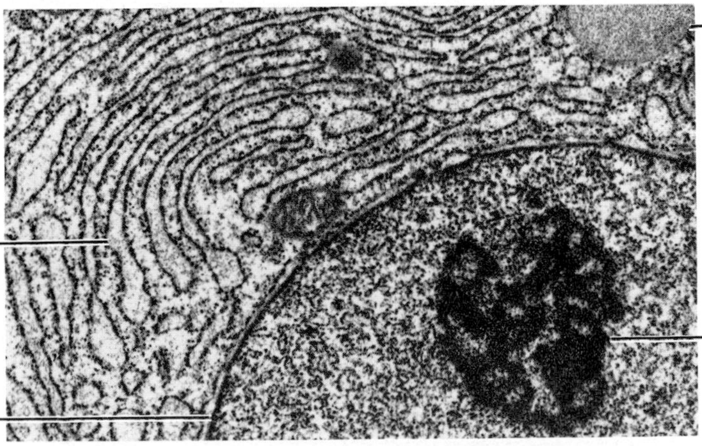

Figure 1-11. Endothelial cell. TEM, ×6000.
Figure 1-12. Intestinal epithelial cell. TEM, ×57,000.
Figure 1-13. Stomach—chief cell. TEM, ×11,000.

1-14

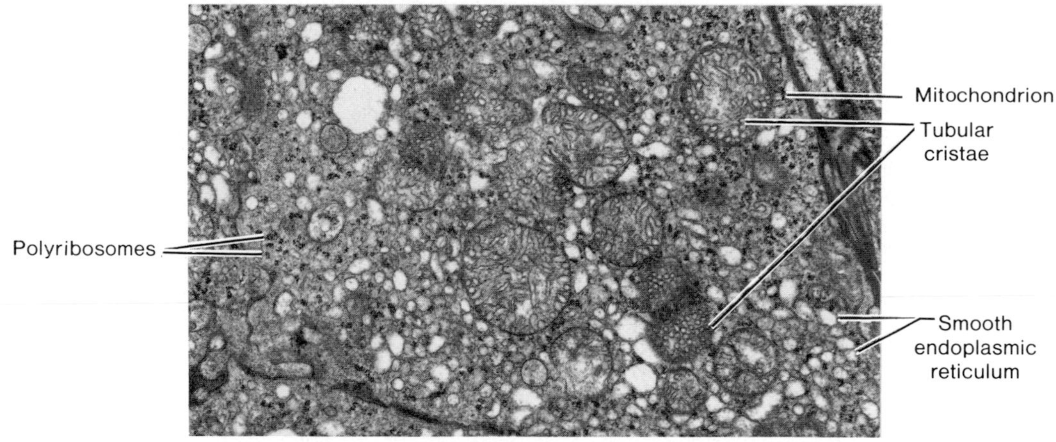

1-15

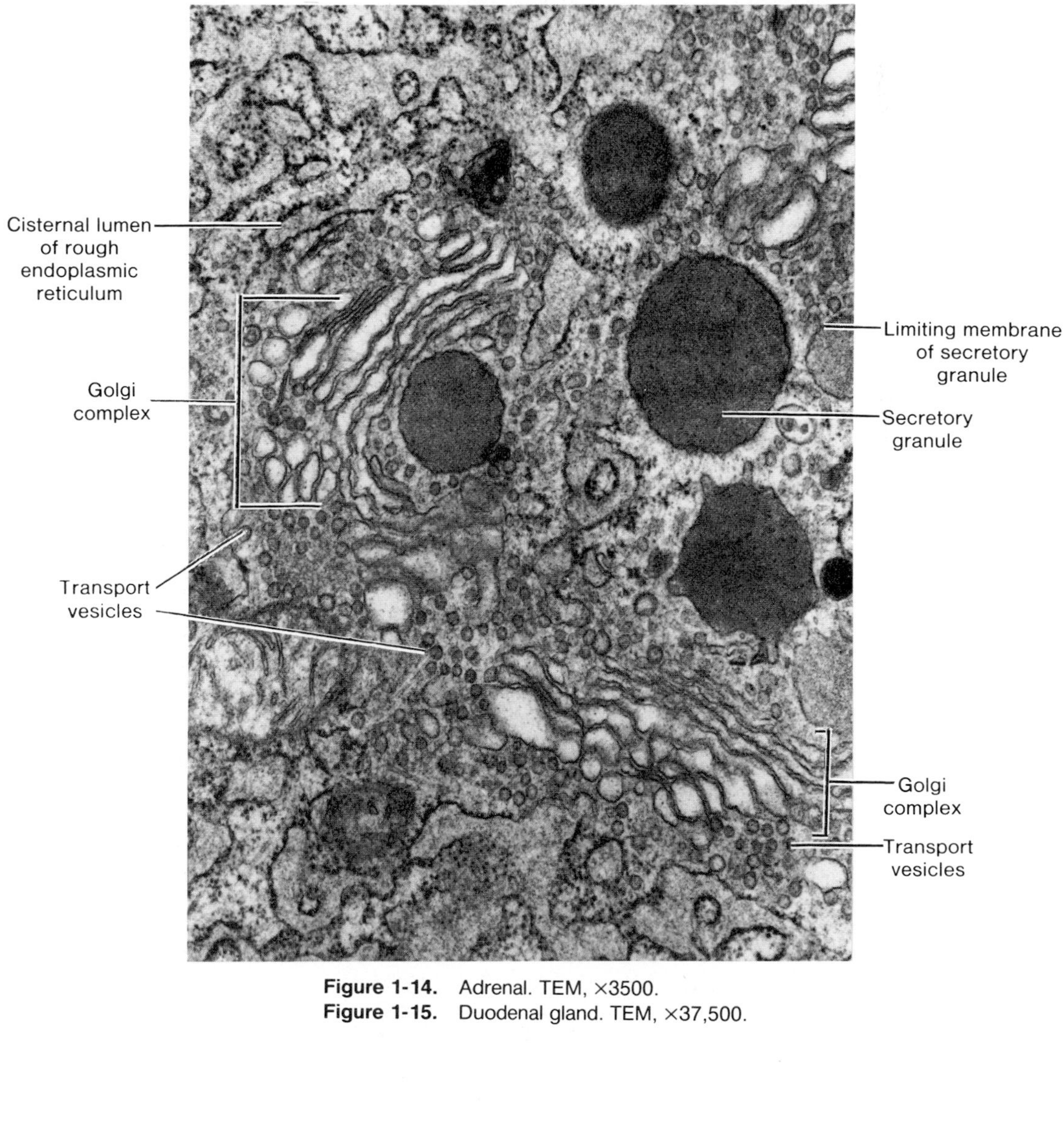

Figure 1-14. Adrenal. TEM, ×3500.
Figure 1-15. Duodenal gland. TEM, ×37,500.

1-16

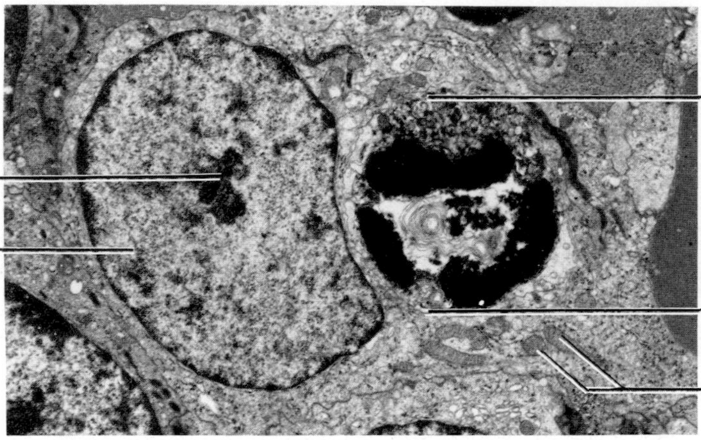

1-17

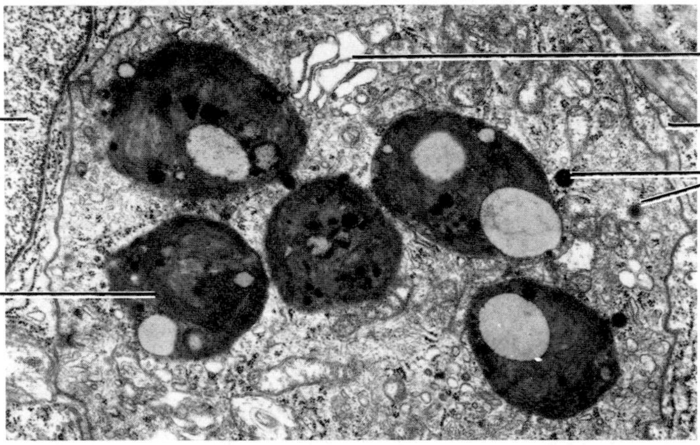

1-18

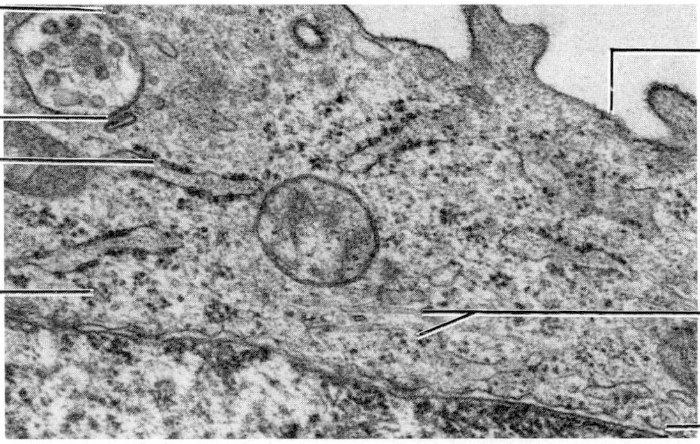

Figure 1-16. Spleen. TEM, ×2500.
Figure 1-17. Stomach. TEM, ×12,000.
Figure 1-18. Kidney. TEM, ×12,000.

1-19

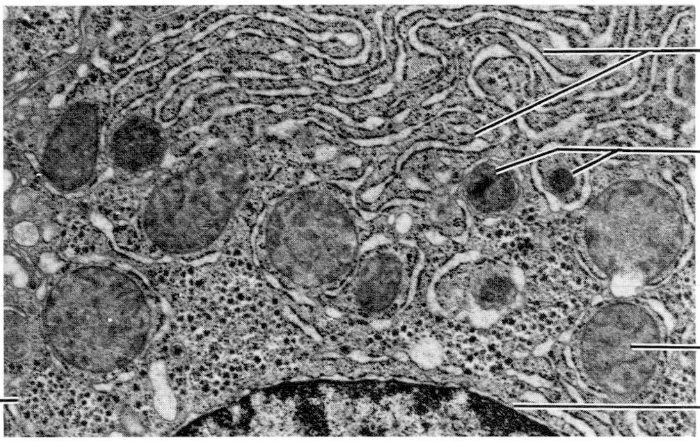

1-20

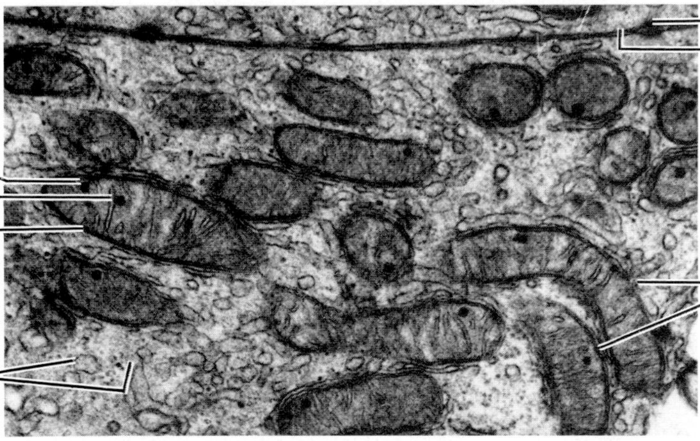

1-21

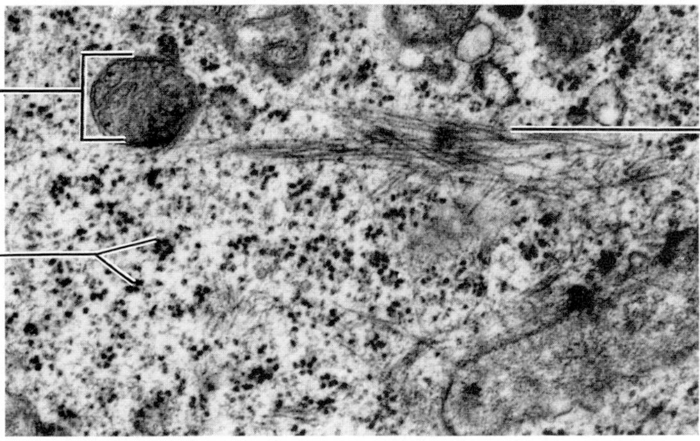

Figure 1-19. Liver. TEM, ×10,000.
Figure 1-20. Intestinal epithelium. TEM, ×10,000.
Figure 1-21. Submandibular gland. TEM, ×50,000.

1-22

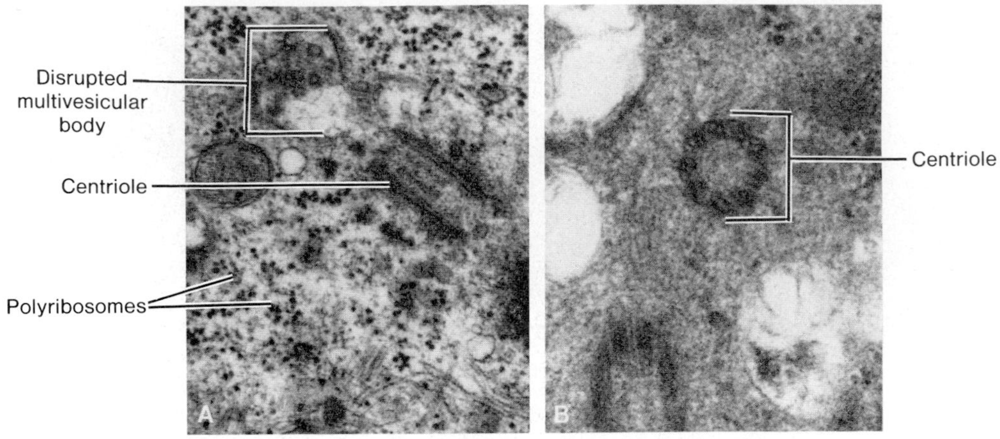

1-23

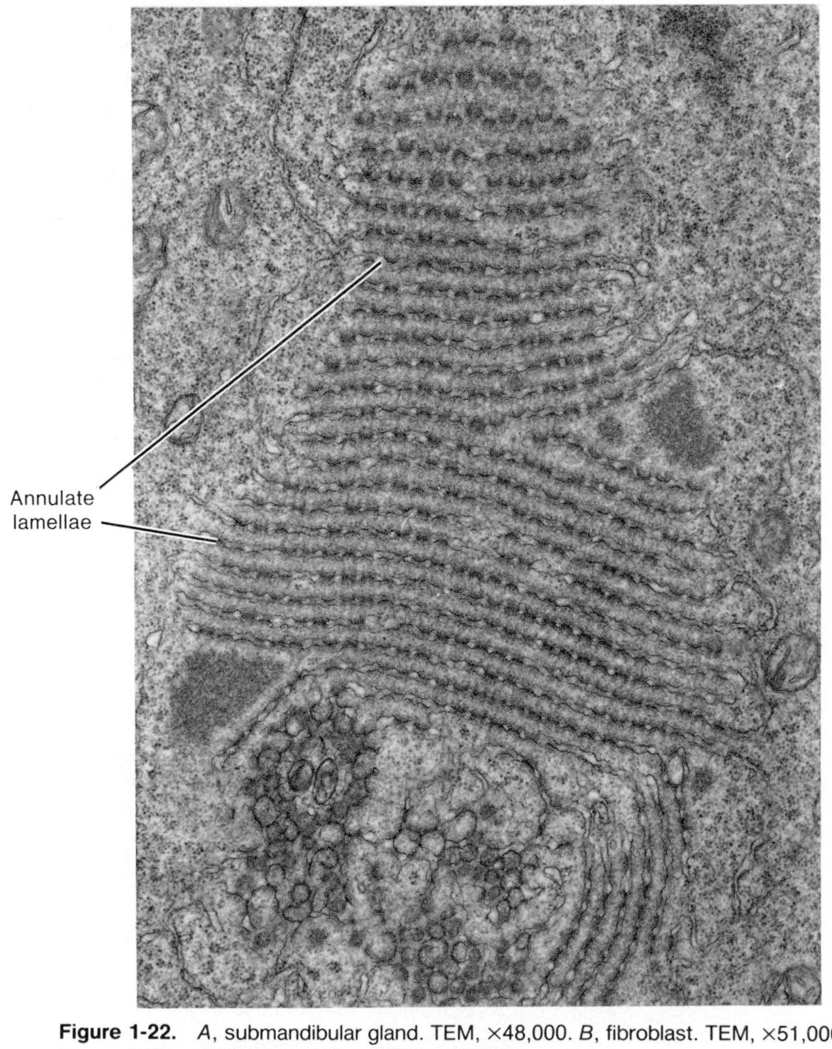

Figure 1-22. *A*, submandibular gland. TEM, ×48,000. *B*, fibroblast. TEM, ×51,000.
Figure 1-23. Annulate lamellae. TEM, ×15,000.

1-24

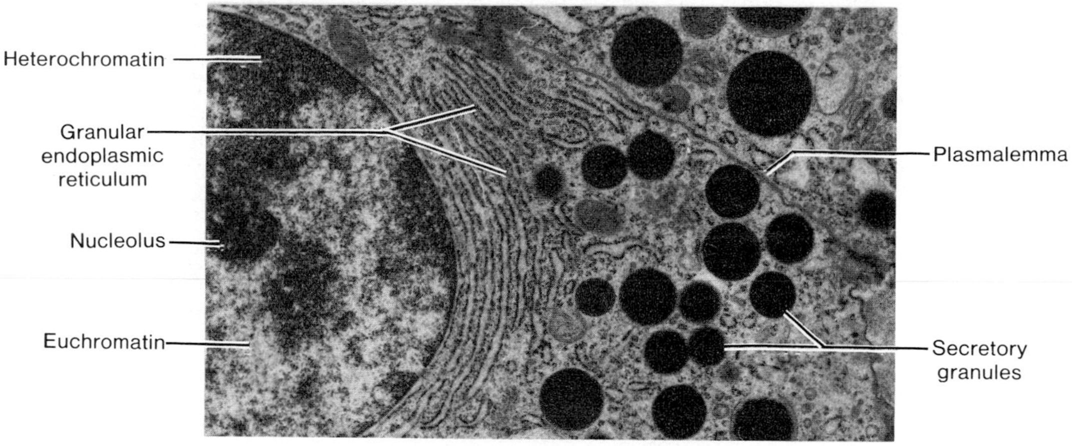

1-25

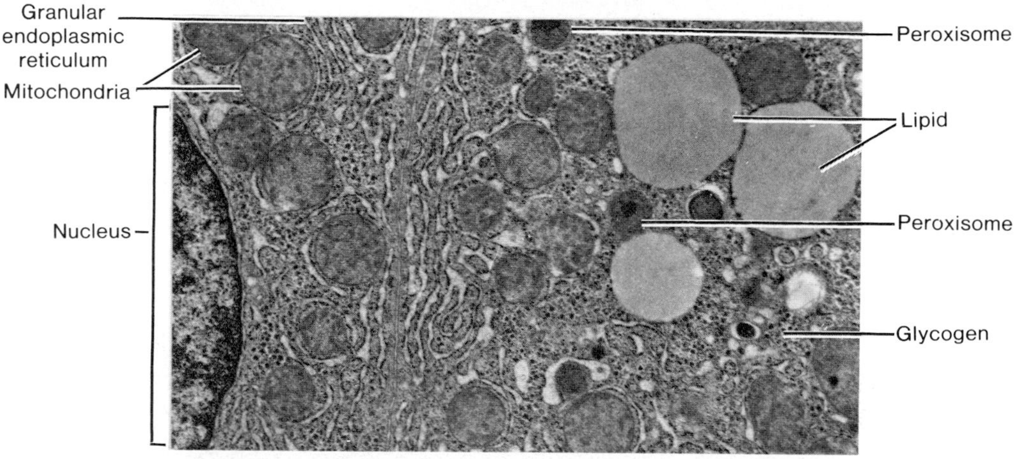

1-26

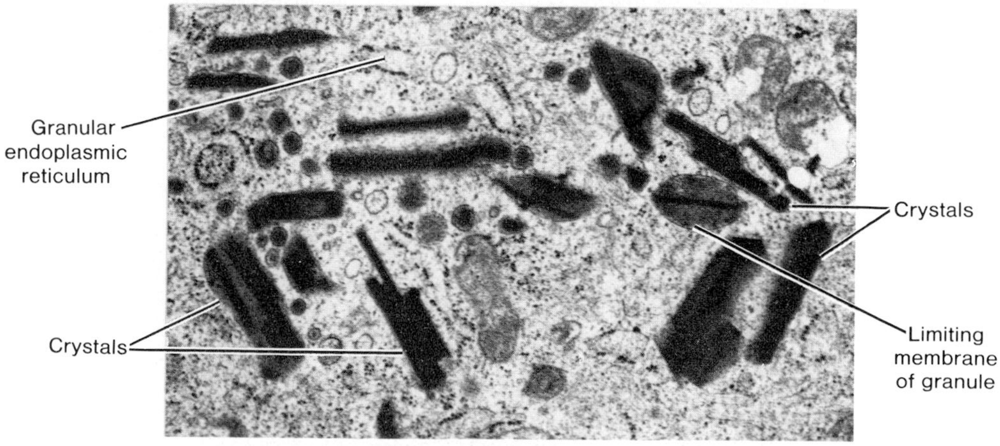

Figure 1-24. Pancreas. TEM, ×8000.
Figure 1-25. Liver. TEM, ×8000.
Figure 1-26. Intestinal epithelium. TEM, ×15,000.

1-27

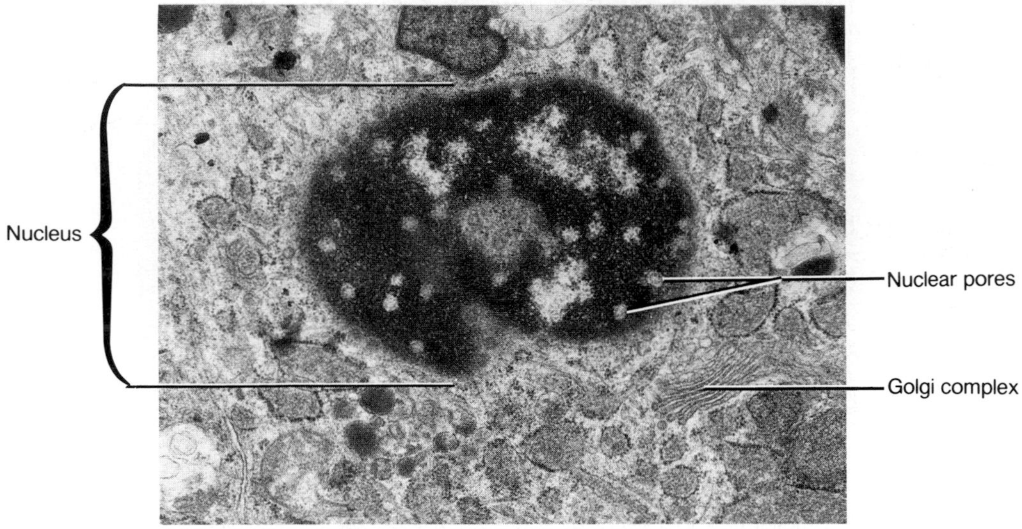

1-28 Mitosis

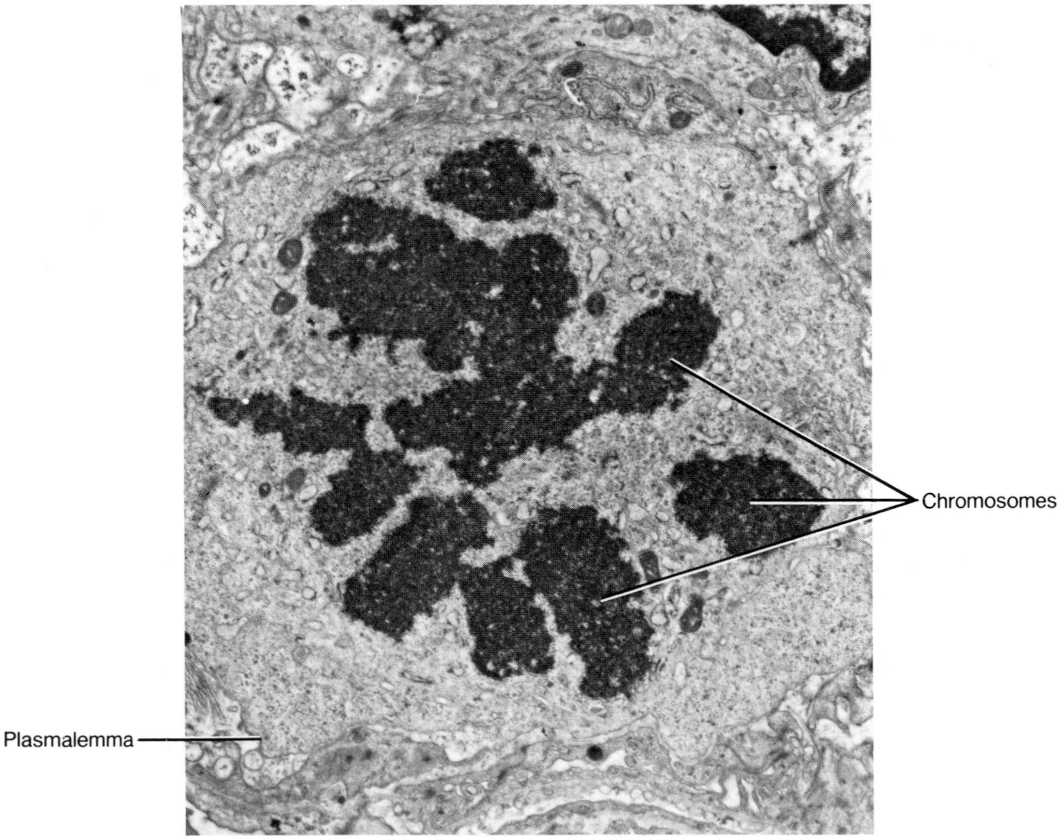

Figure 1-27. From duodenal glands. TEM, ×11,000.
Figure 1-28. Dividing cell. TEM, ×5000.

1-29 Mitosis (Whitefish)

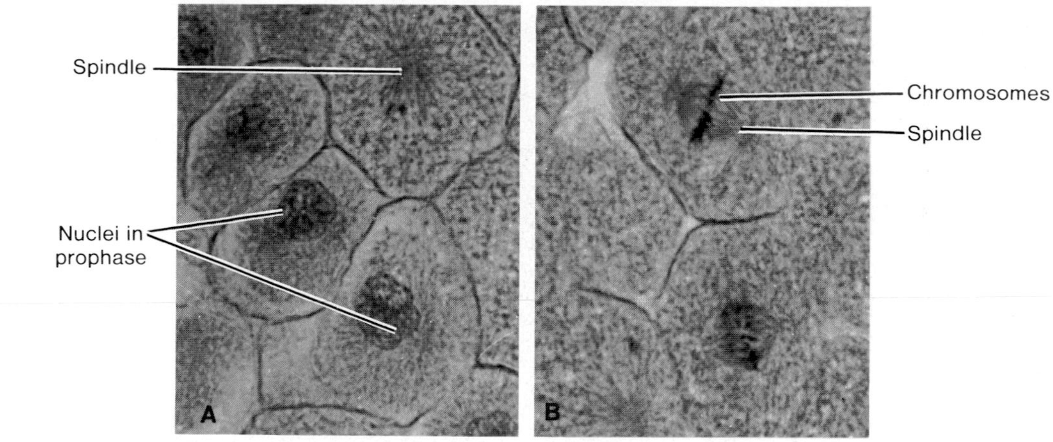

1-30

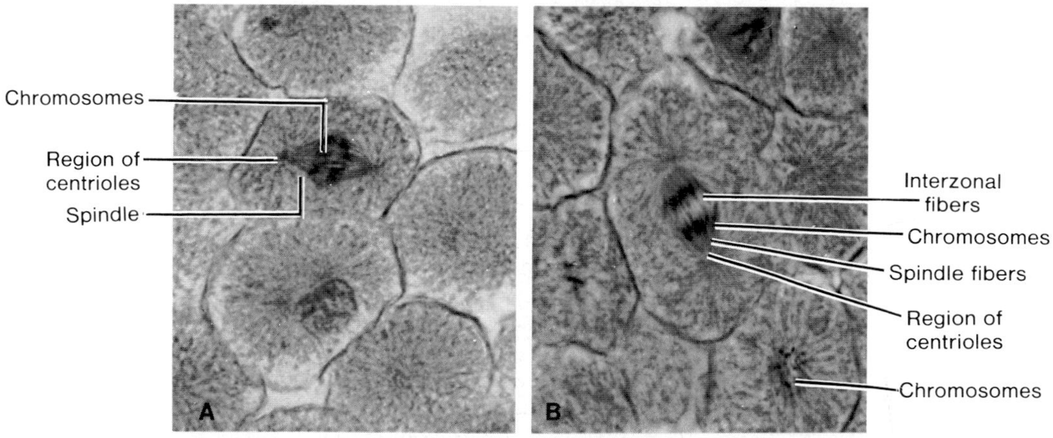

1-31

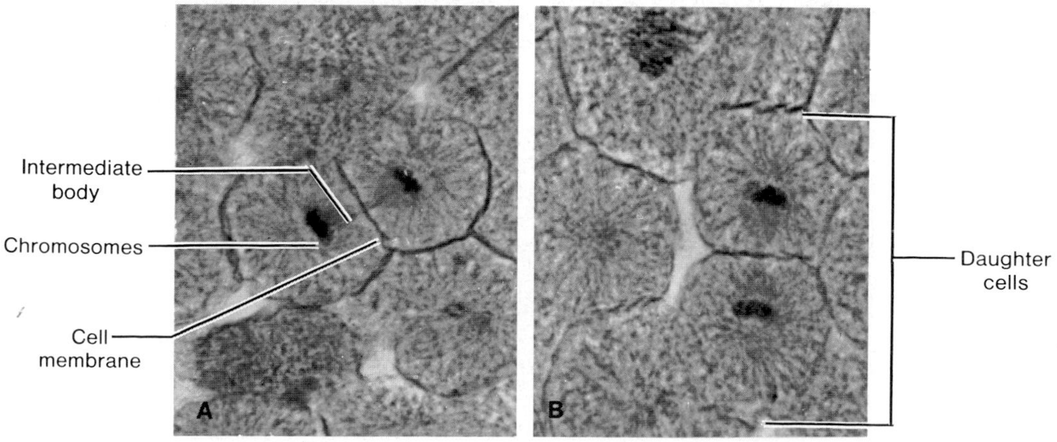

Figure 1-29. *A*, prophase. LM, ×400. *B*, metaphase. LM, ×400.
Figure 1-30. *A*, anaphase. LM, ×400. *B*, telophase. LM, ×400.
Figure 1-31. *A*, telophase. LM, ×400. *B*, telophase. LM, ×400.

2

Epithelium

Epithelium is one of the four basic tissues, the others being connective tissue, muscle and nerve tissue. A basic tissue can be defined as a collection of cells of similar type which, together with their associated extracellular substances, are specialized to perform a common function or functions. Each basic tissue is present, in variable amounts, in the organs that collectively make up the entire organism.

The various epithelia consist of closely aggregated cells with only minimal amounts of intervening intercellular substances.

STRUCTURAL ORGANIZATION

KEY WORDS: sheets, basal lamina, reticular lamina, basement membrane, avascular, glands

The cells of an epithelium form **sheets** that cover the external surfaces of an organism and line the digestive, respiratory, cardiovascular and urogenital tracts. Thus, substances that enter or leave the body must pass through an epithelial layer. Cells within an epithelial sheet are bound firmly together and resist forces that tend to separate them. The space between the membranes of adjacent epithelial cells is narrow (about 20 nm) and contains a small amount of glycosaminoglycan that is rich in cations, chiefly, calcium. The glycosaminoglycan is thought to act as an "intercellular glue" that helps to hold adjacent cell membranes together.

Epithelial cells rest on a **basal lamina** which separates the epithelium from underlying connective tissue. The basal lamina, a product of the epithelial cells, consists of glycoproteins that contain a feltwork of fine filaments. It is reinforced on the connective tissue side by a layer of reticular fibers embedded in proteoglycan. This layer forms the **reticular lamina** and is the product of connective tissue fibroblasts. The basal lamina and reticular lamina together make up the epithelial **basement membrane** that is visible under the light microscope. With but rare exceptions, epithelium is **avascular** and for its nutrition depends on diffusion of substances across the basement membrane.

Epithelial cells also occur in groups to form **glands** specialized for the secretion of various substances.

CLASSIFICATION OF EPITHELIA

KEY WORDS: simple epithelia, stratified epithelia, squamous, cuboidal, columnar

The lining and covering forms of epithelium may consist of a single layer of cells, forming a **simple epithelium**, or multiple layers of cells may be present to form a **stratified** epithelium. In addition, the epithelial cells themselves can be divided into three types according to their geometric shapes: **squamous**—thin, plate-like cells; **cuboidal**—cells in which the height and width are approximately equal; and **columnar**—cells in which the height is greater than the width. Cells somewhat intermediate in height between cuboidal and columnar do occur and frequently are referred to as low columnar.

Simple Epithelia

KEY WORDS: simple squamous, simple cuboidal, simple columnar, pseudostratified columnar, apical surface, basal surface, lateral surface, polarity, mesothelium, endothelium

Epithelium consisting of a single layer of cells can be classed as **simple squamous, simple cuboidal** or **simple columnar,** depending on the shape of the constituent cells. A fourth type of simple epithelium, **pseudostratified columnar,** is composed of more than one type of cell whose nuclei are at different levels, falsely suggesting that the epithelium is made up of two or more layers. While all the cells in this type of epithelium are in contact with the basement membrane, not all extend to the surface.

The surfaces of cells within an epithelial sheet show different orientations. One surface, the **apical surface**, is free while the opposite or **basal surface** is directed toward the underlying connective tissue and the **lateral surfaces** face adjacent epithelial cells. Differences in the orientation of the plasmalemma (i.e., apical, basal or lateral) may be associated with differences in function and, hence, in morphology. Organelles, including the nucleus, frequently take up preferred locations in the cell, in which case the cell is said to show **polarity**. An epithelial cell may be polarized apically, basally or laterally with respect to the distribution of its organelles, depending on the functional organization of the cell.

The term **mesothelium** is the special name given to the simple squamous epithelia that form the serous membranes of the pleura, pericardium and peritoneum. A specific name, **endothelium**, is given to the simple squamous epithelium that lines the cardiovascular and lymph vascular systems.

Stratified Epithelia

KEY WORDS: stratified squamous, stratified cuboidal, stratified columnar, keratinized stratified squamous, nonkeratinized stratified squamous, transitional epithelium, germinal epithelium

Stratified epithelia are classified according to the shape of the superficial (surface) cells, regardless of the shapes of the cells in the deeper layers. Except for those in the basal layer, cells of stratified epithelia are not in contact with the basement membrane and only the most superficial cells have a free surface. In the thicker stratified types, the deeper cells often are irregular in shape. The types of stratified epithelia are: **stratified squamous, stratified cuboidal and stratified columnar.**

In regions where the surface is dry or subject to mechanical abrasion, the outermost layers of cells may be transformed into a nonliving substance called keratin. Keratin is a tough, proteinaceous material that is resistant to mechanical injury and is relatively impervious to bacterial invasion or water loss. This type of stratified epithelium is referred to as a **keratinized stratified squamous** epithelium. The keratinized layer is constantly being shed and replaced. In other regions the stratified squamous type of epithelium is moist, and intact cells rather than keratin are sloughed from the surface. This type of epithelium is called a wet or **nonkeratinized stratified squamous** epithelium.

Two other types, transitional and germinal epithelium, cannot be classified according to the cells of the surface layer. **Transitional epithelium** is restricted to the lining of the urinary passages and extends from the minor calyces of the kidneys to the urethra. Its appearance varies considerably, depending upon the degree of distention to which it is subjected. The superficial cells of a nondistended organ appear rounded or dome-shaped and often show a free convex border that bulges into the lumen. In the distended organ, the superficial cells may vary in shape from squamous to cuboidal.

Germinal epithelium also has a restricted distribution, being found only in the seminiferous tubules of the testes. It is a complex, stratified epithelium that consists of supporting cells and spematogenic cells.

Table 2-1 shows a classification of epithelia and the locations where each type can be found.

Table 2-1.
Classification of Epithelia

Type of Epithelium	Location	Specialization
Simple squamous	Endothelium, mesothelium, parietal layer of Bowman's capsule, thin segment of loop of Henle, rete testis, pulmonary alveoli	
Simple cuboidal	Thyroid, choroid plexus, ducts of many glands, inner surface of the capsule of the lens, covering surface of ovary	
Simple columnar	Surface epithelium of stomach	
	Small and large intestine	Striated border
	Proximal convoluted tubule of kidney	Brush border
	Distal convoluted tubule of kidney	Basal Striations
	Gallbladder, excretory ducts of glands	
	Uterus, oviducts	Cilia
	Small bronchi of lungs	Cilia
	Some paranasal sinuses	Cilia
Pseudostratified columnar	Large excretory ducts of glands, portions of male urethra	
	Epididymis	Sterocilia
	Trachea, bronchi	Cilia
	Eustachian tube	Cilia
	Portions of tympanic cavity	Cilia
Stratified squamous	Buccal surface, esophagus, epiglottis, conjunctiva, cornea, vagina	
	Epidermis of skin	Keratin
	Gingiva, hard palate	Keratin
Stratified cuboidal	Ducts of sweat glands	
Stratified columnar	Cavernous urethra, fornix of conjunctiva, large excretory ducts of glands	
Transitional	Urinary system: renal calyces to urethra	
Germinal	Seminiferous tubules of adult testes	

CELL ATTACHMENTS

In addition to the intercellular matrix, several attachment points or junctions occur between neighboring epithelial cells and are thought to aid in holding adjacent cell membranes in close apposition. They also may serve as anchoring sites for the fine filaments of the cytoskeleton, which assists in stabilizing the cell shape.

Junctional Complexes

KEY WORDS: terminal bars, zonula occludens (tight junction), zonula adherens, macula adherens (desmosome), plaque, tonofilaments, punctum adherens, hemidesmosome

Terminal bars occur along the lateral interfaces of most simple cuboidal and columnar epithelial cells that border on luminal surfaces. They are visible under the light microscope as short dense lines. In electron micrographs the terminal bar is seen to form an area of specialization, the junctional complex, which consists of three distinct regions. Near the free surface, the external laminae of adjacent plasma membranes fuse and the intercellular space is obliterated. This region is the **zonula occludens** or **tight junction**, an area of specialization that forms a zone or "belt" around the perimeter of each cell to create an occluding seal between the apices of adjacent epithelial cells. Materials that pass through the epithelial sheet must traverse the plasma membranes and cannot pass between cells through the intercellular spaces. Tight junctions also have been reported in simple squamous epithelia and in the superficial layers of stratified squamous epithelia.

The second part of the junctional complex, the **zonula adherens**, also forms an adhering belt or zone that surrounds the apex of an epithelial cell, immediately below the zonula occludens. Adjacent plasma membranes are separated by an intercellular space, 15 to 20 nm wide, and in this region the internal laminae of the plasma membranes often are associated with the fine filamentous material of the cytoskeleton.

The third element of the junction is the **macula adherens**, also called the **desmosome.** These small, elliptical disks form spot-like points of attachment between cells. The internal laminae of the adjacent plasma membranes appear dense and thick due to the presence of an amorphous material, called a **plaque**. Cytoplasmic filaments (**tonofilaments**) extend into the plaque, where they appear to form hairpin loops. A thin lamina of moderate density often is seen in the intercellular space of each desmosome. Desmosomes are scattered along epithelial surfaces and are not restricted to regions of tight junctions. They are especially abundant in stratified squamous epithelia, where they are associated with numerous tonofilaments. Desmosome-like junctions that lack attachment plaques and associated tonofilaments also occur between epithelial cells. This type of cell junction has been called a **punctum adherens**.

The basal plasma membrane, although not immediately adjacent to another cell, also shows an attachment, the **hemidesmosome**, which closely resembles one-half of a desmosome. Hemidesmosomes are thought to act as points of adhesion between the basal plasma membrane and the underlying basal lamina. As noted for other junctions, hemidesmosomes also may act as anchoring sites for tonofilaments. The integrity of desmosomes and hemidesmosomes appears to depend upon the presence of calcium ions.

Nexus Junction

KEY WORDS: nexus, gap junction, connexons, connexin, communicating junctions

The **nexus** or **gap junction**, like tight junctions and desmosomes, forms a relatively firm point of attachment between adjacent cells. At a nexus, the plasma membranes are separated by a gap 2 nm wide which is bridged by particles 8 nm in diameter. These particles, the **connexons,** mainly consist of the protein **connexin**. Connexon units are thought to extend through the plasmalemma and cross the intercellular gap to join a corresponding unit from the opposing cell membrane. A hydrophilic channel within the center of each connexon permits intercellular passage of ions, amino acids and nucleotides. The nexus provides an avenue whereby cyclic AMP (c-AMP), released by one cell, can pass to adjacent cells. Thus, the response of a number of cells to a specific hormonal stimulus can be coordinated. Because the nexus junction seems to act as a site of communication between epithelial cells, they often are called **communication junctions**. Nexus junctions also appear to be capable of changing from low to high resistance and, thereby, inhibit cell communication.

Adjacent lateral membranes often do not run parallel to each other but show numerous interdigitations. Such interlocking of cell membranes also is thought to aid in maintaining cell-to-cell adhesion in an epithelial sheet.

SPECIALIZATIONS OF EPITHELIAL MEMBRANES

The cells in an epithelial sheet often show special adaptations of the apical or basal surfaces which may increase the surface area of the cell, constitute motile "appendages" that move material across the surface or have receptor functions. The surface specializations include microvilli, cilia and basal infoldings.

Microvilli

KEY WORDS: striated border, brush border, stereocilia

Microvilli are minute, finger-like evaginations of the apical plasma membrane that enclose cores of cytoplasm. Scattered microvilli occur on the surfaces of most simple epithelial cells, but individually they are too small to be seen with the light microscope. In epithelia such as that which lines the small intestine, microvilli are so numerous, uniform and closely packed that they form a **striated border** which is visible by light microscopy. Microvilli also are numerous on the cells of the proximal convoluted tubules of the kidney. Here they are somewhat longer and less uniform than those in the small intestine and appear as tufts on the cell apices; because of this appearance, they were termed a **brush border**. Microvilli increase the surface area enormously, thereby enhancing the absorptive capacity of epithelial cells.

Epithelial cells that line the epididymis show unusually long, slender, branching microvilli that have been called **stereocilia**. However, stereocilia are not cilia but are true microvilli and also serve to increase the surface area of a cell.

Cilia

KEY WORDS: microtubules, doublets, central pair, (9+2), dynein, basal body, triplets, (9+0), ciliated simple columnar epithelium, ciliated pseudostratified columnar epithelium

Like microvilli, cilia represent appendages of the apical cell membrane but are relatively large and often are motile. They may be single or occur in large numbers and are seen readily with the light microscope. The limiting plasmalemma of the cilium is continuous with that of the cell and encloses a core of cytoplasm containing 20 **microtubules**. Nine pairs of fused microtubules, the **doublets**, form a ring at the periphery of the cilium and surround a **central pair** of individual microtubules. This arrangement has been called the **(9+2)** configuration (Fig. 2-1). Within each doublet, the microtubules are called the A and B microtubules. Microtubule A has two short, divergent arms that project toward tubule B of the adjacent doublet. The arms consist of the protein **dynein**, which has ATPase-like activity. Radial spokes project from the doublets to the central pair of microtubules.

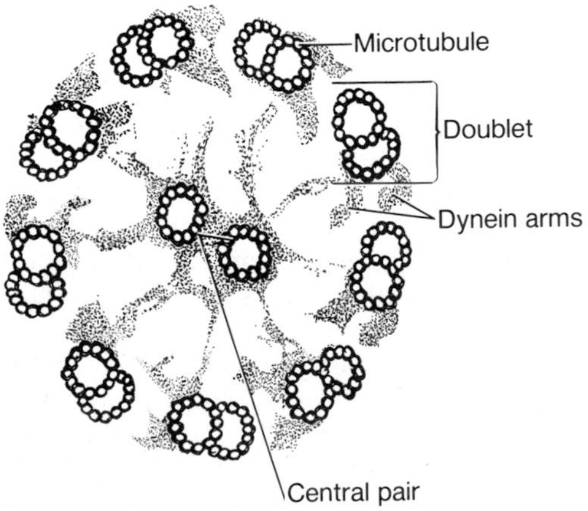

Figure 2.1. Diagrammatic representation of a cilium in cross section.

The microtubules of a cilium originate from a **basal body** in the apical cytoplasm of the cell. The basal body is similar in structure to the centriole and appears as a hollow cylinder, the wall of which consists of nine **triplet** microtubules. Since there are no central microtubules in a basal body, the arrangement of microtubules is expressed as **(9+0)**. Each of the nine doublets in the cilium is continuous with the two innermost microtubules of the triplets in the basal body. The two central microtubules of the ciliary shaft terminate as they reach the basal body and do not join with it.

Ciliary motion is thought to involve a sliding tubule mechanism dependent on the ability of the dynein protein to generate energy through its ATPase-like activity. Cilia are numerous on epithelial cells that line the respiratory tract and parts of the female reproductive tract. Groups of cilia beat in a coordinated, rhythmical fashion to move a thin layer of fluid in one direction across the epithelial surface. In a region such as that of the distal tubules of the kidney, where each cell bears a single cilium, or in the olfactory epithelium, where they occur in small groups on the cells, the cilia are nonmotile and generally are considered to act as chemoreceptors. The most extreme modification of cilia is seen in the formation of the outer segments of the rods and cones of the retina. Here, the modified cilia serve as photoreceptors. Cilia also are found in the maculae and cristae of the inner ear.

The presence of cilia contributes to the classification of epithelia. Where cilia are present on simple columnar epithelial cells, as in the oviduct, the epithelium is called a **ciliated simple columnar epithelium**. Where cilia are associated with pseudostratified epithelium (trachea), the epithelium forms a **ciliated pseudostratified columnar epithelium**.

Basal Infoldings

KEY WORDS: basal plasmalemma, basal infoldings, fluid transport, basal striations

In addition to the apical specializations, some epithelial cells show elaborate infoldings of the **basal plasmalemma**. These are called **basal infoldings** and usually are prominent in epithelia active in **fluid transport** such as in the proximal and distal convoluted tubules of the kidneys and in some ducts of salivary glands. Like microvilli, they greatly increase the surface area of the cell membrane. Mitochondria, which often are numerous in this area of the cell, tend to lie parallel to the infoldings of the plasma membrane. Because of this association, the infoldings are visible with the light microscope and appear as **basal striations**.

GLANDULAR EPITHELIUM

In addition to performing functions such as protection and absorption, the cells of an epithelial sheet may secrete materials also. Epithelial cells adapted specifically for secretion constitute the glands.

Classification of Glands

KEY WORDS: unicellular, multicellular, exocrine, endocrine, type and mode of secretion

Glands can be classified on the basis of their histological organization, possession of ducts, type of material secreted and manner in which material is secreted. Those which consist of only a single cell are called **unicellular**, whereas aggregates of secreting cells form **multicellular** glands. The latter can be divided into **exocrine** and **endocrine** types, according to whether or not they secrete onto a surface. Exocrine glands can be subdivided further on the basis of the branching of their ducts and the configuration of the secretory end piece and on the **type and mode of secretion.**

Unicellular Glands

KEY WORDS: goblet cell, mucin, mucous

The classical example of a unicellular gland is the **goblet cell**, found scattered among columnar epithelial cells, as in the trachea, small intestine and colon. The cell has a narrow base and an expanded apex filled with secretory droplets. Goblet cells elaborate **mucin** which, on hydration, produces a viscous lubricating fluid called **mucus**.

Multicellular Glands

KEY WORDS: secretory sheets, intraepithelial glands

The simplest form of multicellular gland is the **secretory sheet** in which the secreting cells form a continuous epithelial layer. **Intrapithelial glands** are small clusters of cells that lie wholly within an epithelial sheet, clustered about a small lumen.

Exocrine Glands

KEY WORDS: compound, simple, tubules, acini, saccules

Exocrine glands secrete onto an epithelial surface either directly, as in secretory sheets and intraepithelial glands, or by way of a ductal system. If the duct branches, the gland is said to be **compound:** if it does not branch, the gland is **simple**.

The secretory cells may form **tubules, acini** (berry-like end pieces) or **saccules** (dilated, flask-like end pieces). Simple and compound glands can be subdivided on the basis of the shape of the secretory portion. Thus, simple glands can be classed as simple tubular, simple coiled tubular, simple branched tubular or simple branched acinar. Similarly, compound glands are subdivided into compound tubular, compound saccular and compound tubuloacinar types. The initial subdivision into simple and compound is made according to whether or not the ducts branch. Subsequent classification depends on the shape and configuration of the secreting portion (Fig. 2-2 and Table 2-2).

Endocrine Glands

KEY WORDS: lack of ducts, hormones

Like exocrine glands, the endocrine glands arise from an epithelial sheet but during their formation, endocrine glands lose their connections with the surface and thus **lack ducts** (Fig. 2-3). Cells of endocrine glands secrete regulatory material, **hormones**, directly into the blood stream or intercellular spaces. Scattered, solitary endocrine cells occur along the conducting portion of the respiratory tract and in the gastrointestinal tract.

The structure of the large endocrine glands is so diverse that the organs do not readily lend themselves to histological classification. However, some overall structural patterns can be made out and the cells may

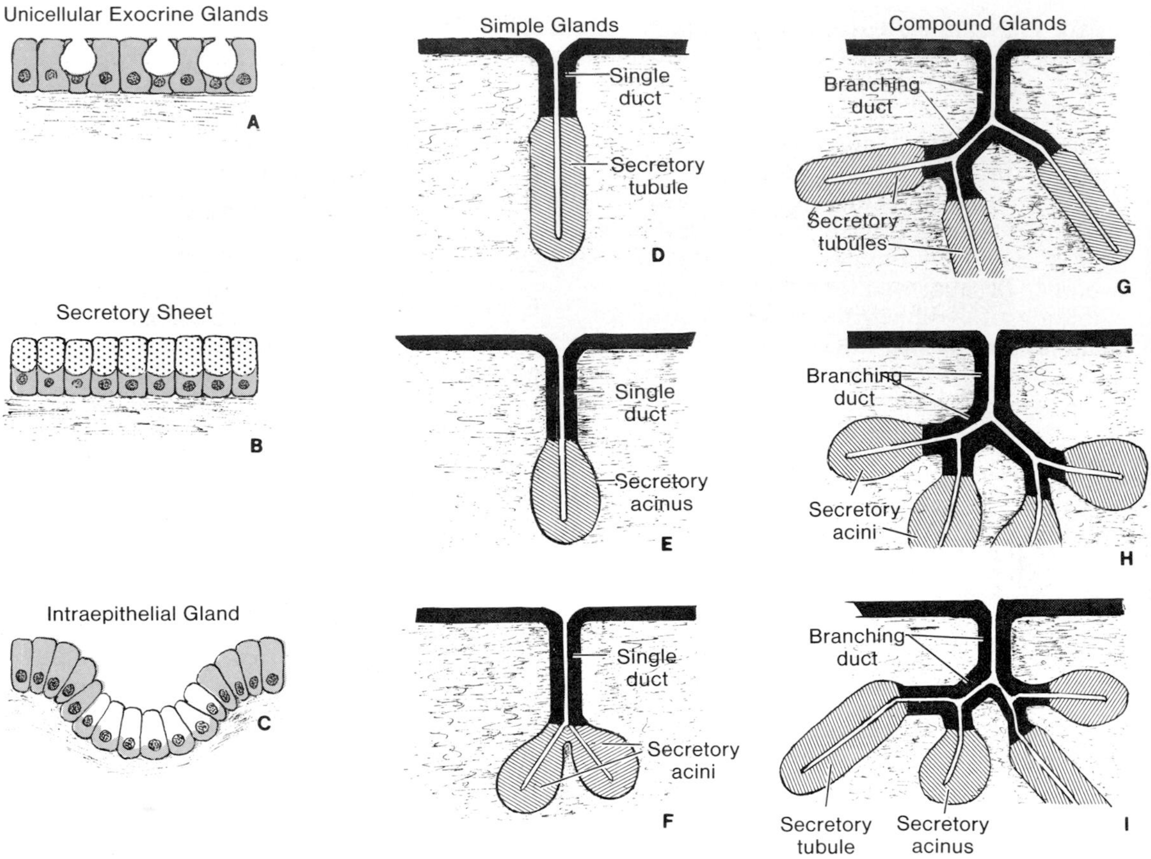

Figure 2.2. A schematic illustrating several glandular forms. *A*, unicellular glands; *B*, secretory sheet; *C*, intraepithelial gland; *D*, simple tubular gland; *E*, simple acinar gland; *F*, simple branched gland; *G*, compound tubular gland; *H*, compound acinar gland; *I*, compound tubuloacinar gland.

be arranged as clumps, cords or hollow spheroidal structures called follicles.

Type and Mode of Secretion

KEY WORDS: mucous, serous, mixed glands, merocrine, holocrine

Glands can be classified as mucous, serous or mixed according to the type of material secreted. Cells of **mucous** glands have pale, vacuolated cytoplasm and flattened, dense nuclei oriented toward the base of the cell. **Serous** cells show spherical nuclei surrounded by a basophilic cytoplasm that contains discrete secretory granules. **Mixed glands** contain variable proportions of serous and mucous cells.

From the mode of secretion, two types of glands can be distinguished. **Merocrine** secretion refers to release of the product through fusion of secretory vesicles with the apical plasmalemma. This is the process identified as exocytosis by electron microscopy, and most exocrine secretion is of this type. **Holocrine** secretion involves release of whole cells (such as sperm from the testes) or the breakdown of an entire cell to form the secretory product (as in sebaceous glands). A third type of secretion, apocrine, has been described in which a portion of the apical cytoplasm was said to be lost along with the secretory material. Electron microscopy has failed to support this mode of secretion except perhaps for the mammary glands. Even here, however, the existence of an apocrine secretion is dubious.

Myoepithelial Cells

The secretory units of some glands are associated with myoepithelial cells, specialized cells located between the glandular cells

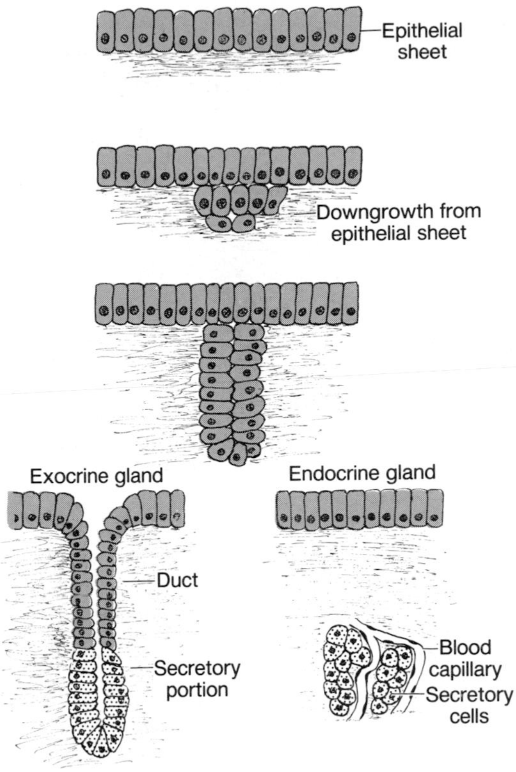

Figure 2.3. Formation of exocrine and endocrine glands. All glands form as an invagination from an epithelial sheet. Glands that retain a connection (duct) to the epithelial sheet of origin are classed as exocrine glands. Those that lose their connection are called endocrine glands and secrete into the blood vasculature.

and the basal lamina. The cytoplasm contains numerous filaments and the cells appear to be contractile. Long cytoplasmic processes extend from the body of the cell to course around the secretory unit. The processes, by their contraction, are thought to aid in expressing products from the secretory units into the ductal system. Myoepithelial cells occur in sweat, mammary and salivary glands and in glands along the bronchi and esophagus.

Development of Epithelium

Epithelium can arise from ectoderm, endoderm or mesoderm. Epithelial sheets derived from these germ layers cover the surface of the developing embryo and line the forming body cavities and tubular structures. Glands form as outpockets of epithe-

Table 2-2.
Classification of Glands

Unicellular Glands	
Goblet cells	Exocrine
G-cell and other endocrine cells of the gastrointestinal mucosa	Endocrine[a]
Multicellular Exocrine Glands	
Type	Example
Secretory sheet	Surface epithelium of gastric mucosa
Intraepithelial glands	Urethra
Simple tubular glands	Intestinal glands
Simple coiled tubular glands	Apocrine sweat glands
Simple branched tubular glands	Esophageal glands
Simple branched acinar glands	Meibomian glands
Compound tubular glands	Glands of gastric cardia
Compound tubuloacinar glands	Pancreas
Compound saccular glands	Prostate

Table 2-3.
Epithelial Derivatives

Epithelial Sheets	
Ectoderm	Epidermis; corneal covering; lining of nasal cavities, nasal sinuses, mouth and anal canal; nails, hair
Endoderm	Covering of posterior one-third of tongue; lining of pharynx, Eustachian tube, larynx, trachea, lungs, gastrointestinal tract, urinary bladder, urethra
Mesoderm	Lining of blood vessels, lymphatics, body cavities; joint cavities, ureter, genital ducts
Glands	
Ectoderm	Sweat, sebaceous, mammary, salivary glands, adenohypophysis
Endoderm	Thymus, thyroid, parathyroids; esophageal, duodenal and intestinal glands; pancreas, liver
Mesoderm	Kidney, gonads, adrenal cortex

lial sheets, from which ductal systems and secretory units develop as the epithelial outgrowth expands. If ductal connections are maintained with the epithelial sheet of origin, an exocrine gland is formed. If the connection is lost, an endocrine gland will develop. A summary of epithelial origins is shown in Table 2-3.

FUNCTIONAL SUMMARY

Epithelium covers the entire body surface and lines the digestive, respiratory, cardiovascular and urogenital systems. Any substance that enters or leaves the body must pass through an epithelial layer. Epithelia protect the organism from mechanical trauma and invasion by organisms, limit fluid loss from underlying connective tissues and prevent dehydration. They also function in absorption, transportation of useful materials and the excretion of wastes. In the form of glands, they secrete products such as hormones which regulate and integrate the activities of many tissues and organs.

Surface specializations—microvilli, stereocilia and basal infoldings—provide a greatly increased cell surface for the absorption and transport of materials into or out of the cells. Cilia provide a mechanism for moving materials across the surface of an epithelium. The nonmotile cilia of olfactory epithelia and kidney tubules serve as chemoreceptors, while the cilia of the inner ear act as mechanoreceptors and the modified cilia of retinal rods and cones are involved in photoreception.

The junctions between adjacent epithelial cells hold the cells together to form a continuous sheet. Desmosomes help maintain these cell-to-cell adhesions and also act as sites where tonofilaments of the cytoskeleton are anchored. Zonula occludens provides a tight seal between cells so that material crossing an epithelium must pass through the membranes of epithelial cells and not through intercellular spaces. Nexus junctions serve as points for intercellular communication and exchange of materials between cells.

Atlas for Chapter 2

Simple Epithelia

2-4

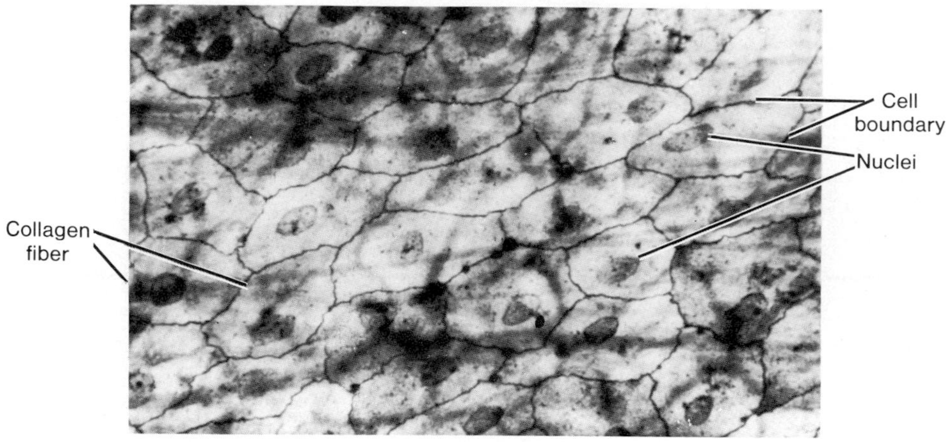

2-5

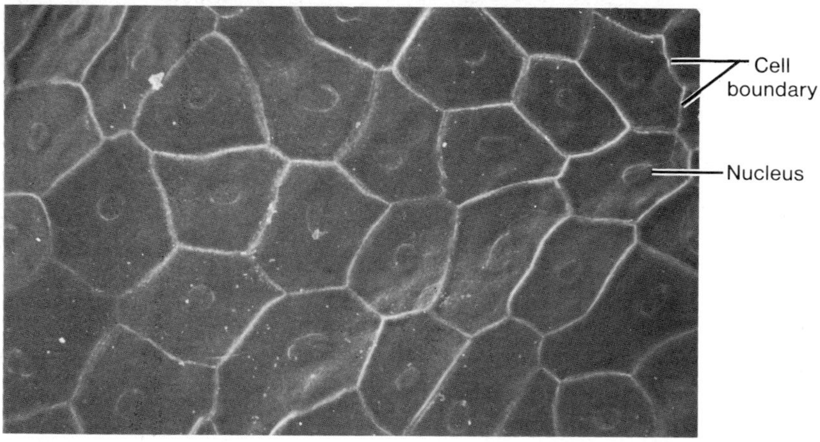

2-6

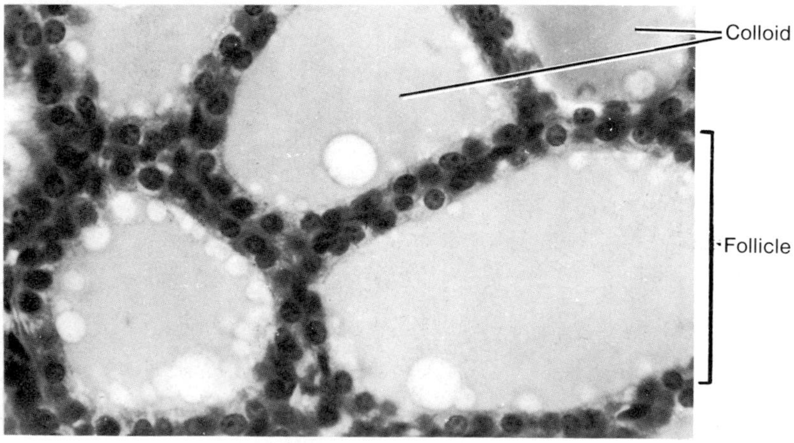

Figure 2.4. Mesentery (squamous). LM, ×400.
Figure 2.5. Periderm (squamous). SEM, ×400.
Figure 2.6. Thyroid (cuboidal). LM, ×300.

2-7

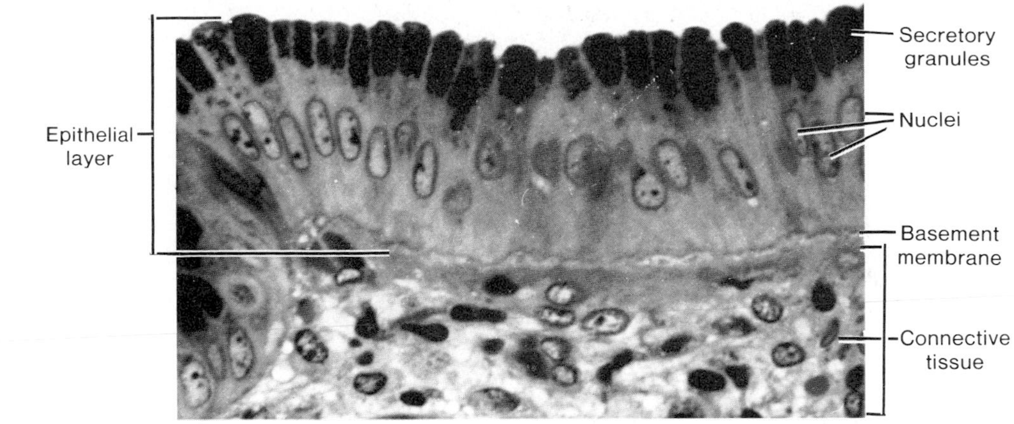

2-8

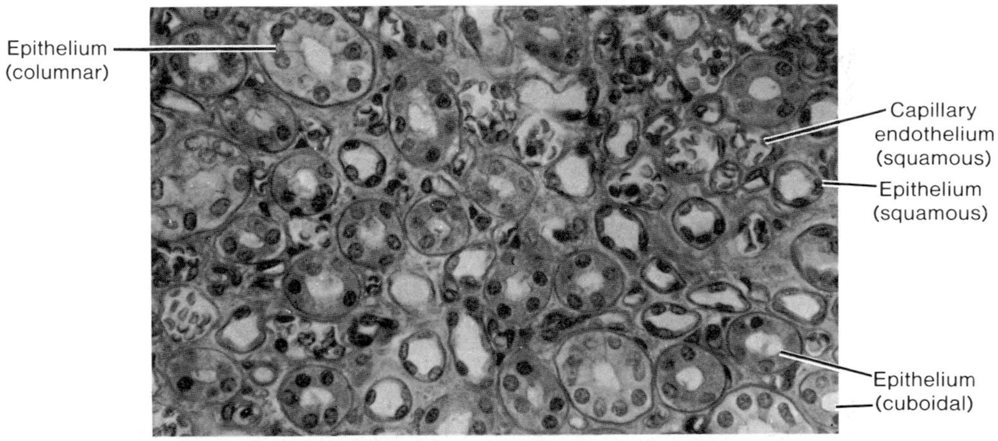

2-9 Pseudostratified and Stratified Epithelia

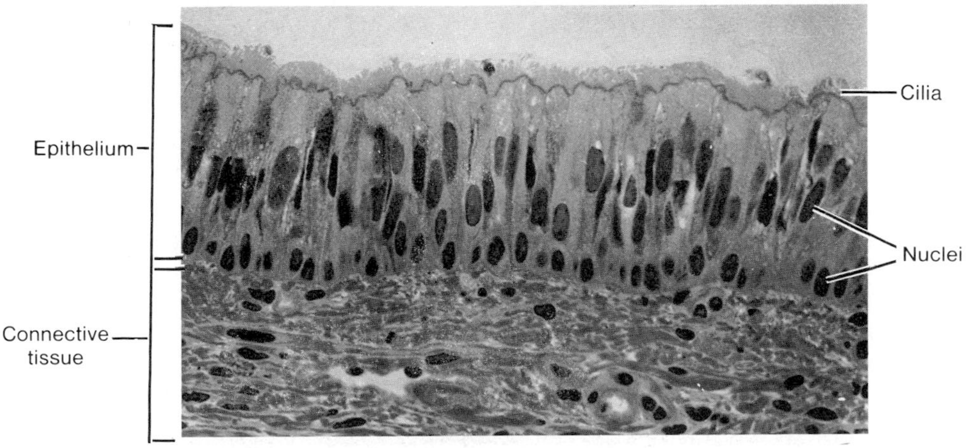

Figure 2.7. Stomach (columnar). LM, ×500.
Figure 2.8. Kidney medulla. LM, ×250.
Figure 2.9. Trachea (ciliated pseudostratified columnar). LM, ×400.

2-10

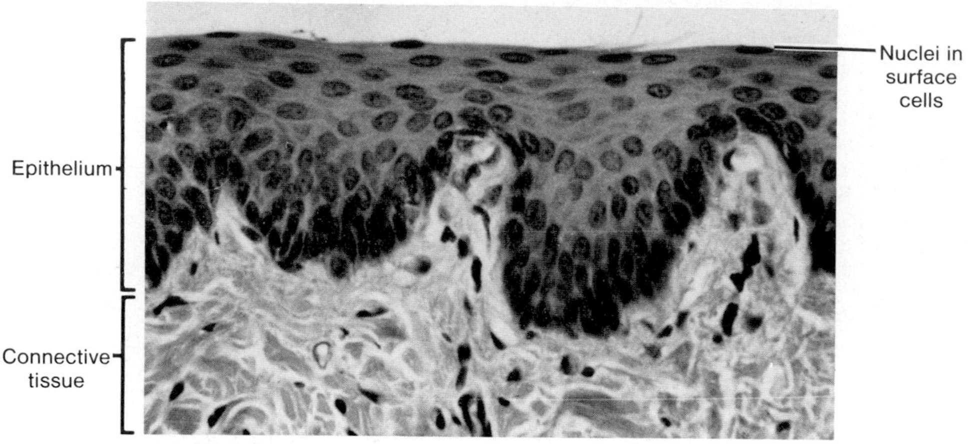

2-11

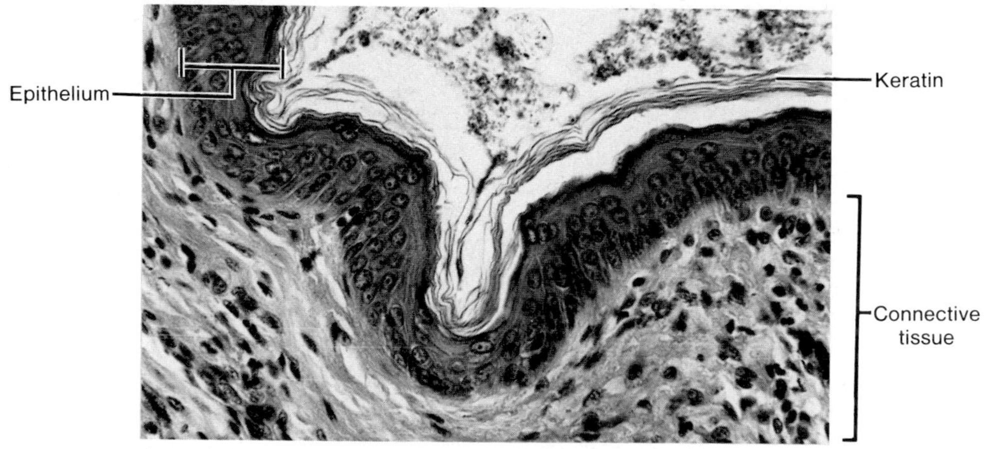

2-12

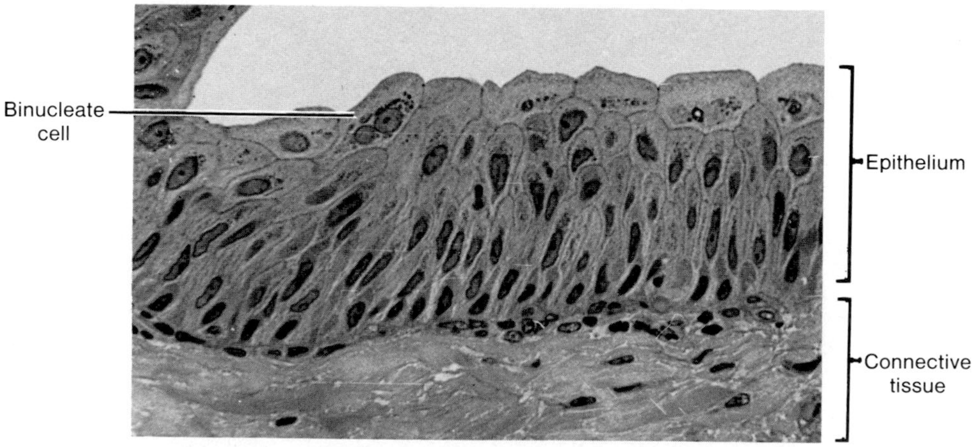

Figure 2.10. Esophagus (nonkeratinized stratified squamous). LM, ×300.
Figure 2.11. Skin (keratinized stratified squamous). LM, ×250.
Figure 12.2. Urinary bladder (transitional), LM, ×300.

2-13 Specializations of Plasmalemma

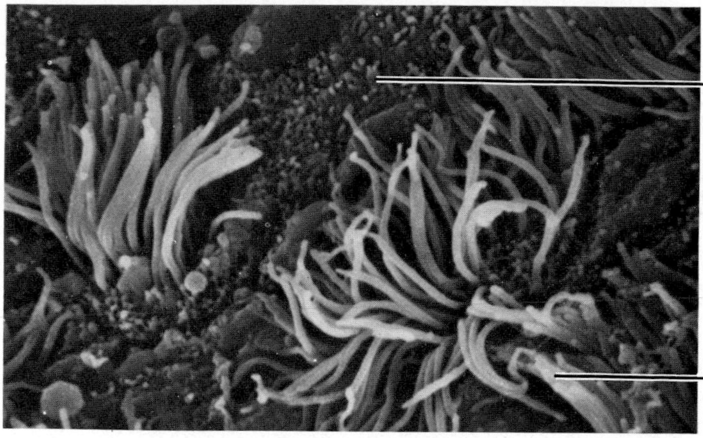

2-14

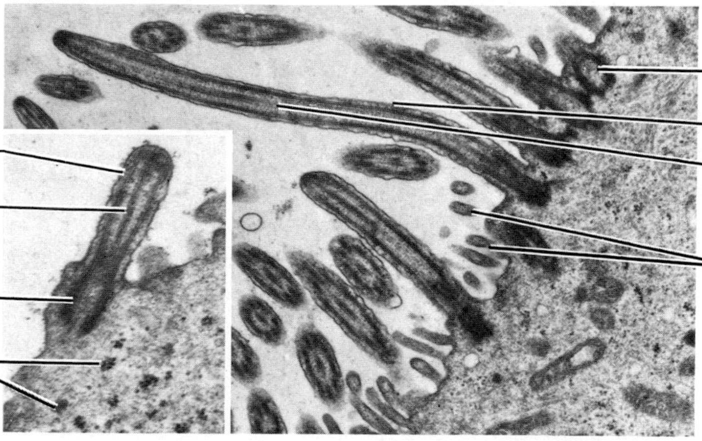

2-15

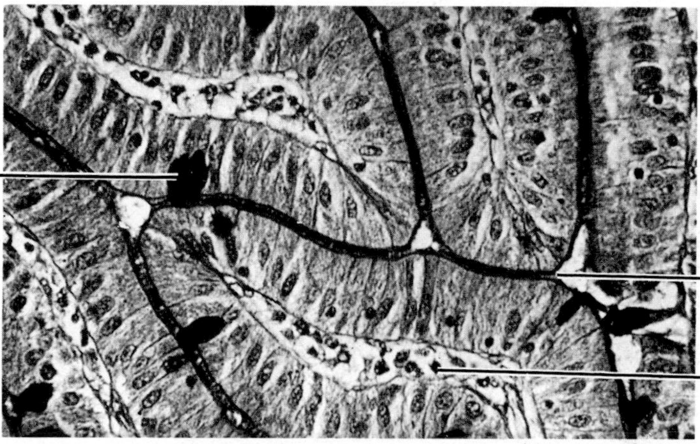

Figure 2.13. Oviduct (ciliated simple columnar). SEM, ×5000.
Figure 2.14. Trachea (ciliated psudostratified columnar.) TEM, ×20,000.
Figure 2.15. Intestine (simple columnar). LM, ×400.

2-16

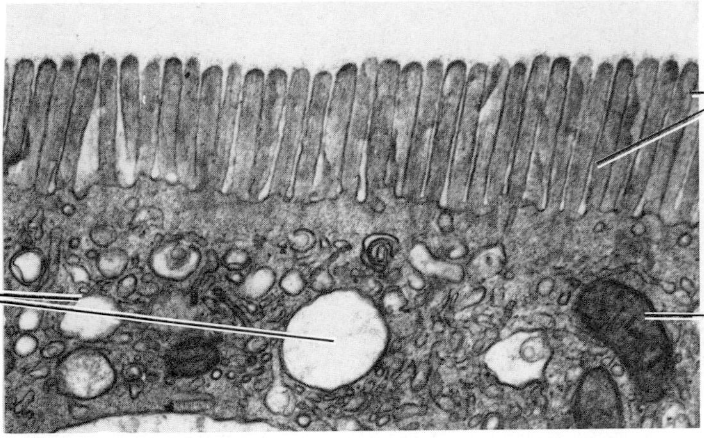

2-17

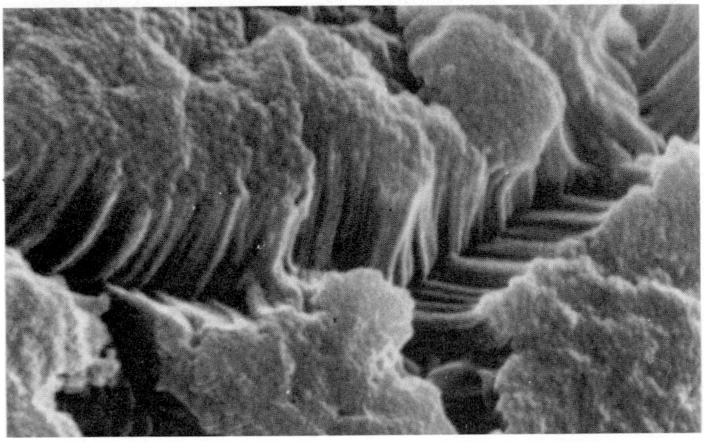

2-18

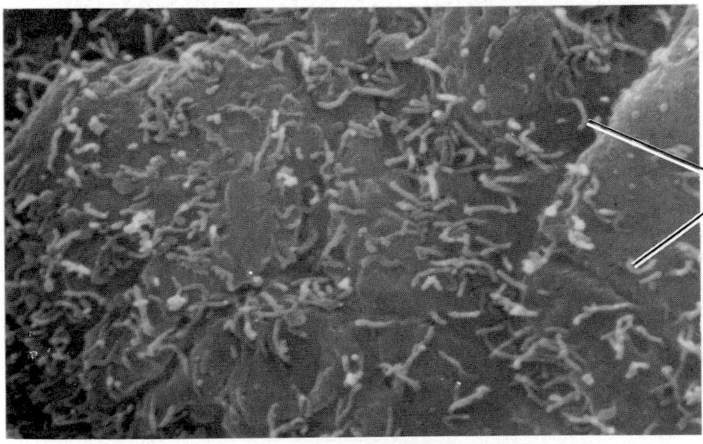

Figure 2.16. Intestine (microvilli, striated border). TEM, ×20,000.
Figure 2.17. Intestine (microvilli), striated border). SEM, ×17,000.
Figure 2.18. Pleura (microvilli). SEM, ×5000.

2-19

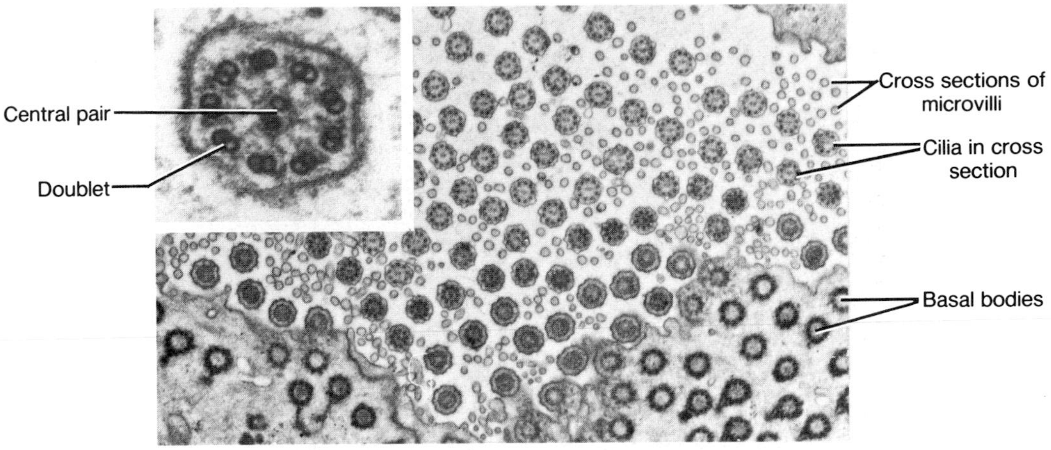

2-20

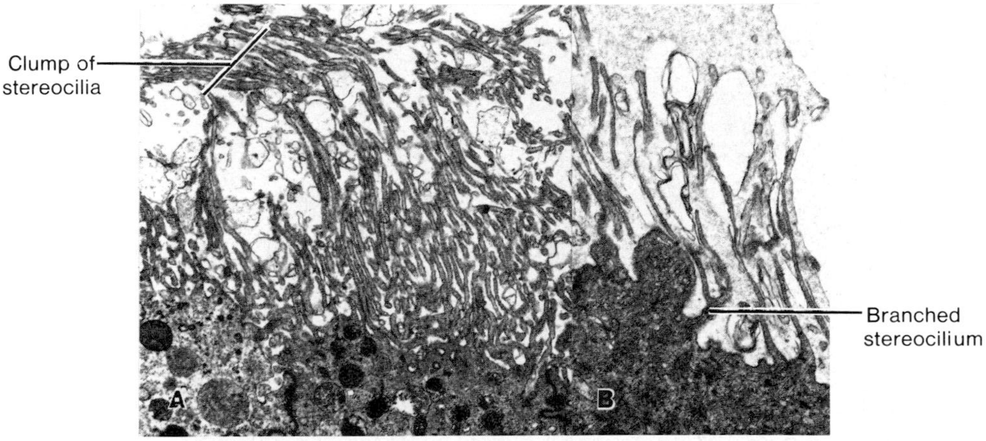

2-21

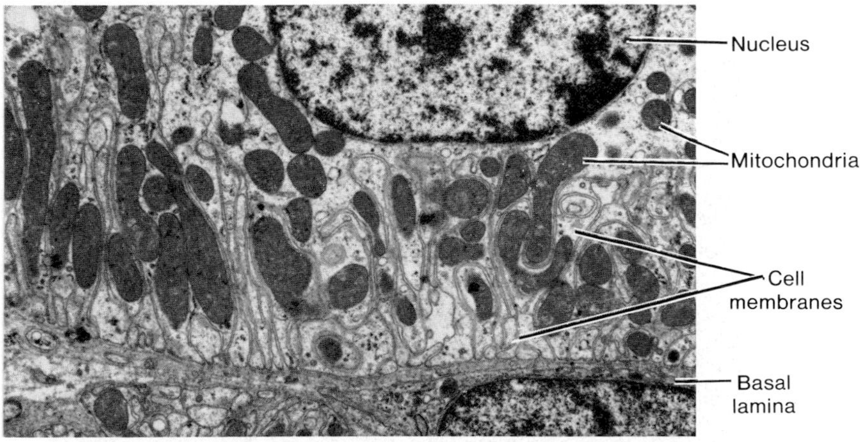

Figure 2.19. Trachea (microvilli and cilia). TEM, ×4000. Inset, ×80,000.
Figure 2.20. Epididymis (stereocilia). TEM, ×4000.
Figure 2.21. Kidney (infolding of basal cell membrane). TEM, ×2000.

2-22 Cell Attachments

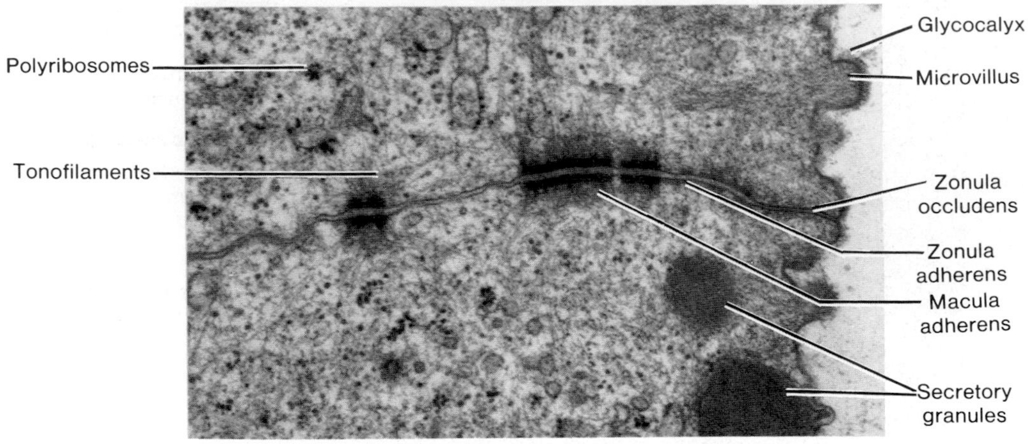

2-23

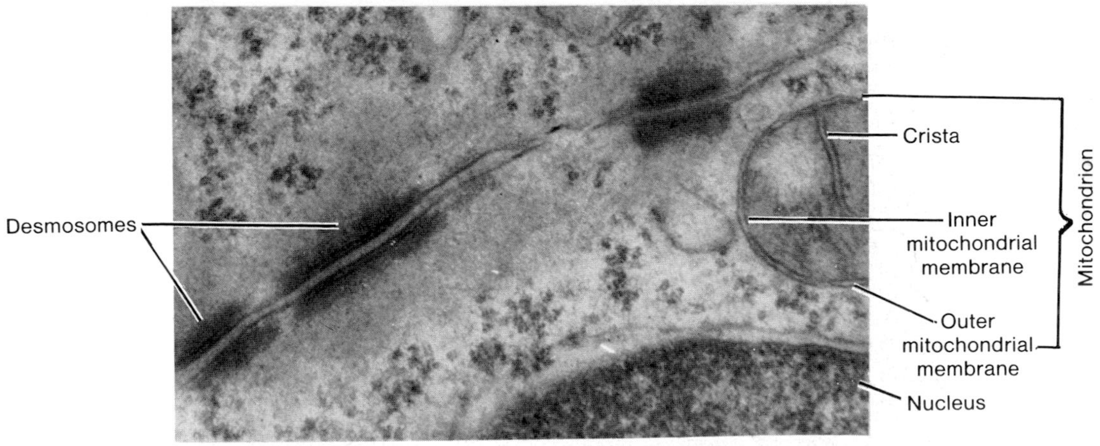

2-24

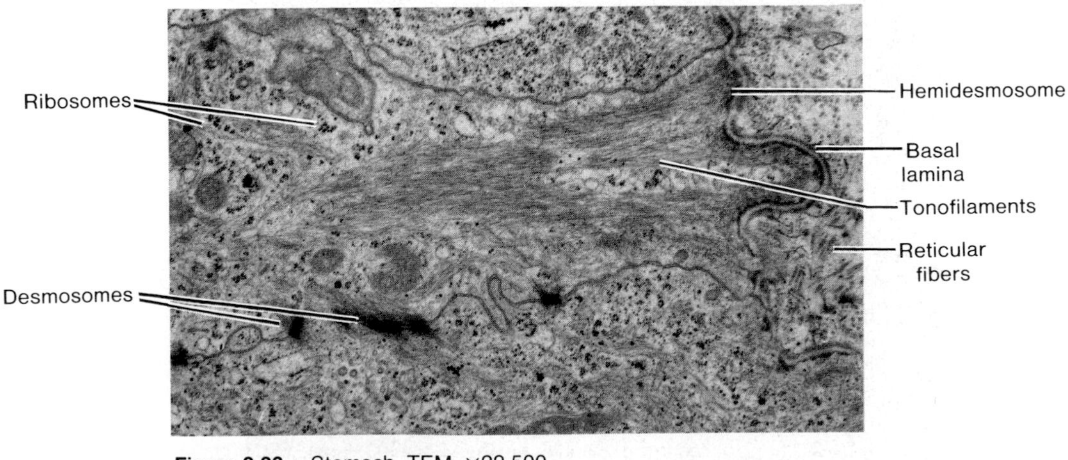

Figure 2.22. Stomach. TEM, ×22,500.
Figure 2.23. Intestinal epithelium (desmosomes, macula adherens). TEM, ×30,000.
Figure 2.24. Epidermis (hemidesmosomes). TEM, ×12,000.

2-25

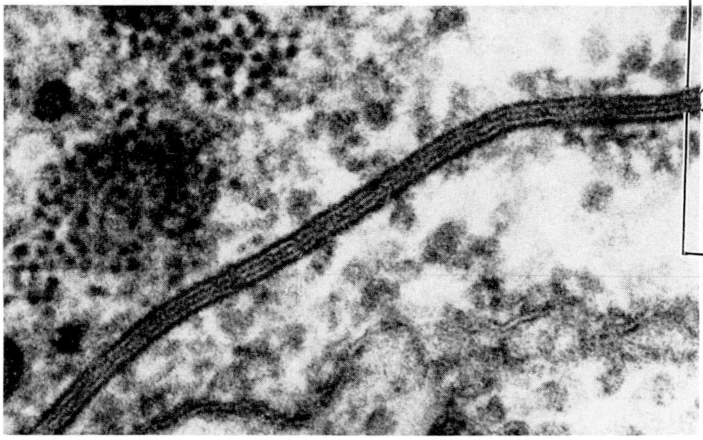

2-26

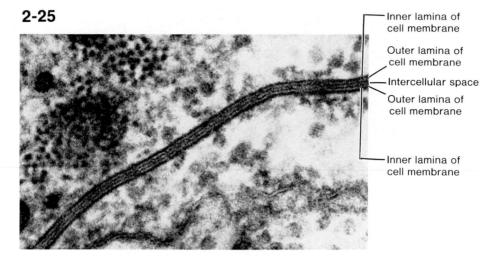

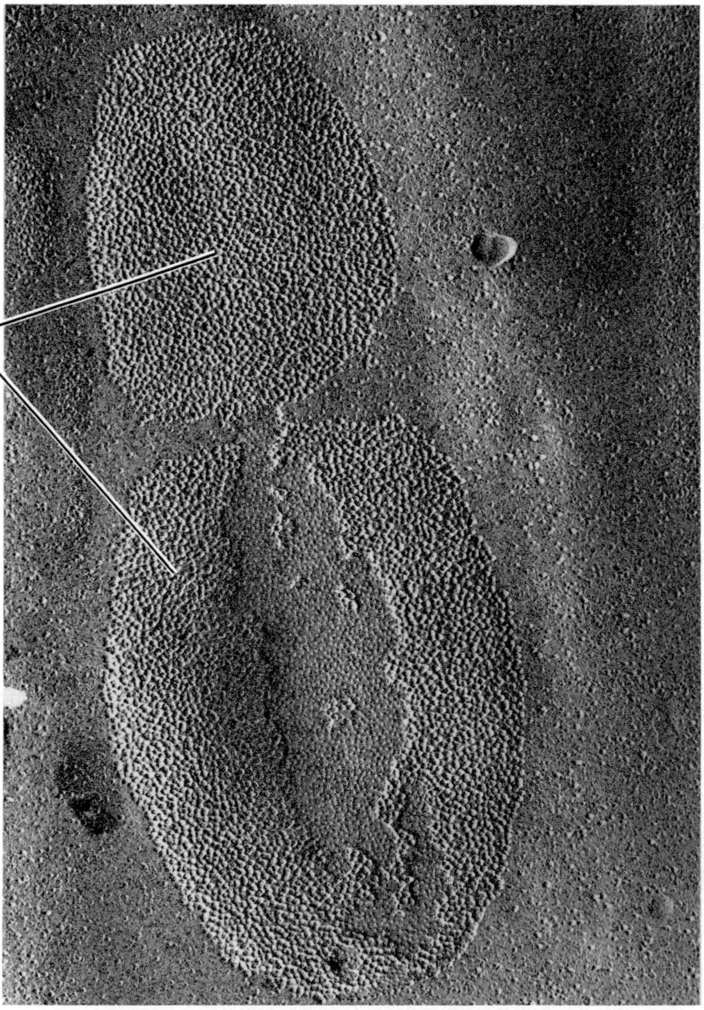

Figure 2.25. Nexus (gap) junction. TEM, ×206,000.
Figure 2.26. Nexus (gap) junction. Freeze-fracture, ×80,000.

Glands

2-27

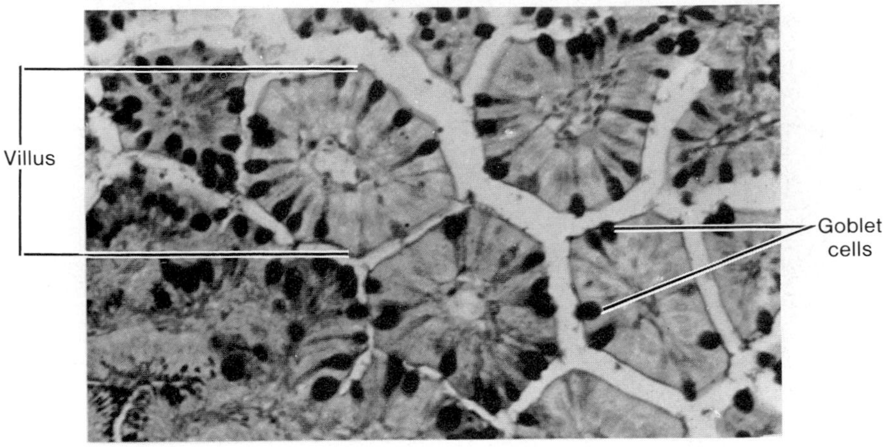

2-28

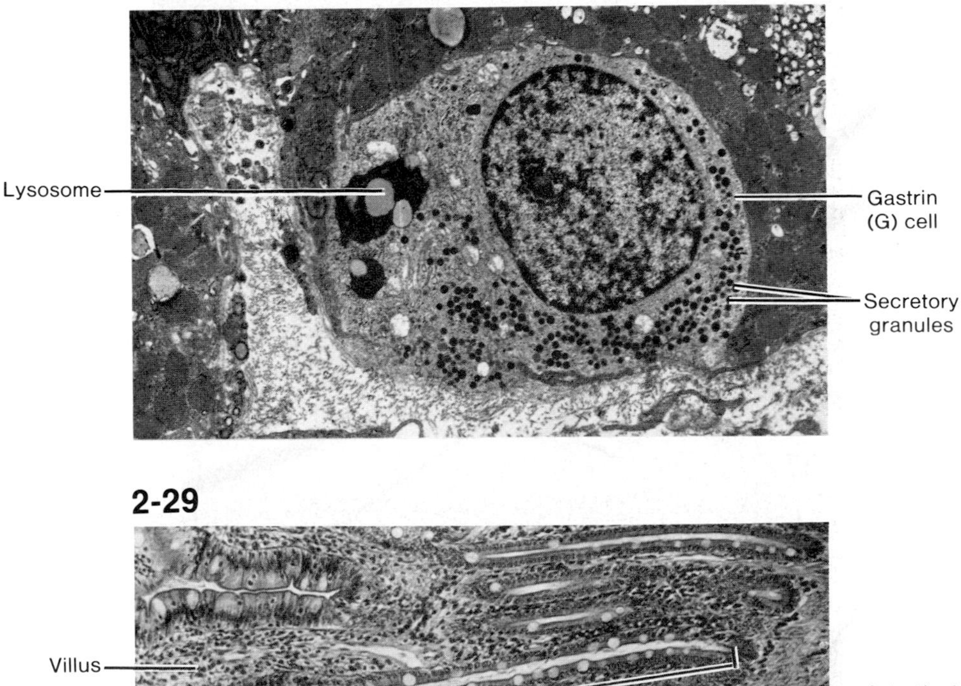

2-29

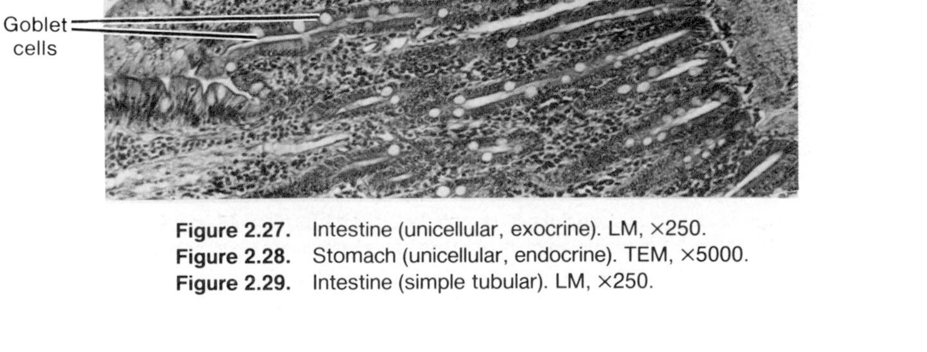

Figure 2.27. Intestine (unicellular, exocrine). LM, ×250.
Figure 2.28. Stomach (unicellular, endocrine). TEM, ×5000.
Figure 2.29. Intestine (simple tubular). LM, ×250.

2-30 Glands

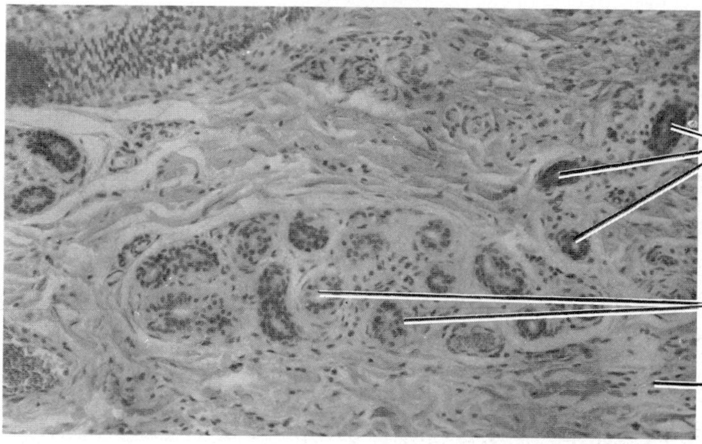

2-31

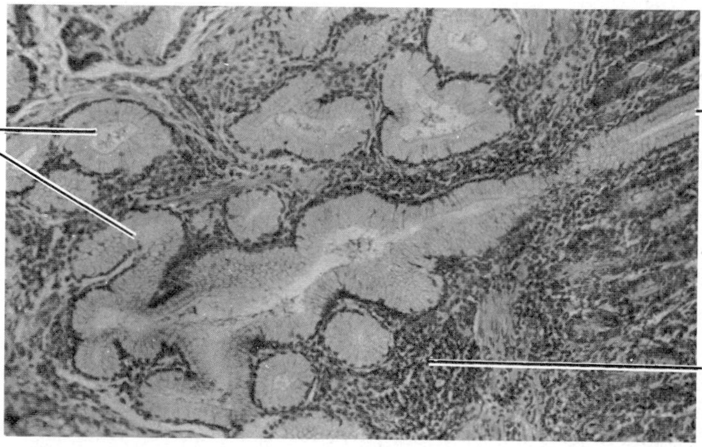

2-32

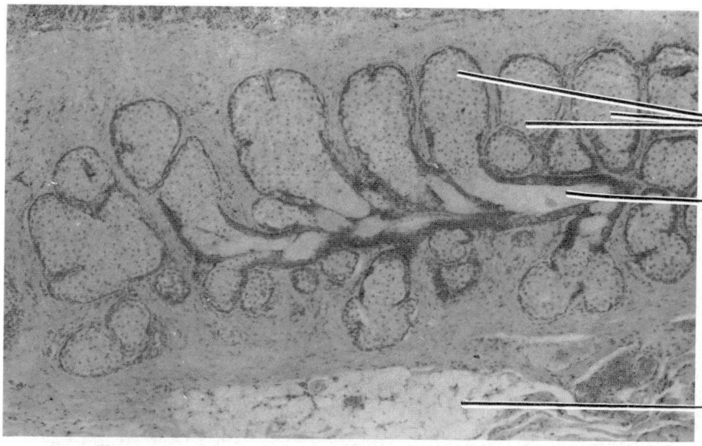

Figure 2.30. Sweat gland (simple coiled tubular). LM, ×250.
Figure 2.31. Duodenal gland (simple branched tubular). LM, ×200.
Figure 2.32. Meibomian gland (simple branched acinar). LM, ×100.

Glands

2-33

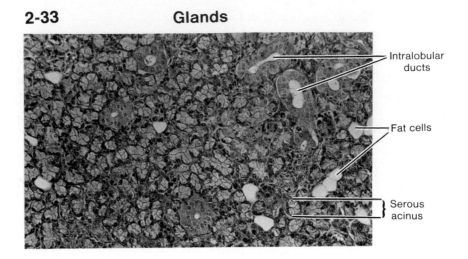

Intralobular ducts
Fat cells
Serous acinus

2-34

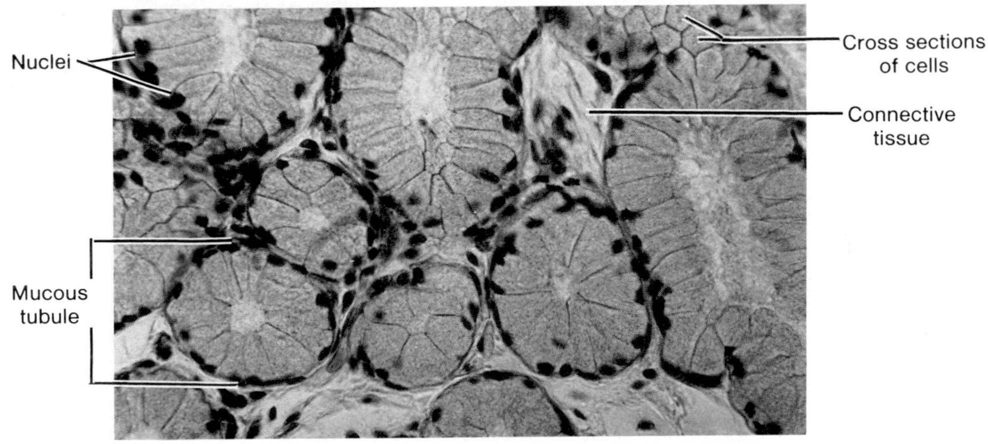
Nuclei
Cross sections of cells
Connective tissue
Mucous tubule

2-35

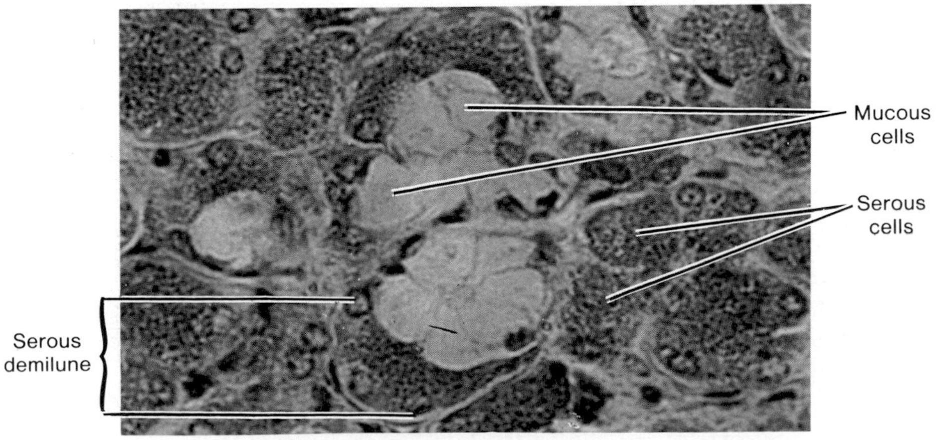
Mucous cells
Serous cells
Serous demilune

Figure 2.33. Parotid gland (compound tubuloacinar). LM, ×100.
Figure 2.34. Esophageal glands (mucous gland). LM, ×300.
Figure 2.35. Submandibular gland. LM, ×300.

2-36 Glands

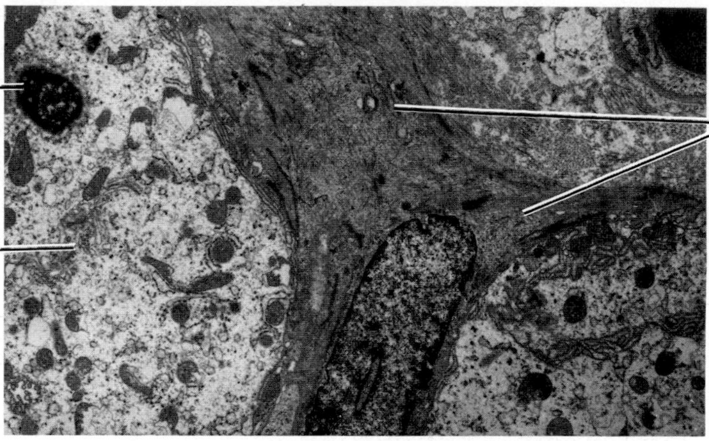

2-37

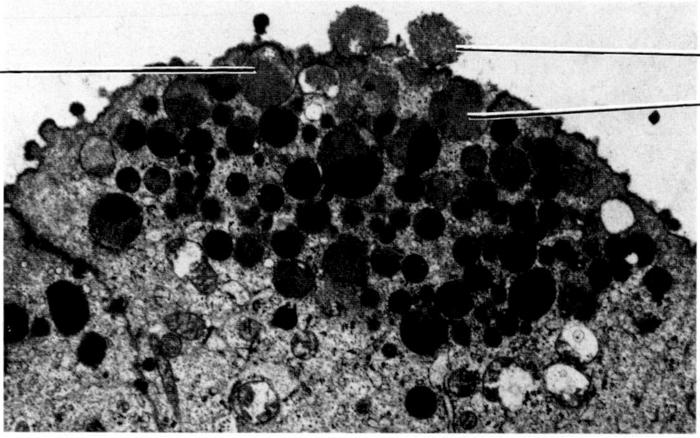

2-38

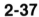

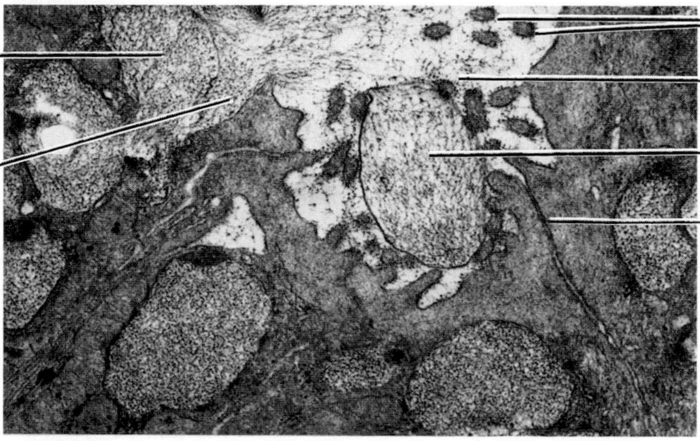

Figure 2.36. Bronchial gland (myoepithelial cell). TEM, ×4500.
Figure 2.37. Stomach (merocrine secretion). TEM, ×5000.
Figure 2.38. Duodenum (merocrine secretion). TEM, ×25,000.

3

General Connective Tissue

Connective tissues comprise a diverse group of tissues derived from mesenchyme and, in keeping with the diversity of types, the connective tissues perform a number of functions. They provide structural elements, serve as a foundation for the support of organs, form a packing material for otherwise unoccupied spaces, provide an insulating blanket (fat) which also serves as a storage depot that can be used to provide energy and they play a vital role in the defense mechanisms of the body. Some are functions of ordinary connective tissue, while others are functions of specialized connective tissue. Connective tissues form the *stroma* of organs, whereas the epithelial components make up the *parenchyma*.

ORGANIZATION

KEY WORDS: cells, intercellular substance, fibers, ground substance, matrix

Like all basic tissues, connective tissues consist of **cells** and **intercellular substances**. The latter consist of **fibers**, **ground substance** and tissue fluid. Unlike epithelium, where the cells are closely apposed with little intervening extracellular material, cells of connective tissue are widely separated by the intercellular fibers and ground substance which form the bulk of these tissues. Collectively, the fibers and ground substance form the connective tissue **matrix**. With only rare exceptions, connective tissue is well vascularized.

Classification

KEY WORDS: extracellular materials, general, special, loose, dense, regular, irregular

Classification of connective tissue into various subgroups is largely descriptive of **extracellular materials** rather than of features of the component cells. Two large categories can be first defined, the **general** and the **special** connective tissues, from which further subdivisions can be made. The general connective tissues are distinguished as **loose** or **dense**, according to whether the fibers are loosely or closely packed. The loose connective tissues can be classified further on the basis of some special properties of their constituents, such as adipose or fatty tissue, reticular tissue, etc. The dense connective tissues can be subdivided into two groups according to whether the fibers are randomly arranged or show an orderly arrangement. Thus, dense connective tissues are classed as **dense irregular** and **dense regular** connective tissue. Table 3-1 provides a classification of the connective tissues and indicates the diversity of their types.

Loose Connective Tissue

This is a common and simple form of connective tissue and can be considered as the prototype of connective tissues. Essentially, all other forms of connective tissues are variants of loose connective tissue in which one or more components have been emphasized to serve specific functions.

Fibers of Connective Tissue

KEY WORDS: collagenous fibers, unit fibrils, tropocollagen, α units, reticular fibers, elastic fibers, microfibrils, elastin

The fibrous intercellular substances consist of collagenous, reticular and elastic fibers. **Collagenous fibers** are found in all connective tissues and, although flexible, have extremely high tensile strength. The fibers vary in thickness from 1 to 10 μm, are of undefined length and run an irregular course with much branching. Ultrastructurally, collagenous fibers consist of parallel fibrils, each of which represents a structural unit. These **unit fibrils** show repeating transverse bands spaced at 64-nm intervals along their length and are composed of **tropocollagen**, in the form of macromolecules that measure approximately 260 nm in length and 1.5 nm in width. The tropocollagen molecules lie parallel to each other and overlap by about one-quarter of their lengths; the overlapping is responsible for the banding pattern. Each molecule of tropocollagen consists of three polypeptide chains, called **α units**, arranged in a helix and linked by hydrogen bonds. The polypeptides are rich in glycine and proline and also contain hydroxyproline and hydroxylysine. However, α units isolated from collagens taken from different sites vary somewhat in the composition and sequence of amino acids.

Nonfibrous collagen molecules are important components of basement membranes also. Five distinct molecular types of collagen have been indentified, all of which consist of three α units arranged in a right-hand helix. They differ mainly in the amino acid constituents of the α chain (Table 3-2).

Reticular fibers do not form bundles, as do collagen fibers, but tend to be present in delicate networks. They are not apparent in routinely prepared tissue sections but can be

Table 3-1
Subdivisions of Connective Tissue

Type	Locations
General connective tissues	
Loose connective tissue	
Mesenchyme	Primarily in the embryo and developing fetus
Mucoid	Umbilical cord
Areolar	A loose packing tissue found in most organs and tissues
Adipose	Omentum, subcutaneous tissue
Reticular	Lymph nodes, bone marrow
Dense connective tissue	
Irregular	Dermis, capsules of organs, periosteum, perichondrium
Regular	
Collagenous	Tendon, ligaments, aponeurosis, cornea
Elastic	Ligamentum nuchae, ligamentum flava
Special connective tissues	
Cartilage	
Hyaline	Costal cartilages, trachea
Fibrous	Symphysis pubis, intervertebral disk
Elastic	External ear, epiglottis
Bone	Skeleton
Blood	Cardiovascular system
Hemopoietic	Bone marrow, lymphatic tissue and organs

Table 3-2
Types of Collagen[a]

Type	Morphological features	Distribution
I	Broad, banded fibrils	Widespread; tendon, bone, dermis, dentin, fascia
II	Small diameter, banded fibrils	Hyaline cartilage, vitreous body, nucleus pulposus, notochord
III	Small diameter, banded fibrils	Corresponds to reticular fibers; prominent in organs with a major smooth muscle component; uterus, blood vessels
IV	Feltwork of nonbanded fibrils	Basal laminae of epithelial cells, glomerular epithelium
V	Thin, nonbanded fibrils	Widespread; pericellular laminae of smooth and striated muscle cells, tendon sheaths

[a] Various types of collagen can be elaborated by cells other than fibroblasts. Collagen is known to be synthesized by chondroblasts, osteoblasts, odontoblasts, and smooth muscle cells.

demonstrated with silver stains and by the periodic acid-Schiff reagent which reacts with the mucopolysaccharide coat of the fibers. In electron micrographs, reticular fibers show the same banding pattern and consist of the same unit fibrils as collagen; they differ principally in the number, diameter, and arrangement of the unit fibrils.

Elastic fibers appear as thin, homogeneous strands which are smaller and of more uniform size than collagen fibers. They cannot be distinguished in routine tissue sections and require special stains to make them visible. As seen with the electron microscope, elastic fibers consist of bundles of **microfibrils** embedded around an amorphous component called **elastin**. The microfibrils measure about 11 nm in diameter and lack crossbanding. During their formation, the microfibrils are laid down first and the elastin is added secondarily, but soon forms the bulk of the fiber. The microfibrillar component tends to have a peripheral location on the fiber.

Elastin, like collagen, contains glycine and proline but has little hydroxyproline and lacks hydroxylysine. It has a high content of valine and contains two amino acids, desmosine and isodesmosine, that are specific to elastin. It is thought that elastin is secreted as a precursor, proelastin. The microfibrillar protein differs from elastin; it contains less glycine and has no hydroxyproline, desmosine or isodesmosine.

Where present, elastic fibers permit connective tissues to undergo considerable expansion or stretching and return to the original shape or dimension when the deforming force is removed. In addition to forming fibers, elastin may be present in fenestrated sheets as in some arterial walls.

Ground Substance

KEY WORDS: gel, glycoproteins and proteoglycans, bound water

The fibers and cells of connective tissue are embedded in an amorphous material called ground substance, which is present as a transparent **gel** of variable viscosity. Ground substance consists of **glycoproteins and proteoglycans** that differ in amount, consistency and type in the different kinds of connective tissues (Table 3-3). Proteoglycans have a bottle brush configuration with long protein cores, to which are attached numerous glycosaminoglycan side chains. Tropocollagen also has been extracted from ground substance but cannot be demonstrated histologically.

Ground substance contains a high proportion of water which is bound to long chain carbohydrates and to proteoglycans; most of the extravascular fluid is in this state. This **bound water** serves as a medium by which nutrients, gases and metabolites can be exchanged between blood and tissue cells. Hyaluronic acid is the principle proteoglycan of loose connective tissue and, because of its capacity to bind water, is primarily

Table 3-3
Types of Proteoglycans

Type	Some locations
Hyaluronic acid	Umbilical cord, vitreous humor, synovial fluid, loose connective tissue
Chondroitin	Cornea
Chondroitin-4-sulfate	Aorta, bone, cartilage, cornea
Chondroitin-6-sulfate	Cartilage, nucleus pulposus, sclera, tendon, umbilical cord
Dermatan sulfate	Aorta, heart valves, ligamentum nuchae, sclera, skin, tendon
Keratan sulfate	Bone, cartilage, cornea, nucleus pulposus

responsible for changes in the permeability and viscosity of this connective tissue. Ground substance also plays an important role in preventing or retarding the spread of microorganisms and various toxic materials elaborated at sites of infections.

Cells

KEY WORDS: fibroblasts, macrophages, system of mononuclear phagocytes, mast cells, heparin, histamine, fat cells, adipose tissue, plasma cells, clock-face nuclei, immunoglobulins

Connective tissues contain a number of different cell types; some are indigenous to the tissues whereas others are transients derived from the blood. The most common and ubiquitous connective tissue cells are the **fibroblasts**. These are large, flattened cells with ellipitical nuclei that contain one or two nucleoli. The cell body is irregular and often appears stellate, with long cytoplasmic processes extending along the connective tissue fibers. The boundaries of the cell are not seen in most histological preparations. The morphology varies with the state of activity; in active cells the nuclei are plump and stain lightly whereas the nuclei of inactive cells appear slender and dense. Ultrastructurally, the active cells show an increase in the amount of granular endoplasmic reticulum. Fibroblasts elaborate the precursors of collagenous, reticular and elastic fibers, produce the amorphous ground substance and maintain these extracellular substances which are continually being removed and renewed.

The peptides of collagen are formed (Fig. 3-1) on the ribosomes of the granular endoplasmic reticulum, from which they are transported to the Golgi complex. A molecular form of collagen (procollagen) is released from the maturing face of the Golgi complex into the surrounding cytoplasm, then outside the cell. An enzyme, procollagen peptidase, converts the procollagen molecule into tropocollagen, which then polymerizes extracellularly to form the unit fibril of collagen.

Macrophages (histiocytes) are almost as abundant as fibroblasts. They are actively phagocytic, ingesting a variety of materials from inert particulate matter to bacteria, tissue debris and whole dead cells. The material ingested is broken down in the usual manner by lysosomal digestion. The macrophage is commonly described as an irregularly shaped cell with blunt cytoplasmic processes and an ovoid or indented nucleus which is smaller and more heterochromatic than that of the fibroblast. In actual fact, macrophages are difficult to distinguish from fibroblasts (especially active fibroblasts) unless the macrophages show evidence of phagocytosis. They can be identified readily in the tissues of animals that have been injected with colloidal materials such as trypan blue or India ink; the phagocytosed particles in the cytoplasm distinguish macrophages from fibroblasts.

The macrophages of loose connective tissue are part of a generalized **system of mononuclear phagocytes** which includes phagocytes of the liver, lung (alveolar macrophages), serous cavities (pleural and peritoneal macrophages), nervous sytem (microglial cells), spleen and lymph nodes. Regardless of where they are found, macrophages have a common origin from precursors in the bone marrow. The monocyte of the blood represents a transit form of macrophage.

Mast cells are present in variable numbers in loose connective tissue and often congregate along small blood vessels. They are large, ovoid cells 20 to 30 μm in diameter with large granules that fill the cytoplasm. In man the granules are membrane-bound and in electron micrographs show a charac-

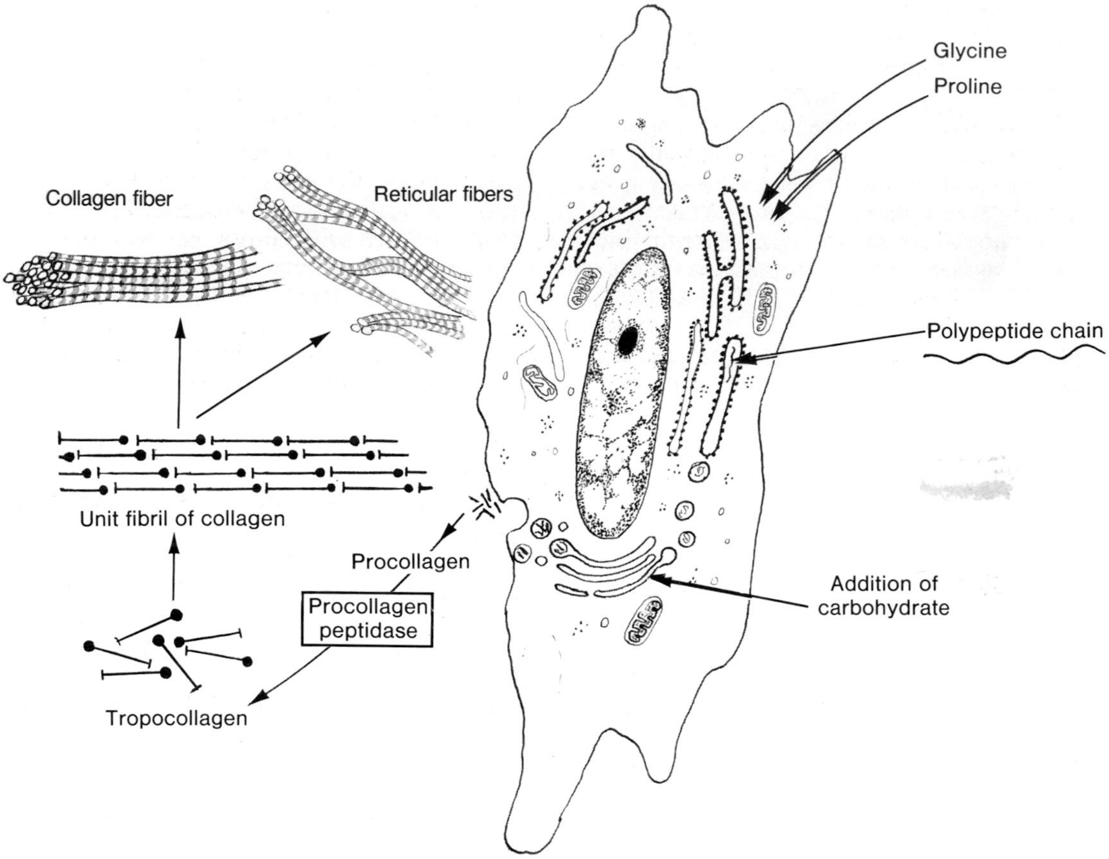

Figure 3-1. Formation of collagen by fibroblasts.

teristic tubular pattern. The granules contain two important biologically active compounds: **heparin**, a potent anticoagulant, and **histamine**, a substance that causes vasodilation and induces an increased permeability of capillaries and venules.

Fat cells are specialized for the synthesis and storage of lipid. Individual fat cells may be scattered throughout loose connective tissue or may accumulate to such an extent that other cells are crowded out and an **adipose tissue** is formed. Individual fat cells acquire so much lipid that the nucleus becomes flattened and pushed to one side; the cytoplasm appears only as a rim around a large droplet of lipid. In routine sections, the fat cells appear empty due to the loss of the lipid: groups of fat cells often have a "chicken wire" appearance because of this.

Plasma cells are not common in most loose connective tissues but may be numerous in the lamina propria of the gastrointestinal tract and are present in lymphoid tissues. Plasma cells appear ovoid in shape with a small, eccentrically placed nucleus in which the chromatin may be distributed along the nuclear envelope in coarse blocks, forming the **"clockface" nucleus.** The cytoplasm is deeply basophilic due to the extensive concentration of the granular endoplasmic reticulum. A pale staining area of the cytoplasm often is found adjacent to one pole of the nucleus and corresponds to a prominent Golgi complex. Plasma cells produce the **immunoglobulins** (antibodies) that form an important defense against infections. Various acidophilic inclusion bodies may be found in the cytoplasm of some plasma cells.

Migratory Cells

KEY WORDS: leukocytes, neutrophils, eosinophils, lymphocytes, monocytes

Variable numbers of **leukocytes** are constantly migrating into the connective tissue from the blood. **Neutrophils** are one type of leukocyte characterized by a lobed nucleus and cytoplasmic granulations. In this particular type, the granules are said to be neutrophilic although in sections they appear faintly pink. The cell is actively phagocytic for small particles. They are especially numerous at sites of local infections and are the major cellular component of pus.

Eosinophils also are characterized by a lobed nucleus and cytoplasmic granules which are larger, more spherical and more discretely visible than those of the neutrophil. As the name implies, the granules stain intensely with acid dyes such as eosin. These cells also are phagocytic and have a special avidity for antigen-antibody complexes.

Lymphocytes belong to the class of leukocytes called mononuclear leukocytes and are characterized by a single, round, nonlobed nucleus. They are the smallest of the cells migrating into connective tissues and measure about 7 μm in diameter. These cells form part of the immunological defense system and may give rise to the antibody-producing cells or elaborate nonspecific cytotoxic agents that destroy foreign cells. They are few in number in normal connective tissues but increase markedly in areas of chronic inflammation.

Monocytes are the blood borne forerunners of the tissue macrophages. Once the monocytes have entered the connective tissues it is difficult, if not impossible, to distinguish them from macrophages. Monocytes can fuse with each other to form multinucleated giant cells in an attempt to engulf or wall off objects that are too large or are otherwise resistant to phagocytosis by a single cell.

Subtypes of Loose Connective Tissue

Mesenchyme is a loose spongy tissue which forms a packing between the developing structures of the embryo. It consists of a loose network of stellate and spindle-shaped cells embedded in an amorphous ground substance that contains only a few fibers. The cells have multiple developmental potentials and can give rise to any of the connective tissues. The presence of mesenchymal cells in the adult long has been advocated to explain the expansion of adult connective tissue cells. However, fibroblasts are capable of sequential divisions and the idea of mesenchymal rests in adults can well be discarded.

Mucoid tissue is found in many parts of the embryo but is particularly prominent in the umbilicus, where it has been called Wharton's jelly. Histologically it resembles mesenchyme: the constituent cells are stellate fibroblasts with long processes that often make contact with those of neighboring cells. The intercellular substance is abundant, soft and jelly-like. It contains thin collagenous fibers which increase with the age of the fetus. Mucoid tissue does not have the developmental potencies of mesenchyme.

Areolar connective tissue is a loosely arranged connective tissue that is widely distributed throughout the body. It contains collagenous fibers and a few elastic fibers embedded in a thin, almost fluid-like ground substance. This type of connective tissue binds organs and organ components together. It also may form a helix around the long axis of expansible tubular structures such as the ducts of glands, the gastrointestinal tract or blood vessels.

Adipose Tissue

KEY WORDS: white fat, unilocular, brown fat, multilocular

Adipose tissue can be subdivided into white fat and brown fat. **White fat** is the more plentiful and is found primarily in the subcutaneous tissue, where it forms the panniculus adiposus, in omenta, in mesenteries, in pararenal tissue and in bone marrow. Adipose tissue differs in two respects from other connective tissues: fat cells and not the intercellular substances are the predominant feature and, unlike other connective tissue cells, each fat cell is surrounded by its own basal lamina. Reticular and collagenous fibers also extend around each fat cell to provide a delicate supporting framework that contains numerous capillaries. White fat is an extremely vascular tissue and also contains numerous nerve fibers. In this type of fat, the cells are filled by a single, large droplet of lipid and white fat is often referred to as **unilocular** fat. The lipid droplet is composed of glycerol esters and fatty acids. The materials within the fat droplet are not static but are in a constant state of flux.

White adipose tissue serves as a storage

depot for calories taken in excess of the body's needs, and fat can be utilized for the production of energy. It also serves as an insulating layer to reduce loss of body heat, acts mechanically as a packing material and forms shock-absorbing pads in the palms of the hands, soles of the feet and around the eyeball.

Brown fat is present in many species, including man, and is prominent in hibernating animals and in the newborn. Brown fat has a restricted distribution, occurring primarily in the interscapular and inguinal regions. The cells show round nuclei and the cytoplasm is filled with numerous small droplets of lipid; hence, this type of fat is referred to as **multilocular** fat. Mitochondria are more numerous and larger than those in cells of white fat, and their content of cytochrome enzymes results in the brown or tan color of brown fat. Each cell of brown fat receives direct sympathetic innervation.

During arousal from hibernation, the lipid within the brown fat is oxidized to produce heat and the release of substances such as glycerol, which are used by other tissues. Because brown fat is even more vascular than is white fat, the temperature of the blood is raised significantly, thus increasing the general body temperature.

Reticular Connective Tissue

KEY WORDS: reticular cells, reticular fibers, fibroblasts

Reticular connective tissue is characterized by a cellular and fibrillar framework as seen in lymphatic tissues and bone marrow. The **reticular cells** are stellate in shape, with the processes extending along the **reticular fibers** to make contact with neighboring cells. The cytoplasm stains lightly and is attenuated and the cell contains a large, palely staining nucleus. The reticular cell is equivalent to the **fibroblast** of other connective tissues and is responsible for the production and maintenance of the fibers. The reticular fibers are identical to those in loose connective tissues.

Dense Connective Tissue

Dense connective tissue differs from the loose variety chiefly in the concentration of fibers and in the reduction of the cellular and amorphous constituents. Two types are identified, the dense irregular and dense regular connective tissues.

Dense irregular connective tissue contains abundant thick collagenous bundles that are irregularly woven into a compact matwork. Among the collagen fibers is an extensive network of elastic fibers.

Dense regular connective tissue also contains a predominance of collagen fibers arranged in bundles, but these show a regular, precise arrangement. The organization of the collagen bundles reflects the mechanical needs of the tissue; in tendons, for example, they are oriented in the direction of pull. Fibroblasts are the only cells present and occur in rows parallel to the collagenous bundles.

Special Connective Tissues

These are connective tissues whose function and histological organization is sufficiently unique to warrant their consideration as distinct and special forms of connective tissues and/or organs. Each will be considered individually in succeeding sections.

DEVELOPMENT OF CONNECTIVE TISSUES

All connective tissues originate from mesoderm, the middle of the three primary germ layers of the early embryo. Mesoderm consists primarily of large stellate mesenchymal cells whose numerous processes are in contact with those of adjacent cells. Initially, only mesenchymal cells and a thin ground substance are present but as development proceeds, an interlacing network of fine collagenous fibers appears. Very early in development the mesodermal layer becomes transformed into a mesenchymal compartment, separated from surrounding epithelium by a basal lamina. Collagen molecules form a major component of such laminae, which are important in determining what substances enter or leave the connective tissue compartments. With further development, the mesenchymal compartment becomes transformed into numerous, irregularly shaped connective tissue passageways that surround neural and muscular tissues or lie between epithelial tissues. The parenchyma of glands and organs develop from invaginations of epithelium that extend into the mesenchymal compartments. Interaction between epithelium and mesenchyme is essential for normal development to occur.

FUNCTIONAL SUMMARY

The functions of connective tissue are mainly passive, but mechanically they are indispensible. They provide the supporting framework for organs and for the body itself and also serve to connect distant structures as, for example, the connection of muscle to bone by tendons. The connective tissues bind organs together and unite the organ components into a functioning unit. Adipose tissue forms an insulating blanket to limit heat loss and forms mechanically protective cushions in the hands and feet and about the eyeball. It also stores excess nutrients in the form of fat which, being labile, can be called upon and used as needed to provide energy.

Collagenous fibers provide tissues with flexibility and high tensile strength; elastic fibers allow considerable deformability of an organ or structure and permit recovery of the shape or size when the force is removed. Collagen molecules also form a major component of basal laminae which determine vascular and epithelial permeability.

The connective tissue also makes a significant contribution to the defense of the body. This is mainly a function of the cellular components as, for example, the phagocytic activity of macrophages and blood granular leukocytes. Also contributing are the antibodies elaborated by plasma cells and cytotoxic agents formed by some lymphocytes. The ground substance also plays an important role in the body's defenses by preventing or retarding the spread of microorganisms and toxic materials elaborated at the site of local infection.

The various connective tissues can be thought of as forming a single vast compartment limited by sheets of epithelia. It is through this compartment that tissue fluid must pass during the exchange of nutrients and waste products between cells and tissues and the blood vasculature. Most immune reactions take place in this compartment. Because the ground substance of loose connective tissue binds water, it can act as the medium by which this exchange is effected.

Atlas for Chapter 3

3-2 General Connective Tissue

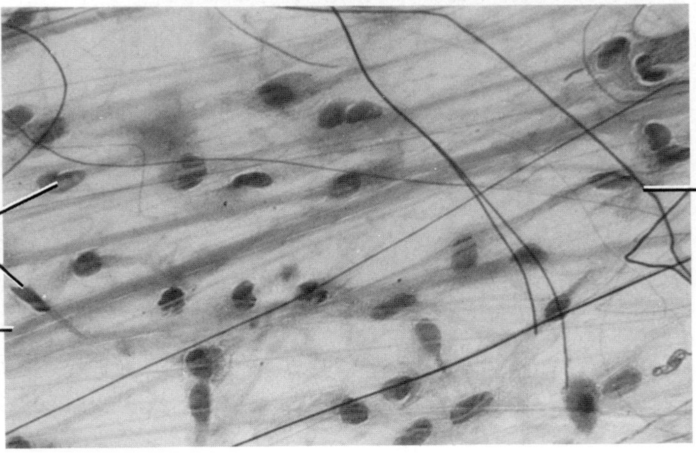

3-3

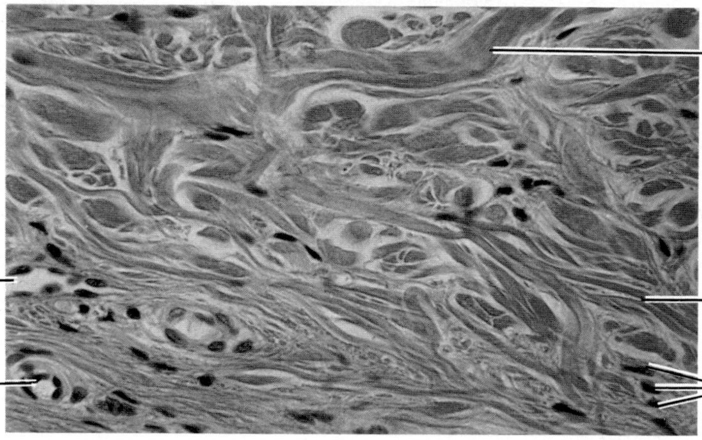

3-4

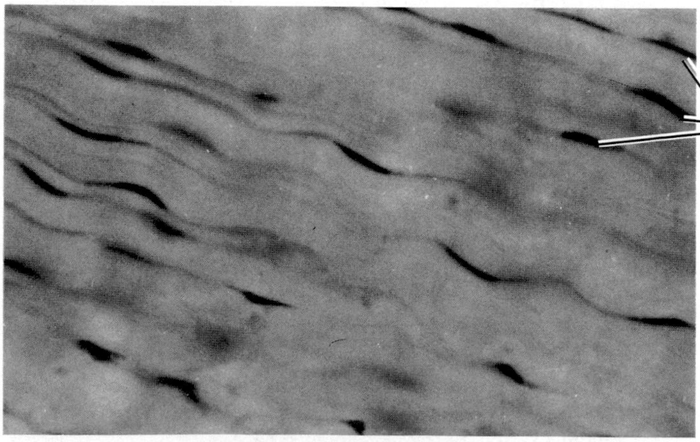

Figure 3-2. Loose connective tissue. LM, ×400.
Figure 3-3. Dermis (dense irregular connective tissue). LM, ×250.
Figure 3-4. Tendon (dense regular connective tissue). LM, ×400.

3-5

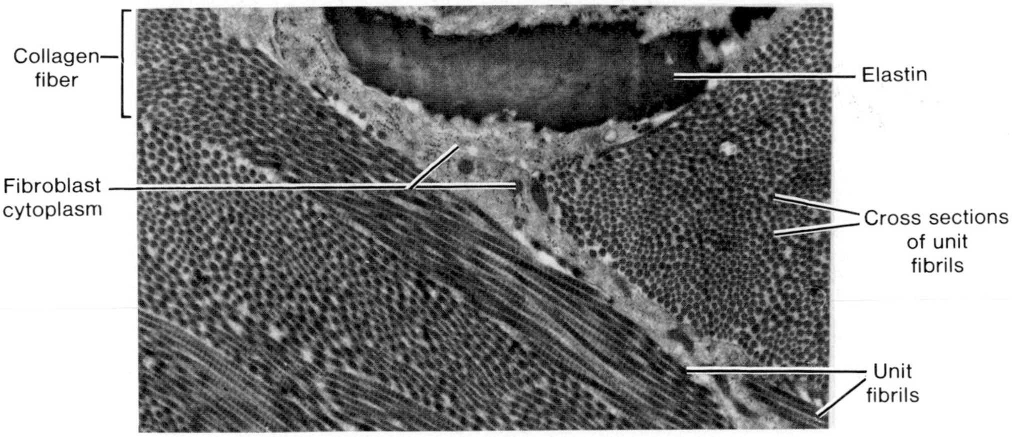

3-6

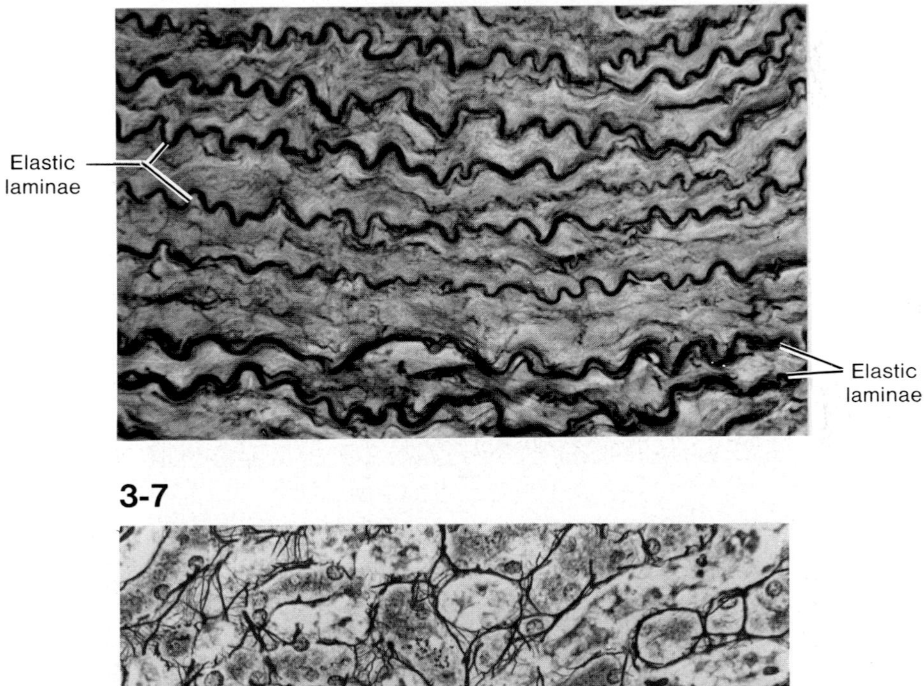

3-7

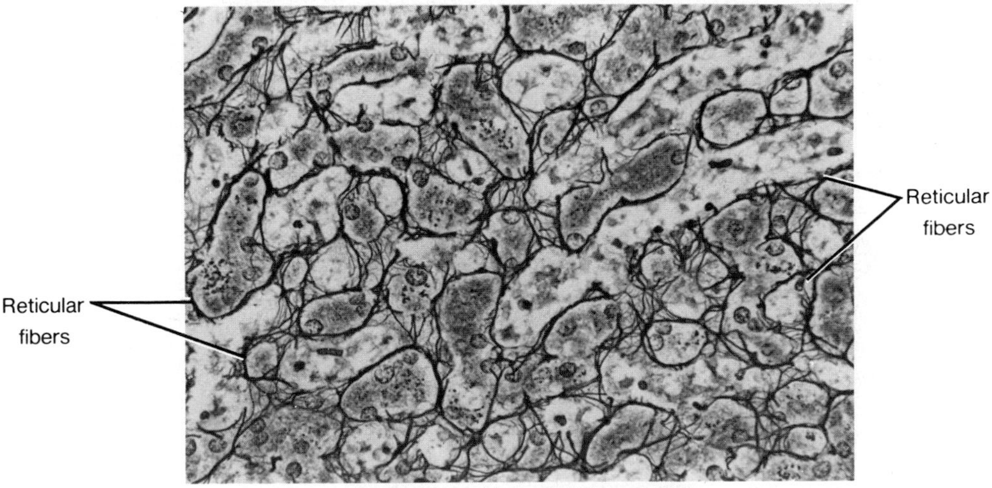

Figure 3-5. Pleura. TEM, ×11,000.
Figure 3-6. Aorta. LM, ×150.
Figure 3-7. Liver. LM, ×200.

3-8

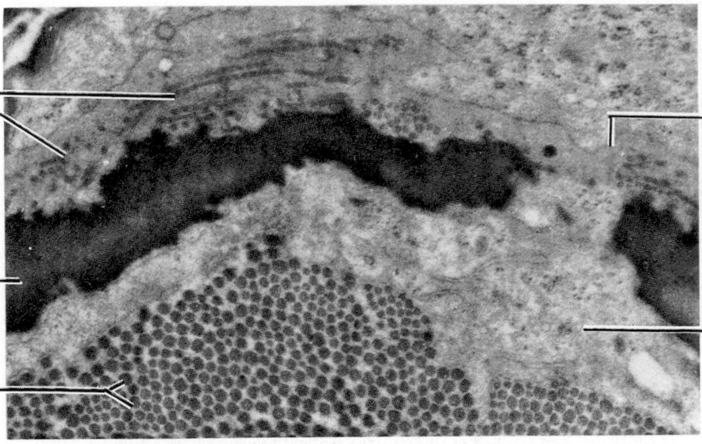

3-9

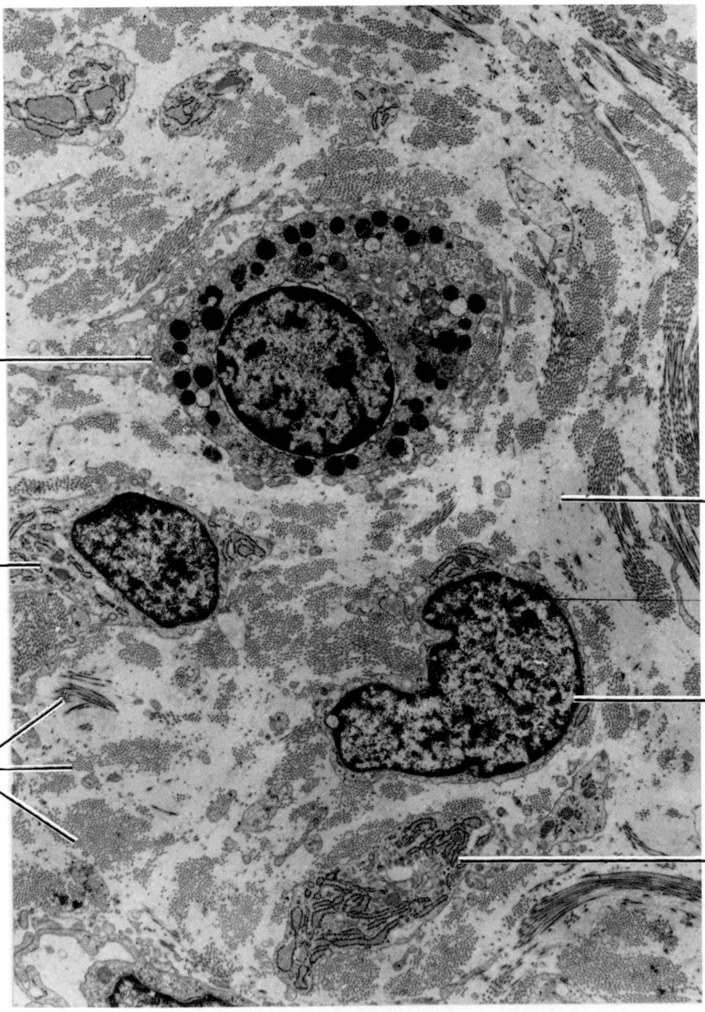

Figure 3-8. Pleura. TEM, ×18,000.
Figure 3-9. Dermis. TEM, ×2000.

3-10

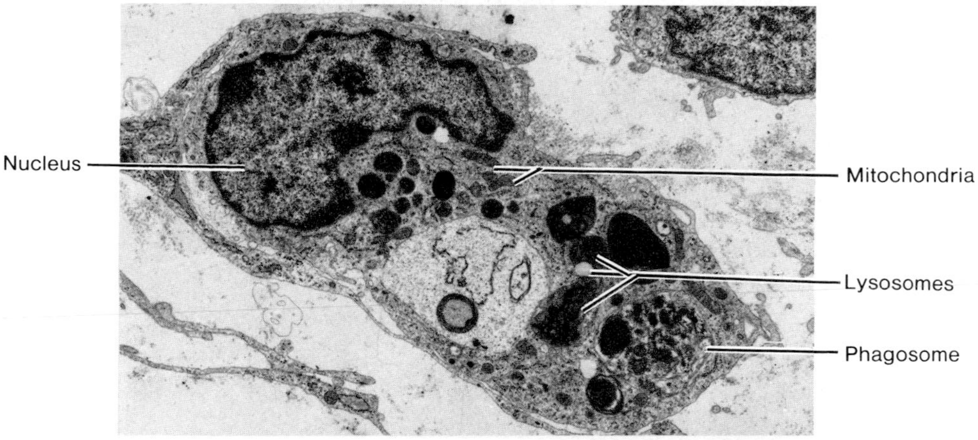

3-11

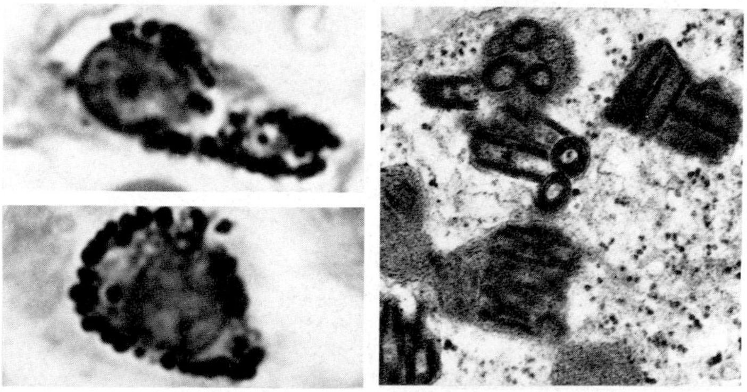

3-12

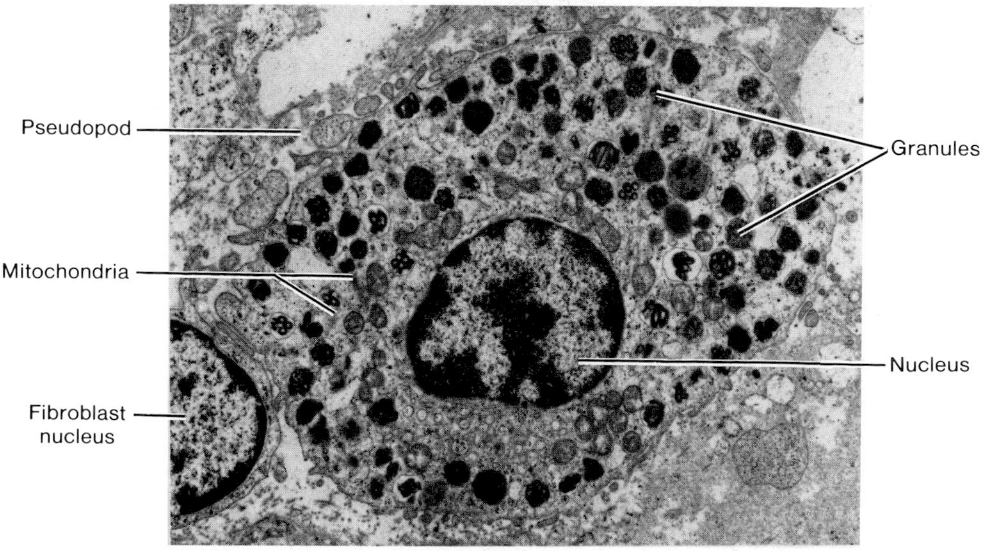

Figure 3-10. Macrophage. TEM, ×4000.
Figure 3-11. Mast cells. LM, ×1100; mast cell granules (human). TEM, ×50,000.
Figure 3-12. Mast cell (human). TEM, ×4000.

3-13

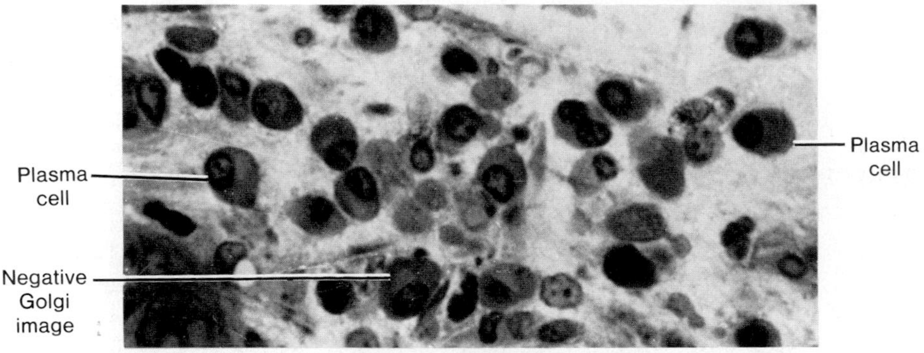

3-14

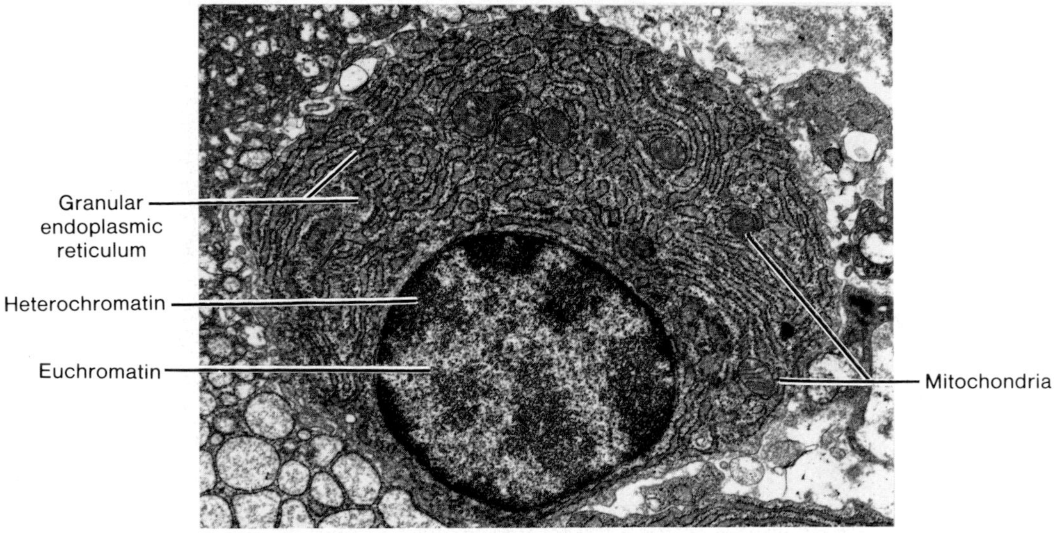

3-15

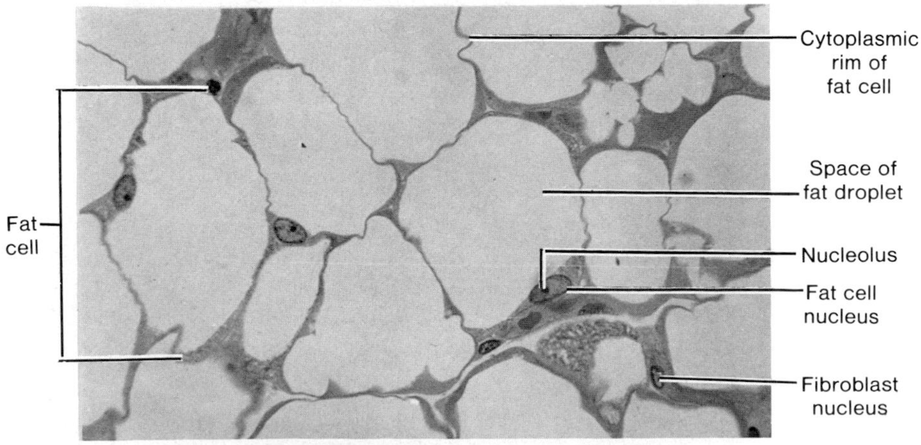

Figure 3-13. Loose connective tissue. LM, ×400.
Figure 3-14. Plasma cell (human). TEM, ×5000.
Figure 3-15. Adipose tissue. LM, ×350.

3-16

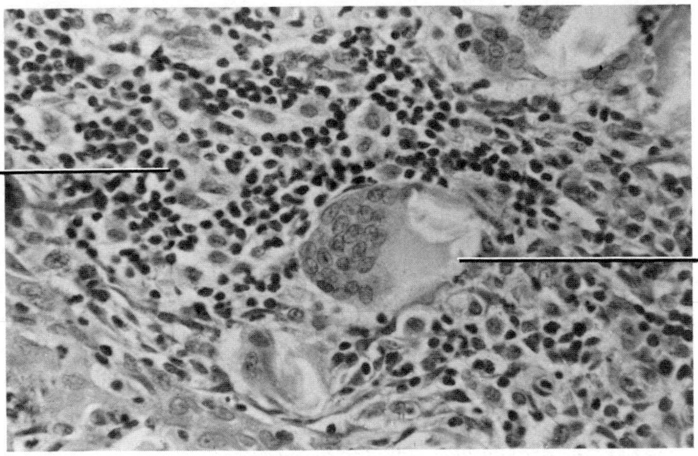

3-17 Development

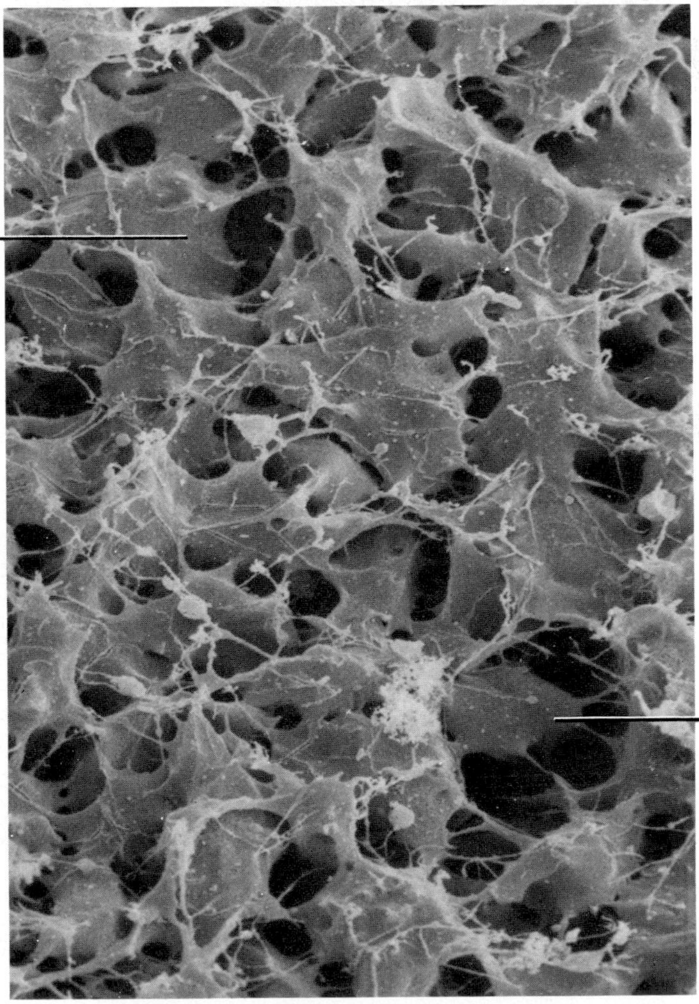

Figure 3-16. Foreign body giant cell. LM, ×250.
Figure 3-17. Mesenchyme. SEM, ×1000.

4

Special Connective Tissue: Cartilage and Bone

CARTILAGE

Cartilage is specially adapted to provide support and contains the usual elements of connective tissues—cells, fibers and ground substance. Together, the fibers and ground substance form the matrix. It is the physical properties of the ground substance that give the firm consistency to cartilage and enable it to withstand considerable pressure and shearing forces. The collagenous and elastic fibers embedded in the ground substance impart tensile strength and elasticity. Cartilage differs from other connective tissues in that it has no nerve or blood supply of its own and lacks lymphatics. Nourishment is derived entirely by diffusion of materials from blood vessels in adjacent tissues. Although of relatively rigid consistency, cartilage matrix has a high content of water and is freely permeable, even to fairly coarse particles.

Classification of cartilage into hyaline, elastic and fibrous types is based upon differences in the abundance and type of fibers that are present within the matrix.

Hyaline Cartilage

KEY WORDS: perichondrium, chondrocytes, lacunae, isogenous groups, chondromucoid, territorial matrix, interterritorial matrix

Of the three types, hyaline cartilage is the most common and forms the costal cartilages, the articular surfaces of bones within joints, and the cartilages of the nose, larynx, trachea, and bronchii and is present in the growing ends of long bones. In the fetus, most of the skeleton is first laid down as hyaline cartilage. Except for the free surfaces of articular cartilages, hyaline cartilage is enclosed within a sheath of dense connective tissue, the **perichondrium.**

The cells of cartilage are called **chondrocytes** and reside in small spaces, **lacunae**, scattered throughout the matrix. The cells generally tend to conform to the shape of the lacunae in which they are contained. Deep within the cartilage the cells and their lacunae are usually rounded, whereas just beneath the perichondrium, they are elliptical with the long axis parallel to the surface.

Chondrocytes often are present in small clusters called **isogenous groups**, and these represent the offspring of a single cell.

In the usual preparations, the cells show an irregular outline and appear shrunken and pulled away from the walls of the lacunae. Electron microscopy reveals that each cell completely fills the lacunar space and sends short cytoplasmic processes into the surrounding matrix, but neighboring chondrocytes do not communicate with each other. The nucleus is round or oval and shows one or more nucleoli. The cytoplasm contains the usual organelles as well as lipid and glycogen inclusions. In growing cartilage, the Golgi complex and endoplasmic reticulum are extensively developed.

Both in the fresh state and in routine histological preparations, the matrix appears relatively homogeneous, since the ground substance and the collagen embedded in it have the same refractive index. The collagen of hyaline cartilage rarely forms bundles but is present as a feltwork of slender fibrils that show variable periodicities or even lack the 64-nm banding. Collagen in cartilage appears to be less polymerized than in other tissues and cartilage is unique in that only type II collagen is present. The ground substance is made up mainly of **proteoglycans** which consist of protein and complex carbohydrates (glycosaminoglycans). The specific proteoglycans of cartilage are chondroitin-4 and chondroitin-6 sulfate, keratan sulfate and a small amount of hyaluronic acid that impart basophilic properties to the ground substance. The matrix around each isogenous group of cells tends to stain more deeply than elsewhere and forms the **territorial matrix.** The less densely stained intervening areas form the **interterritorial matrix.**

The outermost layers of the **perichondrium** consist of well vascularized dense connective tissue that contains elastic and collagenous fibers and fibroblasts. Where it lies against cartilage, the perichondrium is more cellular and passes imperceptibly into cartilage. The slender collagen fibers of the cartilage matrix gradually blend into the wider, cross-banded fibers of the perichondrium. The perichondrial cells adjacent to the cartilage retain the capacity to form new cartilage.

Elastic Cartilage

This essentially is a variant of hyaline cartilage, differing chiefly in the presence of branched elastic fibers in the matrix. Collagenous fibers of the type found in hyaline cartilage also are present. In the deeper portions of the cartilage, the elastic fibers form a dense, closely packed mesh that obscures the ground substance, whereas beneath the perichondrium, the fibers form a looser network and are continuous with those of the perichondrium. Elastic cartilage is more flexible than hyaline cartilage. It is found in the external ear, auditory tube, epiglottis and some of the smaller laryngeal cartilages.

Fibrous Cartilage

Fibrous cartilage (or fibrocartilage) probably is best considered to form a transition between dense connective tissue and cartilage rather than a modified form of hyaline cartilage. It consists of typical cartilage cells enclosed within lacunae, but only a small amount of ground substance is present and that occurs in the immediate vicinity of the cells. The cartilage cells lie singly, in pairs or in short rows between bundles of dense collagen fibers which show the 64-nm banding. Fibrous cartilage lacks a perichondrium and merges into hyaline cartilage, bone or dense fibrous tissue. It occurs in the intervertebral discs, in some articular cartilages, in the symphysis pubis and in sites of attachment of certain tendons to bone.

Development of Cartilage

KEY WORDS: chondroblasts, chondrocytes, interstitial growth, appositional growth

All cartilage arises from mesenchyme and at sites where cartilage is to be formed. The mesenchymal cells lose their processes, round up, proliferate, and crowd together in a dense aggregate. The cells in the interior of the mass differentiate into **chondroblasts** which begin to lay down collagen fibers and ground substance. As the amount of intercellular material increases, the cells become isolated in individual compartments (the lacunae) and take on the characteristics of **chondrocytes.** Continued growth occurs either by expansion of the mass of cartilage from within, or by formation of new cartilage at the surface. These are referred to as interstitial growth and appositional growth, respectively. **Interstitial growth** results from proliferation of young chondrocytes which divide and lay down new matrix to produce an expansion of cartilage from within. Such interstitial growth occurs only in young cartilage that is plastic enough to permit expansion. **Appositional growth** occurs as a result of the activity of the perichondrium, which is derived as a condensation of the mesenchyme surrounding the developing cartilage. The cells of the perichondrium that are immediately adjacent to cartilage divide, and the innermost cells differentiate into chondrocytes, secrete matrix about themselves and add new cartilage to the surface. Although adult perichondrium retains the potential to form new cartilage, the capacity for growth and repair is limited by its avascularity.

BONE

Like cartilage, bone is a connective tissue that is specialized for support. However, in bone, the matrix has become mineralized to form a dense, hard, unyielding substance with high tensile, weight-bearing and compression strength. In spite of its strength and rigidity, bone is a dynamic, living tissue constantly turning over, constantly being renewed and reformed throughout life.

Macroscopic Structure

KEY WORDS: cancellous (spongy) bone, compact (dense) bone, trabeculae, diaphysis, epiphysis, periosteum, endosteum, diploë

Grossly, two forms of bone can be identified: **cancellous** or **spongy bone** and **compact** or **dense bone**. Spongy bone consists of narrow, irregular bars, or **trabeculae**, of bone which branch and unite to form a three-dimensional, interlacing network of boney spicules delimiting a vast system of small communicating spaces which, in life, are filled with bone marrow. Compact bone appears as a solid, continuous mass in which spaces cannot be seen by the naked eye. The two forms of bone are not sharply delimited and the two types merge into one another.

In a typical long bone, the shaft or **diaphysis** appears as a hollow cylinder of compact bone enclosing a large central space, the marrow cavity. The ends of long bones, the **epiphyses**, consist mainly of cancellous bone covered by a thin layer of compact bone. The small intercommunicating spaces in the spongy bone are directly continuous with the marrow cavity of the shaft.

Except over articular surfaces and where tendons and ligaments are inserted, each bone is covered by a specialized, vascular, fibroelastic connective tissue, the **periosteum.** The marrow cavity of the diaphysis and the spaces within the spongy bone are lined by **endosteum** which is similar to periosteum but not as well defined. Both periosteum and endosteum have the ability to form bone under appropriate stimulation.

Flat bones, such as those of the skull, also show compact and spongy bone. The inner, and outer layers (often referred to as the inner and outer tables) consist of thick layers of compact bone. The space between the two plates of compact bone is bridged by spongy bone called the **diploë**.

Microscopic Structure

KEY WORDS: lamellae, lacunae, osteocytes, canaliculi, osteons (haversian systems), interstitial lamellae, cement line, outer and inner circumferential lamellae, haversian canals, Volkmann's canals

The characteristic feature of bone is the arrangement of the mineralized bone matrix into layers or plates called **lamellae.** Small, ovoid **lacunae** are spaced rather uniformly both within and between the lamellae and each is occupied by a single bone cell or **osteocyte.** Radiating from each lacuna are slender tubular passages, or **canaliculi**, which penetrate the lamellae to link up with the canaliculi of adjacent lacunae. Thus, the lacunae are interconnected by an extensive system of exceedingly fine canals.

In compact bone, the lamellae show three common patterns. Most are arranged concentrically around a longitudinally oriented space to form cylindrical units that run parallel to the long axis of the bone. These are the **osteons** (**haversian systems**) and essentially are the unit structure of bone. Osteons vary in size and consist of 8 to 15 concentric lamellae surrounding a wide opening occupied by blood vessels. In longitudinal sections, the osteon appears as plates of boney matrix running parallel to the slit-like space of the vascular channel. Throughout its thickness, compact bone contains a number of osteons running side by side. Other lamellae appear as angular, irregular fragments of lamellar bone that fill the spaces between osteons. These are the **interstitial lamellae.** The osteons and interstitial lamellae are sharply outlined by a refractile line called the **cement line**, which consists of modified matrix. Cement lines are not traversed by canaliculi. At the external surface of the bone, immediately beneath the periosteum, are the **outer circumferential lamellae.** These consist of several lamellae that run about the circumference and extend almost without interruption around most of the shaft of the bone. A similar but less well developed system of lamellae is present on the inner surface, just beneath the endosteum. These form the **inner circumferential lamellae.** Figure 4-1 shows a cross section of bone.

The longitudinally oriented channels at the centers of osteons are called **haversian canals**, and these communicate with each other by means of oblique and transverse connections called **Volkmann's canals** which penetrate the bone from the endosteal and periosteal surfaces, passing perpendicular to the long axis of the bone. Volkmann's canals unite with the haversian canals and provide the means by which the blood vessels within haversian canals communicate with blood vessels of the marrow cavity and, to a lesser extent, with those of the periosteum. Thus, the compact bone contains a vast, continuous network of canals which, with their contained blood vessels, provides for the nutritional needs of the bone. Canaliculi adjacent to an haversian canal open into its cavity, and the canalicular systems bring all of the lacunae into communication with the canal. Volkmann's canals, unlike haversian canals, are not surrounded by concentric lamellae.

Cancellous or spongy bone shows a lamellar structure also, but differs from compact bone in that the trabeculae and spicules of bone are thin and not usually traversed by blood vessels. Therefore, osteons are rare or lacking and spongy bone contains merely angular portions of lamellar bone.

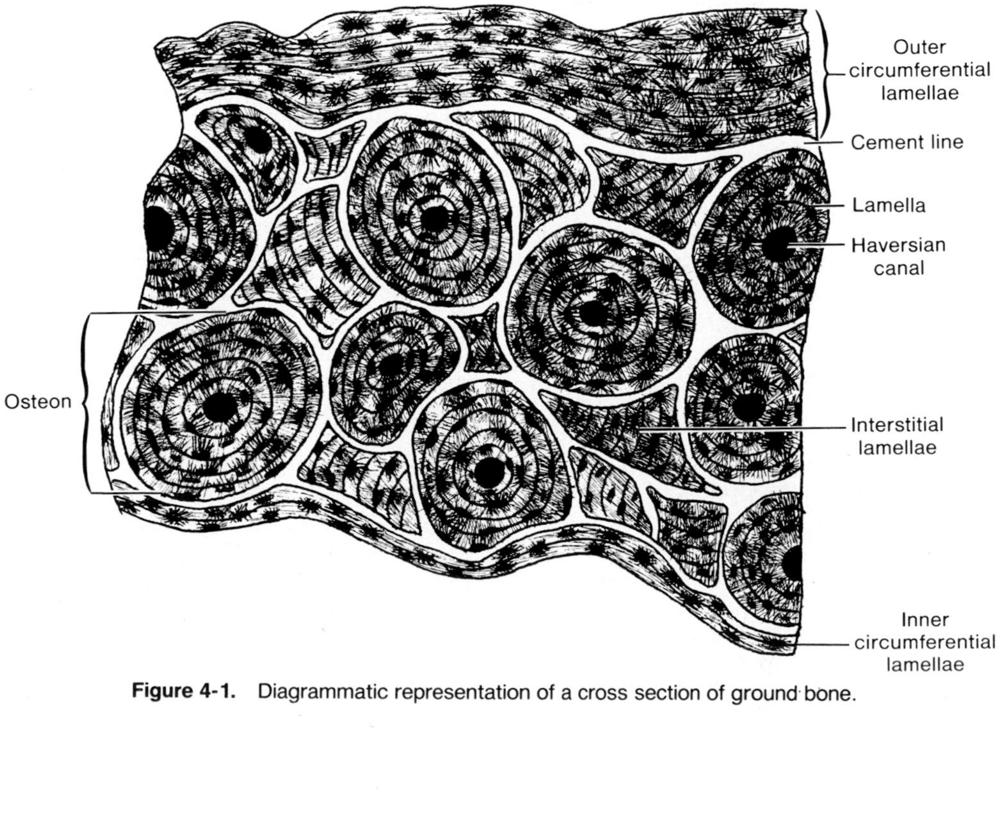

Figure 4-1. Diagrammatic representation of a cross section of ground bone.

Periosteum

KEY WORDS: dense connective tissue, Sharpey's fibers

The outermost layer of the periosteum is a relatively acellular **dense connective tissue** which contains abundant collagenous fibers, a few elastic fibers and a network of blood vessels. Branches of these vessels pass through the thickness of the periosteum to enter Volkmann's canals. The deeper layers of the periosteum are more cellular and consist of a more loosely arranged connective tissue. During development of bone, collagenous fibers of the periosteum become trapped within the circumferential lamellae as **Sharpey's fibers**, which anchor the periosteum to the underlying bone.

Endosteum

The endosteum lines all of the cavities of bone, including the marrow spaces of the diaphysis and epiphysis and the haversian and Volkman's canals. It consists of a single layer of squamous cells with a small and variable content of reticular fibers. In common with the cells of the inner layer of the periosteum, the cells of the endosteum retain osteogenic potential.

Cells of Bone

KEY WORDS: osteocytes, osteoclasts, Howship's lacunae, ruffled border

Osteocytes form the chief cellular component of mature bone and assume the shape of the lacunae in which they are housed. Delicate cytoplasmic processes extend from the cell body and traverse the canaliculi to contact similar processes from neighboring osteocytes. At the points of contact, the apposed cell membranes form junctions of the communicating type (nexus). Thus, the osteocytes are not isolated within their lacunae but are in extensive communication with each other. The osteocyte and its processes are separated from the walls of the lacunae and canaliculi by a thin layer of unmineralized matrix.

Osteocytes contain the usual cell organelles but the Golgi complex is relatively inconspicuous, and the cell contains a low content of endoplasmic reticulum, ribosomes and mitochondria. Although these appearances are consistent with a cell not actively elaborating protein, the osteocyte is not metabolically inert. It is responsible for maintaining bone and plays an active role in regulating the calcium concentration of body fluids.

In areas where bone is being resorbed, large multinucleate giant cells can be found. These are the **osteoclasts** that frequently lie in shallow depressions in the surface of the bone called **Howship's lacunae.** Although the cell may contain 30 or more nuclei, the individual nuclei show no unusual features. They usually are located in the part of the cell farthest from the bone surface. The cytoplasm contains multiple Golgi and centriole pairs and numerous mitochondria and lysosomes. The cell surface adjacent to the bone shows a **ruffled border**, a surface modification that is unique to osteoclasts. The ruffled bolder appears as elaborate folds, 15 nm long, that abut the surface of the bone. A clear zone containing many actin filaments surrounds the ruffled border. Osteoclasts that lack such a border do not seem to participate in bone resorption. Mitochondria tend to accumulate near the ruffled border. The cell surface farthest from the bone shows a smooth contour.

Osteoclasts arise by fusion of monocytes that have emigrated from the blood.

Matrix of Bone

KEY WORDS: amorphous ground substance, collagen fibers, inorganic component

Bone matrix consists of an organic and an inorganic component. The organic component comprises an **amorphous ground substance** in which **collagen fibers** are embedded. The ground substance contains proteoglycans similar to those of cartilage, but in lesser concentration. Most of the proteoglycans of bone lack acidic sulfate groups. The collagen of bone occurs as cross-striated fibers which are highly organized in their arrangement. Within any one lamella the collagen fibers are parallel to each other but take a helical course. The pitch of the helix differs in adjacent lamellae such that the fibers in one form almost a right angle to the fibers in the next lamella. The collagen of bone is exclusively type I.

The **inorganic component** is responsible for the ridigity of bone and consists of calcium phosphate and calcium carbonate with small amounts of calcium and magnesium fluoride. The minerals are present as crystals with an hydroxyapatite structure and are present on and within the collagen at regular intervals along the fibers.

BONE FORMATION

Bone is mesenchymal in origin and develops by replacement of a pre-existing tissue. Depending on the type of connective tissue replaced, two modes of bone formation can be recognized. If bone is formed directly in a primitive connective tissue, the process is called intramembranous ossification, whereas when it occurs by replacement of a preformed cartilaginous model, the process is known as endochondral ossification. The essential process of bone formation is the same in both types, however.

Intramembranous Ossification

KEY WORDS: osteoprogenitor cells, osteoblasts, osteocytes, osteoid

The flat bones of the cranium and part of the mandible of the face develop by intramembranous ossification and are frequently referred to as membrane bones. In the areas where bone is to form, the mesenchyme becomes richly vascularized and the mesenchymal cells show active proliferation. Some cells undergo changes that subsequently lead to bone formation and are regarded as **osteoprogenitor cells.** Structurally, these cells closely resemble the mesenchymal cells from which they arise and identification is chiefly dependent upon their proximity to the site of bone formation.

As bone first forms in the connective tissue bed, the osteoprogenitor cells enlarge to become **osteoblasts** and bars of matrix are laid down. The osteoblasts remain in contact with each other by long tapering processes and, as more and more bone matrix is deposited, the cells and their processes become trapped in the matrix and are then called **osteocytes.** The first matrix laid down consists of ground substance and collagen fibers and, being unmineralized, is soft. At this stage the matrix is called **osteoid** which, after a short lag period, becomes mineralized to form true bone. As the osteoblasts become trapped in the newly deposited matrix and become osteocytes, new osteoblasts are recruited from differentiation of the osteoprogenitor cells.

Bone development occurs in several foci and results in the formation of irregular spicules and trabeculae which increase in size by deposition of new bone at their surfaces. The resulting bone is of the spongy type. In areas that become compact bone, such as the inner and outer tables of the skull, the trabeculae continue to thicken by apposition of bone to their surfaces and the spaces between them are gradually obliterated. Between the plates, where spongy bone persists, thickening of the trabeculae ceases and the intervening connective tissue becomes the blood-forming marrow. The connective tissue surrounding the mass of developing bone condenses to form the periosteum. The osteoblasts on the outer surface of bone assume a fibroblast-like appearance and become incorporated into the inner layer of periosteum, where they persist as the potential bone-forming cells of the periosteum. Similarly, the osteoblasts on the inner surface and those covering the trabeculae of spongy bone become incorporated into the endosteum and also retain their potential for producing bone.

Endochondral Bone Formation

KEY WORDS: primary ossification center, periosteal collar, periosteal bud, zone of reserve cartilage, zone of proliferation, zone of maturation and hypertrophy, zone of calcification and cell death, zone of ossification, zone of resorption, epiphyseal and secondary ossification centers, epiphyseal plate, epiphyseal plate primitive osteon, definitive osteon

The bones of the vertebral column, pelvis, extremities, face and base of the skull develop by formation of bone in a cartilaginous model which must be removed before bone can be laid down. Endochondral bone formation involves both removal of the cartilage model and deposition of bone matrix. These processes are most conveniently studied in a long bone.

The first indications of ossification appear in the center of the cartilage model in the region destined to become the shaft or diaphysis. In this area, called the **primary ossification center**, the chondrocytes hypertrophy and their cytoplasm becomes vacuolated. The lacunae enlarge at the expense of the surrounding matrix and the cartilage between adjacent lacunae becomes reduced to a thin, fenestrated partition. The cartilage matrix remaining in the vicinity of the hypertrophied chondrocytes becomes calcified by the deposition of calcium phosphate. Diffusion of nutrients through the calcified matrix is reduced and the chondrocytes undergo degenerative changes leading to their death.

While these events are occurring in the cartilage, the vascular perichondrium in this area assumes an osteogenic function. A layer of bone, the **periosteal collar**, is formed around the altered cartilage and provides a splint that helps maintain the strength of the shaft. The osteoblasts responsible for development of the bone are derived from the perichondrial cells immediately adjacent to the cartilage. In the region of the bony collar, the perichondrium now has become a periosteum. Blood vessels from the periosteum invade the altered cartilage and form the **periosteal bud.** Contained within the connective tissue sheath accompanying the blood vessels are cells with osteogenic capacities.

With death of the cartilage cells, there is no longer any means of maintaining the cartilage matrix and, aided by the erosive action of the invading blood vessels, the thin partitions between lacunae undergo dissolution. As the adjoining lacunar spaces are opened up, narrow tunnels are formed between spicules of calcified cartilage matrix. Blood vessels grow into the tunnels, bringing with them the osteogenic cells which align themselves on the surface of the cartilage remnants, differentiate into osteoblasts and begin to elaborate bone matrix. At first the matrix is deposited as osteoid but soon becomes mineralized to form true bone. The earliest trabeculae consist of a core of calcified cartilage with an outer shell of bone of variable thickness. These initial trabeculae are soon removed, both by the continued resorption of the calcified cartilage and through activity of the osteoclasts that appear on the bony shell, and an expanding cavity within the developing shaft is opened up. Support for the bone is provided by the continued development of the periosteal collar, which becomes thicker as the periosteum lays down new bone at the surface.

This entire process continues in an orderly wave of activity that extends towards both extremes of the developing bone. Several areas or zones of activity can be distinguished in the cartilage. Beginning at the ends farthest from the primary ossification center, these zones are as follows.

Zone of Reserve Cartilage. This area is composed of primitive hyaline cartilage and initially is a relatively long zone but shortens as the process of ossification encroaches upon it. The cells and their lacunae are randomly arranged throughout the matrix and there is slow growth of this region in all directions.

Zone of Proliferation. In this region active proliferation of chondrocytes occurs and, as the cells divide, the daughter cells become aligned in columns which are separated by only a small amount of matrix. Growth occurs mainly at the ends farthest from the zone of reserve cartilage and the length of the cartilage is increased more than its diameter.

Zone of Maturation and Hypertrophy. Cell division ceases and the cells mature and enlarge; this further increases the length of the cartilage of this region. The lacunae enlarge at the expense of the intervening matrix and the cartilage between adjacent cells in the rows becomes even thinner.

Zone of Calcification and Cell Death. The matrix between the rows of chondrocytes becomes calcified and the cells die, undergo dissolution and leave empty spaces. The thin plates between the cells also undergo dissolution, and the spaces open up to form irregular tunnels bounded by the remains of the calcified cartilage that had been present between the rows of cells.

Zones of Ossification. Vascular connective tissue invades the tunnel-like spaces and provides osteogenic cells which differentiate into osteoblasts; these gather on the surfaces of the calcified cartilage matrix and lay down bone.

Zone of Resorption. Osteoclasts appear on the trabeculae and begin to resorb the bone. Ultimately all of the calcified cartilage and their bony coverings are resorbed and the marrow cavity increases in size.

As these changes occur within the cartilage, the periosteal collar increases in length and thickness, extending toward the end of the developing bone to provide a continuous splint around the area of changing and weakened cartilage.

At about the time of birth, new centers of ossification (**epiphyseal** or **secondary ossification centers**) appear at the ends of the long bones. The cartilage of the epiphyses passes through the same sequences as occurred in the diaphysis but cartilage growth and subsequent ossification spread in all directions from the secondary center, resulting in the formation of a mass of spongy bone. Ultimately all of the cartilage of the epiphysis is replaced by bone except for that at the free ends, which remains as the articular cartilage. Cartilage also persists between the epiphysis and diaphysis as the **epiphyseal plate**, and its continued growth permits further elongation of the bone. Ossification occurs at the diaphyseal side of the plate and, for a time, new cartilage formation and bony replacement continue at about the same rate, so that the epiphyseal plate remains constant in thickness. Eventually, growth in the epiphyseal plate ceases and it becomes completely replaced by bone; increased length of the bone then is no longer possible. Increase in the diameter results from deposition of bone at the outer surface as a result of the activity of the periosteum. At the same time, resorption of lesser amounts of bone occurs at the endosteal surface. Thus, not only is the gross diameter increased, but thickness of the bone and size of the marrow cavity also increase.

Bone formed by the periosteum represents intramembranous bone formation and results in a lattice of irregular bony trabeculae. This is converted to compact bone by a gradual filling in of the spaces between trabeculae. Bone is laid down in ill defined layers which come to surround blood vessels and form the first haversian systems, or **primitive osteons.** These differ from definitive osteons in the organization of collagen in the lamellae. In the first osteons formed, collagen is laid down at random throughout each lamella, whereas in the definitive osteons the collagen is highly ordered and its orientation in successive lamellae is different. As growth of the bone continues, there is a constant remodeling and reconstruction of bone and the primitive osteons are replaced by successive generations of **definitive** or secondary **osteons** (Fig. 4.2).

Replacement of the primitive osteons begins with formation of tunnels within the compact bone as a result of the erosive activity of the osteoclasts. However, there is some evidence that the mature osteocytes also may aid in osteolysis. The cavities enlarge to reach considerable length, whereupon the lytic activity ceases, osteoblasts become active, and bone is deposited on the walls of the cavity until it is refilled to form a typical definitive osteon. The process continues throughout life; resorption cavities continue to form and to be filled in with the

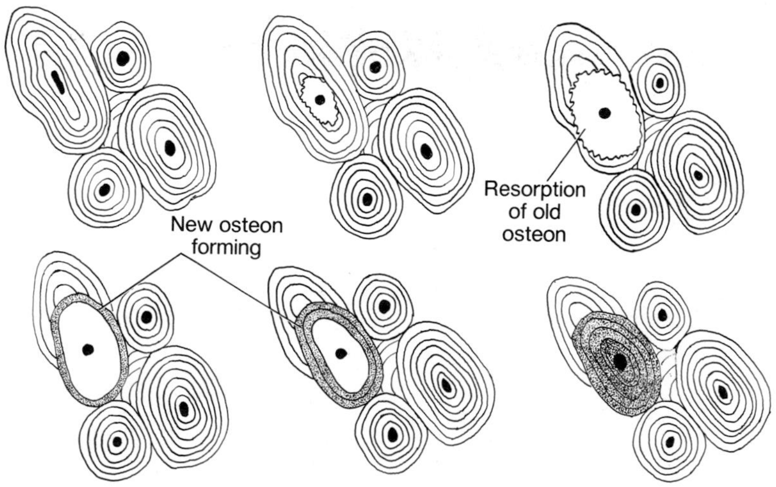

Figure 4-2. Replacement of osteons during remodeling of bone.

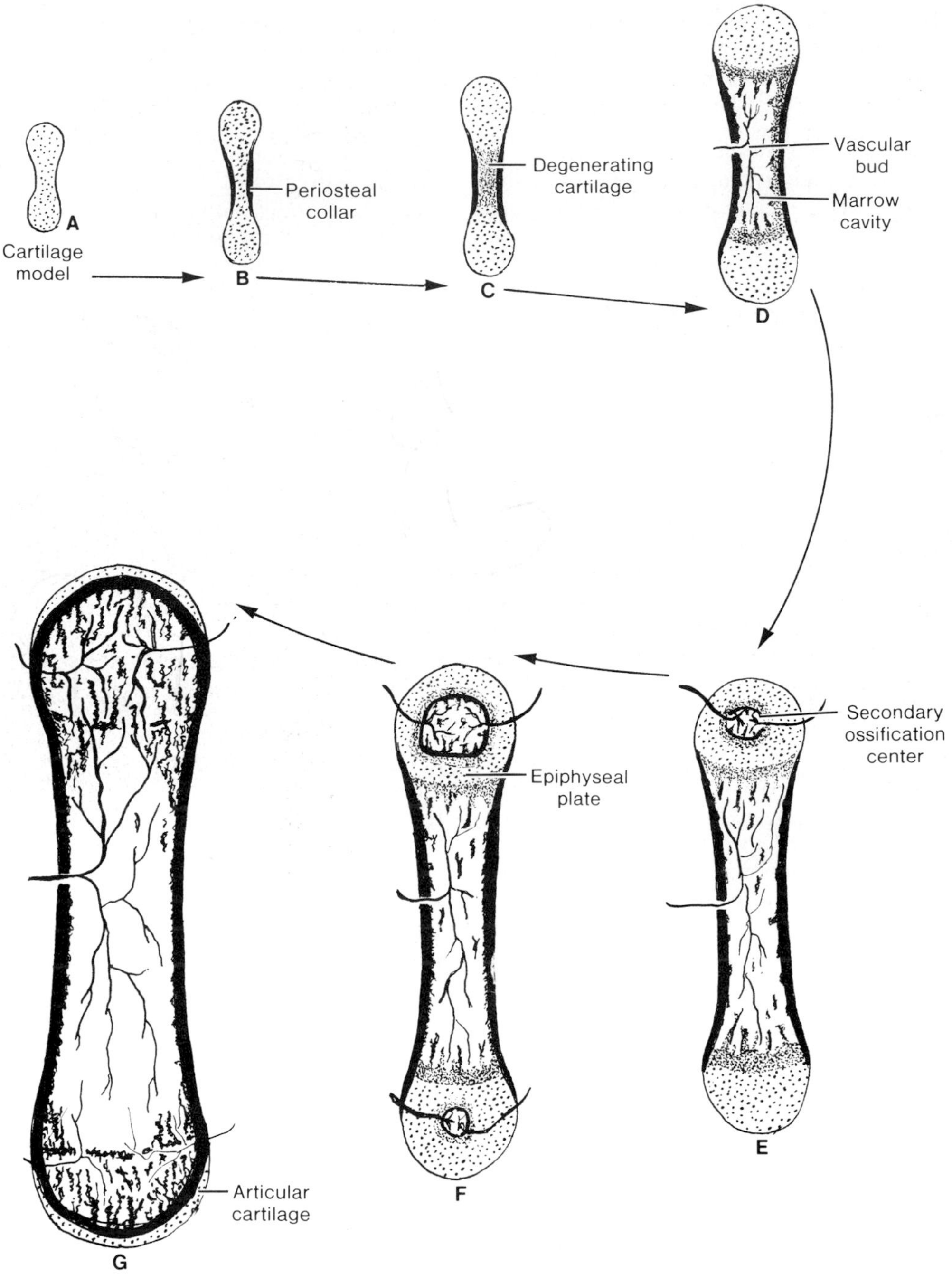

Figure 4-3. Diagrammatic representation of the successive changes during the development of a long bone.

third, fourth and higher generations of osteons. As osteons are replaced, fragments of older osteons remain as the interstitial lamellae. Successive changes during development of a long bone are shown in Figure 4.3.

The cartilage model (*A*) becomes encircled by a periosteal collar in the region that will become the shaft (*B*), and the cartilage in this area begins to calcify and degenerate (*C*). A vascular bud of connective tissue penetrates the altered cartilage which is resorbed, and the cartilage remnants become covered by bone to form irregular trabeculae which in turn are soon resorbed, and an expanding, marrow-filled cavity forms as the process extends toward each end (*D*). Secondary centers of ossification appear in the epiphyses, gradually expanding in all directions to replace the epiphyseal cartilage (*E*). Ultimately cartilage persists at the ends of the bone to form the articular cartilage and, for a time, as the epiphyseal plates from which all further increase in length will occur (*F*). Cartilage in the epiphyseal plate ceases its growth and is replaced by bone. The marrow cavity then becomes continuous throughout the length of the bone (*G*).

FUNCTIONAL SUMMARY

Cartilage serves as a rigid, yet lightweight and flexible supporting tissue. It forms the framework for the respiratory passages and prevents their collapse, provides smooth "bearings" at joints and, as a cushion between the vertebrae, acts as a "shock absorber" for the spine. Cartilage is important in determining the size and shape of bone and in many bones provides the growing area for the lengthening of bones. Its capacity for rapid growth, while maintaining stiffness, makes it suitable for the embryonic skeleton.

About 75% of the water present in cartilage is bound to proteoglycans. These compounds play an important role in the transport of fluids, eletrolytes and nutrients through the cartilage matrix.

Bone forms the principle tissue of support and is capable of bearing great weight. It provides the attachment for muscles of locomotion, carries the joints, serves as a covering to protect vital organs and houses hemopoietic tissues. In addition, bone acts as a store for calcium and phosphorus and aids in maintaining their normal blood and tissue levels.

Atlas for Chapter 4

4-4 Cartilage

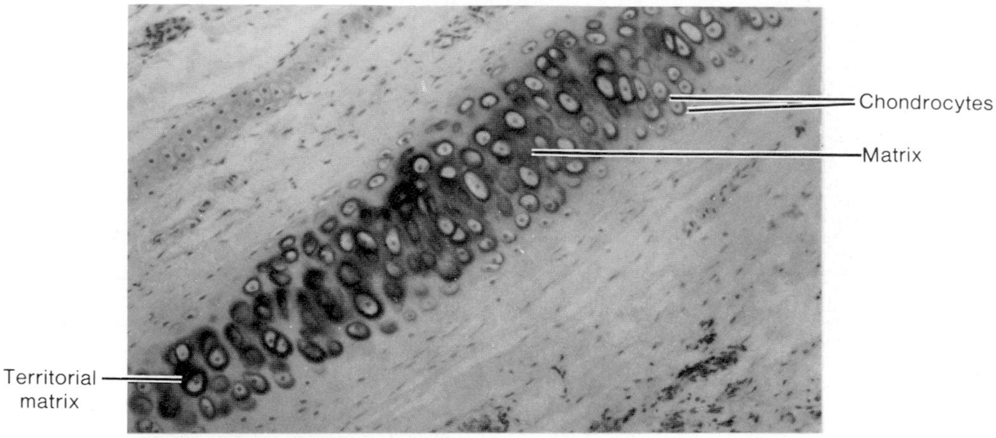

4-5

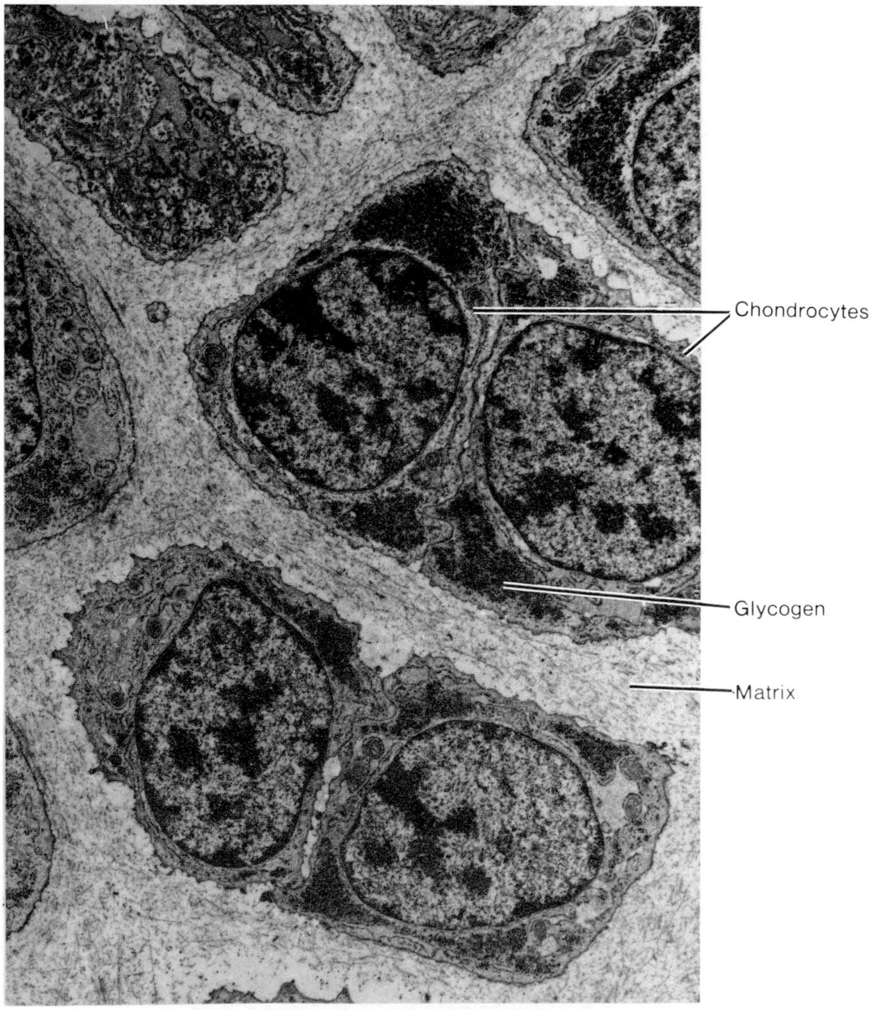

Figure 4-4. Trachea (hyaline cartilage). LM, ×250.
Figure 4-5. Trachea (hyaline cartilage). TEM, ×2500.

4-6

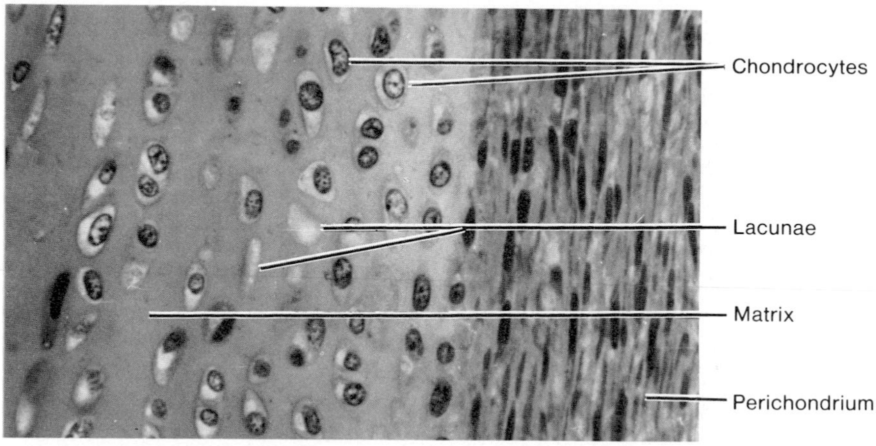

4-7

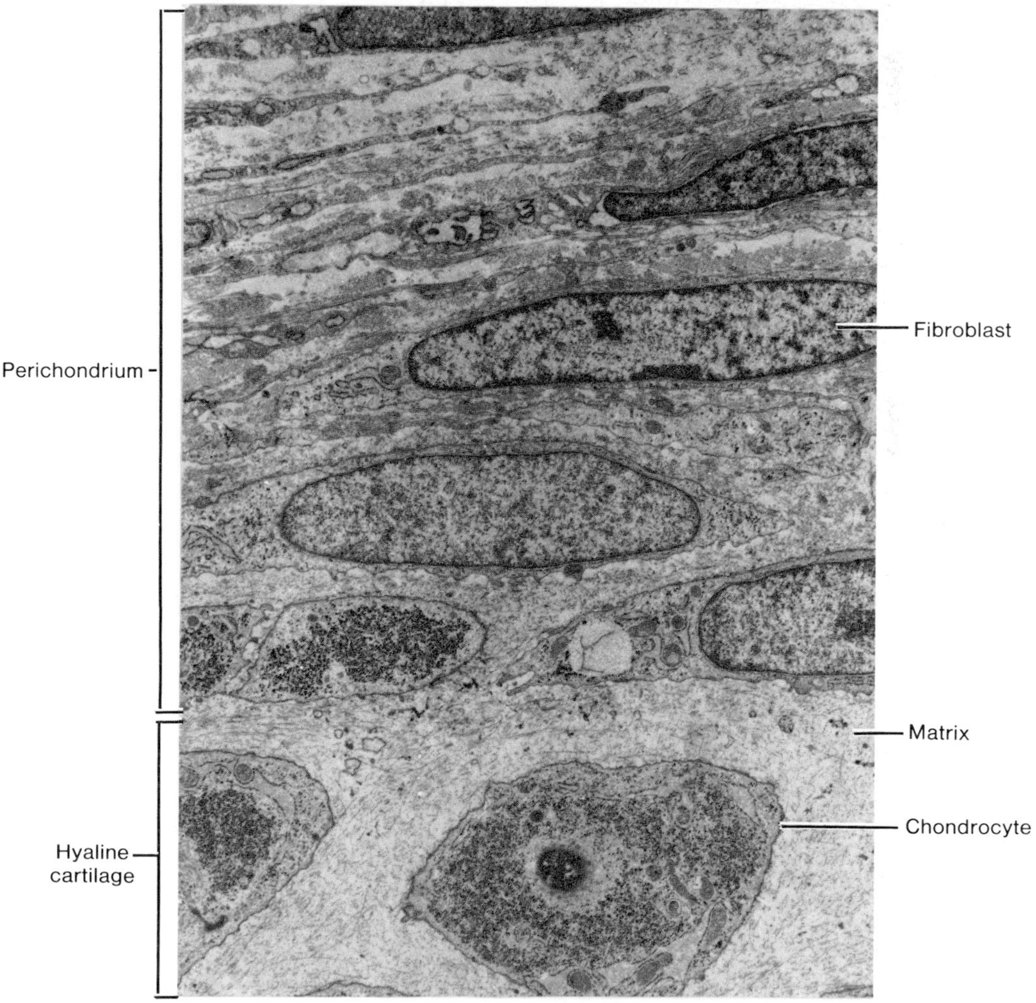

Figure 4-6. Trachea (hyaline cartilage). LM, ×400.
Figure 4-7. Perichondrium. TEM, ×2500.

4-8

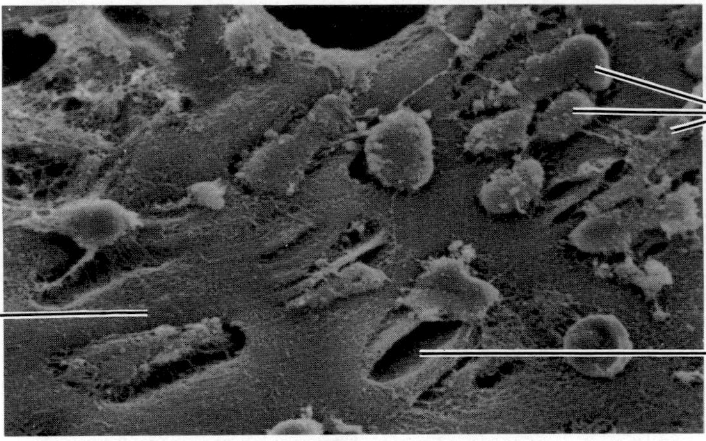

4-9

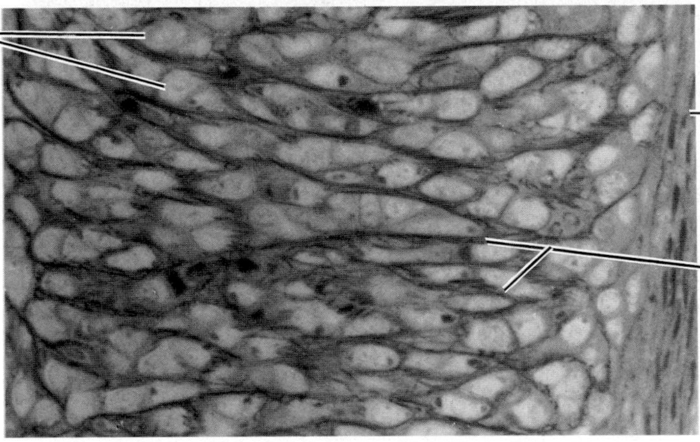

4-10

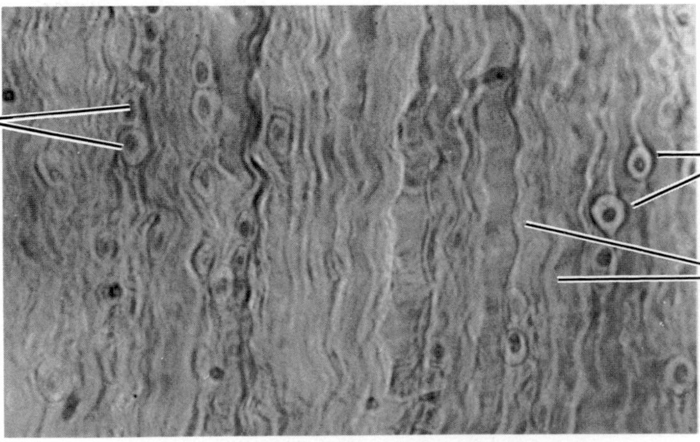

Figure 4-8. Trachea (hyaline cartilage). SEM, ×1000.
Figure 4-9. External ear (elastic cartilage). LM, ×250.
Figure 4-10. Symphysis pubis (fibrocartilage). LM, ×300.

4-11 Bone

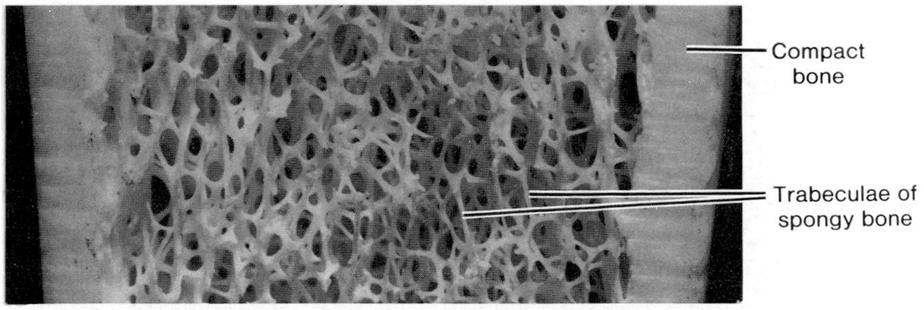

4-12

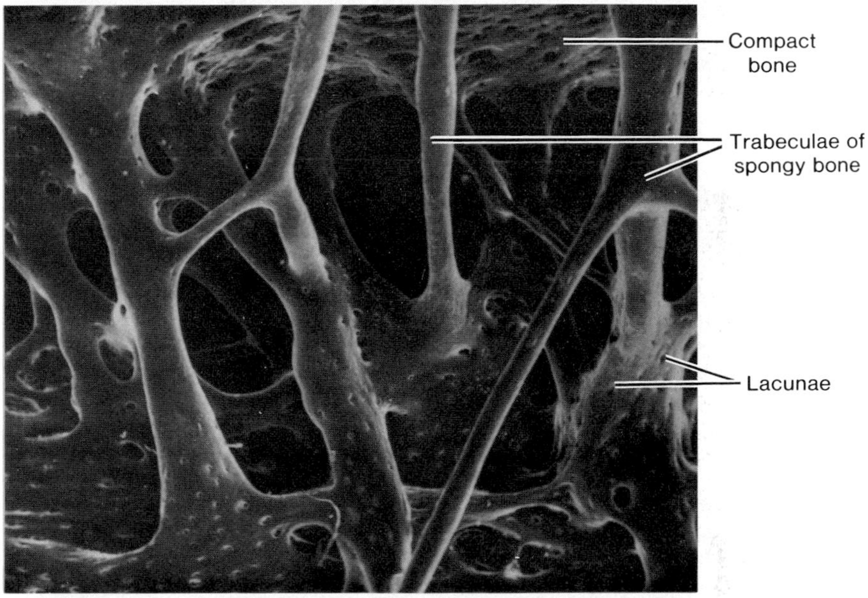

4-13

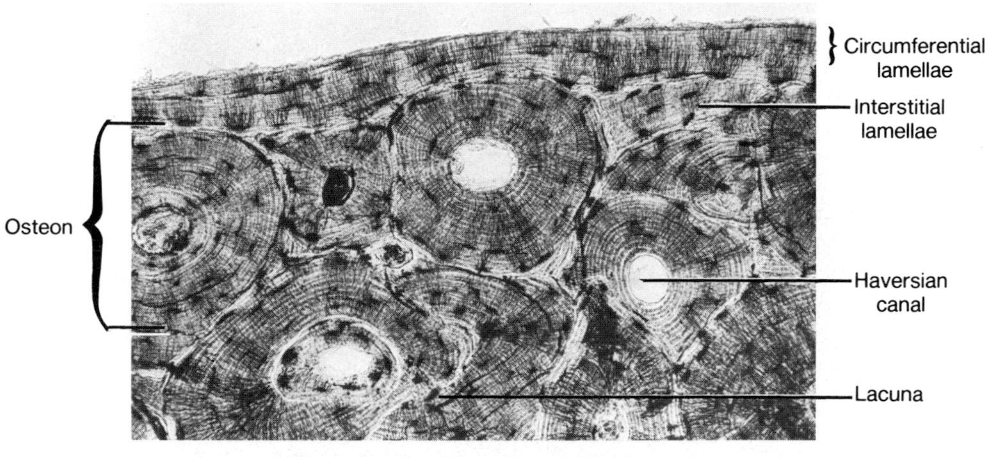

Figure 4-11. Cut shaft of long bone. ×5.
Figure 4-12. Spongy bone. SEM, ×50.
Figure 4-13. Compact bone. LM, ×250.

4-14

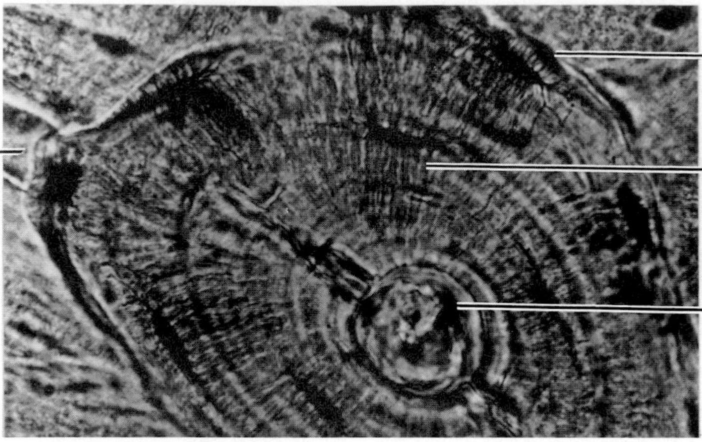

4-15

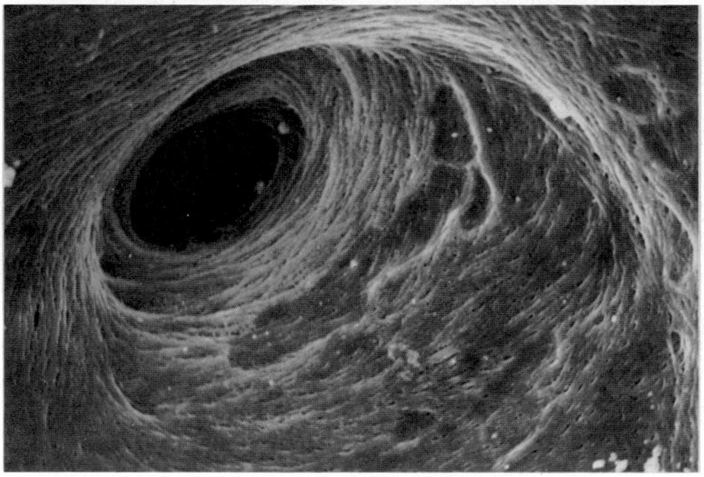

4-16

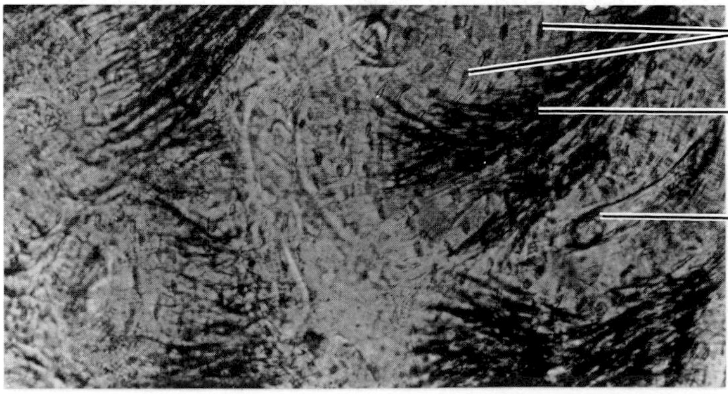

Figure 4-14. Haversian system or osteon. LM, ×400.
Figure 4-15. Haversian canal. SEM, ×500.
Figure 4-16. Sharpey's fibers. LM, ×250.

4-17 Bone Formation

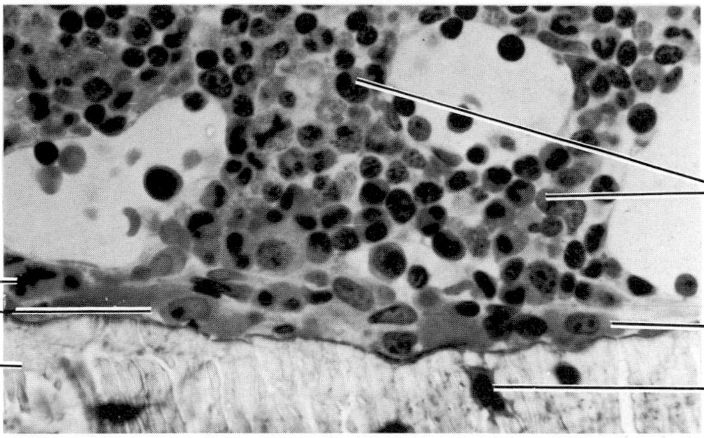

4-18

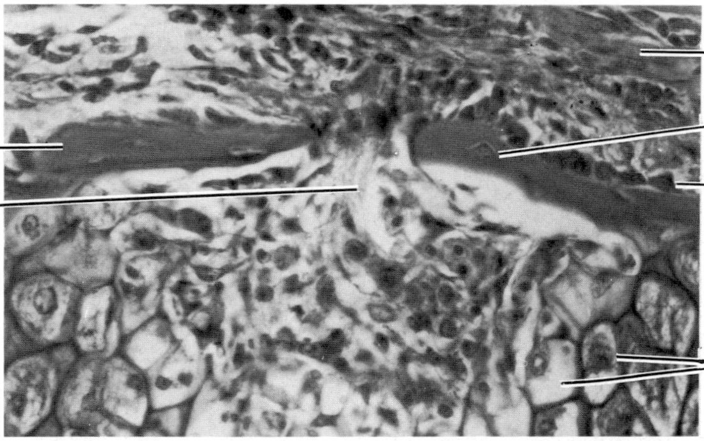

4-19

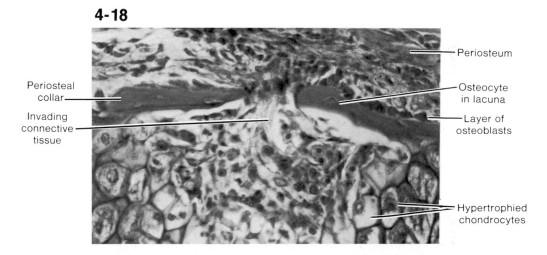

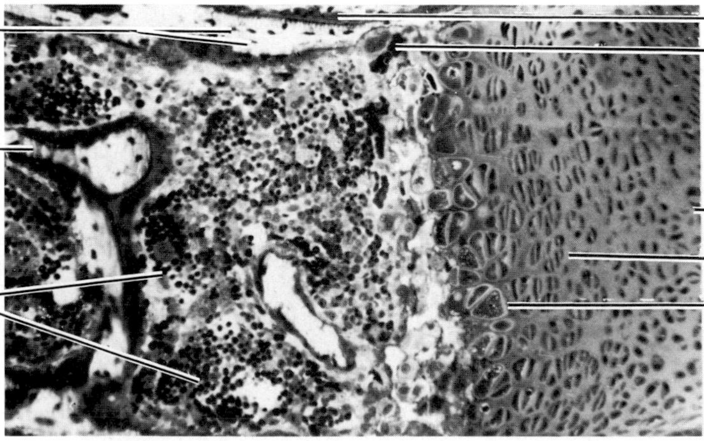

Figure 4-17. Osteoblasts. LM, ×400.
Figure 4-18. Osteogenic bud. LM, ×250.
Figure 4-19. Endochondral bone formation. LM, ×100.

4-20

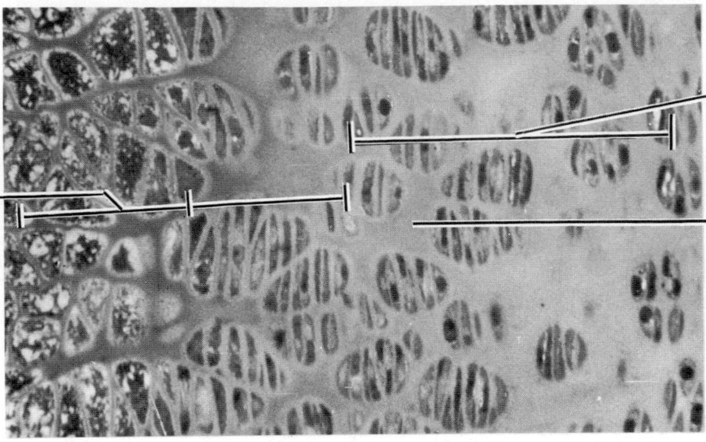

4-21

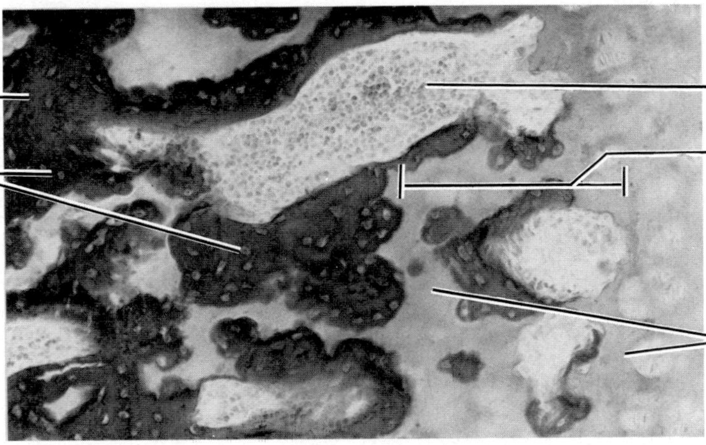

4-22

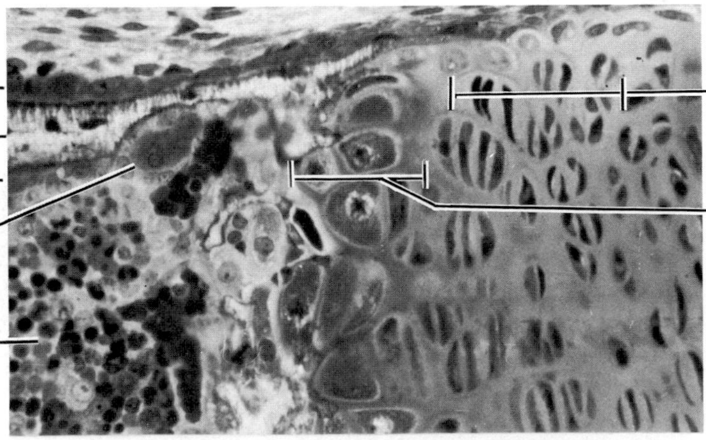

Figure 4-20. Endochondral bone formation. LM, ×300.
Figure 4-21. Endochondral bone formation. LM, ×250.
Figure 4-22. Endochondral bone formation. LM, ×300.

4-23

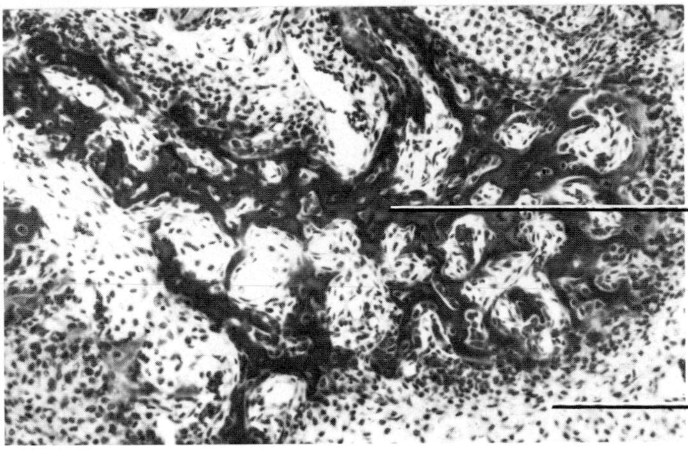

4-24

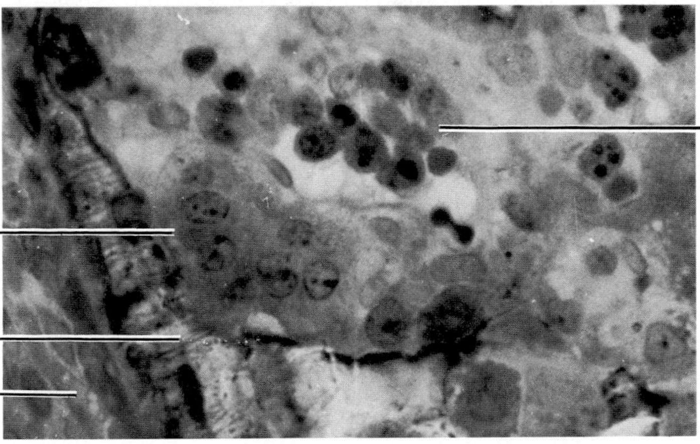

4-25

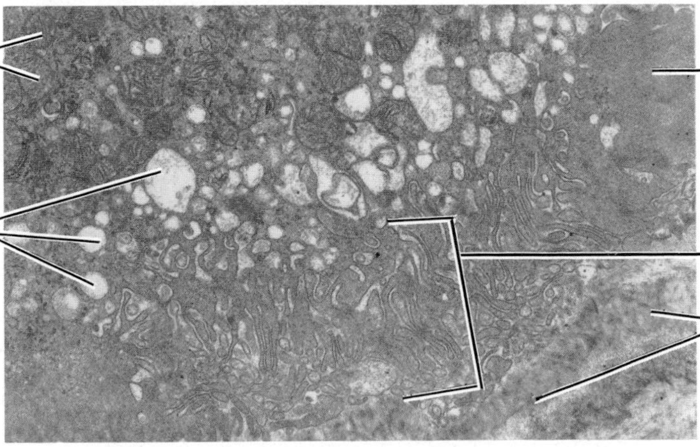

Figure 4-23. Intramembranous bone formation. LM, ×100.
Figure 4-24. Osteoclast. LM, ×500.
Figure 4-25. Ruffled border of osteoclast. TEM, ×12,000.

5

Special Connective Tissue: Blood

Blood usually is defined as a special connective tissue in which the intercellular substance is a fluid. Unlike other connective tissues, however, the intercellular substance of blood lacks a fibrous component and most of the intercellular protein is produced by cells in other tissues (especially the liver) and not by the blood cells. In mammals, many of the formed elements of blood consist not of true cells but anucleated elements (erythrocytes) and fragments of cytoplasm (platelets). True cells (leukocytes) constitute only a small part of the formed elements, are present as transients and use the blood only as a vehicle for their dissemination to other organs and tissues into which they migrate to carry out their functions. Only the erythrocytes and platelets function within the blood vascular system. None of the formed elements replicate within the blood; as they are lost, new elements are added from special blood-forming tissues located outside the circulation.

Regardless of the species, the total quantity of blood forms a rather constant proportion of the body mass, generally accounting for 6 to 8% of the body weight. In man the volume is about 5 liters, or approximately 7.5% of body weight.

COMPONENTS OF BLOOD

KEY WORDS: formed elements, erythrocytes, platelets, leukocytes, plasma, hematocrit, buffy coat, albumin, fibrinogen, globulin, serum

Blood consists of the **formed elements** which comprise the **erythrocytes, platelets**, and **leukocytes**, and a fluid intercellular substance, the **plasma**. These can be separated by centrifugation and, when carried out in calibrated tubes, the result (the **hematocrit**) gives an estimate of the volume of the formed elements. The heaviest components, the erythrocytes, form the lower layer and in man make up about 45% of the blood volume. Leukocytes and platelets are present in the **buffy coat**, a grayish-white layer immediately above the erythrocytes, and form about 1% of the total blood volume. The uppermost layer consists of the plasma, which contains three major types of protein—albumin, globulin, and fibrinogen. **Albumin**, the most abundant and smallest of the plasma proteins, is formed in the liver, as is **fibrinogen**, an essential component of the clotting mechanism. The **globulins** include several proteins of different sizes, among which are immunoglobulins (antibodies), synthesized by cells of the lymphatic organs and tissues. Plasma and serum are not equivalent, although both represent the fluid portion of the blood. Plasma is obtained from blood after treatment with an anticoagulant and contains all the components of the fluid portion. **Serum** is obtained from clotted or defibrinated blood and does not contain fibrinogen but does contain other components elaborated during the process of blood clotting.

Erythrocytes

At rest, the average human consumes about 250 ml of oxygen and produces about 200 ml of carbon dioxide per minute. With activity these quantities may increase by as much as 10- to 20-fold. Gases are carried and exchanged by the erythrocytes, which transport the gases with great efficiency. Exchange of gases occurs in the blood capillaries of the lung, and erythrocytes pass through the capillaries in slightly less than 1 second; yet, in less than this, gaseous exchange is completed.

Structure

KEY WORDS: anucleate, hemoglobin, erythroplastid, absence of organelles

In smear preparations and tissue sections, the mammalian erythrocyte appears as an **anucleate**, uniformly acidophilic body devoid of any internal structures. The bulk of the cell consists of a pigment, **hemoglobin**, which makes up about 95% of the dry weight. The term **erythroplastid** more aptly describes these elements, but custom and usage have given the terms "erythrocyte" and "red cells" the status of proper terminology. Electron microscopy confirms the **absence of organelles** in the mammalian red cell. In fishes, amphibia, reptiles, and birds, the red cells retain a nucleus; some of the cells also show mitochondria, a Golgi complex, and vestiges of endoplasmic reticulum. The purpose of the nucleus in these species is uncertain since it appears to be inert and nonfunctioning. At the other extreme, is the icefish, which has no erythrocytes at all. It inhabits the cold waters of the Antarctic, carries out a rather sluggish existence and transports gases in the plasma.

Shape and Size

KEY WORDS: biconcave disk, central depression, cell membrane, spectrin

The mammalian erythrocyte usually is described as a **biconcave disk**, and while this shape is seen in man and some other mammals, it is less obvious in many other species in which the cells appear as flat disks. Face on, the red cell usually presents a smooth, rounded contour with, in the biconcave forms, a **central depression**. Elliptical or cigar-shaped erythrocytes are characteristic of the camel, alpaca and llama and small spherical cells are present in the chevrotain (mouse deer).

The diameter varies widely between species but is maintained within close limits within a species and in the individuals of a species. In man, erythrocytes seen in smears average 7.6 μm in diameter, being slightly smaller in tissue sections (6.5 to 7.0 μm) and slightly larger (about 8 μm) in fresh blood. The largest red cells are the nucleated cells of *Amphiuma*, which measure 70 μm in their greatest diameter and 37 μm in their least diameter. Among mammals, the smallest red cells are found in the mouse deer while the largest occur in the Indian elephant. Despite the wide variations in diameter, the thickness of the red cell (about 2 μm) is remarkably consistent in all species, and apparently this is the optimum distance from the cell surface for the functioning of hemoglobin.

Erythrocytes are enclosed by a typical **cell membrane**, the flexibility and elasticity of which allows the red cell to accomodate to passage through small capillaries. In vivo the cells often assume a cup shape as they pass through blood vessels. The flexibility of the cell membrane would seem to exclude it from having a prominent role in maintaining the shape of the cell. No internal cytoskeleton has been identified, but it has been suggested that proteins may form a molecular network that acts as a cytoskeleton. A subplasmalemmal network of a protein (**spectrin**) has been described which may maintain the biconcave shape and still provide flexibility. Hemoglobin might play a role, since marked changes in shape are associated with the abnormal hemoglobin of sickle cell anemia.

In fish, birds, reptiles and amphibia, a bundle of microtubules encircles the perimeter of the flattened cell and serves as a cytoskeletal element. Similar structures are not found in mammalian erythrocytes.

Number and Survival

The number of circulating red cells also varies with species and while the correlation is not absolute, there appears to be an inverse relationship between cell size and numbers. In *Amphiuma*, with its huge nucleated cells, the blood contains only 20,000 to 30,000 red cells/mm^3 of blood, while in the goat, whose red cells average only 4.5 μm in diameter, the same volume of blood contains 12,000,000 to 20,000,000 erythrocytes. Some mammals show consistent sex differences in the number of red cells. For humans, values of 4,500,000 to 6,000,000/mm^3 in the male and 3,800,000 to 5,000,000/mm^3 in the female are considered normal.

In general, the survival time of red cells is related to the metabolic rate of the species. Survival time is longer in animals with a low metabolic rate and is increased during hibernation. In man the survival time is about 120 days. Although the red cells generally are removed as they age and wear out, a variable degree of random destruction also occurs. The presence of a nucleus does not appear to offer an extension of survival times and some of the shortest-lived erythrocytes occur in species with nucleated red blood cells.

As erythrocytes age, they use up most of the enzymes associated with ATP production and are unable to maintain themselves. By the end of their life span, the cells have become rather rigid due to degradation of protein and its cross linkage with calcium. These aged red cells are trapped and destroyed by phagocytes in the spleen mainly, but also in the liver and bone marrow. Iron in hemoglobin is recovered, stored and recycled into new red cells.

Reticulocytes

KEY WORDS: polychromatophilic, ribonucleoprotein

Although most red cells stain an orange-pink with the usual blood stains, a small number take on a bluish or slate gray tint. These **polychromatophilic** cells are erythrocytes that have not fully completed their maturation. They contain a small amount of **ribonucleoprotein** which, when stained with brilliant cresyl blue or new methylene blue, precipitates as a web or network, and thus the cells are called reticulocytes. Their numbers in peripheral blood form a rough index of erythrocyte production. Normally, reticulocytes make up only 1 to 2% of the red cells in man, about 1% in the dog and 0.1% in cats. Reticulocytes are not found in equine blood.

Rouleaux

Mammalian erythrocytes tend to adhere to each other by their broad surfaces and from stacks called rouleaux. The tendency is more pronounced in some species; ruminants generally show little rouleaux formation, while in equine species, the tendency may be extreme. Rouleaux formation depends upon changes in the blood plasma rather than in the red cells. Any condition which increases the net positive charge in the plasma results in changes in the surface charge on the erythrocytes, allowing them to adhere to each other more readily. Increased rouleaux is reflected in an increase in the rate at which the red cells settle out or sediment. Rouleaux formation is a temporary phenomenon, may occur intravascularly, and does no harm to the red cells.

Abnormalities

KEY WORDS: anisocytosis, macrocytes, microcytes, poikilocytosis, crenations, sickling, hypochromia, target cells, Howell-Jolly bodies

Departures from the normal size, shape or staining properties of erythrocytes can be important indicators of disease but to much less a degree some of these abnormalities may be found in healthy individuals also. **Anisocytosis** describes abnormal variations in the size of the red cells, which may be **macrocytes** (larger than normal) or **microcytes** (smaller than normal). Irregularity in shape is called **poikilocytosis** and the cells show blunt, pointed or hook-shaped projections from their surfaces. A special form of poikilocytosis occurs in normal cells placed in a hypertonic solution; water is abstracted from the cell, leaving it shrunken and bearing numerous projections from its surface.

Such a red cell is said to be **crenated**. The process is reversible and the cell resumes its normal appearance when returned to an isotonic milieu. One of the most severe changes in shape occurs during **sickling** of red cells in sickle cell anemia, in which the erythrocytes take on the form of crescents, holly leaves or even tubes.

Hypochromia denotes a decrease in the intensity of staining and indicates a lessened amount of hemoglobin; it frequently accompanies microcytosis. Cells which are thinner than normal often appear as **target cells** in which the staining appears as a central disk and an external ring separated by an unstained band.

Howell-Jolly bodies are nuclear fragments left over from the nucleated precursors of the red cell and appear as one or two rounded or rod-shaped basophilic granules. An increase in the number of reticulocytes is considered an abnormality, but the cell itself is not an abnormal erythrocyte.

Hemoglobin

Gas transport in mammals is accomplished by hemoglobin, an iron-containing respiratory pigment that imparts the red color to mammalian blood. Many invertebrates possess respiratory pigments for gas transport which are totally unlike hemoglobin. In Crustacea, for example, the pigment is a copper-containing hemocyanin which, when combined with molecular oxygen, assumes a blue color. Hemocyanin is not contained within corpuscular elements, however.

Structure

KEY WORDS: heme, α and β chains, γ chain, sickle hemoglobin (hemoglobin S)

Hemoglobin is one of a group of catalytic compounds which possesses an iron porphyrin prosthetic group, **heme**, attached to a protein, globin. Structurally, hemoglobin is a symmetrical molecule formed by two equal, mirror image halves. Each half molecule consists of two different peptide chains, the **α and β chains**, each bearing a heme group around which the chain is coiled. Thus, each molecule of hemoglobin contains two α chains and two β chains and four heme groups. The heme groups form the functional component; the peptide chains form the globin portion of the molecule. The amino acid composition and sequences in the peptide chains confer species specificity to the whole molecule and determine the type of hemoglobin present. In man, for example, the hemoglobin present in fetal red cells differs from that of adult red cells in the amino acid arrangement and composition of the β chains. Indeed, the fetal β chain differs so greatly that it is designated a **γ chain**. Even minor modifications of the peptide chains can result in gross changes in the entire molecule, as demonstrated by the **sickle hemoglobin (hemoglobin S)** associated with sickle cell anemia. The only deficit in the whole molecule is the replacement, in the sixth position of the β chains, of the glutamic acid in normal hemoglobin by a valine in the sickle hemoglobin.

Platelets

Platelets are the second most numerous of the formed elements of blood and are found only in mammals. In other vertebrates they are represented by a somewhat different element, the thrombocyte. Like erythrocytes, platelets are not true cells but represent fragments of cytoplasm derived from a large precursor cell in the bone marrow.

Structure

KEY WORDS: granulomers (chromomere), hyalomere, microfibrils, marginal bundle

Platelets appear as small, anucleate bodies that range in size from 2 to 5 μm. In stained smears, platelets show a granular portion, the granulomere and a pale granule free part, the hyalomere. The **granulomere (chromomere)** frequently occupies the central region of the platelet and may be so compact as to suggest a nucleus but like red cells, platelets lack nuclei. However, separation into two distinct zones is not seen in circulating platelets or in those fixed instantaneously by drawing blood directly into fixative. Under these conditions, the granulomere material remains evenly distributed. Electron micrographs reveal that the granulomere consists of lysosomes, mitochondria, dense granules that contain serotonin, ADP, ATP and calcium, and α particles which contain platelet-specific proteins, fibrinogen and other clotting factors. Mitochondria are small, few in number and have few cristae. Variable numbers of glycogen granules also are present. Each platelet is bounded by a typical cell membrane.

The **hyalomere** represents the cytoplasmic matrix and appears as a homogeneous, finely granular background. A crisscross arrangement of **microfibrils** is present immediately beneath the plasmalemma and may serve as a cytoskeleton. A narrow peripheral zone remains free of granulomere elements and is the site of a system of microtubules that forms the **marginal bundle**. This structure has been described as a single, coiled tubule that acts as a stiffening element to help maintain the discoidal shape.

Number

The number of platelets varies widely, not only with species but also for individuals. The variations reflect the difficulties in obtaining accurate counts, due to physiological factors that affect the numbers, and to certain properties of the platelets themselves. A characteristic feature of platelets is their propensity to stick to foreign surfaces and to each other to form clumps. When in contact with a foreign surface, platelets spread to cover an area several hundred times that of their initial surface. Although platelet levels in man usually are given as 250,000 to 400,000/mm^3 of blood, some estimates extend the range to 900,000/mm^3. Transient fluctuations in platelets have been associated with variation in oxygen concentration, exposure to periods of cold and food intake. Strangely, highly spiced foods have been reportd to result in a significant decrease in circulating platelets. Emotional states such as fear and rage result in markedly elevated counts in some animals, especially the cat. A progressive decrease occurs in women during the two weeks prior to menstruation, with a rapid return to normal thereafter.

Thrombocytes

In birds, fishes, amphibia and reptiles, platelets are represented by nucleated cells, the thrombocytes. Although size varies somewhat, the general morphology of thrombocytes is similar in different species. The nucleus generally conforms to the shape of the cell, which may be rounded, ovoid or spindle-shaped, depending upon the species examined. Specific granules, mitochondria, scattered ribosomes and vesicles and tubules of endoplasmic reticulum are present. As in mammalian platelets, mitochondria are scarce, small and of simple structure, containing only 2 to 3 cristae. Thrombocytes readily stick to each other and often appear in small clusters. The cells function in blood coagulation.

Leukocytes

The leukocytes or white blood cells (WBC) are true cells that possess nuclei and cytoplasmic organelles and are capable of ameboid movement. They migrate from the blood into the tissues whey they perform their main functions.

Classification

KEY WORDS: granular, agranular, polymorphonuclear, mononuclear, neutrophils (heterophils), eosinophils, basophils, pseudoeosinophils, lymphocytes, monocytes

Leukocytes can be divided into **granular** and **agranular** types on the basis of cytoplasmic granulation, or into **polymorphonuclear** and **mononuclear** according to the shape of the nucleus. The granular leukocytes contain multilobed nuclei and thus the terms granular leukocyte and polymorphonuclear leukocyte denote the same class of cells.

Granulocytes can be subdivided into **neutrophils (heterophils), eosinophils** and **basophils** according to the color of the granules after the usual blood stains. Heterophil granules do not stain the same in all species and the term is used inclusively for this type of granular leukocyte, regardless of staining reaction or species. The term **neutrophil** refers to the heterophil of man. In fish and birds, heterophil granules are rod-shaped and eosinophilic, while in rabbits and guinea pigs the homolog of the human neutrophil contains coarse, rounded eosinophilic granules. To distinguish these from true eosinophils, the heterophils of rabbits and guinea pigs have been called **pseudoeosinophils**.

The agranular leukocytes consist of the **lymphocytes** and **monocytes** which possess inconspicuous or no granules, and a single nonlobed nucleus. The distinction between granular and agranular leukocytes is not absolute: Monocytes regularly show fine cytoplasmic granules and lymphocytes may contain a few granules also. The distinction is an old one based on the staining appearance with less refined dyes but remains useful since the granules in the granular leukocytes are specific, distinctive and prominent.

Neutrophil (Heterophil)

KEY WORDS: lobes, filaments, band forms, nuclear appendages, drumstick, specific granules, lysozyme, lactoferrin, phagocytin, azurophil granules, lysosomes

The heterophil granulocyte (neutrophil in man) is characterized by the shape of the nucleus, which contains small **lobes** connected by thin **filaments**. The number of lobes varies but in man 2 to 4 are usual. The lobes in a given cell do not change with age and the leukocyte appears to retain the same degree of lobation throughout its life. Excessive lobation occurs in some diseases or as an inherited anomaly in man, and several species normally show up to 7 or 8 nuclear lobes. In rodents such as the rat and mouse, the nucleus frequently forms a ring (annular nucleus) which may be twisted and assume the form of a figure 8. In other species lobation is not as distinct as in man and the thin filaments are replaced by coarse narrowings of the nucleus.

The nucleus stains deeply and the chromatin is aggregated into clumps that form a patchy network. Nucleoli are absent. A simple, elongated, nonlobed nucleus is regularly seen in a small number of granulocytes; called **band forms**, they represent cells recently released from the bone marrow. In addition to the nuclear lobation, **nuclear appendages** in the shape of hooks, hand racquets, clubs or **drumsticks** may be present. Only the drumstick has any significance; it represents the female sex chromatin and is found on a terminal lobe in about 2 to 3% of the neutrophils.

The cytoplasm of human neutrophils contains two types of granules. The most numerous are the **specific granules**, which are small and take on a pinkish hue. These granules contain **lysozyme**, an enzyme complex that acts against components of bacterial cell walls; **lactoferrin,** another antibacterial substance; and a several other rather poorly characterized basic proteins (**phagocytins**) that also have bactericidal activity. **Azurophil granules** are less numerous, somewhat larger and stain a reddish purple. They contain lysozyme as well as a battery of lysosomal enzymes and are considered to be modified **lysosomes**.

Electron micrographs show the granules to be scattered throughout the cytoplasm, except in a narrow peripheral zone. This region contains fine filaments and microtubules that appear to function in cell movement. A small Golgi complex and a pair of centrioles are situated centrally in the cell. Rare profiles of endoplasmic reticulum, a few mitochondria and ribosomes are present also. Azurophil granules are large and homogeneous, whereas the smaller, less dense, specific granules may contain a crystalloid body.

Neutrophil granulocytes are the chief type of leukocyte in man, forming 55 to 70% of the circulating white blood cells. In other species, the heterophils may be less numerous and lymphocytes predominate. Neutrophils range from 12 to 15 μm in diameter but are slightly smaller in fresh blood.

Eosinophil Leukocytes

KEY WORDS: diurnal variations, nuclear lobulation, crystalloid, internus, lysosomes, peroxidase

Eosinophils form only a small proportion of the total leukocytes and in man normally account for 1 to 3% of the circulating white blood cells. Their number in blood bears some relation to the activity of the adrenal gland and a decrease in the number of eosinophils is seen in the alarm reaction. This may account for the wide range of values reported, even in the same animal. For example, the percentage of eosinophils reported in the blood of the cow has ranged from 0 to 30 and similar values have been recorded for monkeys and cats. Distinct **diurnal variations** occur in many animals, including man, and appear to be related to activity cycles.

The eosinophil is about the same size as the neutrophil and also is characterized by **nuclear lobulation**. Although often described as having a bilobed nucleus, cells with three and four nuclear lobes are not uncommon and conditions that produce hypersegmentation of the neutrophil nucleus also produce excessive lobulation in the eosinophil granulocyte. Annular nuclei are seen in rodents.

The distinctive feature of eosinophils is the closely packed, uniform spherical granules that stain a brillant red or orange-red. The granules are membrane bound and show an internal structure that has been called **crystalloid** or **internus**. In man the crystalloid assumes various forms and may be multiple, while in the cat the structures are cylindrical and show concentric lamellations. The crystal is embedded in a finely granular matrix. The eosinophil granules are **lysosomes** and contain the usual lysosomal enzymes. They show a higher content of **peroxidase** than do the azurophil granules of neutrophils and lack lysozyme and phagocytin.

Basophil Leukocytes

KEY WORDS: lobes, filaments, metachromatic

Basophil granulocytes rarely make up more than 1% or at most 2% of the leukocyte count, although an exception to this is the rabbit in which values as high as 9% are not uncommon. In man, basophils comprise only about 0.5% of the total leukocytes. They are slightly smaller than the heterophil granulocytes and in blood smears measure 10 to 12 μm in diameter.

Nuclear **lobes** are less distinct and more poorly defined than in neutrophils or eosinophils. More than 2 to 3 lobes are rare. The **filaments** between lobes tend to be short and broad and rarely form the threadlike structures seen in neutrophils. Annular nuclei are sometimes seen in the rat and mouse and can be found in the opossum also. The nuclear chromatin is relatively homogeneous, stains less deeply than that of other granulocytes and nucleoli are absent.

The cytoplasm contains prominent, rather coarse granules that stain a deep violet with the usual blood stains and **metachromatically** with toluidine blue or thionine. In the human, well-preserved granules are spherical and uniform but being soluble in water and glycerin, they frequently appear irregular in size and shape in fixed preparations. In the rat the granules are more ovoid, while in the guinea pig they are distinctly oval and larger than in humans. The granules are scattered unevenly throughout the cytoplasm, often overlie and obscure the nucleus, and are neither as numerous nor as densely packed as the granules of the eosinophil leukocyte. Electron microscopy reveals an internal pattern of structure that varies with the species. In man, a regular striation of the granule has been described, while in the mouse, the granules show a finely reticulated pattern. A complex lamellation is seen in the basophil granules of the guinea pig, giving to them a honeycomb appearance. The granules contain glycosaminoglycans, eosinophil chemotactic factors, prostaglandins and a platelet-activating factor.

Lymphocytes

KEY WORDS: agranulocyte, small lymphocyte, mononuclear, short-lived lymphocytes, long-lived lymphocytes, T lymphocytes, cell-mediated immunity, B lymphocytes, humoral immunity, bursa of Fabricius, mitogens, null cells

Lymphocytes are present in all classes of vertebrates and cells of similar morphology have been described in nonvertebrates also. In some mammals (rodents, opossum) they are the dominant type of leukocyte, while in others they are second only to the heterophils. In all species they are the predominant type of **agranulocyte**. In man the lymphocyte accounts for 20 to 35% of the circulating leukocytes.

Blood lymphocytes show a spectrum of sizes from the **small lymphocyte** with a diameter of 6 to 8 μm to larger forms measuring 10 to 12 μm in diameter. The large lymphocytes or lymphoblasts (14 to 15 μm) of lymphatic tissues are rarely found in normal blood and the small lymphocyte is the most common form. The small lymphocyte is a **mononuclear** leukocyte that contains a single, deeply stained, rounded or slightly indented nucleus surrounded by only a thin rim of lightly basophilic cytoplasm. Nucleoli usually are not seen in blood smears but are visible in living cells and in electron micrographs. A few nonspecific azurophil granules may be present and a small Golgi apparatus, centrioles, a few mitochondria, some ribosomes and profiles of smooth endoplasmic reticulum can be seen. The larger forms of lymphocytes are identified by a more abundant cytoplasm, an increased number of ribosomes and mitochondria, a greater amount of endoplasmic reticulum and an increase in the size of the Golgi apparatus.

Although morphologically indistinguishable, at least two groups of small lymphocytes are known which differ in their life span, background and functions. Some small lymphocytes live only a few days while for others survival is measured in months and years: these constitute **short-lived** and **long-lived lymphocytes**, respectively. The long-lived cells are thought to be "memory cells." On the basis of their background and functions, small lymphocytes can be classed as T lymphocytes and B lymphocytes. **T lymphocytes** are those that have been processed by the thymus and programmed to take part in **cell-mediated immune responses** in which the cells elaborate nonspecific, cytolytic agents. **B lymphocytes** play a central role in **humoral** or antibody-mediated **immune responses**. The organ involved in conditioning B lymphocytes is unknown in mammals but may be the bone marrow. In aves, conditioning of B lymphocytes occurs in the **bursa of Fabricius**, an appendix-like diverticulum of the cloaca.

T and B cells can be distinguished by the presence of cytochemical markers on their surfaces. A third class of lymphocyte, the **null cell**, has been described and consists of cells that lack T or B cell markers.

Small lymphocytes are not simple "end cells." They respond to a number of **mitogenic agents** and, when cultured with one of these substances (phytohemagglutinin, concanavalin A, etc.), undergo progressive enlargement, nucleoli become visible and ribosomes increase in number. Within 48 to 72 hours, the cells assume the appearance of lymphoblasts and begin to divide, mature and differentiate into plasma cells. A small number, however, remain as small lymphocytes. The mechanism of this reaction is unknown but it appears to mimic in vitro the response of small lymphocytes to antigens in vivo. The large lymphocytes of the blood may be lymphocytes that have been stimulated antigenically and represent the first indications of an immune response.

Monocytes

KEY WORDS: mononuclear leukocyte, azurophil granules, ground-glass cytoplasm, primary lysosomes, mononuclear phagocyte system

Monocytes constitute the second type of **mononuclear leukocyte** normally found in blood. Their proportions are fairly consistent throughout various species and monocytes regularly form 3 to 8% of the circulating leukocytes. The cells vary from 10 to 15 μm in diameter and contain a fairly large nucleus that may be rounded, kidney-shaped or horseshoe-shaped. Segmentation of the nucleus with filament formation never occurs, but coarse constrictions with blunt broad lobes may be present. The chromatin is more loosely dispersed than in the lymphocyte and the nucleus therefore stains less densely. Two to three nucleoli sometimes can be seen. The blue-gray cytoplasm is more abundant and contains numerous, fine **azurophil granules** that impart an opacity of the cytoplasm which has been described as having a "**ground-glass**" appearance. Ultrastructurally, the nucleus shows one or two nucleoli, and the cytoplasm contains a small amount of granular endoplasmic reticulum, ribosomes and polyribosomes. Small, elongated mitochondria are present and the Golgi apparatus is well formed. The azurophil granules represent **primary lysosomes** and appear as dense homogeneous structures.

Monocytes are part of the **mononuclear phagocyte system** and represent the cells of this system that are in transit. They have little function while in the blood but emigrate into various organs and tissues throughout the body, where they differentiate into the macrophages. In addition to serving as tissue scavengers, monocytes also have a role in processing antigen in the immune response.

Total Leukocyte Count

KEY WORDS: leukocytosis, leukopenia

Like all the formed elements, the total number of leukocytes tend to fall within a relatively stable range in normal individuals but vary widely in disease and with species. In the human, the normal range is from 5,000 to 12,000 leukocytes/mm^3 of blood. An increase above normal is termed a **leukocytosis** and may be due to disease or to emotional or physical stress. In man a leukocytosis reaching 25,000 to 35,000/mm^3 has been reported following severe exercise. These values reflect the flushing out into the circulation of leukocytes sequestered in capillary beds and marginated at the periphery of the blood stream. Decreases in leukocyte numbers are termed a **leukopenia**. Diurnal variations of greater or lesser degree are associated with activity cycles and have been reported in a number of animals, including man. Sex differences have been noted in some animals, with higher values occurring in males, but there appear to be no significant sex differences in the leukocyte counts in man.

FUNCTIONAL SUMMARY

Blood has important functions in transporting various materials throughout the body, in maintaining the acid-base balance and in providing various defense mechanisms. Transport functions include carriage of oxygen from the lungs to all the cells of the body, transport of nutrients, and removal of the waste products of cell metabolism. It aids in regulating body temperature by dissipating the heat formed during metabolism, and distributes hormones, thus serving to integrate the functions of the endocrine system. Through its buffering capacities, blood helps maintain the acid-base balance and ensures an environment in which tissue cells may function normally.

Transport of oxygen to tissues and return of carbon dioxide to the lungs is a function of erythrocytes and their contained hemoglobin. Packaging of hemoglobin into cells allows for a local environment in which hemoglobin can function most effectively and also prevents the oxidation of hemoglobin to useless forms. This is achieved not only by mechanical packaging but also by provision of enzyme systems within the erythrocyte that prevent irreversible oxidation of hemoglobin. The retention of hemoglobin within the cell allows for an increased concentration of the pigment without increasing the viscosity of blood. The anucleate red cells of mammals are more efficient in gas transport than their nucleated counterparts.

Platelets have several rather diverse functions concerned with maintaining the integrity of the blood vasculature. Because of their ability to stick to each other and to foreign surfaces, platelets can temporarily repair small gaps in vessels. They have an important role in blood clotting and release clot-initiating factors but also appear to contain fibrinolytic factors which dissolve clots. Thus, platelets may aid in maintaining the fluidity of blood. They are essential for clot retraction which results in formation of a firm dense clot. When platelets are reduced in numbers, the clot is soft and friable. Although not synthesized by platelets, they contain epinephrine and 5-hydroxytryptamine, which are vasoconstrictors. While probably contributing little to the body's defense, platelets are able to phagocytose small particles, viruses and bacteria.

Neutrophils are avidly phagocytic and are part of the first line of defense against bacterial infections. The azurophil granules are lysosomes and phagocytosis by granulocytes is associated with fusion of the ingested material in the usual manner of lysosomal digestion. They also contain lysozyme that hydrolyses glycosides in bacterial cell walls, and peroxidase which complexes with hydrogen peroxide to release activated oxygen, an antibacterial agent. The specific granules also contain a number of antibacterial agents, including lysozyme, lactoferrin which binds iron (required by bacteria) and cationic compounds.

Eosinophils appear to have a special affinity for antigen-antibody complexes which tend to bind complement and induce cell lysis. Phagocytosis of completed antigen-antibody by eosinophils may suppress these events in normal tissues. Eosinophils may regulate allergic responses by degrading histamine and histamine-like substances. They also have a major role in control of certain parasitic infestations. A basic protein (MBP) in the crystalloid core of the granule enhances the antibody-mediated destruction of parasites.

Basophil granules contain heparin, an anticoagulant, and vasodilation agents, histamine and slow-reacting substance (SRS). Histamine induces a prompt and transient vasodilation, whereas that induced by SRS is more sustained and occurs after a latent period. Both increase vascular permeability.

Lymphocytes are concerned primarily with the immune responses, of which there are two major

types, humoral and cellular. The basis of humoral immunity is the production of antibodies and their diffusion throughout the body fluids. As antigen enters the body, it is complexed on the surface of B lymphocytes, becomes internalized and triggers cell proliferation and differentiation into plasma cells. This results in production of a clone of plasma cells which synthesizes the immunogloblins and additional B lymphocytes which do not differentiate but remain as memory cells. On second exposure to the same antigen, the memory B cells rapidly divide and give rise to plasma cells which then synthesize the antibody. The process of humoral antibody production is highly specific and only those antigens that fit receptors on the surface of B lymphocytes will trigger the response.

Cellular immunity depends upon T lymphocytes. In response to antigen, the T cells proliferate and release factors that act over a short range. Among these are substances that inhibit the migration of macrophages from sites of antigen concentration, macrophage-activating factor that stimulates macrophage activity, lymphotoxin which destroys nonlymphoid cells, and various other specific and nonspecific agents. With most antigens that evoke a humoral response, stimulation of B cells also requires the participation of T lymphocytes and macrophages. How the T cells interact with B lymphocytes is poorly understood; they may recognize the antigen and concentrate it on their surfaces before presenting it to the B cells, or elaborate substances that activate the B lymphocyte.

Monocytes leave the blood and differentiate into tissue macrophages. They not only serve as tissue scavengers, ingesting and removing particulate matter, tissue debris and infective agents, but also play a role in the immune responses. Their exact role in immunity is not known, but macrophages may retain antigen on their surfaces long enough to stimulate lymphocytes to antibody production, or they may release partially processed antigen for lymphocyte stimulation. Macrophages also appear to have secretory functions and liberate antiviral agents (interferon), as well as a number of enzymes that digest collagen, elastin and fibrin.

Atlas for Chapter 5

Peripheral Blood

5-1

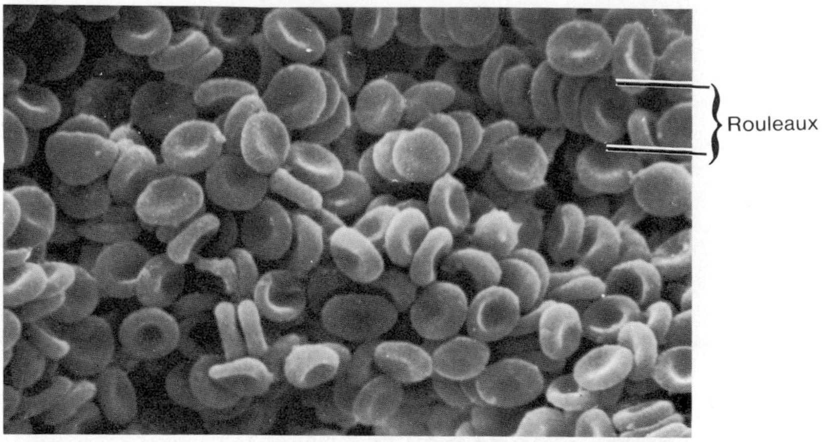

5-2

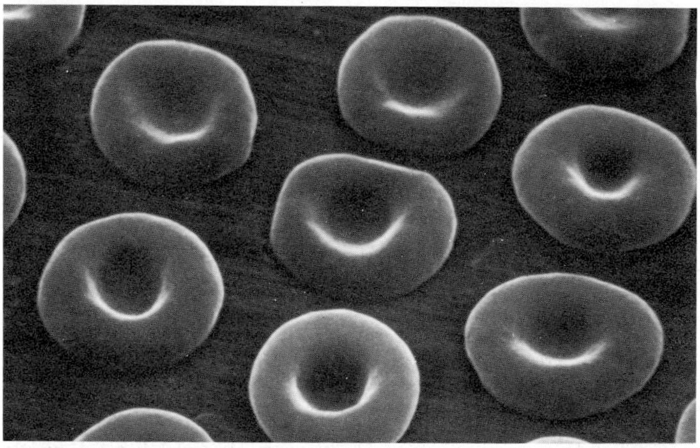

5-3

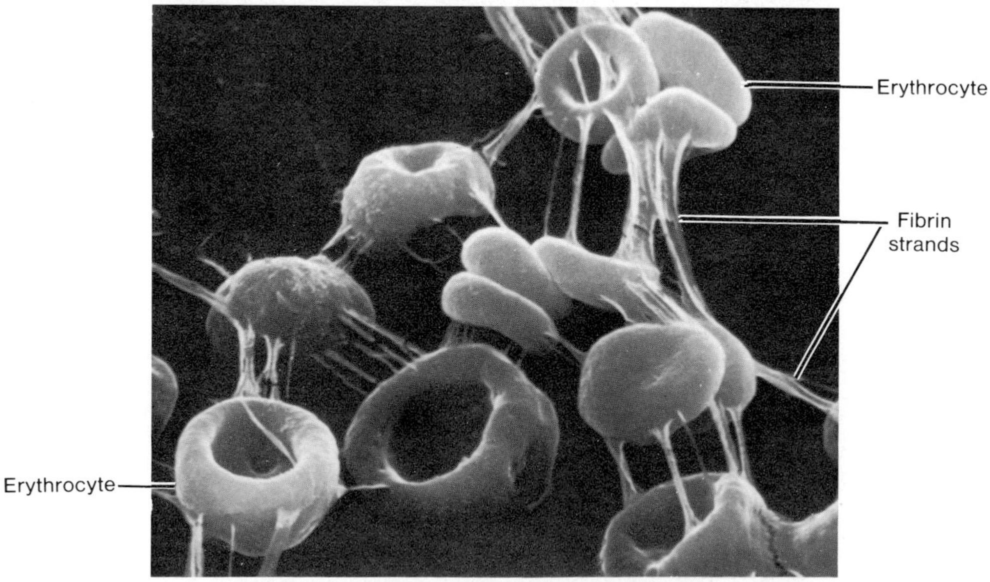

Figure 5-1. Erythrocytes (human). SEM, ×2000.
Figure 5-2. Erythrocytes (human). SEM, ×5000.
Figure 5-3. Blood clot (human). SEM, ×500.

5-4

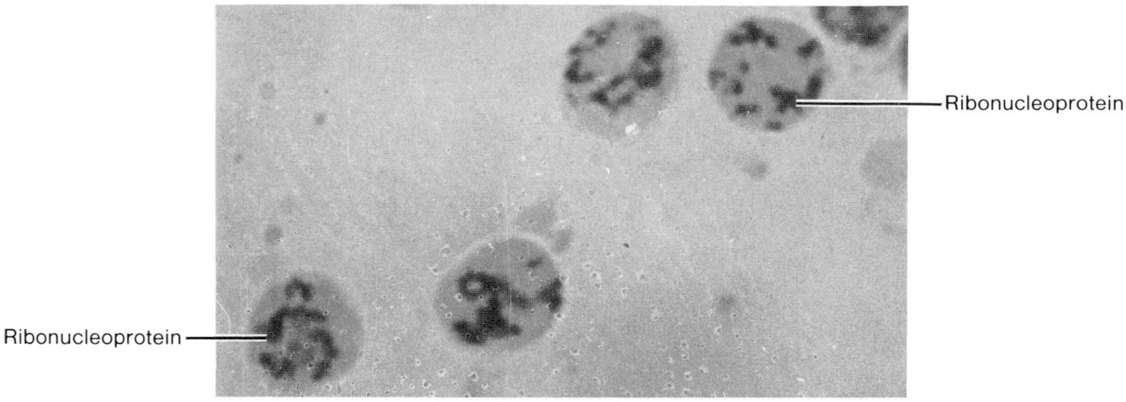

5-5

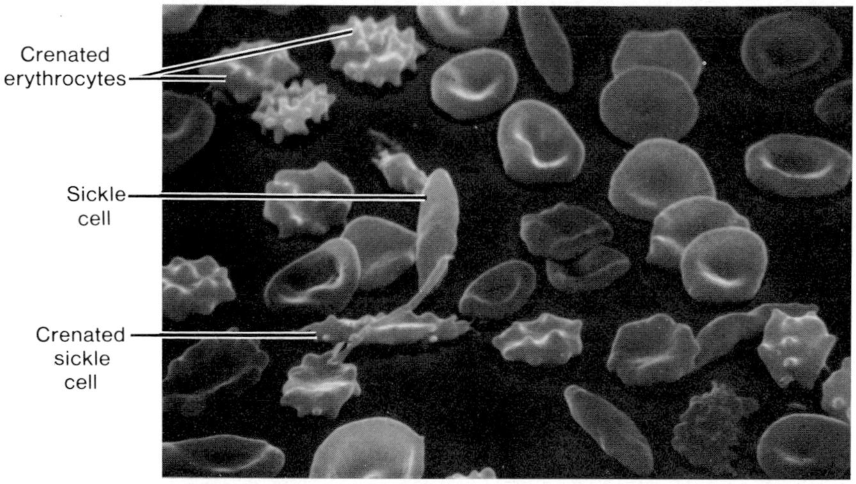

5-6

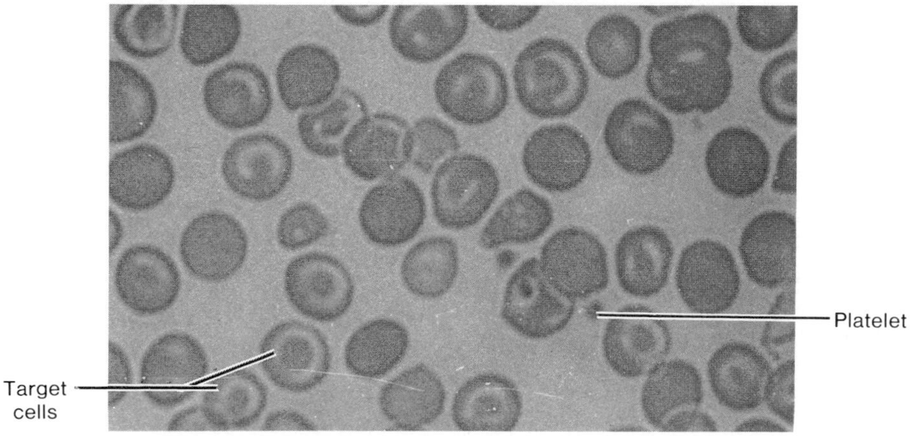

Figure 5-4. Reticulocytes. LM, ×1000.
Figure 5-5. Erythrocytes (human sickle cell anemia). SEM, ×5000.
Figure 5-6. Target cells. LM, ×1000.

5-7

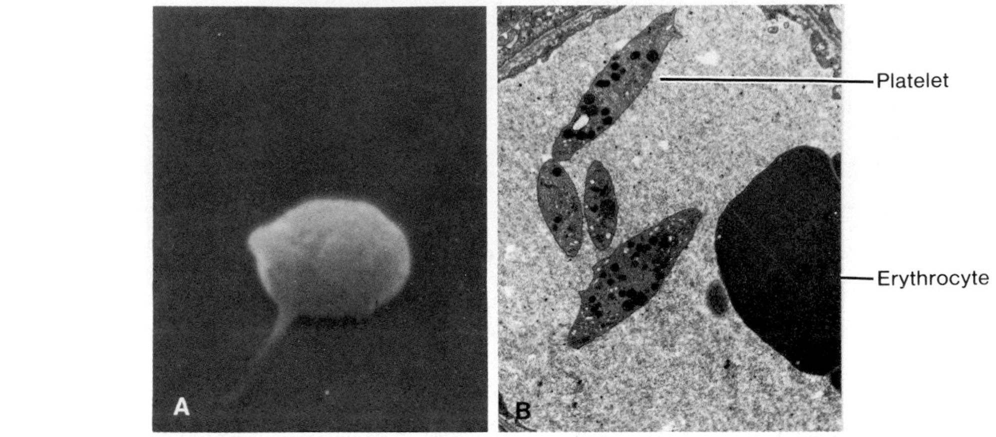

5-8

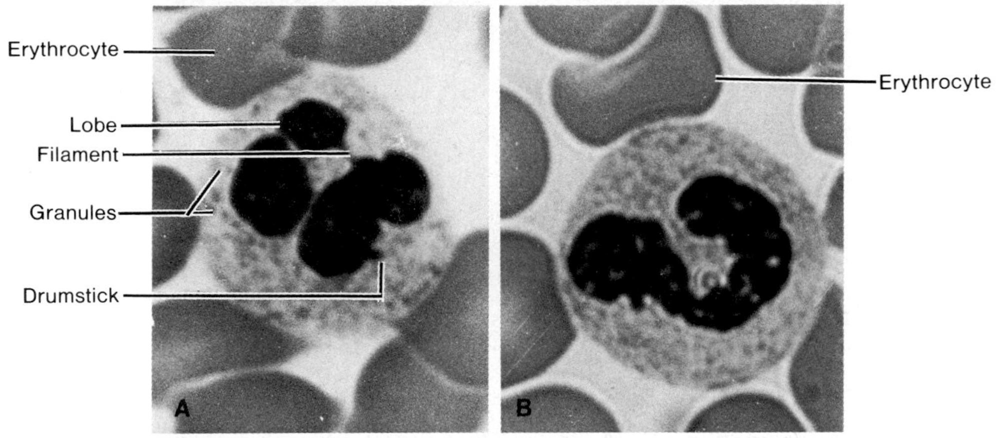

5-9

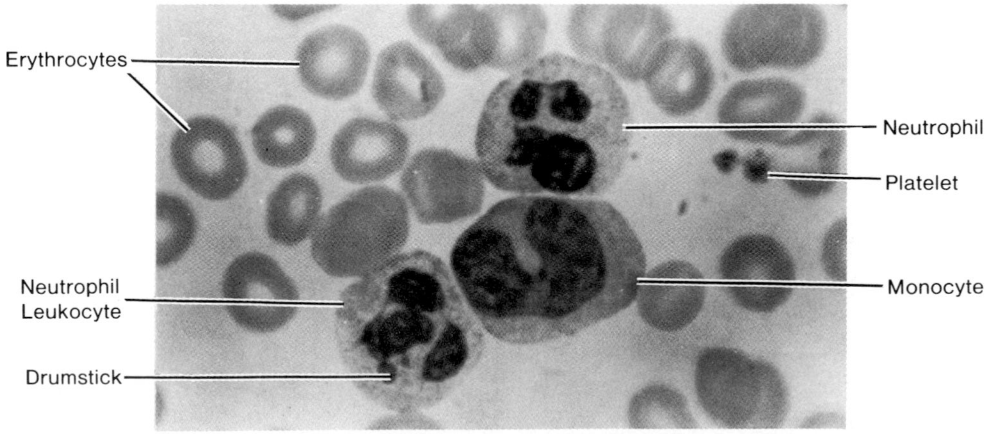

Figure 5-7. *A*, platelet (human). SEM, ×10,000. *B*, platelets. TEM, ×6000.
Figure 5-8. *A*, neutrophil. LM, ×15,000. *B*, neutrophil (band form). LM, ×1500.
Figure 5-9. Leukocytes (human). LM, ×1000.

5-10

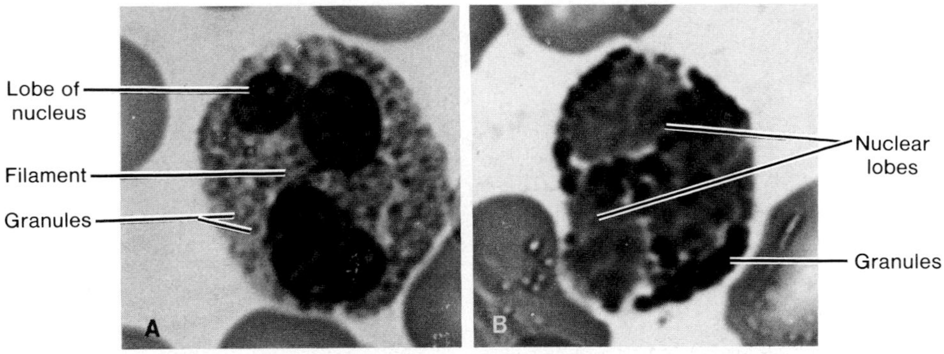

5-11

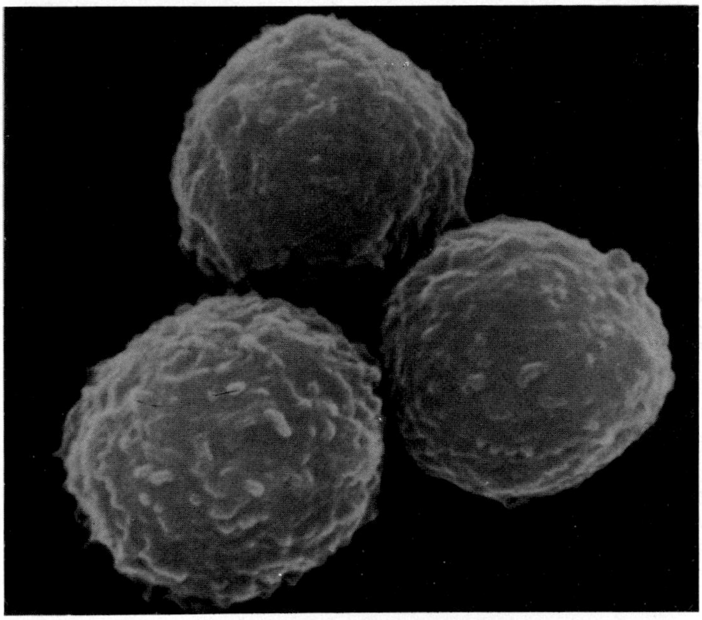

5-12

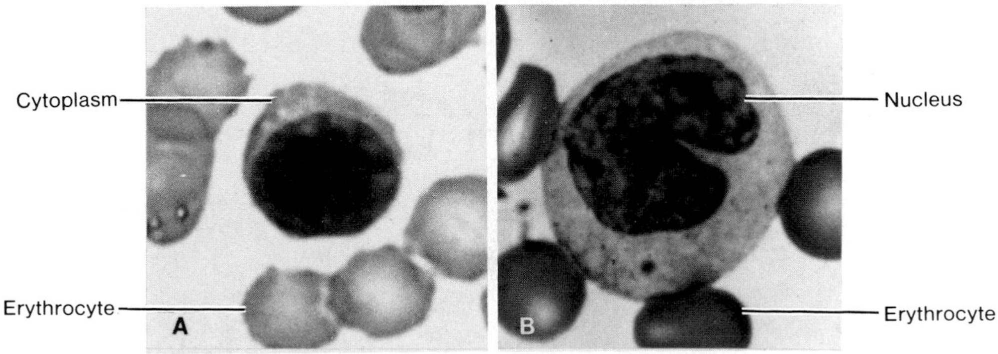

Figure 5-10. *A*, eosinophil (human). LM, ×1500. *B*, basophil (human). LM, ×1500.
Figure 5-11. Lymphocytes (human). SEM, ×10,000.
Figure 5-12. *A*, lymphocyte (human). LM, ×1200. *B*, monocyte (human). LM, ×1200.

5-13

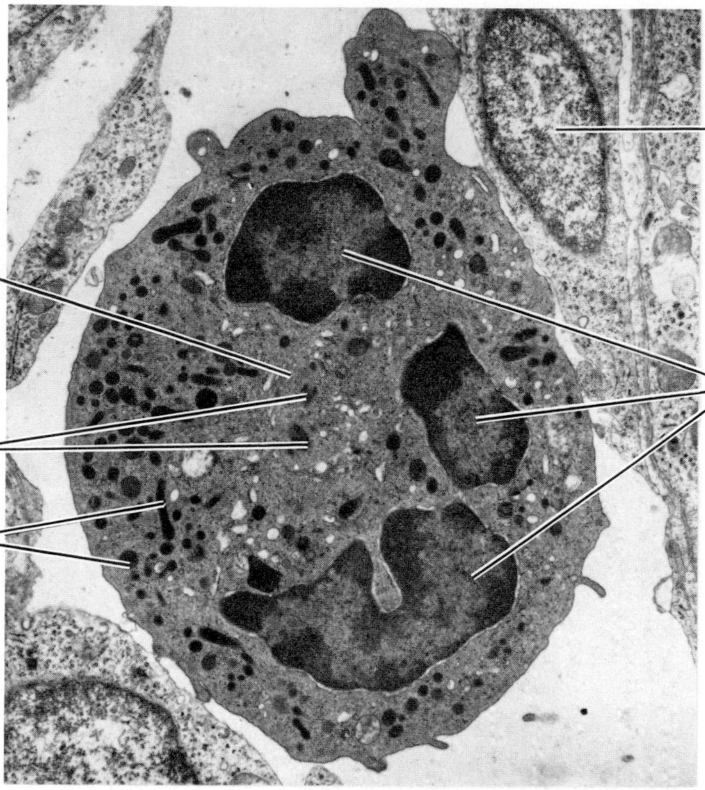

5-14

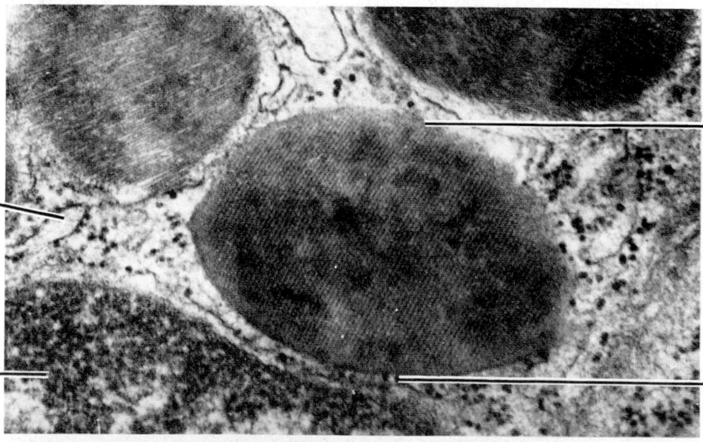

5-15

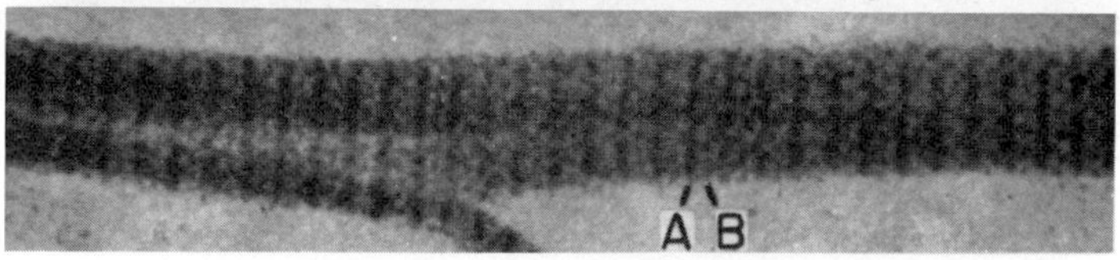

Figure 5-13. Neutrophil leukocyte. TEM, ×6000.
Figure 5-14. Granules of basophil leukocyte. TEM, ×25,000.
Figure 5-15. Fibrin. TEM, ×186,000.

5-16

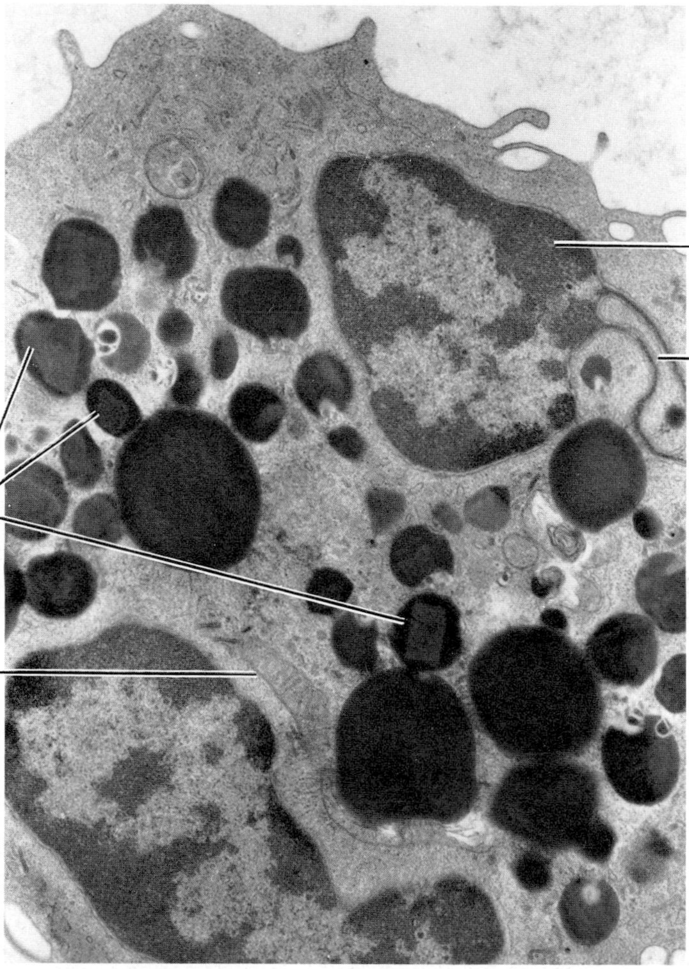

5-17

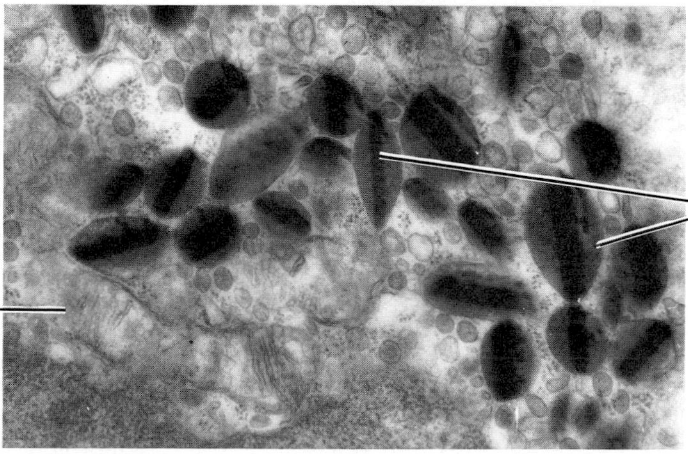

Figure 5-16. Eosinophil (human). TEM, ×15,000.
Figure 5-17. Eosinophil granules (rat). TEM, ×20,000.

6

Special Connective Tissue: Hemopoietic Tissue

Since the formed elements of blood are not self-replicating, their numbers in circulation must be maintained by continuous replacement from other sources. These specialized centers are the blood-forming or hemopoietic tissues which, in higher vertebrates, consist of the bone marrow, spleen, lymph nodes and thymus. In lower animals other organs may be involved in the formation of blood cells. For example in fishes, blood formation may occur in the kidney capsule, liver, wall of the digestive tract, heart, genital organs or cranial capsule, depending on the species. Reptiles appear to represent a class in which a transition to bone marrow is occurring as the major site of blood formation. In some, such as the horned toad, the chief hemopoietic organ is the spleen, which produces erythrocytes, monocytes, lymphocytes and thrombocytes, while the bone marrow is the organ of granulocyte formation. In other reptiles, such as the turtle, the spleen and marrow share the task of hemopoiesis, while in the lizard the bone marrow is the active site for production of granulocytes, red cells and thrombocytes.

EMBRYONIC AND FETAL HEMOPOIESIS

In adult mammals the hemopoietic tissue is restricted to the bone marrow and lymphoid tissues, but in embryonic and fetal life, blood cell formation occurs successively in the yolk sac, liver, spleen and bone marrow. Some residual formation of erythrocytes and platelets normally continues in the spleen in adult rats, mice, rabbits, hamsters, and opossums. In some pathological conditions, the human liver and spleen may resume a role in hemopoiesis.

Yolk Sac

KEY WORDS: blood islands, primitive erythroblasts

Blood development in the embryo is virtually the same for all mammals and begins soon after formation of the germ layers. It first appears in the walls of the yolk sac with the development of the **blood islands.** The mesenchymal cells of the yolk sac proliferate to form solid masses of cells which soon become endothelial lined spaces that contain developing blood cells. Most of these first hemopoietic cells differentiate into **primitive erythroblasts** that synthesize hemoglobin and become the nucleated erythrocytes characteristic of the embryo. In the human, yolk sac erythropoiesis begins about 19 days after fertilization and continues until the end of the 12th week.

Hepatic Hemopoiesis

KEY WORDS: definitive erythroblasts

The liver is the second important blood-forming organ of the embryo, and in the human this phase of hemopoiesis begins during the 6th week. Erythropoiesis dominates and there is considerable formation of platelets and macrophages (monocytes), but granulocyte production is minor. The liver is the principal site of red cell formation from the 3rd to 6th months of gestation. Formation of red cells in the liver continues, in decreasing amount, until birth. Hepatic erythropoiesis resembles that in adult bone marrow and the red cell precursors in the liver have been called **definitive erythroblasts** since they ultimately give rise to non-nucleated red cells. The developing cells form islands of hemopoietic tissue between the cords of hepatic cells. Granular leukocytes and megakaryocytes appear in the liver during the 2nd month.

Splenic Hemopoiesis

A minor level of splenic hemopoiesis overlaps that of the liver and contributes to the production of erythrocytes mainly, but also of platelets and granulocytes. Formation of these cells wanes as the bone marrow takes over these functions, but the spleen remains active in production of lymphocytes throughout life. In some animals, erythrocytes and megakaryocytes continue to be produced by the spleen even in the adult.

Myeloid Phase

The myeloid phase of hemopoiesis begins when ossification centers develop in the cartilaginous models of the long bones. Occasional hemopoietic cells may be found in the clavicle of the human fetus at 2½ months; foci of erythropoietic cells are found by 4 months; and by 6 months the bone marrow is an important source of circulating blood cells. During the last 3 months of pregnancy, the bone marrow is the chief blood forming organ of the fetus.

BONE MARROW

In the adult mammal the major organ for hemopoiesis is the bone marrow, which produces the erythrocytes, platelets, granular leukocytes and monocytes. Many of the lymphocytes also are produced in the bone marrow and take up residence in the lymphatic tissues secondarily. In toto the bone marrow constitutes an organ that rivals the liver in weight and in man has been estimated to account for between 4 and 5% of the body weight.

Types

KEY WORDS: red marrow, active, hemopoietic marrow, yellow, fatty marrow, inactive, extramedullary hemopoiesis

Bone marrow is an extremely cellular connective tissue that fills the hollow cavities of bone (the medullary cavities) and on gross inspection may appear either red or yellow in color. **Red marrow** is that which is actively engaged in the production of blood cells and forms the **active** or **hemopoietic marrow.** Its red color is due to the content of erythrocytes and their pigmented precursors. **Yellow** or **fatty marrow** is **inactive** and the principal cellular components are fat cells. In addition to the gross areas of fatty marrow, fat cells also are scattered throughout the red marrow.

The amount and distribution of fatty marrow varies with age, the requirement for blood cells and the species. All bones contain active marrow in the late fetus and neonate but in large animals, including man, there is a gradual replacement of active marrow by the fatty type, with aging. Beginning in the shafts of the long bones, fat gradually replaces the red marrow so that in the adult, almost all of the marrow in the limbs is of the fatty type. Active marrow remains at the ends of the long bones and in the ribs, sternum, clavicles, vertebrae, pelvis and skull. Gross areas of fatty marrow are not found in small animals, but fat cells are scattered throughout the active marrow. In these animals fatty marrow makes up about 10% of the total marrow, whereas in humans it forms about 50%.

Although not hemopoietic, fatty marrow is very labile and is easily replaced by red marrow. In dogs that have been made anemic, transition from fatty marrow to red marrow may occur within 48 hours. The yellow marrow serves as a reserve space for the expansion of active marrow under conditions of increased demand for blood. The active marrow first replaces the scattered fat cells within the red marrow itself but, if demands for blood remain high or are increased, red marrow gradually encroaches into the gross areas of fatty marrow. In those animals with little yellow marrow, increased demands for blood are met by replacement of the scattered fat cells and closer packing of the hemopoietic marrow cells. Prolonged or increased demands for blood cells then are met by expansion of hemopoietic activity into other organs and tissues such as the spleen, liver and lymph nodes. Blood formation by tissues other than the bone marrow is termed **extramedullary hemopoiesis** and occurs in humans in certain pathological states.

Structure

KEY WORDS: reticular connective tissue, reticular cells, reticular fibers, hemopoietic cells, free cells, fixed cells, nutrient artery, central nutrient (longitudinal) artery, sinuses, central longitudinal vein, extravascular blood formation

Bone marrow is a specialized form of connective tissue which, on the basis of its fiber content, can be classed as a **reticular connective tissue.** A loose spongy network of **reticular cells** and associated **reticular fibers** fills the medullary cavities of bone and provides a supporting framework for the **hemopoietic cells.** The network of fibers and cells is continuous with the endosteum of the bone and also is intimately associated with the blood vessels that pervade the marrow. Within the meshes of the reticular network are all of the cell types normally found in blood and their precursors, phagocytes, fat cells, plasma cells and mast cells. These constitute the **free cells** of the marrow. The reticular cells are **fixed cells** that have no special phagocytic powers and do not give rise to the precursor cells of the hemopoietic marrow. They are responsible for the formation of the reticular fibers. In sections, reticular cells have large, palely stained nuclei and irregularly branched cytoplasm that extends along the reticular fibers.

The marrow contains an extensive vascular system derived from the **nutrient artery** to the bone. In long bones this artery enters about midshaft and gives off the **central nutrient** or **central longitudinal** branches which run centrally in the marrow cavity toward the ends of the bone. Other arterial branches enter the cavity from the epiphysis. Along its course, the central nutrient artery provides numerous branches that pass toward the bony wall. Some of these arterioles enter the bone to supply osteons, whereas others turn back and unite with venous **sinuses** (sinusoids) that are scattered throughout the marrow. The sinuses pursue a radial course toward the center of the marrow cavity, where they empty into the **central longitudinal veins.**

Sinuses are thin walled vessels of wide bore (60 to 75 μm diameter) that run a tortuous course through the marrow and anastomose freely to form a complex vascular network. The endothelial lining consists of attenuated, flattened squamous cells that rest upon a thin, discontinuous basement membrane. The adjacent cells are tightly apposed and united by zonula adherens and gap junctions. Surrounding the structure, to a variable extent, is a loose coating of reticular cells which are continuous with those of the reticular network. The hemopoietic elements lie outside the sinuses and form irregular cords between them. These cords of developing blood cells collectively form the hemopoietic compartment of the marrow, while the sinuses and arteries are referred to as the vascular compartment.

In smears, the marrow cells appear to be randomly distributed, but in serial sections some ordering of the cells can be seen. Fat cells, though generally scattered, tend to be concentrated toward the center of the marrow, where they cluster about blood vessels. The hemopoietic cells are largely confined to an area adjacent to the endosteum. The erythrocytes develop in small islets close to the sinuses and there is some ordering of the cells within an islet according to their state of development. The most mature cells occupy the outer rim of the islet. The cells which give rise to platelets (megakaryocytes) also are closely applied to the walls of the sinuses and frequently can be seen to discharge platelets through apertures in the sinusoidal wall. Developing granulocytes form nests of cells that tend to be located at some distance from the sinuses.

Formation of blood cells occurs **extravascularly:** the cells form outside the blood vessels, and in order to reach the circulation, newly formed cells must pass through the wall of a blood vessel. The site of penetration of the blood cells into the vascular lumen is the sinus. The mechanism that controls the passage of cells across the sinus wall and regulates the number of cells delivered to the circulation is not known. To gain access to the lumen of the sinusoid, the blood cells must penetrate the outer investment of reticular cells and cross the endothelial lining. In areas of active passage of cells into the lumen of the sinus, the reticular sheath is much reduced and in this area the vessel appears to consist only of an endothelium. The blood cells penetrate the endothelial cells through fenestrations or apertures in the cytoplasm and not by insinuating themselves between adjacent endothelial cells. The openings are relatively large, 1 to 3 μm in diameter, and appear to develop only in relation to, and during, the actual passage of cells, and are absent at other times.

Stem Cells

KEY WORDS: stem cells, pluripotent stem cell, spleen colony, colony forming unit (CFU), restricted stem cell, candidate stem cell

The hemopoietic cells of the marrow encompass the various developmental stages of the blood cells from a primitive **stem cell** to the mature elements found in the circulation. A stem cell can be defined as a cell capable of maintaining itself through cell replication and able to differentiate into a more mature cell type. There is much evidence that the bone marrow contains a **pluripotent stem cell** capable of giving rise to all of the different types of blood cells. Mice that have received a lethal dose of irradiation soon die because of the loss of all of their blood cells due to destruction of the hemopoietic organs. However, if a transfusion of bone marrow cells is given soon after exposure to irradiation, death is averted and both the bone marrow and lymphatic tissues are reconstituted with functional cells derived from the transfused marrow. During recovery, macroscopic nodules, the **spleen colonies**, appear in the spleen and these represent islands of proliferating hemopoietic cells. The number of colonies formed is directly proportional to the number of donor marrow cells injected. The cells in the inoculum that give rise to the spleen colonies are called **colony forming units (CFU).**

The colonies contain both undifferentiated and maturing cells. Some colonies consist only of cells of the erythrocyte line, while others contain only developing granulocytes or developing megakaryocytes. Many, however, are mixed colonies and contain developing cells of all three types. Evidence for the unicellular origin of mixed colonies has been obtained by using donor cells that have been irradiated just sufficiently to induce unique chromosome markers. When these cells form spleen colonies, all of the constituent cells of the mixed colonies bear the same distinctive markers and therefore must have arisen from the same colony forming unit. Cultures of cells from granulocytic and mixed colonies produce monocytes and macrophages which also carry the same marker chromosomes.

Although most investigators have not described lymphocytic colonies in the spleen, mice injected with irradiated marrow show the same chromosomal marker in cells that are repopulating the thymus, lymph nodes and bone marrow. The reconstituted marrow of these animals, when injected into new, irradiated recipients, produce spleen colonies that also carry the same marker chromosomes. The cells from a spleen colony are capable of completely restoring all of the hemopoietic tissues, indicating that the colony forming unit has the potential of forming cells of lymphatic lineage.

Spleen colonies, which arise from a single colony forming unit, give rise to new spleen colonies when injected into irradiated animals. Even those colonies that appear to be purely erythropoietic or granulocytic can give rise to colonies of all types. Thus, the colony forming unit is capable not only of differentiation but also of self-renewal and fulfills the definition of a stem cell. The bone marrow then must contain a pluripotential stem cell capable of feeding into the erythrocyte, granular leukocyte, megakaryocyte, monocyte and lymphoid lines.

In addition to the pluripotent stem cell, it appears that bone marrow also contains stem cells whose capacity for development is more restricted. These form the **restricted stem cells** that are committed to the development of one specific cell line. Experimental evidence supports the existence of restricted stem cells for erythrocytes, neutrophils, megakaryocytes, eosinophils and monocytes, although some studies suggest a common precursor for neutrophils and monocytes. These restricted stem cells arise from the pluripotent stem cell and are rapidly proliferative, but have limited capacity for self renewal. The pluripotent stem cells, although capable of extensive replication, are only very slowly proliferative and actually represent a reserve cell. It is the restricted stem cell that provides for the immediate, day-to-day replacement of the blood cells.

Although the existence of a pluripotent stem cell has been established, its morphology has not been determined with certainty. There is, however, evidence that it may be similar to the lymphocyte. Fractionation of bone marrow on sedimentation columns has shown that the colony forming units (stem cells) are contained in a fraction whose cells have a size and weight comparable to that of lymphocytes. Further, the number of stem cells in bone marrow can be increased by administering antimitotic drugs that destroy those hemopoietic cells capable of division. Since pluripotent stem cells are only slowly proliferative, they are unaffected by the drug and their relative numbers in the donor marrow are greatly increased. The stem cells then can be further enriched by density gradient centrifugation. As shown by the ability to produce spleen colonies, cells of lymphoid appearance increase in proportion to the increase in the number of stem cells. These lymphocyte-like cells have been called **candidate stem cells.** While similar to lymphocytes, some differences in their morphology have been described. The nucleus is more irregularly shaped than that in most lymphocytes and is less deeply indented, and the chromatin is more finely dispersed. Mitochondria, few in both types of cell, are smaller and more numerous in the candidate stem cell than in lymphocytes, and free ribosomes, but no rough endoplasmic reticulum or lysosomes, are present in the candidate stem cell.

The origin of the stem cell remains controversial. It appears unlikely that it arises from the reticular cells of bone marrow. The earliest hemopoietic cells are those of the blood islands of the yolk sac and there is evidence that undifferentiated cells from the yolk sac circulate in the fetus and successively occupy the liver, spleen and bone marrow. As hepatic hemopoiesis declines, the number of circulating stem cells increases, suggesting a possible large scale migration of stem cells into the marrow. Cells of the blood islands contain colony forming units and can completely restore all of the hemopoietic organs in an irradiated animal.

Development of Erythrocytes

KEY WORDS: erythropoiesis, proerythroblast, basophilic erythroblast, polychromatophilic erythroblast, acidophilic erythroblast (normoblast), reticulocyte

Production of erythrocytes is called **erythropoiesis** and during this process the erythrocyte undergoes a continuous progression of changes that involves both the cytoplasm and the nucleus. The cell as a whole becomes progressively smaller and its cytoplasm becomes increasingly acidophilic as it accumulates hemoglobin and loses its organelles. The nucleus becomes smaller, more heterochromatic and condensed and ultimately is lost from the cell.

Although it is possible to describe various "stages" in the developmental sequence, the process of erythropoiesis does not occur in a stepwise fashion. Rather, the process is a continuous one in which, at several points, the cells show distinctive, recognizable morphological features. Unfortunately, the nomenclature of the red cell precursors is confused by the multiplicity of terms applied by different workers to the different stages in the maturational series. The terms used here are in common usage, but alternative nomenclature, including that approved by an international committee for the standardization of blood cell terminology, is provided.

Proerythroblast (Pronormoblast, Rubriblast). The proerythroblast is the earliest recognizable precursor of the red cell line and is derived from the pluripotent stem cell by way of a restricted stem cell. The cell is relatively large, having a diameter between 15 and 20 μm. The nongranular, basophilic cytoplasm frequently stains unevenly and shows patches that are relatively poorly stained, especially in a zone around or close to the nucleus. The basophilia of the cytoplasm is an important point in the identification of this early form of the red cell. Synthesis of hemoglobin has begun in the proerythroblast, but its presence is obscured by the basophilia of the cytoplasm. The nucleus occupies almost three-quarters of the cell body, and its chromatin is finely and uniformly granular or stippled in appearance. Two or more nucleoli are present and may be prominent. In electron micrographs the proerythroblast shows poor development of the endoplasmic reticulum and the Golgi complex, but free ribosomes are present and polyribosomes are scattered throughout the cytoplasm.

Basophilic Erythroblast (Basophilic Normoblast, Prorubricyte). The proerythroblast undergoes several divisions to give rise to basophilic erythroblasts. These generally are smaller than the proerythroblast and range in size from 12 to 16 μm in diameter. The nucleus still occupies a large part of the cell, but the chromatin is more coarsely clumped and deeply stained. Nucleoli usually are not visible. The cytoplasm is evenly and deeply basophilic, often more so than that of the proerythroblast. Electron microscopy shows only a few or no profiles of endoplasmic reticulum, but an abundance of free ribosomes and polyribosomes. Hemoglobin can be recognized as fine particles of low electron-density but, as in proerythroblasts, is not discernible by light microscopy because of the intense cytoplasmic basophilia.

Polychromatophilic Erythroblast (Polychromatic Normoblast, Rubricyte). The basophilic erythroblast also is capable of several mitotic divisions, its progeny forming the polychromatophilic erythroblasts. The nucleus occupies a smaller part of the cell body and shows a dense chromatin network with scattered coarse clumps of chromatin. The cytoplasmic staining varies from a deep bluish-gray to a light slate gray and reflects the changing proportions of ribosomes and hemoglobin. When the nucleolus disappears, no new ribosomes are formed and the changing staining characteristics of the cytoplasm are the result of a decreasing concentration of ribosomes (which accept the blue component of the blood stains) and the progressive accumulation of hemoglobin (which binds the eosin component). Cell size varies considerably but generally is less than that of the basophilic erythroblast. The polychromatophilic erythroblasts encompass several generations of cells, the size reflecting the number of cell divisions that have occurred. It is sometimes convenient to divide these cells into "early" and "late" stages, the subdivisions being made on the basis of the size of the cell and the intensity of the cytoplasmic basophilia.

Acidophilic (Orthochromatic) Erythroblast (Acidophilic Normoblast, Metarubricyte). These cells also are commonly referred to as **normoblasts.** At this stage the cells have acquired almost their complete complement of hemoglobin and the cytoplasm takes on a distinctly eosinophilic color. The nucleus is small, densely stained and pyknotic and frequently assumes an eccentric position in the cell. Electron micrographs reveal a uniformly dense cytoplasm devoid of organelles, except for a rare mitochondrion and widely scattered ribosomes. The cell no longer undergoes division and the nucleus is finally extruded from the cell, along with a thin film of cytoplasm.

Reticulocyte. The newly formed erythrocytes contain a small number of ribosomes but in only a few cells (less than 2%) are they sufficient to produce coloring of the cytoplasm. These form the polychromatophilic erythrocytes which, after the usual blood stains, have a grayish tint instead of the clear pink of the more mature forms. When stained with brilliant cresyl blue, the residual ribosomal nucleoprotein appears as a web or reticulum. The reticulum decreases with increasing maturity of the cell and so varies from a rather prominent network to only a few granules or threads. Reticulocytes are about 20% larger in volume than the normal mature red cells. Following loss of the nucleus, the red cell is held in the marrow for an additional 2 to 3 days until fully mature. Unless there are urgent demands for new erythrocytes, the reticulocyte is not released, except in very small numbers. In man, it has been estimated that these young red cells form a marrow reserve equal to about 2% of the number of cells in circulation. Figure 6-1 illustrates the changes in cell morphology during red cell formation.

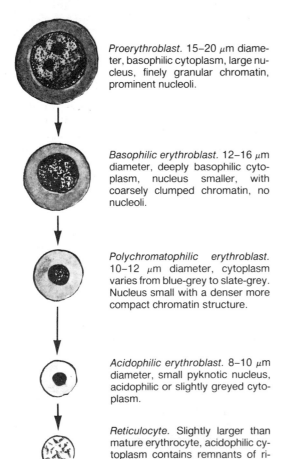

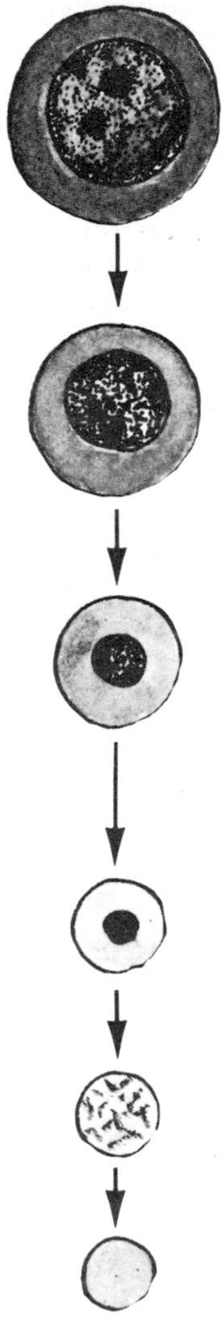

Proerythroblast. 15–20 μm diameter, basophilic cytoplasm, large nucleus, finely granular chromatin, prominent nucleoli.

Basophilic erythroblast. 12–16 μm diameter, deeply basophilic cytoplasm, nucleus smaller, with coarsely clumped chromatin, no nucleoli.

Polychromatophilic erythroblast. 10–12 μm diameter, cytoplasm varies from blue-grey to slate-grey. Nucleus small with a denser more compact chromatin structure.

Acidophilic erythroblast. 8–10 μm diameter, small pyknotic nucleus, acidophilic or slightly greyed cytoplasm.

Reticulocyte. Slightly larger than mature erythrocyte, acidophilic cytoplasm contains remnants of ribonucleoprotein stainable as a network or web.

Red blood corpuscle.

Figure 6-1. Cytological changes during development of erythrocytes.

Loss of Nucleus

Ordinarily the nucleus is lost just before the cell enters the sinus. Just prior to loss, the nucleus assumes an eccentric position in the cell. Active expulsion of the nucleus by the normoblast has been seen in vitro and may involve some contractile protein, possibly spectrin. Enucleation of erythrocytes also has been described as the cells pass through the pores in the sinusoidal lining. The flexible cytoplasmic portion is able to squeeze through the pore but the rigid nucleus is held back and stripped from the cell, along with a small amount of cytoplasm. The nuclei, whether lost by this method or by active expulsion by the cell itself, are rapidly engulfed and destroyed by phagocytes.

Formation of Granular Leukocytes

KEY WORDS: granulocytopoiesis, myeloblast, promyelocyte, azurophilic granules, myelocyte, specific granules, metamyelocyte, band form

The maturational changes that lead to production of the mature granular leukocytes are called **granulocytopoiesis.** In this process the cells accumulate granules, and the nucleus becomes flattened and indented, finally assuming the lobulated form seen in the mature cell. During the process of maturation, several definite stages of development can be identified. However, as with the red cell series, the maturational changes that occur during the development of granulocytes are continuous and cells of intermediate morphology are often found. The stages commonly identified are: myeloblast, promyelocyte, myelocyte, metamyelocyte, band form and polymorphonuclear or segmented granulocyte. An alternative nomenclature substitutes the stem "granulo" for "myelo" and the series becomes: granuloblast, progranulocyte, granulocyte, metagranulocyte, band form and polymorphonuclear granulocyte.

Myeloblast. This is the first recognizable precursor of the granular leukocytes and represents a restricted stem cell committed to granulocyte production. It is present in the bone marrow only in low numbers. The myeloblast is relatively small and ranges in size from 10 to 13 μm in diameter. The cytoplasm is distinctly basophilic but less so than the proerythroblast and lacks granules. The round or oval nucleus occupies much of the cell, stains palely and presents a somewhat vesicular appearance. Multiple nucleoli are present. Electron microscopy reveals abundant free ribosomes in the cytoplasm but relatively little rough endoplasmic reticulum. Mitochondria are numerous and are relatively small.

Promyelocyte. The promyelocyte is somewhat larger and measures between 15 and 20 μm in diameter. The nucleus may be slightly flattened, show a slight indentation, or retain the rounded or oval shape; the chromatin is dispersed and lightly stained, and multiple nucleoli still are present. The basophilic cytoplasm contains a variable number of purplish-red **azurophilic granules**, the number of which increases as the promyelocyte continues its development. Electron micrographs show abundant rough endoplasmic reticulum, free ribosomes, numerous mitochondria and a well developed Golgi apparatus. The azurophil granules are formed *only* during the promyelocyte stage and are produced at the inner or concave face of the Golgi complex by the fusion of dense-cored vacuoles.

Myelocytes. Divergence of granulocyte development into the three distinct lines has occurred at the myelocyte stage with the appearance of the **specific granules.** Thus, neutrophil, eosinophil and basophil myelocytes can be distinguished. Myelocytes are smaller than the promyelocyte and measure from 12 to 18 μm in diameter. The nucleus is more deeply indented and the chromatin is more condensed. Some myelocytes may still show a nucleolus outlined by a condensation of chromatin, whereas in others the nucleolus is poorly defined or marked only by an irregular mass of condensed chromatin. The myelocyte is the last cell of the granulocytic series capable of mitosis.

Neutrophil Myelocytes. The cytoplasm contains two populations of granules—the azurophil granules produced at the promyelocyte stage and the specific neutrophil granules that are formed by the myelocyte. Although both types of granules arise by fusion of dense-cored vacuoles derived from the Golgi complex, the specific granules are produced at the outer or convex face of the Golgi body rather than at the concave face as with the azurophil granules. With successive divisions of the myelocytes, the number of azurophil granules in each cell is progressively reduced and specific granules soon outnumber the azurophil type. During maturation of myelocytes, the cytoplasm becomes less basophilic and there is an associated decrease in free ribosomes and rough endoplasmic reticulum.

The specific neutrophil granules stain lightly in routine smear preparations, take up a delicate lilac pink color and are too small to be individually resolved with the light microscope. The azurophil granules are larger and take on a purplish-red coloration with the usual blood stains but are less numerous. With the electron microscope, azurophil granules appear larger and more dense than the neutrophil granule. The contents of the granules also differ; azurophil granules are lysosomes and possess a complex of enzymes, among which aryl-sulfatase, acid phosphatase, β-galactosidase, β-glucuronidase, esterase, nucleotidase and peroxidase have been identified. The specific neutrophil granules contain alkaline phosphatase and proteins with antibacterial properties.

Neutrophil Metamyelocytes. The myelocytes eventually reach a stage at which they no longer divide. They then mature into the metamyelocyte. This cell shows all of the cytological characteristics of the myelocyte, except that the nucleus is deeply indented into a horseshoe shape and shows a dense chromatin network with numerous well defined chromatin masses. Two types of granules still are present, but specific granules constitute 80 to 90% of the granule population.

Neutrophil Band. The **band form** neutrophil presents the same general morphology as the mature polymorphonuclear cell, except that the nucleus forms a variously curved or twisted band. It may be irregularly segmented, but not to the extent that definite lobes and filaments have formed.

The stages of maturation of the eosinophil granulocytes are the same as for the neutrophil. The specific eosinophil granule usually is identifiable soon after it appears but at first may have a purplish-blue color, becoming progressively more orange. The eosinophil granule may be identified as early as in the promyelocyte state. The granules are much larger than the neutrophil type and in electron micrographs are only slightly less dense and smaller than the azurophil granules.

As the cells mature, the cytoplasm becomes less basophilic and the nucleus more and more indented, but the mature eosinophil does not show the degree of lobulation seen in the neutrophil granulocytes. In the later stages of myelocyte formation and in the metamyelocyte, the granules show a crystallization of their contents. Thus, some granules reveal a crystal of varying shape occupying the center of the granule, surrounded by a matrix of lower density. Other granules remain dense and homogeneous. Eosinophil granules are lysosomes and contain the usual battery of lysosomal enzymes.

The basophil granulocytes also pass through the same maturational sequences and the first definitive granules may appear at the promyelocyte stage. Initially they are truly basophilic but then become metachromatic and with toluidine or methylene blue stain a violet rather than a blue color. In addition to chemotactic and platelet factors, the granules contain heparin, histamine and several enzymes, including diaphorase, dehydrogenases, peroxidases and histidine-decarboxylase, which converts histidine to histamine.

The maturational changes and stages of development in the granular leukocytes are depicted in Figure 6-2.

Formation of Platelets

KEY WORDS: thrombopoiesis, megakaryocytes, perinuclear, intermediate and marginal zones, demarcation membranes, megakaryoblast, polyploidy, promegakaryocyte

Thrombopoiesis (or thrombocytopoiesis) refers to the formation of the mammalian platelets or, in other vertebrates, to thrombocytes. In the mammal, platelets are derived from a giant bone marrow cell, the **megakaryocyte**, which may measure 100 μm or more in diameter. Those vertebrates that possess thrombocytes in place of platelets do not have megakaryocytes. In humans, megakaryocytes are found only in the bone marrow but in rodents and opossums they also are present in the spleen, even in adults.

The nucleus of the megakaryocyte is large, convoluted and contains multiple irregular lobes of variable size, interconnected by constricted regions. The coarsely patterned chromatin stains deeply. The cytoplasm is abundant, irregularly outlined and often has blunt pseudopods projecting from the surface. In smears, the cytoplasm appears homogeneous and contains numerous azurophil granules. Ultrastructurally a variable degree of zonation of the cytoplasm is apparent. Immediately about the nucleus a narrow **perinuclear zone** contains a few mitochondria, the Golgi complex, rough endoplasmic reticulum, numerous polyribosomes and some granules. A large **intermediate zone** is indistinctly separated from the perinuclear zone and contains granules, vesicles of different size and shape, components of the Golgi element, mitochondria and ribosomes. Depending upon the degree of development of the megakaryocyte, the granules may be uniformly distributed or gathered into small clusters outlined in variable degree by a system of membranes. The outermost, or **marginal zone**, is finely granular, of variable width and lacks organelles but contains packets of microfilaments.

Platelets are formed by segmentation of the megakaryocyte cytoplasm through the development of a system of **demarcation membranes.** Clustering of the azurophil granules occurs, accompanied by the simultaneous appearance of small vesicles which become aligned in rows between groups of granules. The vesicles initially are discontinuous, but subsequently elongate and fuse to form a three-dimensional system of paired membranes. The narrow spaces between the membranes form clefts which surround each future platelet, and as they are shed, the platelets separate along the narrow clefts. The demarcation membranes are continuous with the plasmalemma and thus each platelet is bounded by a typical trilaminar cell membrane. The megakaryocyte delivers platelets through apertures in the wall of the sinusoid, either as individual platelets or as ribbons of platelets that separate into individual elements within the sinusoidal lumen. Following the shedding of platelets, the megakaryocyte consists only of a nucleus surrounded by a thin rim of cytoplasm bounded by an intact cell membrane. It generally is assumed that such megakaryocytes are unable to restore their cytoplasm and degenerate, with new generations of

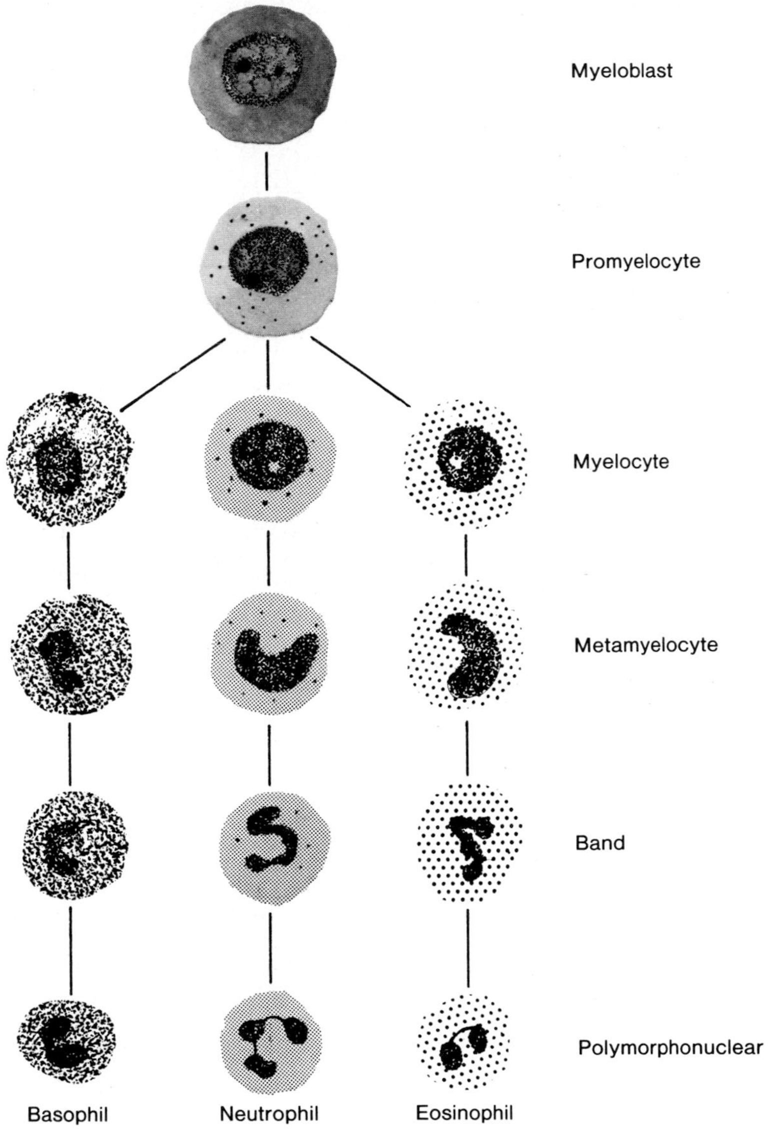

Figure 6-2. Maturational sequences of granular leukocytes.

megakaryocytes being formed to replace them. Degenerate megakaryocytes can be found in the circulation, especially in the capillaries of the lungs, where they may remain for some time.

Megakaryocytes originate from stem cells, the first recognizable precursor being a large cell, 20 to 30 μm in diameter, with a single round or oval nucleus. The chromatin shows a finely granular pattern and the basophilic cytoplasm is free of granules. This cell has been called the **megakaryoblast.** The nucleus undergoes a series of replications and centrioles divide, but cytoplasmic division does not occur. At metaphase, the chromosomes become aligned in several planes on a complex multipolar spindle. With subsequent reconstitution of the nucleus, the groups of chromosomes are incorporated into a large, lobulated nucleus. Thus, a series of **polyploid** cells arises which in man and rabbits reaches 64n. In other animals (guinea pig, rat, opossum), a lesser degree of ploidy is shown, and even in man and rabbits 16n nuclei are the most frequent. In general the cell and nuclear size are proportional to the degree of ploidy. The intriguing suggestion has been made that the segmentation of the cytoplasm by the demarcation membranes represents a delayed and modified cytokinesis.

Cells of 4n to 8n ploidy measuring 30 to 45 μm in diameter frequently are called **promegakaryocytes.** The fully formed, but as yet nonfunctional, megakaryocyte consistently shows the clear outer or marginal zone, whereas in the platelet-forming megakaryocyte this zone disappears.

The nucleated thrombocytes are derived from a mononuclear stem cell of the marrow, not from megakaryocytes. Maturation of the thrombocytes is attended by the clumping of the nuclear chromatin, the appearance of cytoplasmic granules, the elongation of the cell and a decrease in the cytoplasmic basophilia. The thrombocyte retains its nucleus and remains as a distinct, complete cell, in contrast to the mammalian platelet which is a cytoplasmic fragment.

Development of Monocytes

KEY WORDS: promonocytes, tissue macrophages

It now is generally accepted that the monocytes take their origin from a pool of precursors in the bone marrow. What remains in doubt is the identity of the precursor cells. There is some evidence that the monocytes may arise from the same restricted stem cell as the granular leukocytes, since on culture, the cells of granulocytic spleen colonies sometimes yield monocytes as well as granulocytes.

The immature monocytes of the bone marrow (the **promonocyte**) appear to be rare and difficult to distinguish. They range from 8 to 15 μm in diameter and possess large round to oval nuclei with evenly dispersed chromatin and several nucleoli. The cytoplasm is fairly abundant and contains numerous free ribosomes but only scanty endoplasmic reticulum. The prominent Golgi complex is associated with numerous small granules that represent the formative stages of azurophilic granules. The mature monocytes of the bone marrow closely resemble those of the blood, are somewhat smaller than the promonocyte (9 to 11 μm diameter) and contain fewer ribosomes and larger and more abundant azurophil granules. The latter contain a variety of hydrolytic enzymes and are primary lysosomes. Following release into the blood, the monocyte continues its maturation in the circulation and additional azurophilic granules are formed.

Monocytes migrate into a variety of tissues, where they complete their maturation by transforming into peritoneal macrophages, alveolar macrophages of the lung, Kupffer cells and the **macrophages** of other **tissues.**

Formation of Lymphocytes in the Marrow

Lymphocytes arise from the pluripotential stem cells of the marrow from which they migrate to populate the lymphatic organs. Restricted stem cells that reach the thymus proliferate there and differentiate into the T lymphocytes. After being released from the thymus, T cells migrate to the spleen, where they complete their maturation and are released as long-lived small lymphocytes. The B lymphocytes also originate in the marrow from stem cells and, in birds, migrate to the bursa of Fabricius, where they differentiate into B lymphocytes. The equivalent of the bursa in mammals has not been identified, but the bone marrow itself may be the organ of differentiation. B cells also appear to complete their development in the spleen. Both B and T cells circulate and recirculate through the blood, lymph and lymphatic organs.

Control of Blood Formation

KEY WORDS: erythropoietin, hypoxia, renal erythropoietic factor (erythrogenin), granulopoietin, thrombopoietin

Erythropoiesis is under humoral control and is regulated primarily by means of the specific erythropoiesis stimulating factor, **erythropoietin.** The fundamental stimulus for red cell production is **hypoxia**, the rate of production of erythropoietin being inversely related to the oxygen supply of the tissues. Erythropoietin is a glycoprotein hormone produced by the interaction of precursors formed by the kidney. There is evidence that the kidney produces an enzyme, **renal erythropoietic factor (erythrogenin)** that activates a blood-borne precursor. The kidney is not the sole source of erythropoietin since it can be produced in animals from which the kidneys have been removed. The sites of extrarenal production of erythropoietin have not been determined but small amounts of an erythropoietic active substance have been detected after perfusion of the liver.

Erythropoietin appears to induce hemoglobin synthesis and in doing so initiates the differentiation of the committed (restricted) stem cell. It also appears to accelerate hemoglobin synthesis in those more differentiated cells that still are capable of synthesizing RNA and appears to promote the release of reticulocytes from the marrow.

Whether there are individual hemopoietic hormones for each of the cell types of the bone marrow is not known. There is considerable evidence, however, for the existence of other circulating poietins which control the differentiation of granulocytes and megakaryocytes. These factors, **granulopoietin** and **thrombopoietin**, have not been characterized, nor has the site of production been determined.

LYMPHATIC TISSUES

Scattered throughout the body are various lymphoid elements that form part of the body's defense system. Generally disposed so that noxious agents entering the body soon come in contact with them, lymphatic tissues are prominent in the connective tissue coats of the gastrointestinal, respiratory and urogenital tracts. Lymphatic structures also are inserted into the lymphatic drainage and into the blood circulation, where they serve to filter the lymph and blood. Eventually all of the body fluids are filtered through some form of lymphatic structure.

Lymphatic elements may be spread throughout the connective tissues to form the lymphatic tissues, or they may be organized into more discrete structures to form lymphatic organs.

Classification

KEY WORDS: reticular connective tissue, hemopoietic tissue, diffuse lymphatic tissue, nodular lymphatic tissue

Lymphatic tissue represents a specialization within the connective tissue compartment and, like all tissues, can be classified according to the type of fiber that is present. On this basis, lymphatic tissue can be defined as a **reticular** connective tissue. It also can be considered a **hemopoietic tissue** since it contributes cells (lymphocytes) to the blood. In common with bone marrow, the cellular content exceeds the intercellular materials. Subdivision of lymphatic tissues into **diffuse** and **nodular** depends on the arrangement and concentration of the cells, not on differences in fiber type.

Cells of Lymphatic Tissues

KEY WORDS: fixed cells, reticular cells, free cells, small, medium and large lymphocytes, plasma cells, macrophages

The cells of lymphatic tissue are present either as fixed or as free cells. The **fixed cells** are the **reticular cells** responsible for the formation and maintenance of the reticular fibers. These two elements of the reticular network are intimately related and the fibers frequently reside in deep clefts or grooves in the cytoplasm of the reticular cells. By light microscopy, the reticular cells appear as elongated or stellate elements with round or oval, palely stained nuclei and scant, lightly basophilic cytoplasm. However, the cytoplasm is more voluminous than is apparent under the light microscope, since the bulk of it is thinly spread along the reticular fibers. Electron microscopy reveals a variable amount of endoplasmic reticulum and a moderately well developed Golgi element: other organelles are relatively inconspicuous. Reticular cells are not undifferentiated cells and they are incapable of giving rise to other cell types. Although a phagocytic function frequently is ascribed to some of these cells, the reticular cells show no special capacity for phagocytosis.

The remaining cells of lymphatic tissue are contained within the spaces of the reticular network and constitute the **free cells.** The bulk of these are lymphocytes but macrophages and plasma cells also are present in variable numbers. The term lymphocyte includes a spectrum of cells that possess some general, common features. As a class they show a rounded, centrally-placed nucleus and lack specific granules. The cytoplasm, shows variable degrees of basophilia. The lymphocyte population customarily is divided into **small, medium** and **large lym-**

phocytes on the basis of their size, nuclear morphology and intensity of cytoplasmic staining. Although such a subdivision is useful for purposes of description, it is somewhat artificial. The three types are not sharply separated and cells of intermediate size and morphology do occur. The lymphocyte family consists of a continuum of cell sizes and morphologies between the small and large types.

Small lymphocytes are the most numerous type. As seen in lymphatic tissues, they vary from 4 to 8 μm in diameter and possess a deeply-stained nucleus surrounded by a thin rim of cytoplasm that may be slightly expanded at one side of the cell. Although rounded in shape when in a fluid medium such as blood or lymph, in tissues the cells are crowded together and assume various polyhedral shapes due to mutual compression. The nucleus is rounded or slightly indented and contains a nucleolus that is barely distinguishable unless thin sections are examined. The chromatin is present as scattered masses of heterochromatin with some intervening, paler-staining euchromatin. Electron microscopy reveals a small Golgi complex and centrioles located at the region of the nuclear indentation, and a few mitochondria are present in this area also. A moderate number of free ribosomes are scattered singly throughout the cytoplasm: granular endoplasmic reticulum is sparse. A few lysosomes also are present.

The **medium lymphocytes** range from 8 to 12 μm in diameter. The nucleus is somewhat larger, more palely-stained because of greater dispersion of the chromatin, and nucleoli are larger and more easily seen. The cytoplasm is more voluminous and shows greater basophilia because of an increased number of free ribosomes. These cells also are referred to as prolymphocytes.

Large lymphocytes (lymphoblasts) range in size from 15 to 20 μm. Occasionally, even larger forms (25 to 30 μm) may be found and some authors reserve the term lymphoblast for these larger cells. The nucleus is rounded, palely-stained, contains one or two prominent nucleoli and the chromatin has a fine, more or less uniformly dispersed character. The cell possesses abundant basophilic cytoplasm in which are large numbers of free ribosomes and polyribosomes. The centrosomal region and Golgi apparatus are more highly developed and mitochondria are more abundant, but granular endoplasmic reticulum remains scanty.

In the development of lymphocytes, it generally is accepted that the direction of maturation is from large (lymphoblast) to small. However, this progression is complicated by the ability of the small lymphocyte to respond to antigenic agents, reassume a blast-like appearance and character and reproduce additional small lymphocytes and plasma cells.

Plasma cells (plasmocytes) vary in size from 6 to 20 μm in diameter. By light microscopy, the cell presents a rounded, somewhat elongated or polyhedral form, depending upon its location. The nucleus is rounded or oval and usually is eccentrically placed; this is most obvious in the elongated cells, and in rounded cells the nucleus may be only slightly eccentric in its placement. The nuclear chromatin is dispersed in coarse heterochromatic blocks spaced along the nuclear membrane, giving the nucleus a clock face or wheel spoke appearance. Occasionally, binucleate cells may be seen. The cytoplasm is deeply basophilic, except for a prominent pale area adjacent to the nucleus. This pale area represents a negative image of the Golgi apparatus.

Occasionally, plasma cells contain prominent inclusions in their cytoplasm which take the form of various globular or crystalline deposits. Perhaps the best known of these are the Russell's bodies, round or ovoid acidophilic inclusions of variable size which give positive staining reactions both for protein and carbohydrate.

The characteristic feature of the cell in electron micrographs is the extensive development of the granular endoplasmic reticulum which almost completely fills the cytoplasm. The cisternae may be flat and parallel or may be distended with flocculent material. Free ribosomes also are numerous. Electron microscopy confirms a well developed Golgi apparatus in the paranuclear area, which also contains the centrioles. Russell's bodies, when present, are seen to be contained within distended cisternae of the granular endoplasmic reticulum.

The **macrophages** of lymphatic tissues are part of a system of mononuclear phagocytes widely spread throughout tissues and organs. The cells vary from 10 to 20 μm in diameter and possess an oval, kidney or horseshoe-shaped nucleus in which one or more nucleoli are present. The cytoplasm is abundant and lightly basophilic and may be vacuolated or contain ingested material. Unless the cytoplasm does contain phagocytosed matter, the macrophage is difficult to distinguish from other large mononuclear cells. In electron micrographs, the cytoplasm shows numerous folds, processes and invaginations of the surface and contains the usual assembly of organelles. The Golgi apparatus is conspicuous and lysosomes are numerous. Residual bodies may be prominent. Like macrophages elsewhere, those found in lymphatic tissue are derived from blood monocytes.

Diffuse Lymphatic Tissue

KEY WORDS: reticular fibers, reticular cells, lymphatic cells

This form of lymphatic tissue is a constituent part of lymphatic organs and also is widely dispersed along mucous membranes. It appears as a rather loose aggregate of cells and shows no distinct demarcation from the surrounding tissues with which it gradually blends. Basically, diffuse lymphatic tissue consists of a three-dimensional array of **reticular fibers** and their closely associated **reticular cells** that form a sponge-like framework pervaded by large numbers of cells, chief of which are the **lymphatic cells**.

Diffuse lymphatic tissue is particularly prominent in the connective tissue that underlines the epithelium of the intestine. Here the lymphatic tissue, in association with the lining epithelium, produces antibody that bathes the luminal surface. Any antigen that penetrates the epithelial lining induces an immune response in the lymphatic tissue the cellularity of which is related to the bacterial content in the lumen of the intestines.

Nodular Lymphatic Tissue

KEY WORDS: solitary nodules, confluent nodules, primary nodules, germinal centers, secondary nodules, dark pole, light pole, cap, Peyer's patches

Nodular lymphatic tissue contains the same structural elements as diffuse lymphatic tissue and differs only in that the components are organized into compact, somewhat circumscribed structures. They may occur anywhere in connective tissue but are prominent along the digestive and respiratory tracts. Lymphatic nodules, also called follicles, may be present singly as **solitary nodules** or in masses forming **confluent nodules**, as in the appendix and Peyer's patches of the ileum. Lymphatic nodules also form prominent structural components of lymphatic organs such as the tonsils, lymph nodes and spleen.

In ordinary histological sections, some nodular lymphatic tissue appears as rounded collections of densely-packed small lymphocytes and this type of nodule is called a **primary nodule.** Other lymphatic nodules contain a lightly staining central area surrounded by a deeply stained cuff or cap of closely packed small lymphocytes. The pale region has been called a **germinal center** and the whole structure a **secondary nodule.**

Reticular fibers are scarce within the germinal center and the free cells are supported in the meshes of a cellular framework that consists of stellate reticular cells. The numerous processes of these cells are joined by desmosomes. Reticular fibers are present in the cuff of cells at the periphery of the germinal center, where they form a concentric envelope around the structure.

Germinal centers are organized into dark and light poles. The light pole contains a few scattered small lymphocytes and reticular cells, and is densely populated with large and medium lymphocytes. Mitotic figures, pyknotic nuclei of degenerating cells and macrophages also are present. Surrounding the center is a zone of small lymphocytes (the mantle, crescent or corona) which usually is thicker at one pole of the center, where it forms the **cap**. The poles of the center have definite orientations, the light poles always being oriented toward superficial or surface structures.

Germinal centers appear to be sites where lymphocytes are formed, but many of the newly-formed cells die there. They also are sites of antibody formation and each germinal center appears to represent clones derived from an antigen-stimulated lympho-

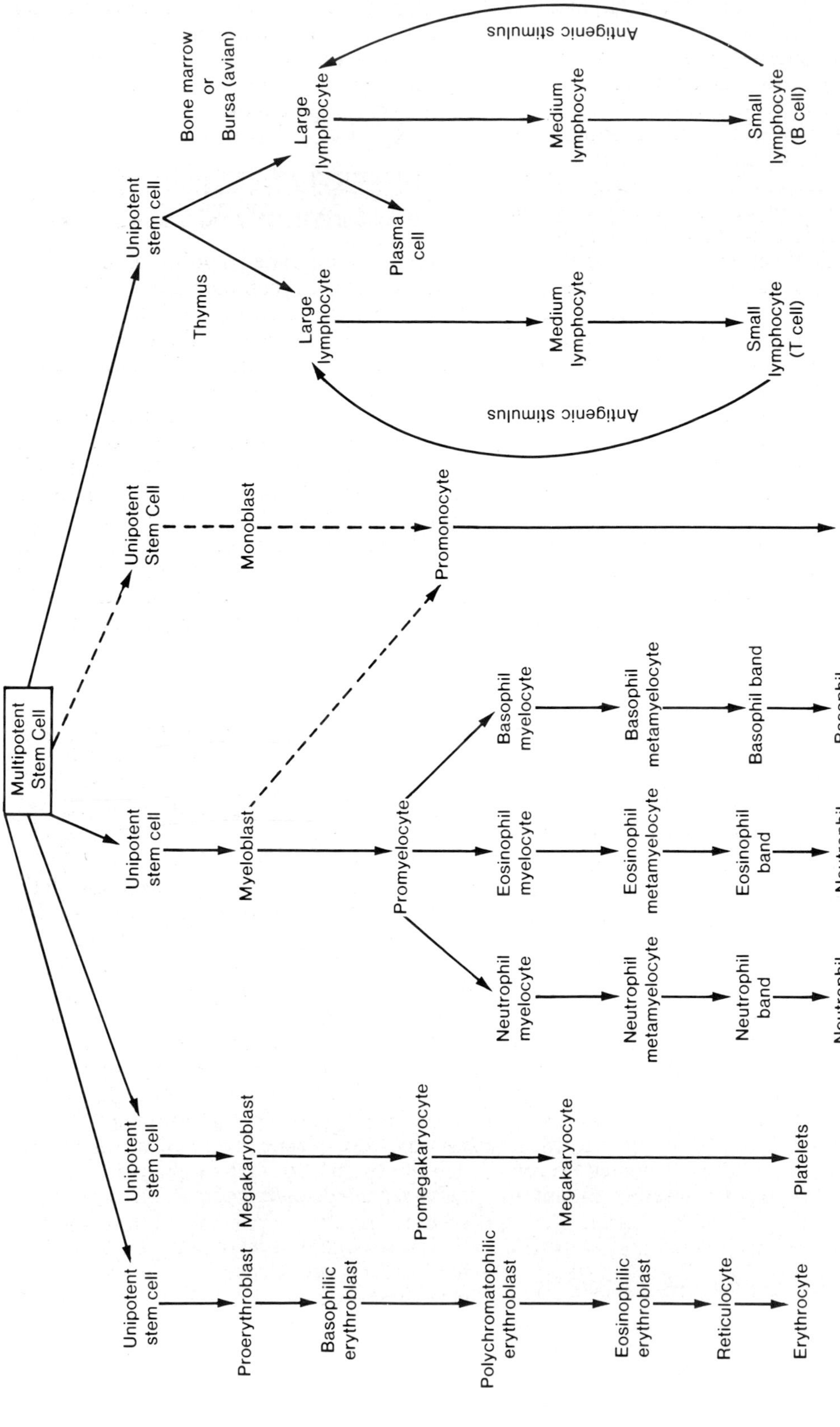

Figure 6-3. Interrelationships of hemopoietic cell lines.

cyte. The lymphocytes in secondary nodules belong to the B class.

Germinal centers appear only after birth in response to antigenic stimuli and are absent in animals born and raised in a germ-free environment. Following a primary exposure to antigen, germinal centers form de novo, then regress in the absence of the antigen. Upon second stimulation by the antigen, there is a rapid and marked production of germinal centers which precedes the rise in circulating antibody. It has been suggested that germinal centers arise as the result of repeated contact with antigen and may be involved in the long-term memory of antibody response.

Aggregate or confluent lymphatic nodules are exemplified by the **Peyer's patches** found in the lower half of the small intestine and occur also in the appendix. Peyer's patches consist of many secondary nodules massed together to form grossly visible, oval structures that underlay the intestinal epithelium. The light poles of the germinal centers are directed toward the surface epithelium. The individual nodules may be quite discrete and well defined, but frequently they coalesce and can be defined only at their apices and by their germinal centers. Peyer's patches are prominent in children but undergo gradual regression with aging.

INTERRELATIONSHIPS OF THE HEMOPOIETIC CELLS

The current understanding of the interrelationships between the various blood cell lines is illustrated in Figure 6-3. A pluripotent stem cell, present in the bone marrow and capable of unlimited self-renewal, gives rise to several types of unipotent stem cells. The latter have a limited capacity for self-renewal and each is committed to but one line of development. Thus, there is a unipotent stem cell for each of the cell types seen in blood which gives rise to the morphological stages that can be recognized in any of the lines of development. Neither the multipotent nor the unipotent stem cells have been characterized morphologically.

FUNCTIONAL SUMMARY

The obvious function of the hemopoietic tissues is to provide the blood with continuous replacement of cells. Separation of the replicating cells from their end products in the blood and sequestering them in specific hemopoietic tissues permits the establishment of environments best suited for each of the tissues. It ensures that the replicating cells are not unduly influenced by the activities of other organs and tissues, as would occur if the replicating cells also were circulating. In addition, it provides the blood with small cells that can more easily circulate through the fine capillary beds of the tissues and organs. Since there is no necessity to set aside, within the circulation, a population of cells concerned with replication, all of the cells of the blood are functional and can serve the body. The further subdivision of the hemopoietic tissue into its bone marrow and lymphatic components permits the conditioning of populations of cells (such as the T lymphocytes) without at the same time exposing the remainder of the hemopoietic cells to these same conditioning factors.

Within the bone marrow, the yellow or fatty marrow fills unoccupied space within the bone but being extremely labile is readily replaced by active marrow when demands for blood become insistent. The sinusoids of the marrow, because of their thin walls, provide sites at which the newly formed blood cells gain access to the circulation. Additional maturation of cells occurs within the sinusoids and the cells held here serve as a reserve which can be called upon under conditions of increased need for blood cells.

Atlas for Chapter 6

6-4 Fetal Hemopoietic Tissue

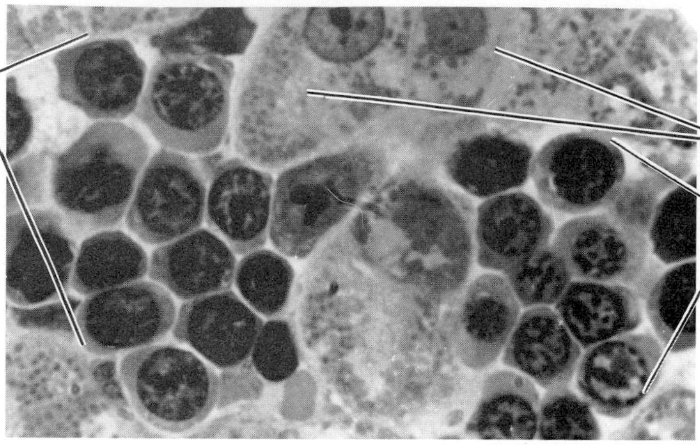

6-5

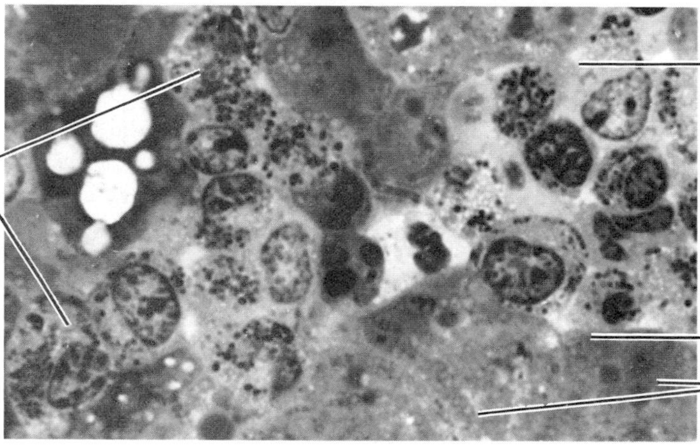

6-6

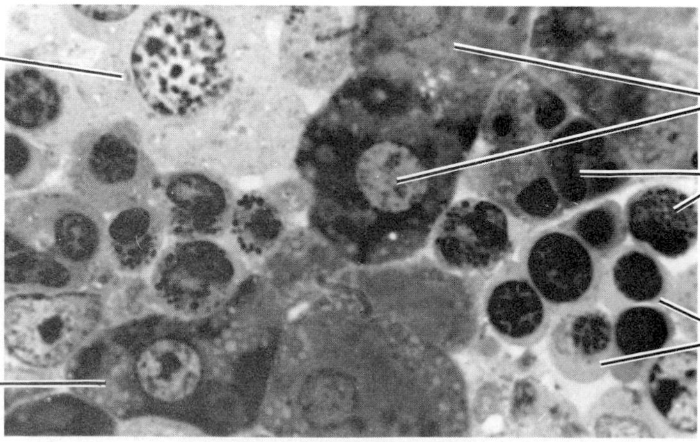

Figure 6-4. Liver. LM, ×1000.
Figure 6-5. Liver. LM, ×1000.
Figure 6-6. Liver. LM, ×1000.

6-7 Bone Marrow

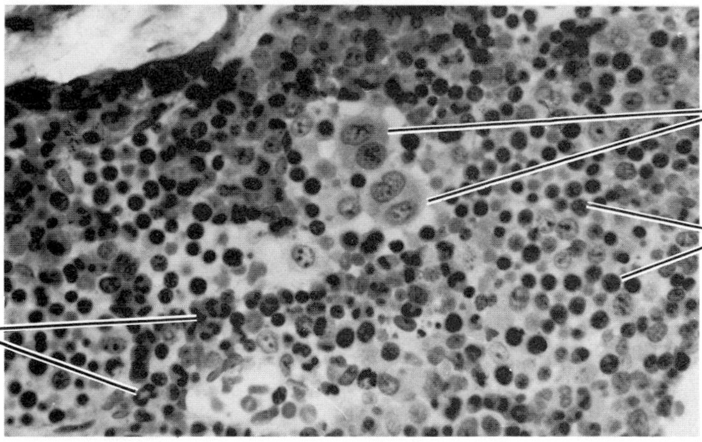

6-8

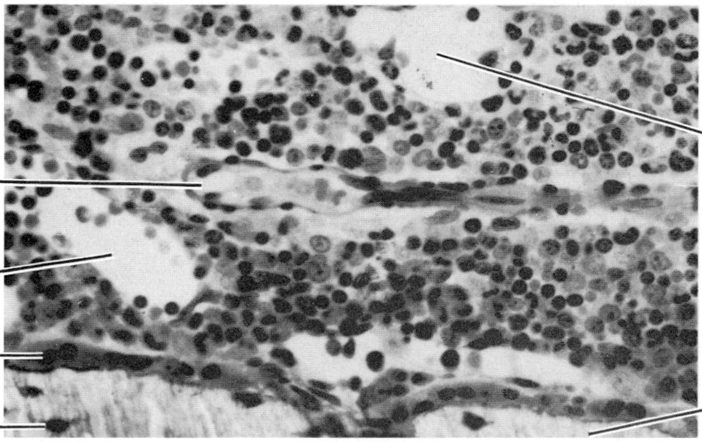

6-9

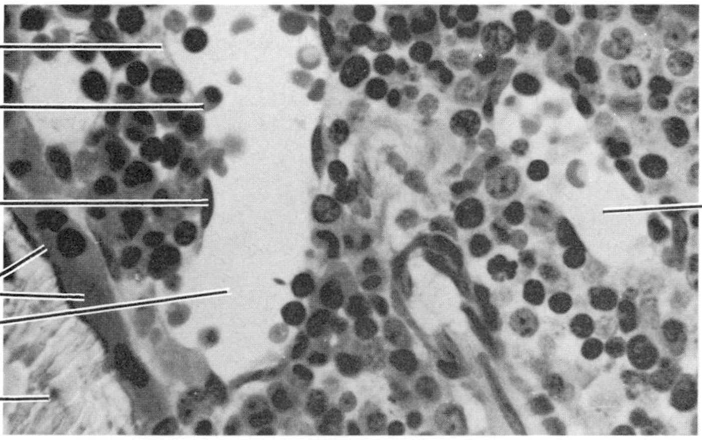

Figure 6-7. Hemopoietic tissue. LM, ×250.
Figure 6-8. Hemopoietic tissue. LM, ×250.
Figure 6-9. Hemopoietic tissue. LM, ×400.

6-10 Hemopoietic Tissue

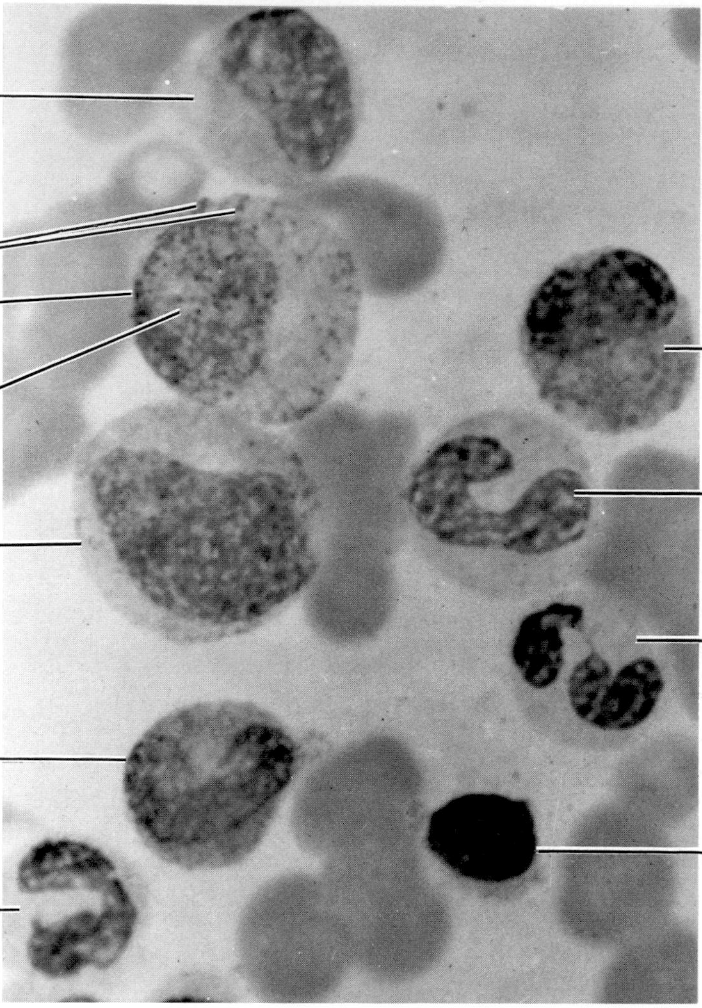

6-11

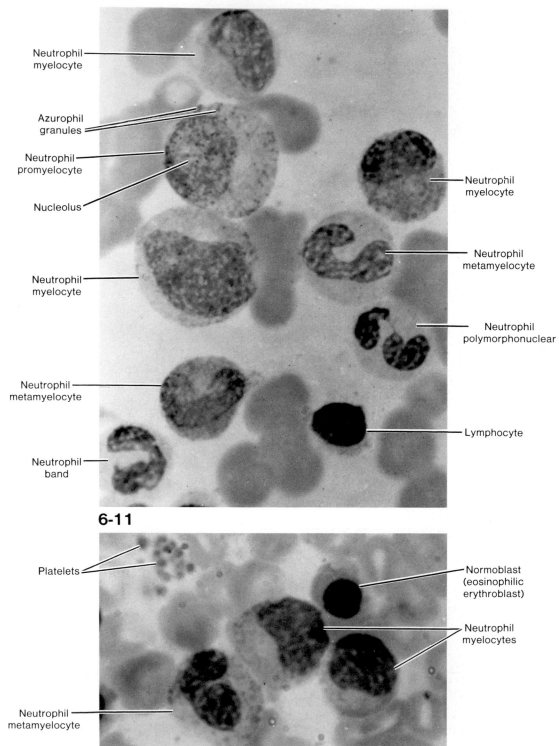

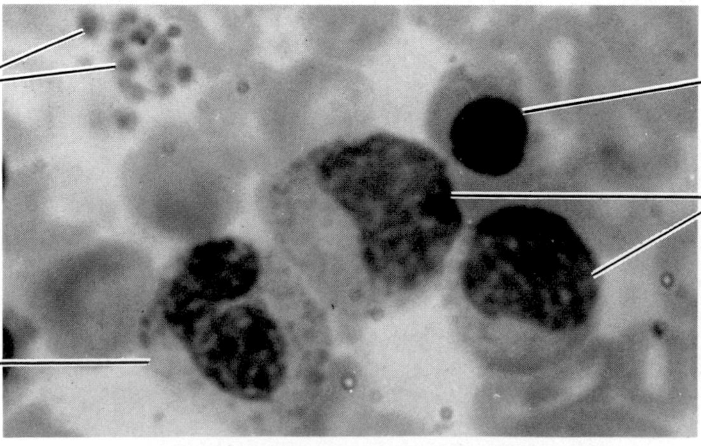

Figure 6-10. Bone marrow (human). LM, ×1200.
Figure 6-11. Bone marrow (human). LM, ×1100.

6-12

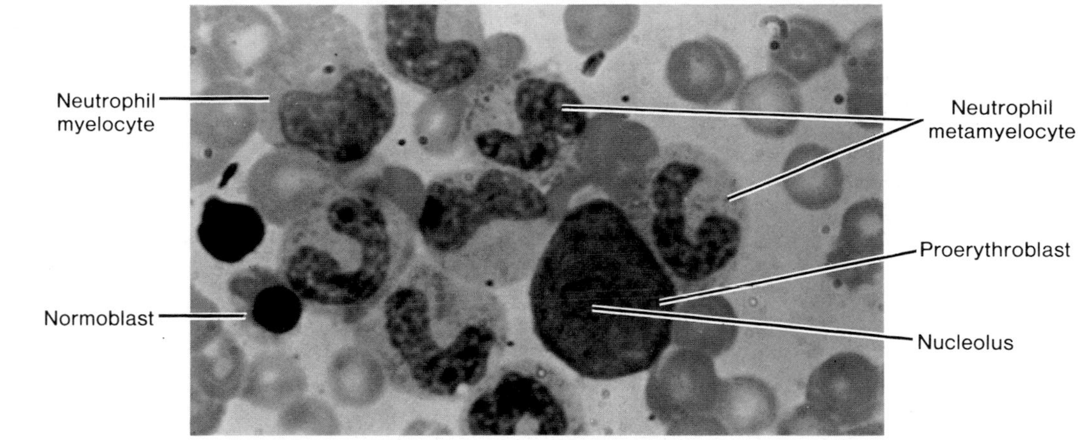

6-13

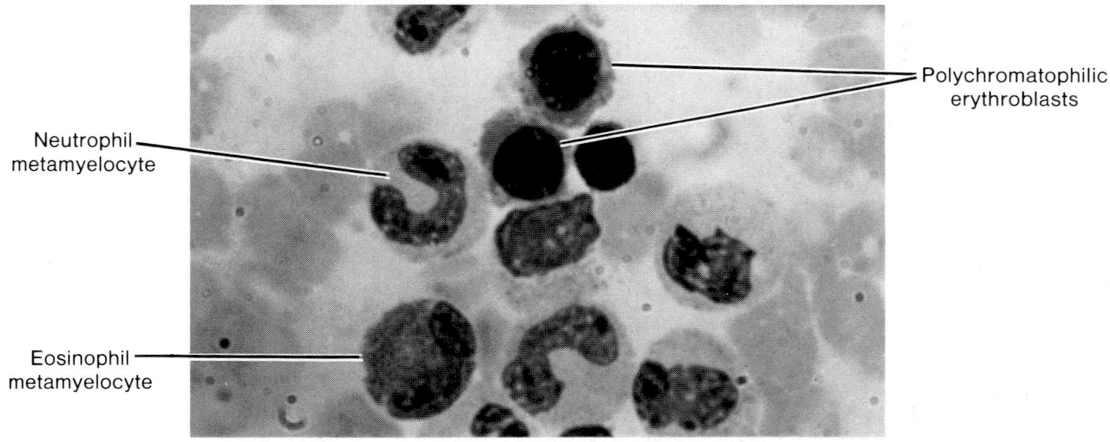

6-14

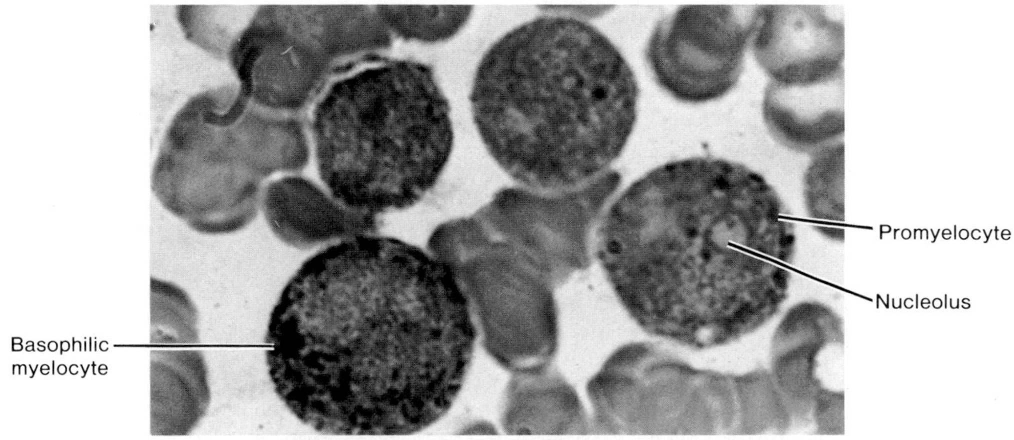

Figure 6-12. Bone marrow (human). LM, ×1000.
Figure 6-13. Bone marrow (human). LM, ×1000.
Figure 6-14. Bone marrow (human). LM, ×1000.

6-15

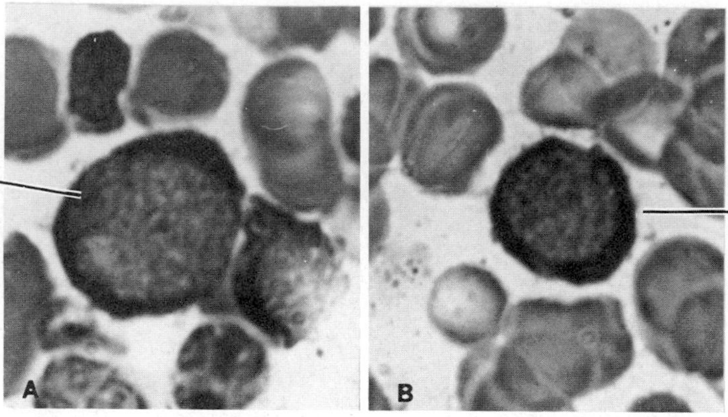

6-16

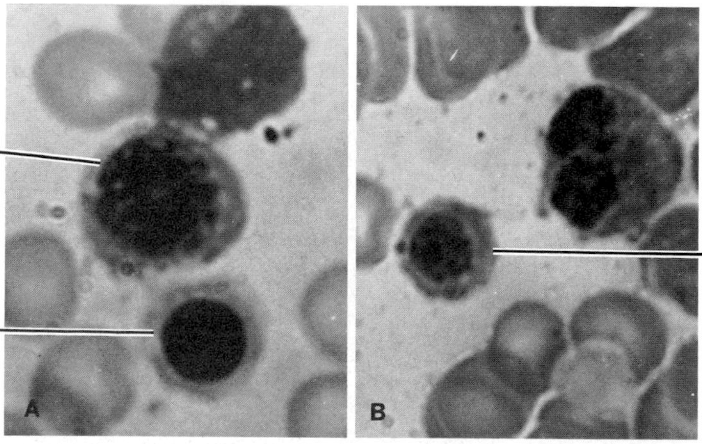

6-17

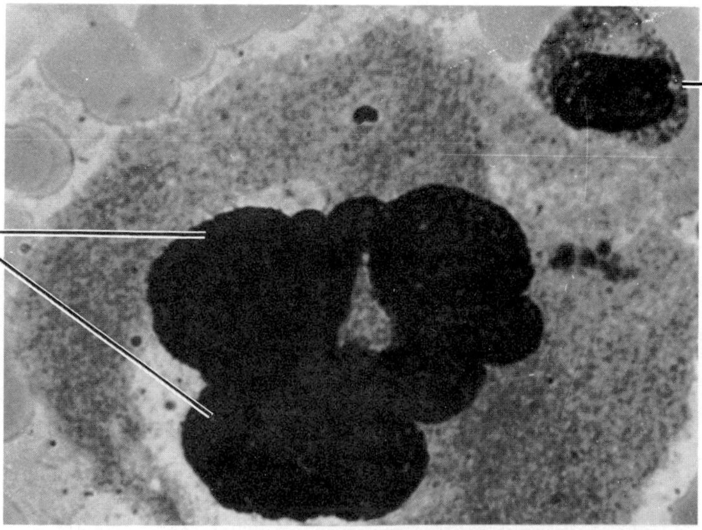

Figure 6-15. *A*, bone marrow (human). LM, ×1000. *B*, bone marrow (human). LM, ×1000.
Figure 6.16. *A*, bone marrow (human). LM, ×1000. *B*, bone marrow (human). LM, ×1000.
Figure 6-17. Megakaryocyte (human). LM, ×1000.

6-18

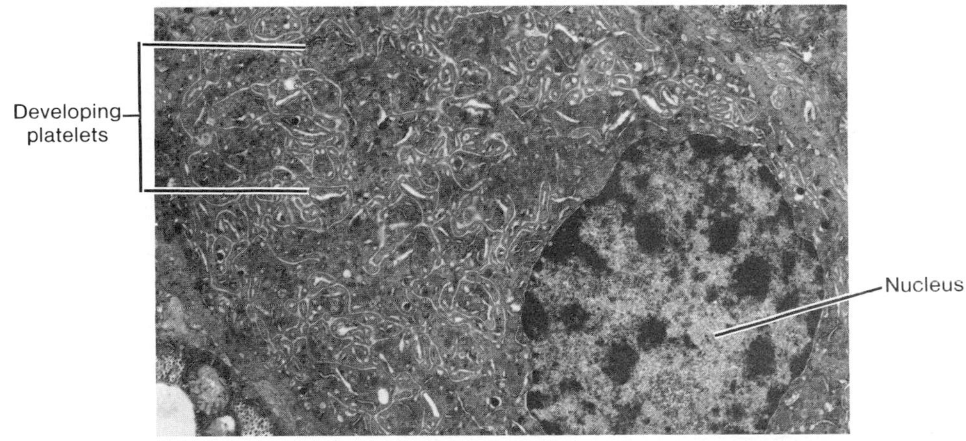

6-19

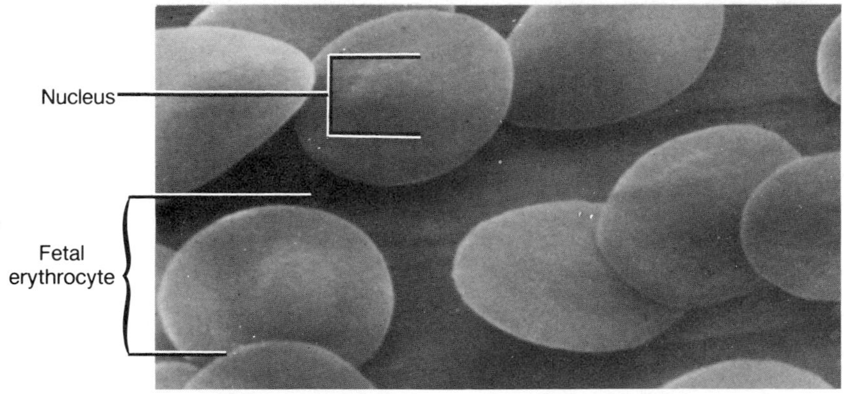

6-20

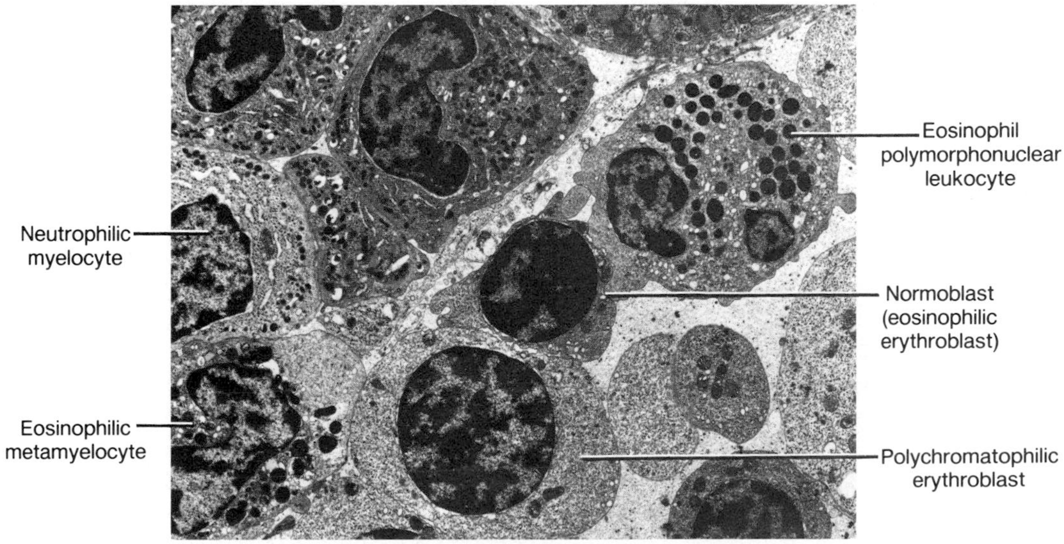

Figure 6-18. Megakaryocyte. TEM, ×5000.
Figure 6-19. Fetal erythrocytes. SEM, ×600.
Figure 6-20. Hemopoietic tissue (liver). TEM, ×2000.

6-21

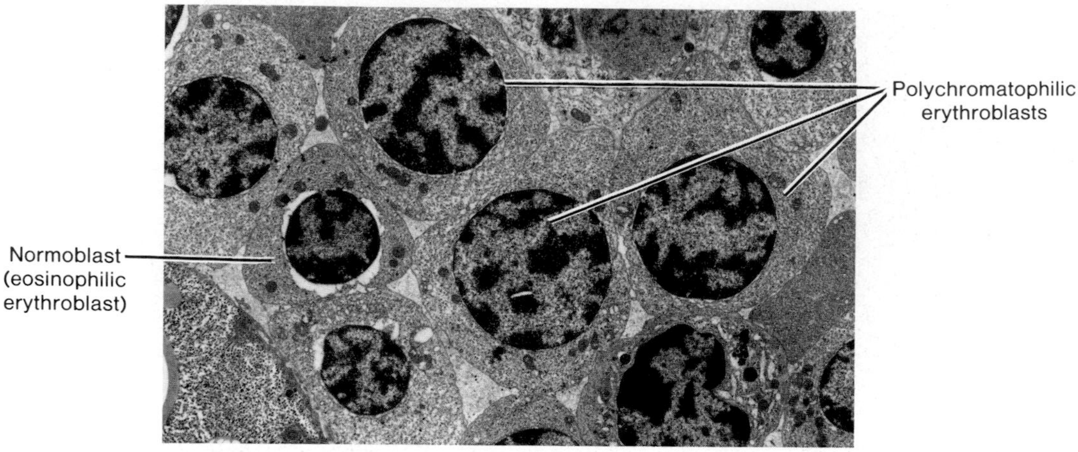

6-22 **Lymphatic Tissue**

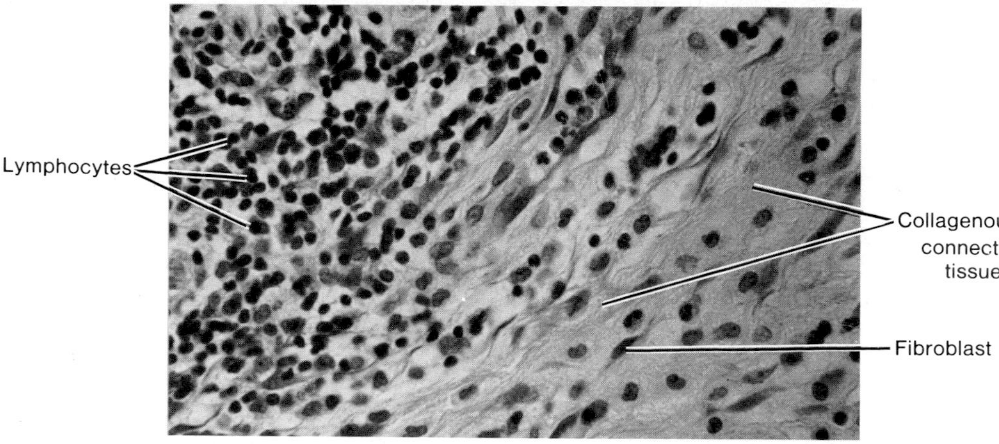

6-23

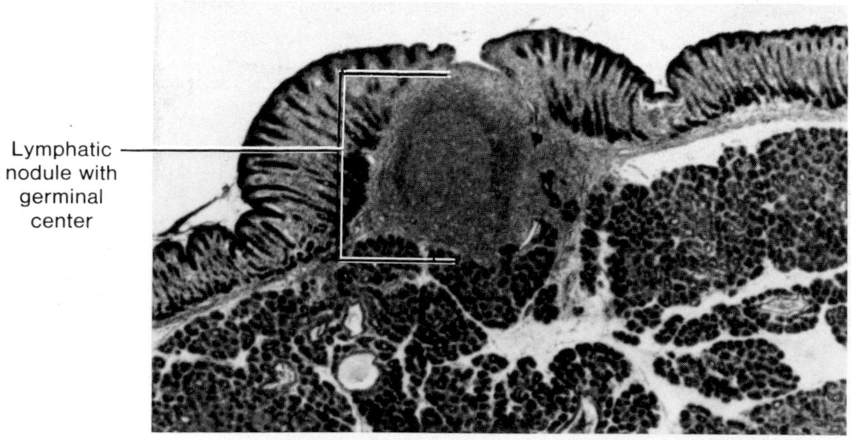

Figure 6-21. Hemopoietic tissue (liver). TEM, ×2000.
Figure 6-22. Diffuse lymphatic tissue (eyelid). LM, ×250.
Figure 6-23. Gastric mucosa. LM, ×40.

7

Muscle

Of the four basic tissues, muscle is that in which the property of contractility has been emphasized. The purposeful movements of the body as a whole and the maintenance of posture are the result of contractions of muscles attached to the skeleton. Muscle contraction also is responsible for the beating of the heart, breathing, constriction of blood vessels, peristaltic movements of the intestines, emptying of the bladder and other vital processes. The unit of structure of all muscles is the muscle cell which, because of its elongated shape, also is called a fiber. Functionally, the shape of the cell is important since a greater unidimensional contraction can be achieved by an elongated cell than by a rounded cell of the same volume. Within a muscle mass, the fibers are oriented in the direction of movement.

CLASSIFICATION

KEY WORDS: striated muscle, skeletal muscle, cardiac muscle, smooth muscle, visceral muscle, voluntary muscle, involuntary muscle

In vertebrates, three kinds of muscle can be distinguished on the basis of their morphology and function. Some muscles show a regular pattern of alternating light and dark bands that extend across the width of the fiber and thus have been called **striated muscle.** This kind of muscle is associated with the skeleton and heart and forms **skeletal muscle** and **cardiac muscle,** respectively. **Smooth muscle**, which lacks cross striations, occurs in the walls of viscera and often is referred to as **visceral muscle.** Functionally, muscle is either **voluntary** (under control of the will) or **involuntary** (not controlled by the will). The striated skeletal muscle is voluntary; smooth muscle is involuntary; and cardiac muscle is involuntary striated muscle.

Skeletal Muscle

Skeletal muscle is the most abundant tissue in the vertebrate body and forms those structures generally referred to as "the muscles." It permits a wide range of voluntary activities, from the intricate and skilled movements involved in writing to the rapid, powerful forces associated with jumping, or throwing a ball. The power that can be generated by skeletal muscle is illustrated by the speed attained by a thrown ball which, at the moment of leaving the fingertips, has been clocked at over 90 miles/hour.

Organization

KEY WORDS: fiber, multinucleated cell, fascicle, muscle, epimysium, perimysium, endomysium

The smallest independent unit of striated muscle visible with the light microscope is the **fiber**, which is a long, **multinucleated cell.** Large numbers of fibers arranged in parallel are grouped together to form the **fascicles** that can be seen with the naked eye. Groups of fascicles in turn make up an entire **muscle.** The fasicles vary in size with different muscles and, in general, are small in muscles associated with fine movements and large in muscles that perform actions demanding greater power.

At all levels of organization, muscle is associated with connective tissue (Fig. 7-1). The entire muscle is surrounded by a connective tissue sheath called the **epimysium** and from the deep surface of the epimysium, septa pass into the muscle to invest each fascicle as the **perimysium.** In turn, delicate extensions of the perimysium envelop each fiber as the **endomysium.** Although given different names according to its association with the different structural units of a muscle, the connective tissue is continuous from one part to another. It consists of collagenous, reticular and elastic fibers and contains several cell types, including fibroblasts, macrophages and fat cells. The endomysium consists mainly of reticular fibers and fine collagenous fibers; it carries blood capillaries and small nerve branches. The larger blood vessels and nerves lie within the perimysium. The connective tissue not only binds the muscle units together but also acts as a harness and aids in transmitting the force of and integrating their contraction. The amount of connective tissue varies from muscle to muscle and is relatively greater in muscles that are capable of finely graded movements. Elastic tissue is most abundant in muscles that attach to soft parts such as the muscles of the tongue and face.

The Muscle Fiber (Cell)

KEY WORDS: banding, cross striations, A bands, I bands, Z line, H band, M line, sarcomere

As a generality, skeletal muscle fibers do not branch, but in some animals the muscles of the tongue and face may branch where the fibers insert into the mucous membrane or skin. The fibers of skeletal muscle are

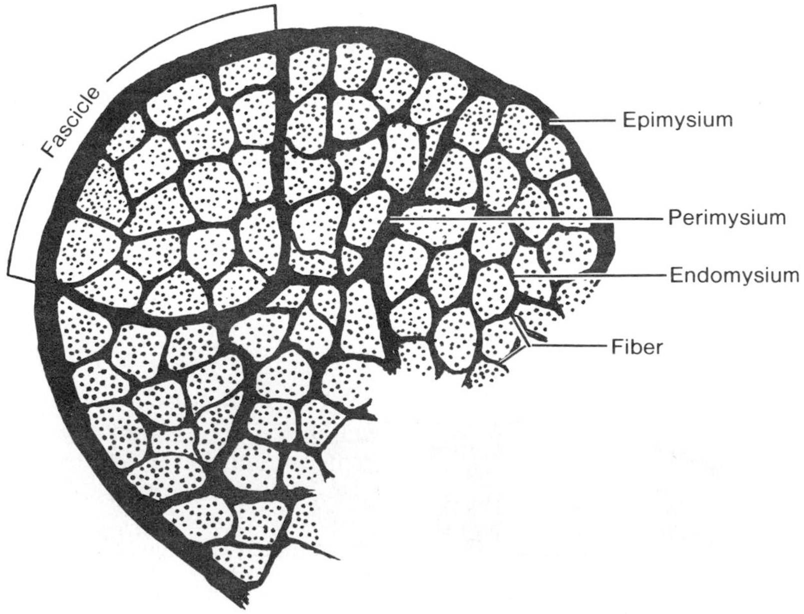

Figure 7-1. Portion of a muscle in transverse section to show the structural organization and the relationships of the connective tissue.

elongated tubular cells which vary in shape and length. Some are cylindrical with rounded ends and appear to extend throughout the length of a muscle; others are spindle-shaped with narrowly tapering ends and apparently do not run the length of the muscle. One end of the fiber may attach to a tendon while the other unites with connective tissue in the belly of the muscle, or both ends may lie within the muscle mass. In transverse sections of fresh muscle the fibers are round or ovoid, but in fixed material appear irregularly polyhedral.

The diameter of the fibers ranges between 10 and 100 μm. The size varies with the class of animal, decreasing through fish, amphibia, reptiles, mammals and birds and also varies from muscle to muscle and within the same muscle. There are indications that the longer fibers have the greater diameters and are associated with the more powerful muscles. Some spatial arrangement of the fibers within a muscle has been noted, the fibers of larger diameters tending to be located more centrally. The size of the fibers changes with use; fibers may hypertrophy (increase in size) in response to continued use or atrophy (decrease in size) with disuse.

The most outstanding feature of skeletal muscle fibers is the presence of alternating light and dark segments which result in the **banding** or **cross striations** (Fig. 7-2) that are seen when the fiber is viewed in longtitudinal section. Under polarized light, the dark bands are anisotropic and are called the **A bands**, whereas the light bands are isotropic and, thus, are called the **I bands.** Running transversely through the center of the I band is a narrow dense line, the **Z line** or Z disk. In good preparations, a pale narrow region, the **H band**, can be seen transecting the A band, with a dark **m line** within it.

The relative length of each band depends upon the state of contraction of the fiber. The length of the A bands remains constant, whereas the I band is prominent in a stretched muscle and short in a contracted muscle. The contractile unit of the fiber is called a **sarcomere** and is defined as the distance between two successive Z lines. Within the sarcomere, as the I band becomes shorter, the Z lines approach the ends of the A bands.

Fiber Types in Skeletal Muscle

KEY WORDS: red fibers, white fibers, intermediate fibers, slow twitch, fast twitch

Some skeletal muscles appear redder than others when seen grossly and muscles frequently are divided into red and white types. The appearances reflect the kind of muscle fiber present and these have been designated as red, white and intermediate fibers. Red muscles contain a preponderance of small **red fibers** which contain abundant myoglobin (a pigment with properties similar to those of hemoglobin), have numerous mitochondria and are rich in oxidative enzymes but poor in phosphorylases. The mitochondria possess many closely packed cristae and are aggregated beneath the sarcolemma and form rows between the myofibrils. This type of fiber also is characterized by the thickness of the Z line. In white muscle, the **white fiber** is the predominant type and is distinguished by the larger size, the smaller number of mitochondria and the narrower Z line. The white fiber is poor in oxidative enzymes but rich in phosphorylases and contains less myoglobin. The **intermediate fibers** show features midway between those of red and white fibers; they are prevalent in red muscle.

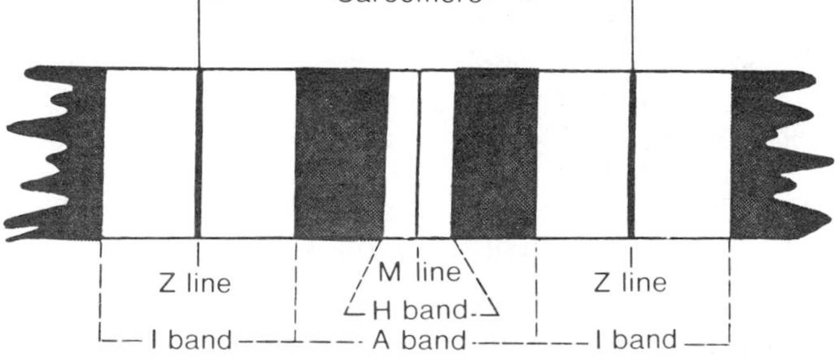

Figure 7-2. Banding pattern of striated skeletal muscle.

Physiologically, the red fibers appear to represent **slow twitch** fibers adapted to slow, repetive contractions seen in postural muscles. White fibers, on the other hand, have been considered to represent **fast twitch** fibers adapted to rapid, short-lived forces. The distinctions are not entirely clear-cut, however, and the pattern of fiber distribution appears to be regulated by the nervous system. Alterations in distribution and in the chemical and physiological properties of the fiber type have been demonstrated experimentally after cross innervation or following stimulation of specific motor neurons. There is evidence that different types of muscle fibers correspond to different types of motor units with different contraction times.

Differences in fiber types can be demonstrated after histochemical staining for various enzymes. The slow-contracting red fibers, for example, stain weakly for adenosine triphosphatase at pH 9, whereas the fast-contracting fibers show a marked staining reactivity; conversely, the slow-acting fibers stain intensely for nicotinic acid dehydrogenase and succinic acid dehydrogenase, whereas the fast twitch fibers show weak to intermediate reactivity. Such histochemical studies, especially on nonhuman muscles, have suggested that a complex system of fiber types may exist; by using a battery of histochemical reactions, as many as eight distinct fibers types have been identified in some species.

Structure of the Muscle Fiber

KEY WORDS: sarcolemma, multinucleated, peripheral nuclei, sarcoplasm, myofibrils, intermediate filaments, desmin, vimentin, sarcoplasmic reticulum, sarcotubules, terminal cisternae, T-tubule, triad, T system, junctional feet

Each muscle fiber is an elongated cell invested by a delicate membrane which, by electron microscopy, can be resolved into the plasmalemma and an adherent, outer coat of glycoprotein. The plasmalemma of muscle cells is referred to as the **sarcolemma** but is no different from the limiting membrane of any other cell. The outer glycoprotein layer is associated with delicate reticular fibers and corresponds to a basal lamina. The fine reticular fibers of this layer mingle with the reticular fibers of the surrounding endomysium.

The striated muscle fiber is **multinucleated.** The nuclei are elongated in the direction of the long axis of the fiber and, in adult mammalian muscle, have a **peripheral location**, immediately below the sarcolemma. The chromatin tends to be distributed along the inner surface of the nuclear membrane and one or two nucleoli usually are present. The nuclei are spaced fairly evenly along the fiber but become more numerous and more irregularly distributed in the area of attachment of the muscle to a tendon. Although the cytoplasm of the muscle cell is called the **sarcoplasm**, it corresponds to that of any cell. Many small Golgi bodies are present, located near the nuclei at one pole, and lysosomes also usually have a juxtanuclear position.

Myofibrils are elongated, thread-like structures which run the length of the muscle fiber within the sarcoplasm. At 1 to 2 μm in diameter, the myofibrils are the smallest units of contractile material that can be identified with the light microscope. In cross sections, myofibrils appear as small dots and in longitudinal section, produce a longitudinal striation of the fiber. Each myofibril shows a banding pattern identical to that of the whole fiber. Indeed, the banding of the fiber is the result of the bands on the component myofibrils being in register. The cross striations are restricted to the myofibrils and do not extend across the sarcoplasm between adjacent myofibrils. However, the striations on adjacent fibrils are kept in alignment by a system of **intermediate filaments** composed of the proteins **desmin** and **vimentin.** The filaments apparently interconnect the Z discs of adjacent myofibrils.

Associated with each myofibril is the **sarcoplasmic reticulum**, a modification of the smooth endoplasmic reticulum seen in other cells. The organelle consists of an extensive and continuous system of membrane-bound tubules, the **sarcotubules**, that form a mesh work around each myofibril. At each junction of A and I bands, a pair of dilated sarcotubules, the **terminal cisternae**, pass around each myofibril and become continuous with the terminal cisternae of adjacent myofibrils. One of the terminal cisternae serves the A band; the other serves the I band. From each of the terminal cisternae, narrow longitudinally oriented sarcotubules extend over the A and I bands, respectively. In the A bands, the tubules form an irregular anastomosis in the region of the H band, while in the I band a similar confluence occurs in the region of the Z line. Thus, each A and I band is covered by a "unit," or segment of sarcoplasmic reticulum. Each unit consists of the terminal cisternae at the A-I junction, joined by longitudinally oriented sarcotubules which anastomose in the region of the H band and Z lines of their respective A and I bands.

The pairs of terminal cisternae at the A-I junction are separated by a slender tubule, the **T tubule.** The three structures, the T tubule and the two terminal cisternae, are referred to as the **triad** of skeletal muscle. In amphibia the triad occurs at the Z line of each band rather than at the A-I junction as in mammals. The T tubules are inward extensions of the sarcolemma and penetrate deeply into the muscle fiber to surround each myofibril. The T tubules of one myofibril communicate with those of adjacent myofibrils to form a complete network across the fiber. The lumen of the T tubule does not open into the cisternae but does communicate with the extracellular space at the surface of the sarcolemma. The T tubules are distinct from the sarcoplasmic reticulum and collectively form the T system (Fig. 7-3).

The **T system** serves for the rapid transmission of impulses from the exterior of the fiber to the myofibrils throughout the cell,

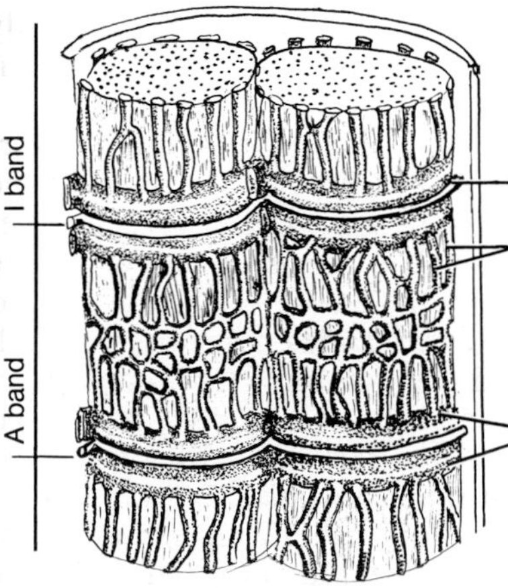

Figure 7-3. Diagrammatic representation of the sarcoplasmic reticulum and system of T-tubules in skeletal muscle.

thereby producing a coordinated response. The T tubules and terminal cisternae are closely apposed and **junctional feet** span the narrow gap between T tubules and terminal cisternae, forming areas of low resistance through which the impulse passes to the sarcoplasmic reticulum. In electron micrographs, the terminal feet appear as regularly spaced densities extending from the T tubules to the terminal cisternae. These are matched by evenly spaced dimples in the cisternal membranes, corresponding to sites where the feet are located. Passage of the electrical impulse to the endoplasmic reticulum results in the release of free calcium ions from the reticulum into the neighboring contractile elements, bringing about their contraction.

Structure of Myofibrils

KEY WORDS: myofilaments, thick filaments, myosin, thin filaments, actin, light meromyosin, heavy meromyosin, tropomyosin, troponin

Under the electron microscope, the myofibril is seen to consist of longitudinally arranged, fine **myofilaments.** Two types of myofilaments have been identified, differing in size and chemical composition. **Thick filaments** are 10 nm in diameter and are composed largely of **myosin** while the **thin filaments** measure 5 nm in diameter and consist primarily of **actin.** The thick, myosin filaments are 1.5 μm in length, with a slightly thicker middle portion and tapering ends. The middle portion is smooth, whereas the ends are studded with many short projections. Myosin filaments can be dissociated further into their constituent molecules, of which there are about 180 per filament, each consisting of a tailpiece and a head. The tails of the molecules lie in parallel and are so arranged that the middle smooth portion consists of the tails only. The heads project laterally from the filament along its tapered ends and form a helical pattern along the filament. Most of the tail consists of **light meromyosin**, whereas the heads, with part of the tail, consist of **heavy meromyosin.**

The thin filaments are about 1 μm in length and are composed of globular subunits of actin attached end to end to form two longitudinal strands wound about each other in a loose helix. A second protein, **tropomyosin**, lies within the groove between the two actin strands; still another protein, **troponin**, is bound to the tropomyosin at intervals of 40 nm.

The globular heads on the myosin filaments contain the enzyme ATPase that splits adenosine triphosphate to yield the energy for muscle contraction; the reaction is stimulated by calcium ions released from the sarcoplasmic reticulum. Troponin on the thin filament appears to be the calcium receptive protein of the contractile system.

The arrangement of the thick and thin myofilaments is responsible for the banding pattern of the myofibrils. The I band consists only of thin filaments that extend in both directions from the Z line. The filaments on one side are offset from those of the other and connecting elements appear to run obliquely across the Z line creating a zigzag pattern. The structure and chemical composition of the Z line and the attachments of the thin filaments to it are not well understood. As the actin filament approaches the Z line, it becomes continuous with four slender threads, each of which appears to form a loop within the Z line and join a thread from an adjacent actin filament. A protein, α actin, has been identified in the Z line.

The A band consists principally of the thick filaments with slender cross connections at their midpoints which give rise to the M line. Actin filaments extend into the A band between the thick filaments; the extent to which they penetrate determines the width of the H band (which consists only of thick filaments) and depends upon the degree of contraction of the muscle (Fig. 7-4). At the ends of the A bands, where the thick and thin filaments interdigitate, the narrow space between the filaments is traversed by cross bridges formed by the heads of the myosin molecules.

The arrangement of the filaments also establishes the ultrastructural basis of the contractile mechanism (Fig. 7-5). During contraction, the A band remains constant in length, the I band and H bands both decrease, and the Z lines approach the ends of the A bands. The changes are the result of an alteration in the relative positions of the thick and thin filaments. No change in the lengths of the filaments is involved; the actin filaments slide past the thick myosin filaments to penetrate more deeply into the A band and, as a consequence, the I and H bands become shorter. The Z lines are drawn closer to the ends of the A bands, thereby decreasing the length of each sacromere (the distance between successive Z lines) to produce an overall shortening of the myofibril.

The sliding action of the filaments results from repeated "make and break" attachments between the heads of the myosin molecules and the neighboring actin filaments. The attachments are made at sites progres-

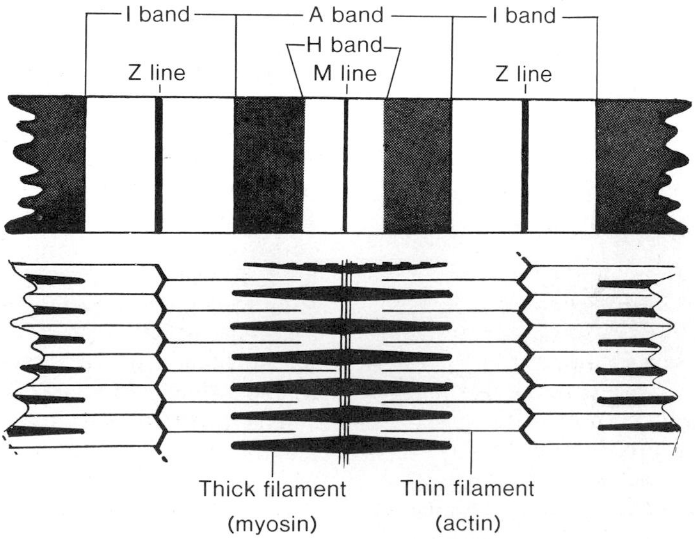

Figure 7-4. Relationship of crossbanding to the arrangement of thin and thick filaments.

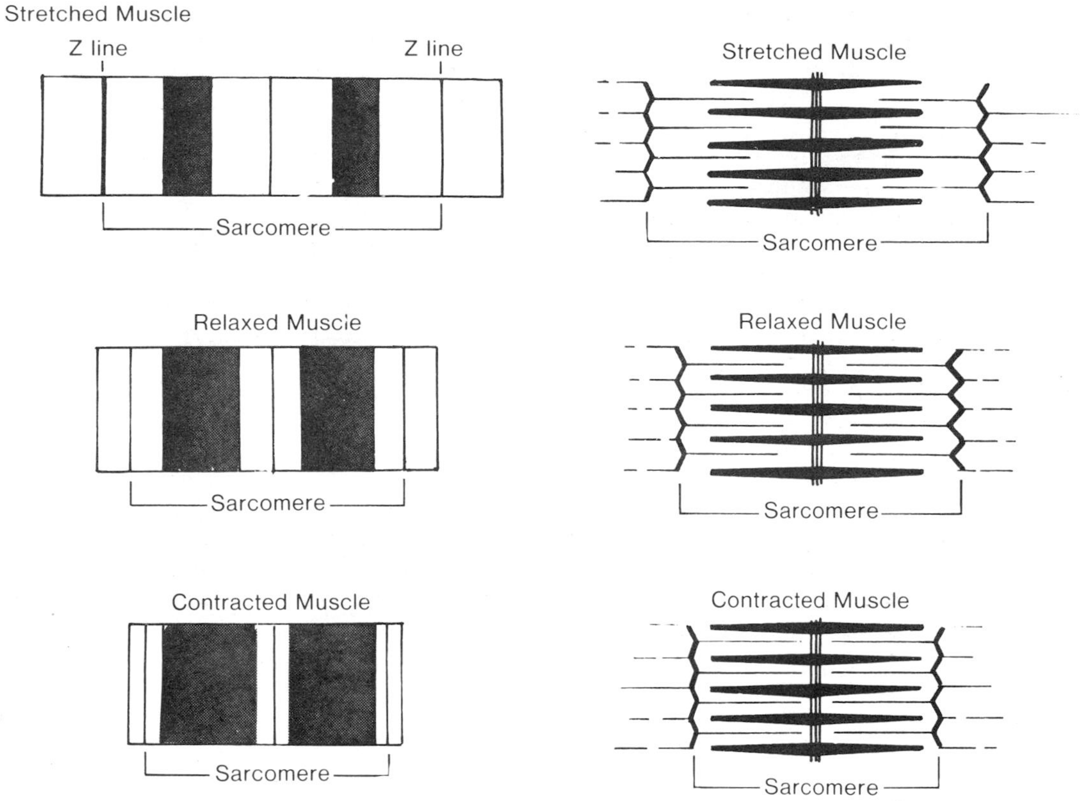

Figure 7-5. Banding pattern and arrangement of thick and thin filaments in stretched, relaxed and contracted muscle.

sively further along the actin filaments, causing the filaments to slide past each other. It is postulated that the force resulting in the movement of the filaments is generated as the globular heads of the myosin actively change their angle of attachment to the actin filaments.

Motor Nerve Endings

KEY WORDS: motor unit, motor end plate, myoneural junction, synaptic troughs, primary synaptic clefts, secondary synaptic clefts, junctional folds, synaptic vesicles, acetylcholine

Each muscle is supplied by one or more nerves which contain both motor and sensory fibers. A motor neuron and the muscle fibers supplied by it constitute a **motor unit.** The size of the motor unit is determined by the number of muscle fibers served by a single nerve fiber and varies between muscles; it is small where precise control of muscle activity is required and large in muscles showing coarse activities. In the intrinsic muscles of the eye, every muscle fiber is supplied by a nerve fiber (thus forming a small motor unit), whereas in the major muscles of the limb, a single nerve fiber may supply 1500 to 2000 muscle fibers—a large motor unit.

Branches of the motor nerve terminate on the muscle fiber at a specialized junctional region called the **motor end plate** or **myoneural junction** (Fig. 7-6). The junction appears as a slightly elevated plaque on the muscle fiber, associated with an accumulation of nuclei. As the nerve approaches the end plate, it loses its myelin covering and terminates in a number of bulbous expansions, the outer surfaces of which are covered by a continuation of the Schwann cells. The nerve endings lie in shallow recesses, the **synaptic troughs** or **primary synaptic clefts,** in the surface of the muscle fiber; additional invaginations of the sarcolemma lining these clefts form numerous **secondary synaptic clefts** or **junctional folds.** Acetylcholinesterase receptor is present on the outermost

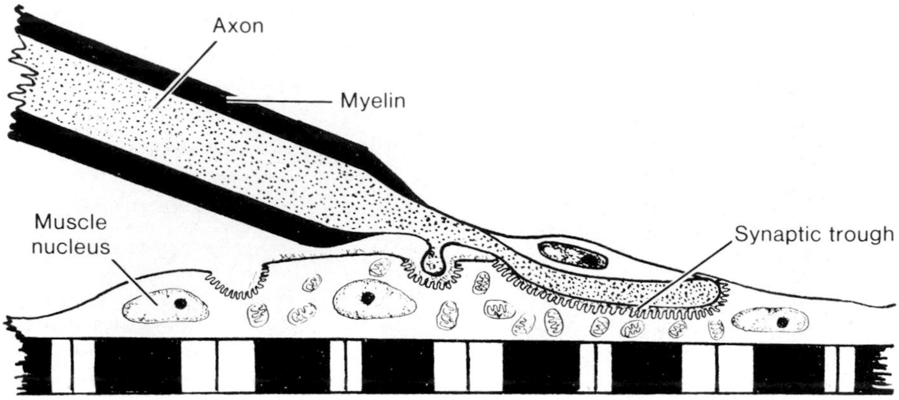

Figure 7-6. Motor end plate.

edges of the secondary cleft, while acetylcholinesterase itself is located along the inner surface of the secondary clefts and is present in the sarcolemma in this region. Although the nerve and muscle fibers are intimately related at the junctions, their cell membranes remain separated by a glycoprotein layer derived from fusion of the basal laminae of the muscle fiber, nerve fiber and Schwann cells. This layer not only extends along the primary synaptic cleft, but also dips into each secondary cleft. The sarcoplasm underlying the nerve terminal contains numerous large, vesicular nuclei and abundant mitochondria, ribosomes and rough endoplasmic reticulum. The nerve terminals contain many mitochondria and a large number of **synaptic vesicles** that appear to be the storage sites of **acetylcholine**, a neurotransmitter agent.

Sensory Nerve Endings

KEY WORDS: muscle spindle (neuromuscular spindle), intrafusal fibers, extrafusal fibers, nuclear bag fibers, nuclear chain fiber, annulospiral endings, flower spray endings, motor end plates, trail endings

Skeletal muscles contain numerous sensory endings, some of which are simple spiral terminations of nonmyelinated nerves that wrap around the muscle fibers, whereas others are highly organized structures called **muscle (neuromuscular) spindles** (Fig. 7-7). Each muscle spindle consists of an elongated, ovoid connective tissue capsule that encloses a few thin modified striated muscle fibers associated with sensory and motor nerves. The modified muscle fibers traverse the capsular space from end to end and are called the **intrafusal fibers** to distinguish them from the ordinary muscle fibers, the **extrafusal fibers**, outside the capsule.

Two distinct types of intrafusal fibers are present. Both are striated over most of their lengths, but midway along the fibers the striations are lost and replaced by an aggregation of nuclei. One type of intrafusal fiber is larger and the nonstriated region is occupied by a cluster of nuclei that produces a slight expansion of the fiber in this region; these fibers have been called the **nuclear bag fibers.** The second type of fiber is thinner and the nuclei in the central region form a single row; this type of fiber is called the **nuclear chain fiber.** The nuclear bag fibers extend beyond the capsule to attach to the endomysium of surrounding extrafusal fibers. Nuclear chain fibers are the more numerous and are shorter; they attach to the capsule at the poles of the spindle or to the sheaths of the nuclear bag fibers. Since the central areas of the intrafusal fibers lack myofibrils, these regions are noncontractile.

Each spindle receives a single, thick sensory nerve fiber that provides several nonmyelinated branches which terminate in a complex system of spirals and rings at the central regions of the intrafusal fibers. These **annulospiral endings** run beneath the basal lamina in a groove in the sarcolemma. **Flower spray endings** are cluster or spray-like terminations of smaller sensory nerves that occur mainly on the nuclear chain fibers. The intrafusal muscle fibers also receive small motor nerve fibers that terminate either as **motor end plates** or as long, diffuse

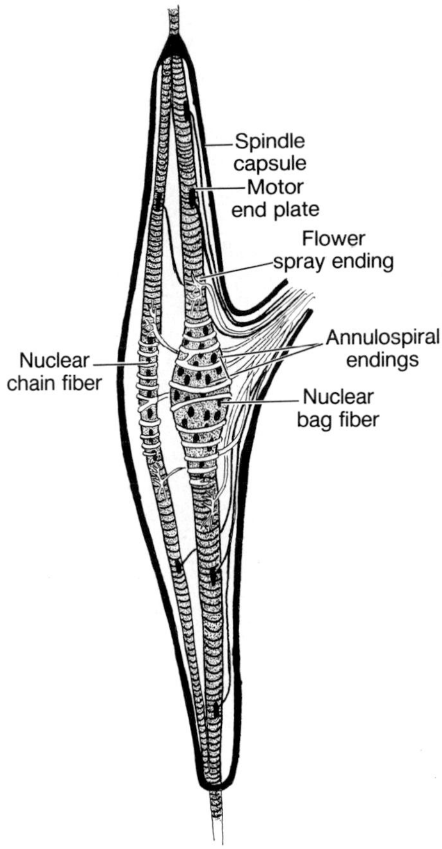

Figure 7-7. Muscle spindle.

trail endings which ramify over the intrafusal fibers, making several contacts with them.

Muscle spindles serve as stretch receptors and are found mainly in slow-contracting extensor muscles that are involved in maintaining posture. They also are present in muscles that show fine movements. Activity of the motor nerves maintains tension on the intrafusal fibers, resulting in a stretching of their nonstriated segments. The degree of stretch is sufficient to maintain the sensory nerve endings in this region in a state of excitation that is close to their thresholds. Stretching of a muscle as a whole produces an increased tension on the intrafusal fibers and a further stretching of their nonstriated regions, resulting in the discharge of impulses by the sensory nerve endings. With contraction of the muscle, tension on the spindle is reduced and the sensory nerve endings cease firing. The frequency of the discharge by the nerve endings is proportional to the tension on the intrafusal fibers and, together with the number of active spindles, ensures a degree of muscle contraction appropriate to the stimulus.

Tendon and Tendon-Muscle Junctions

KEY WORDS: collagen bundles, endotendineum, fascicles, peritendineum, epitendineum, fibroblasts, tendon organs

Tendons consist of thick, closely packed **bundles of collagenous fibers.** Surrounding each bundle is a small amount of loose fibroelastic connective tissue, the **endotendineum.** Variable numbers of collagen bundles are collected into **fascicles**, which are wrapped in a somewhat coarser connective tissue called the **peritendineum.** Groups of fascicles form the tendon itself, which is enveloped in a thick layer of connective tissue, the **epitendineum.** The only cells present are **fibroblasts**, which are arranged in columns between the collagenous bundles.

Where muscle and tendon join, the connective tissue of the endomysium, perimysium and epimysium becomes strongly fibrous and blends with the connective tissue of the tendon. On the muscle side of the junction, the connective tissue fibers extend into indentations of the sarcolemma and are firmly attached to the basal lamina, to which the sarcolemma also is adherent. Within the muscle fiber, the actin filaments of the last sarcomere are anchored to the plasmalemma at the end of the fiber. Thus, contraction of the muscle fiber is passed to the sarcolemma, the basal lamina and then by way of the connective tissue sheaths to the tendon.

Tendon organs are encapsulated sensory receptors found at musculotendinous junctions. The organ consists of a fibrous capsule traversed by specialized collagenous bundles that are continuous with those outside the capsule. A single large sensory nerve pierces the capsule and gives rise to several nonmyelinated branches whose terminations entwine among the collagenous bundles. The tendon organs sense the stresses produced by muscle contractions, preventing them from becoming excessive.

Cardiac Muscle

Cardiac muscle occurs only in the heart, where it forms the muscle wall (the myocardium). It bears some resemblances both to skeletal and smooth muscle; like skeletal muscle, cardiac muscle is striated but, like smooth muscle, it is involuntary. However, cardiac muscle differs from both in many of its structural details and is unique in that its contractions are automatic and spontaneous and require no external stimulation.

Organization

KEY WORDS: branching fibers, endomysium, perimysium

Like skeletal muscle, the histological unit of structure of cardiac muscle is the cell (fiber), but in cardiac muscle they are associated end to end to form long tracts, each about 80 μm long by 15 μm wide. The **fibers** may divide at their ends and **branch** to connect with adjacent fibers and thus form a network. Between the fibers is a web of collagenous and reticular fibers corresponding to an **endomysium**, but it is more irregular than that of skeletal muscle, because of the branching of the cardiac muscle fibers. Larger bundles of fibers are wrapped in a coarser connective tissue of collagenous and reticular fibers, forming a **perimysium,** much, as in skeletal muscle.

Fibers

KEY WORDS: sarcolemma, central nuclei, A, I, M, H, and Z bands, actin and myosin filaments, sarcoplasmic reticulum, T tubules, Z lines, diads, peripheral couplings (subsarcolemmal cisternae)

Each cell or fiber is enclosed in a **sarcolemma**, external to which is an outer lamina associated with fine reticular cells. The **nuclei** are located **centrally** in the fiber and there are only one or two per fiber (cell). The same banding pattern seen in skeletal muscle is present on cardiac fibers, and **A, I, M, H** and **Z bands** can be distinguished but are not as conspicuous as in skeletal muscle. The banding patterns are due to the arrangement of **actin** and **myosin filaments**, but the aggregation of the filaments into myofibrils is not well defined, and bundles of myofilaments often become confluent with those of adjacent bundles or are separated by rows of mitochondria. The bundles of myofilaments diverge around the nucleus to leave a fusiform area of sarcoplasm at each pole. These areas are occupied by small Golgi elements and numerous mitochondria which are large and have closely packed cristae. Glycogen is a prominent feature of cardiac muscle.

The **sarcoplasmic reticulum** (Fig. 7-8) is neither as extensive nor as well developed as that in skeletal muscle. The sarcotubules are continuous over the length of the sarcomere and anastomose freely to give a plexiform pattern, with no special anastomosis at the H band. Terminal cisternae are lacking, and the reticulum makes contact with **T tubules** by means of small, irregular expansions of the sarcotubules. Since most T tubules are apposed to only one cisterna at any point, these couplings of T tubule and sarcoplasmic reticulum have been called **diads.** The T tubules are located at the **Z lines**, rather than at the A-I junctions, and their lumina are much wider than in the T tubules of skeletal muscle. The luminal surfaces of the cardiac T tubules are coated by a continuation of the basal lamina of the sarcolemma. The sarcotubules at the periphery of the cell may also be closely apposed to the sarcolemma, and these couplings have been called the **peripheral couplings** or **subsarcolemmal cisternae.** As in skeletal muscle, the functional unit of cardiac muscle is the sarcomere, demarcated by two successive Z lines.

Intercalated Disks

KEY WORDS: desmosomes, fascia adherens, nexus (gap junction)

At their end to end associations, the cardiac muscle cells (fibers) are united by spe-

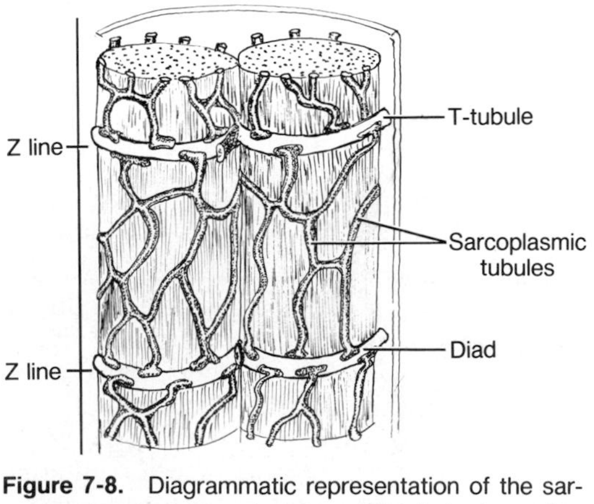

Figure 7-8. Diagrammatic representation of the sarcoplasmic reticulum and system of T tubules in cardiac muscle.

cial junctions which are visible under the light microscope as dark lines, the intercalated disks. These cross the fibers in stepwise fashion at the level of the Z lines and so have transverse and longtitudinal parts. Along the transverse parts, the opposing cells are extensively interdigitated and at points are united by **desmosomes.** For the most part, the junction between cells is more extensive than that of a desmosome and so is called a **fascia adherens.** The sarcoplasm immediately below the cell membrane contains a mat of filamentous material into which the actin filaments insert, thus binding the ends of the myofilaments to the sarcolemma. At irregular sites along the junctions, the membranes of opposing cells are united by **nexus** or **gap junctions.**

The longitudinal part of the intercalated disk is continuous with the transverse portion and also shows gap junctions which, however, are much more extensive. The gap junctions represent areas of low electrical resistance that serve for rapid spread of excitation from cell to cell.

Smooth Muscle

Smooth muscle is widely distributed throughout the body and plays an essential role in the function of organs. It forms the contractile portion of the walls of blood vessels and of hollow viscera such as the digestive, respiratory, urinary and reproductive tracts. Smooth muscle also is present in the skin, where it forms small muscles attached to hair follicles and in the iris and ciliary body of the eye, in the erectile tissue of the clitoris and penis and in the stroma of the ovary and prostate.

Smooth Muscle Fibers

KEY WORDS: cell, single central nucleus, myofibrils, filaments, dense bodies, basal (external) lamina, gap junctions (nexuses), attachment plaques

Each smooth muscle fiber is an elongated, slender **cell** with an expanded central region and tapering ends. The fibers vary in length in different organs, from 20 μm in small blood vessels to 500 or 600 μm in the pregnant uterus. A **single, centrally placed nucleus** occupies the wide portion of the fiber about midway along its length, elongated in the long axis of the fiber. In a contracted fiber, the nucleus has a wrinkled or pleated outline. The fibers lack cross striations and, in the usual histological preparations, appear homogeneous. However, longitudinal striations can be seen after maceration of the fibers in acid; these represent the **myofibrils.**

In electron micrographs the sarcoplasm in the region of the nucleus shows long, slender mitochondria, a few tubules of granular endoplasmic reticulum, clusters of free ribosomes and a small Golgi complex at one pole of the nucleus. There is no sarcoplasmic reticulum, unlike cardiac and skeletal muscle. The bulk of the cytoplasm contains closely packed, fine **filaments** arranged in bundles that run parallel to the long axis of the fiber. Mitochondria and glycogen granules are interspersed between the myofibrils, and scattered throughout the sarcoplasm are a number of oval **dense bodies** into which the myofilaments appear to insert.

The sarcolemma is covered externally by a thick extracellular **basal** or **external lamina** consisting of proteoglycans with numerous fine collagenous and reticular fibers that blend with the surrounding connective tissue. In certain regions, the basal lamina is lacking and the membranes of neighboring cells are closely related in **gap junctions,** through which excitation impulses spread from one fiber to another. Areas of increased density, similar to the dense bodies, occur at intervals along the inner aspect of the sarcolemma and become more numerous along the ends of the fibers. These dense regions appear to be sites of attachment of myofilaments to the cell membrane and thus have been called **attachment plaques.** Between these areas, the sarcolemma shows numerous caveoli, indicative of micropinocytosis.

Myofilaments

KEY WORDS: thick filaments, thin filaments, myosin, actin, labile myosin

Both **thick** and **thin filaments** have been demonstrated in smooth muscle by electron microscopy, and **myosin** and **actin** have been identified biochemically. However, myosin filaments have been difficult to identify in standard electron microscopic preparations. It has been suggested that in smooth muscle, **myosin** is **labile** and aggregates into filaments only prior to contraction. Myosin and actin of smooth muscle are capable of interaction as in striated muscle, and it appears that the sliding filament mechanism accounts for contraction of smooth muscle also.

Organization

Smooth muscle cells may be present as isolated units or small bundles in ordinary connective tissue, as in the intestinal villi, the dartos tunic of the scrotum or in the capsule and trabeculae of the spleen. They also form prominent sheets, as in the walls of the intestine, in which the fibers all run in the same direction but are offset so that the thick portions of the fibers lie adjacent to the tapering ends of neighboring fibers. Thus, in transverse sections, the outlines of the fibers vary in diameter according to where along its length the fiber was sectioned. Nuclei are few and are present only in the largest profiles, which represent sections through the expanded areas of the cell. A thin connective tissue with few fibroblasts and consisting of fine collagenous, reticular and elastic fibers extends between the smooth muscle cells and becomes continuous with a more dense connective tissue which binds the muscle cells into bundles or sheets. This latter connective tissue contains more abundant fibroblasts, collagenous and elastic fibers, and a network of blood vessels and nerves. The traction produced by contracting fibers is transmitted to the reticuloelastic sheath about the cells and then to the denser connective tissue, permitting a uniform contraction throughout the smooth muscle sheet. Reticular and elastic fibers and the external lamina of the reticuloelastic sheath are products of the smooth muscle cells.

DEVELOPMENT OF MUSCLE

Skeletal Muscle. Skeletal muscle arises from mesenchyme in various parts of the embryo. Muscles of the trunk are derived from myotomal mesenchyme; those of the limbs develop from somatic mesenchyme. Muscles of the face, pharynx, larynx and those involved in mastication all arise in the mesenchyme of the branchial arches.

Initially, the precursor muscle cells or myoblasts are rounded, noncontractile cells with single, centrally-placed nuclei. As they develop, the cells become spindle-shaped and synthesize myofilaments which assume a peripheral position in the cell and aggregate into myofibrils. All components of the sarcomere are present. The cells fuse to one another, end to end, to form groups of multinucleated cylinders called primary myotubules. New generations of muscle cells develop from undifferentiated mononuclear cells that lie along the walls of the primary myotubules. The new cells form new myotubules or are added to the ends of older myotubules to form a fiber containing from 50 to 100 nuclei which at first are centrally-placed. The nuclei later move to their characteristic positions just beneath the sarcolemma.

Cardiac Muscle. Cardiac muscle develops from mesenchyme (the myoepithelial mantle) that envelops the endocardial tube of the early embryonic heart. The cells are stellate at first and joined by desmosomes. Unlike skeletal muscle cells, primitive cardiac muscle cells divide repeatedly. With the synthesis of myofilaments, the cells elongate and become myoblasts which soon begin rhythmical contractions. Cell division continues into postnatal life but subsequently gives way to hypertrophy as the means of growth. The sites of desmosomal unions between cells transform into the intercalated discs.

Formation of T tubules characterizes the final stage of differentiation of mammalian cardiac muscle. The tubules arise from invaginations of the sarcolemma, late in the prenatal period in guinea pigs, sheep and cattle, but develop postnatally in the rat, mouse, and opossum. However, when considered relative to development of the external form, rather than the chronological age, the time at which cardiac T tubules develop is the same for all mammals.

Smooth Muscle. Smooth muscle arises from the mesenchyme at various sites in the embryo where smooth muscle ordinarily will occur in the adult. The stellate mesenchymal cells synthesize contractile proteins, assume a fusiform shape and continue to increase in size. There is evidence that even in the adult, new muscle cells may arise by mitotic division, as in the uterus. Generally however, adult growth of smooth muscle is the result of hypertrophy. The smooth muscle of the iris is commonly held to be derived from cells near the margin of the optic cup and therefore is of ectodermal origin.

FUNCTIONAL SUMMARY

Nerve impulses reaching the myoneural junctions of skeletal muscles cause release of acetylcholine contained within the synaptic vesicles. This neurotransmitter diffuses across the synaptic trough, the surface area of which is greatly increased by the junctional folds. Acetylcholine causes depolarization of the sarcolemma at the end plate, from which an excitation wave sweeps over the surface of the muscle fiber and, by means of the T system, to all of the myofibrils throughout the fiber. At the triads, the impulse is passed to the endoplasmic reticulum, causing release of calcium ions from the sarcotubules. Free calcium ions activate the myosin-actin interaction, apparently through the intervention of tropomyosin and troponin. Troponin is the calcium receptive protein which, in the presence of increased calcium ion, is thought to undergo structural changes bringing about the interaction of myosin and actin. The energy for the cross bridging between myosin and actin is obtained from the breakdown of adenosine triphosphate by ATPase contained on the myosin filaments. As the actin filaments slide past the myosin filaments to penetrate more deeply between them, the length of each sarcomere is reduced, resulting in an overall shortening of each myofibril and thus of each fiber. The tension generated is transmitted in succession to the sarcolemma, the external lamina, the connective tissue and then to a tendon or other muscle attachment. Muscle spindles serve as stretch receptors and coordinate the degree of muscle contraction with the extent of the stimulus. Tendon organs sense the stresses produced by muscle contractions and prevent them from becoming excessive.

The duration of the excitation wave at the myoneural junction is limited by the rapid breakdown of acetylcholine by the enzyme acetylcholinesterase that is associated with the junctional folds. With termination of the excitation wave, calcium is rebound on the sarcoplasmic reticulum, and ATPase activity and actin-myosin interactions cease, with a consequent relaxation of the muscle.

Contraction of cardiac muscle occurs spontaneously, i.e., it contracts in the absence of an external stimulus. However, the mechanism of contraction is identical to that of skeletal muscle and involves the interaction of actin and myosin filaments. Cardiac muscle has a greater dependency upon calcium than does skeletal muscle, which may relate to the relatively poorer development of the sarcoplasmic reticulum; the poorer development of this organelle also may reflect the relatively slower contraction time of cardiac muscle. The high content of mitochondria and glycogen is related to the constant, rhythmic expenditure of energy which typifies cardiac muscle. Cardiac muscle fibers have an inherent capacity to conduct impulses and, because of the numerous gap junctions between cardiac muscle cells, electrically the tissue acts as though there were no membranes between cells. Rapid distribution of impulses throughout cardiac muscle is aided also by the numerous branchings which provide unions between adjacent fibers.

Although thick and thin myofilaments have been identified in smooth muscle cells, the filaments appear to be packed in random fashion and not in the precise and orderly fashion seen in skeletal and cardiac muscle. This is said to permit the unhindered generation of a steady tension over a wide range of fiber lengths. The contraction of smooth muscle is somewhat unique in that forceful contractions can be sustained for long periods without fatigue of the muscle. An example of such contractions are those of the uterine muscle during parturition. This type of contraction differs from that of skeletal muscles, which are unable to sustain contractions without becoming fatigued, or with cardiac muscle, which shows inherent, intermittent contractions. The absence of an

organized endoplasmic reticulum in smooth muscle is related to the slow contractions exhibited by smooth muscle.

The presence of nexus junctions permits the free passage of impulses and, as in cardiac muscle, smooth muscle frequently acts electrically as though there were no cell boundaries. Thus, a few motor nerves can control large numbers of smooth muscle cells. The connective tissue between and around smooth muscle bundles serves to transmit the forces generated by individual cells into a coordinated force transmitted throughout the entire tissue.

Atlas and Table of Key Features for Chapter 7

Table 7-1
Key Histological Features of Muscle Types

Type	Cell Shape	Nuclei	Diameter	Striations	Other
Smooth	Small spindles	Central, single	Small with marked variation	Absent	Packed tightly, little connective tissue between fibers
Cardiac	Short branching cylinders	Central, usually single, may be double	Large, moderate variation	Present	Intercalated disks
Skeletal	Long cylinders	Peripheral, multiple	Large, uniform	Present	

7-9 Skeletal Muscle

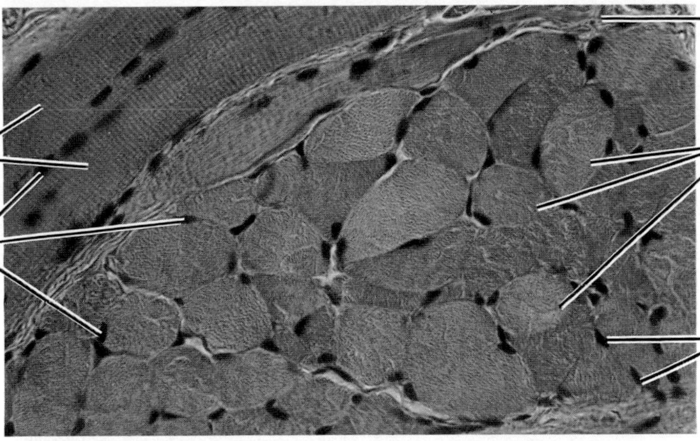

7-10

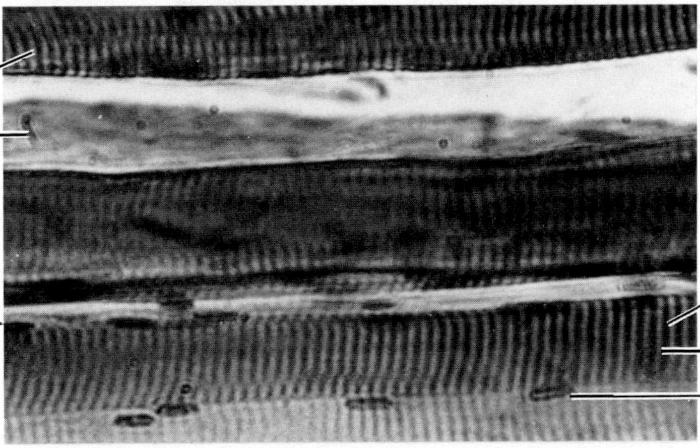

7-11

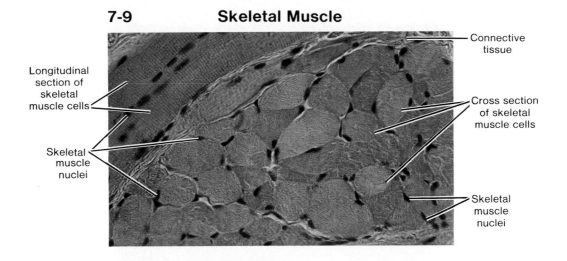

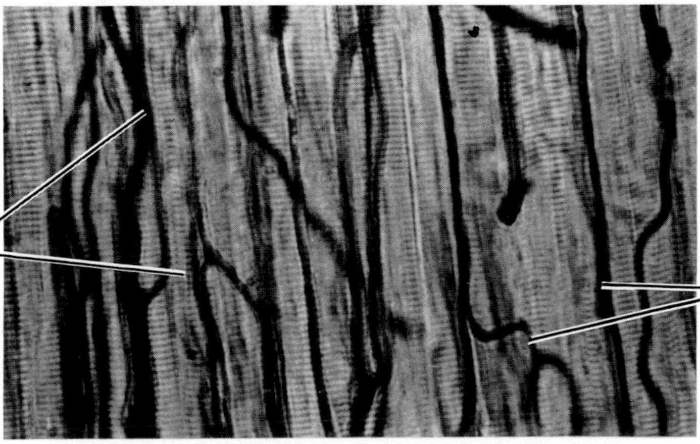

Figure 7-9. Longitudinal and cross section. LM, ×300.
Figure 7-10. Longitudinal section. LM, ×1000.
Figure 7-11. Vasculature of skeletal muscle. LM, ×250.

7-12

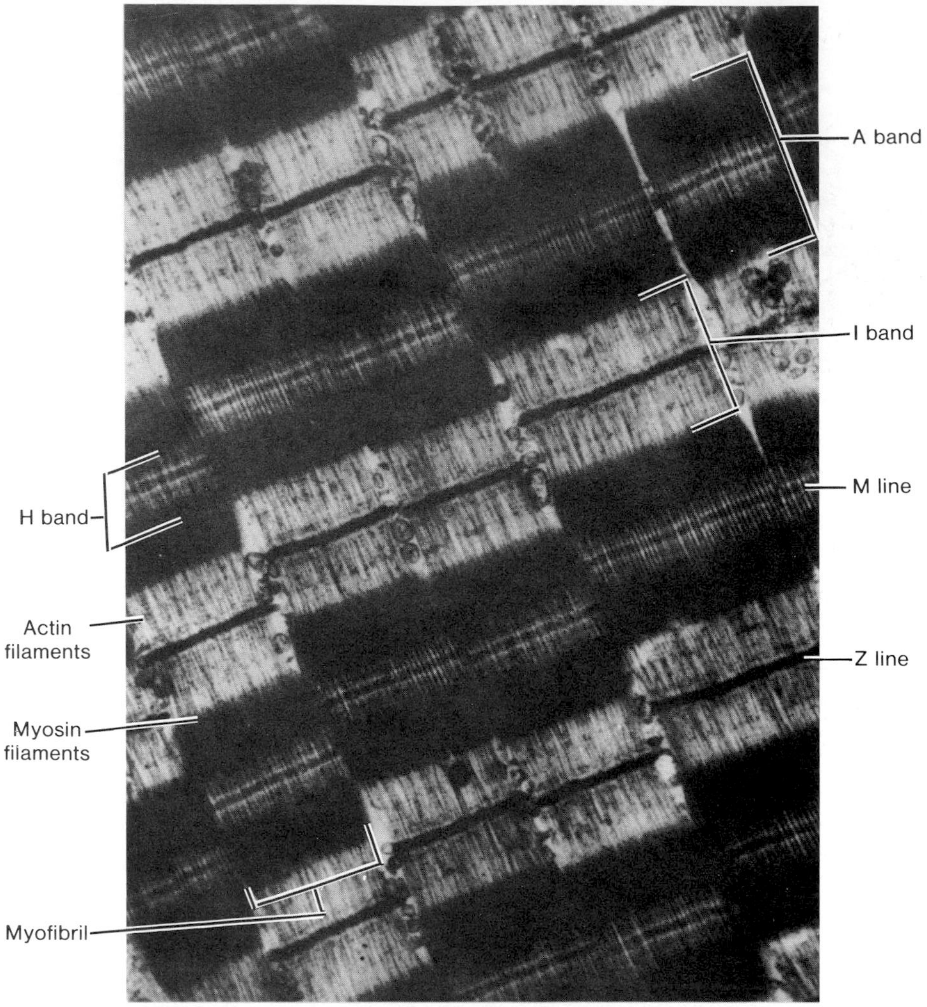

7-13

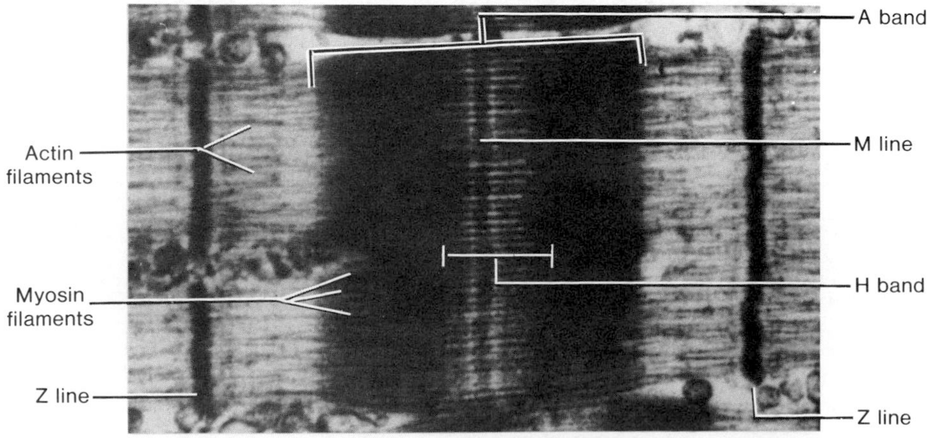

Figure 7-12. Skeletal muscle. TEM, ×26,000.
Figure 7-13. Skeletal muscle (sarcomere). TEM, ×40,000.

7-14

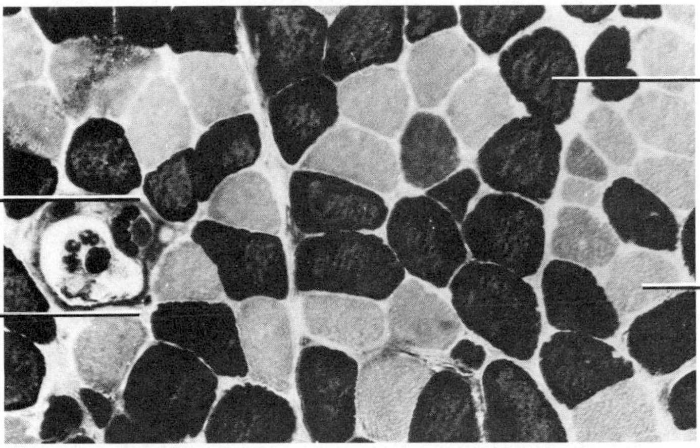

7-15

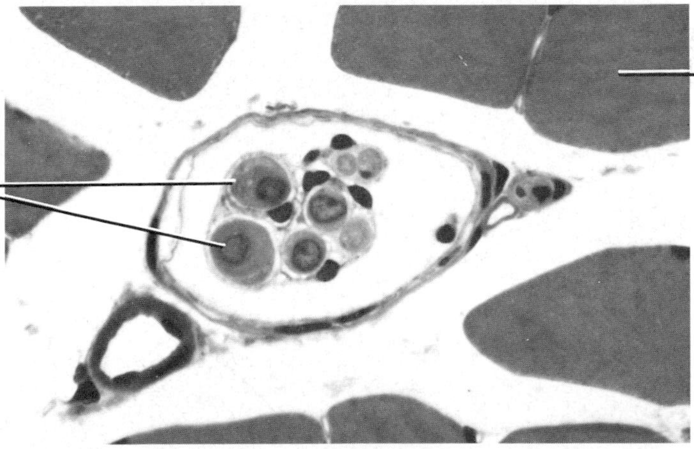

7-16 Development

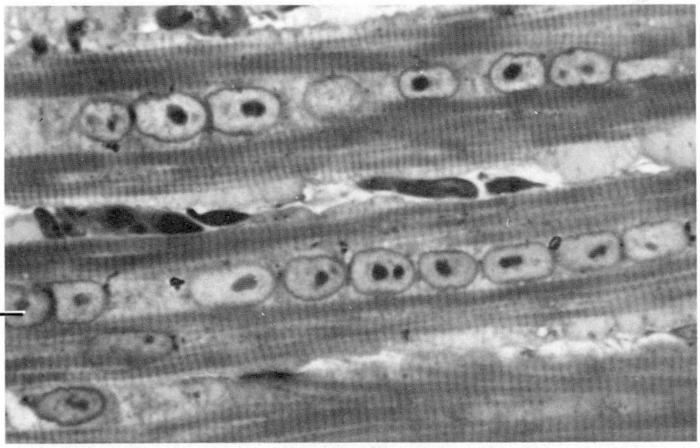

Figure 7-14. Skeletal muscle, ATPase (pH 10.4). LM, ×250.
Figure 7-15. Muscle spindle. LM, ×400.
Figure 7-16. Skeletal muscle. LM, ×400.

7-17 Cardiac Muscle

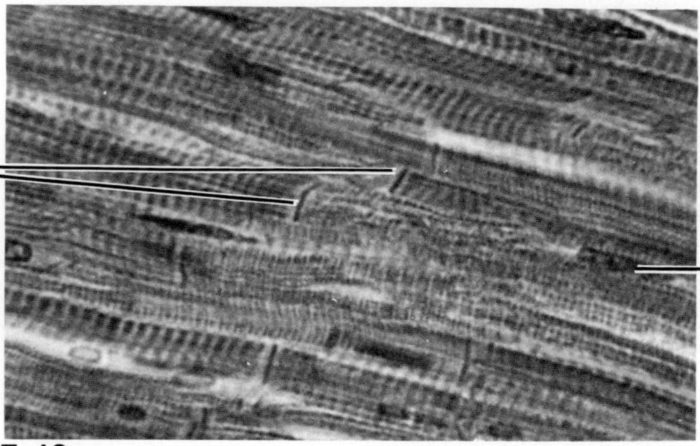

7-18

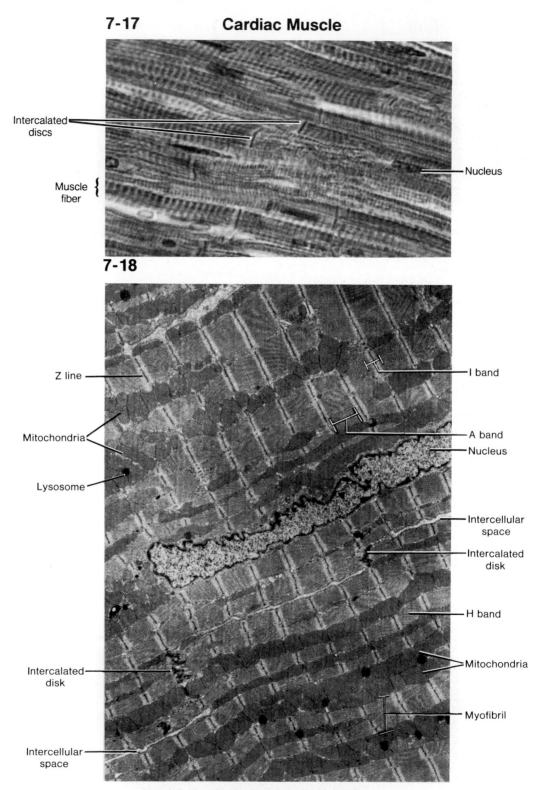

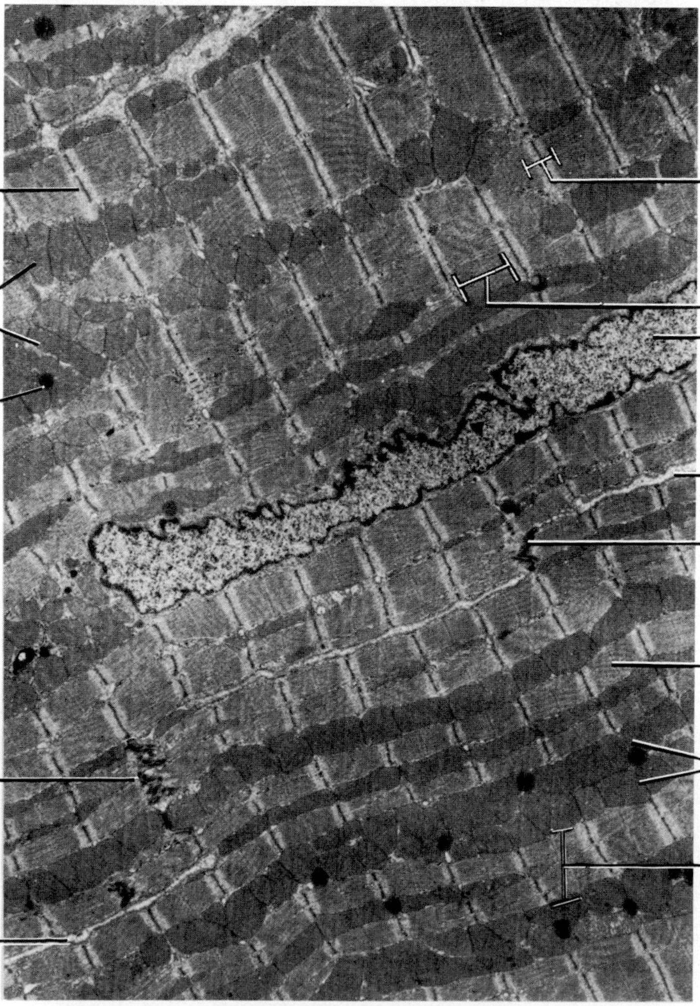

Figure 7-17. Longitudinal section. LM, ×400.
Figure 7-18. Two cardiac muscle cells. TEM, ×6000.

7-19

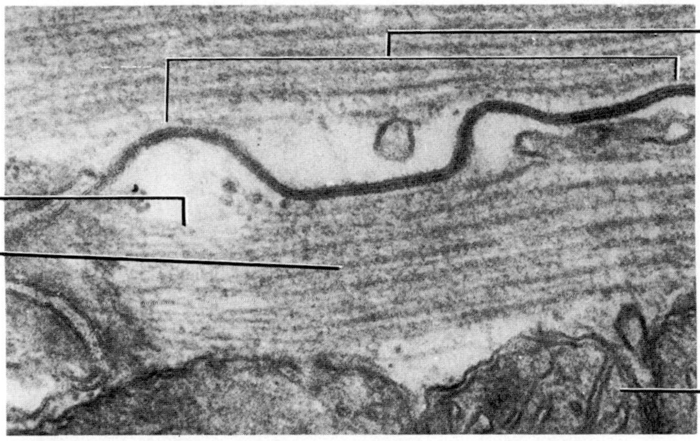

7-20

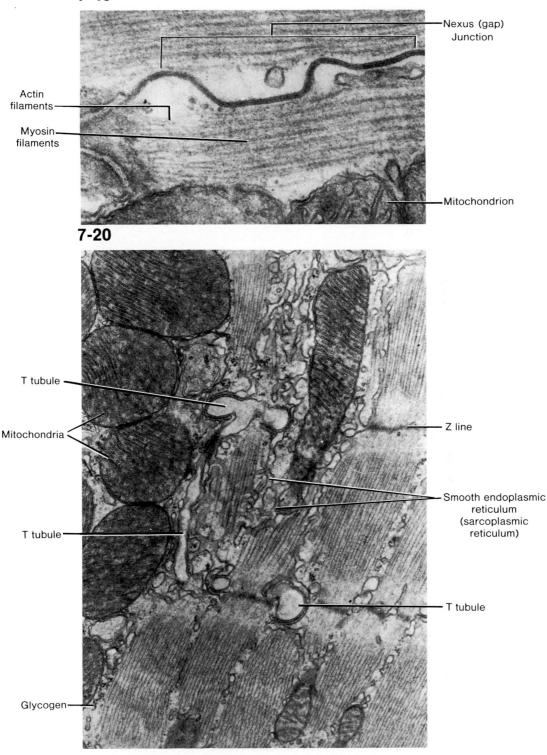

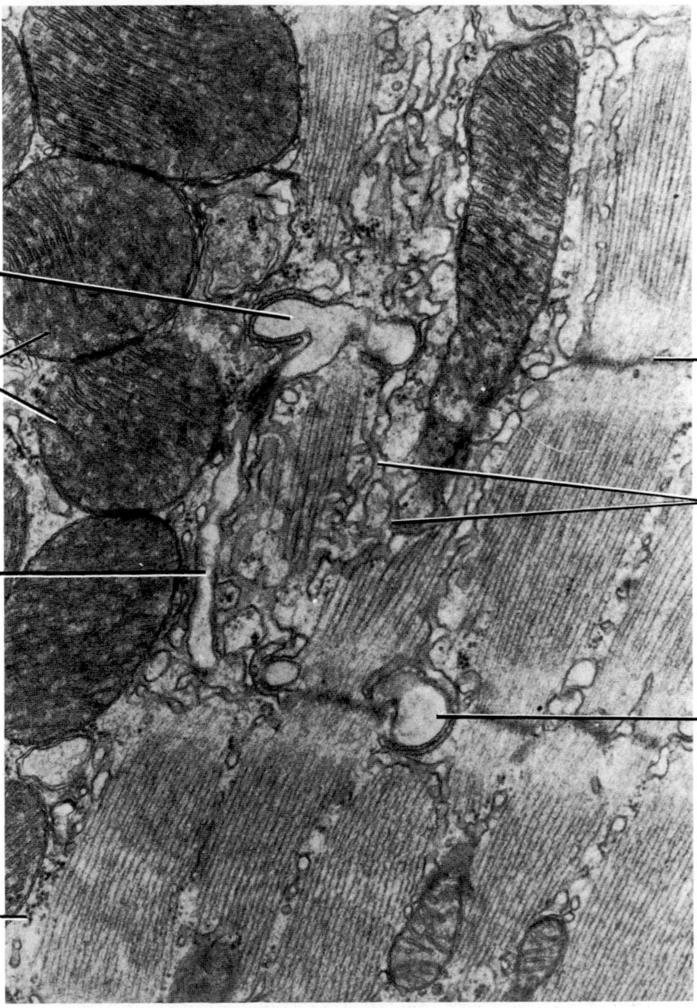

Figure 7-19. Gap junction between cells. TEM, ×100,800.
Figure 7-20. Heart ventricle. TEM, ×26,950.

7-21

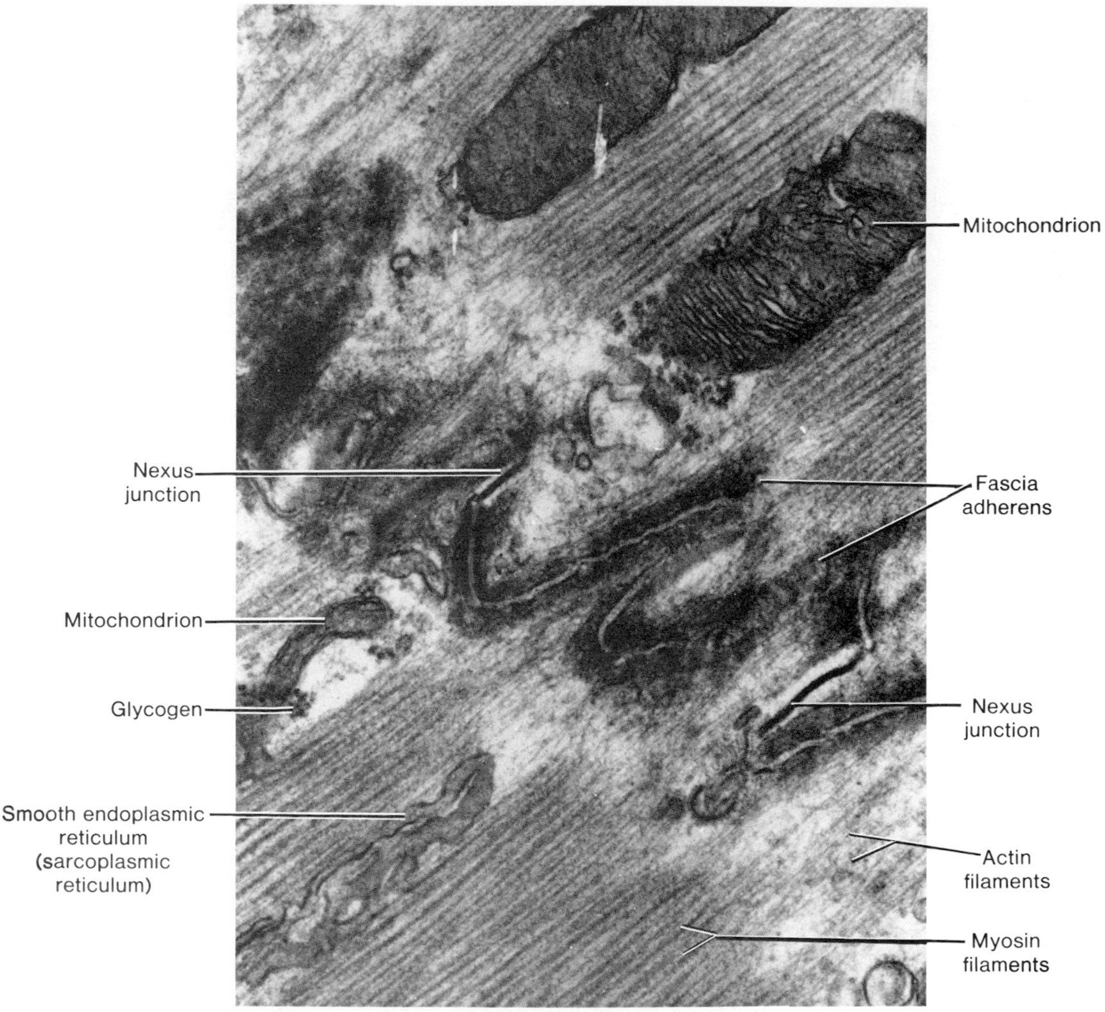

7-22 Smooth Muscle

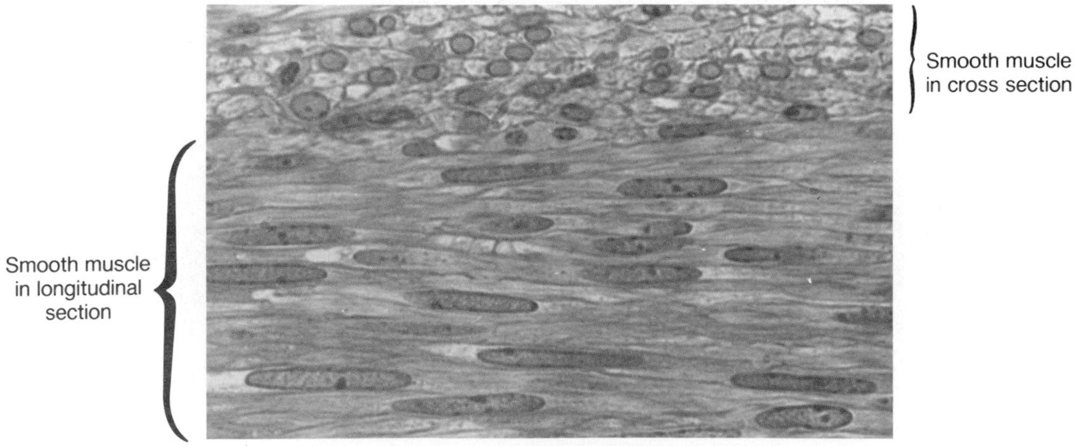

Figure 7-21. Intercalated disk. TEM, ×52,800.
Figure 7-22. Oviduct. LM, ×400.

7-23

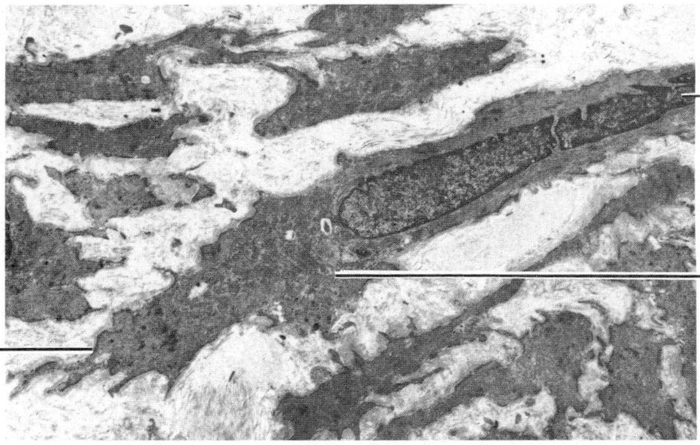

7-24

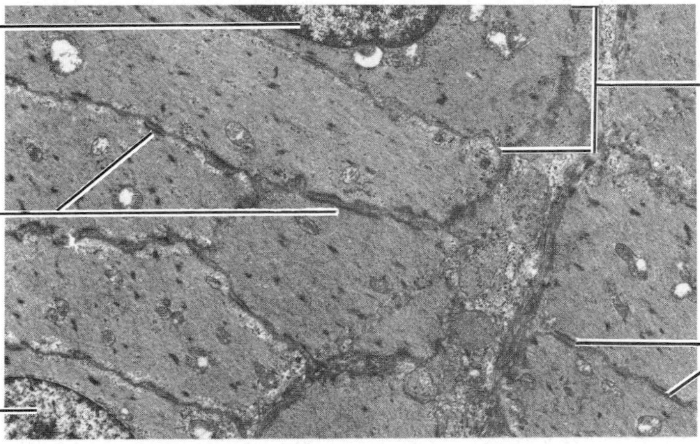

7-25

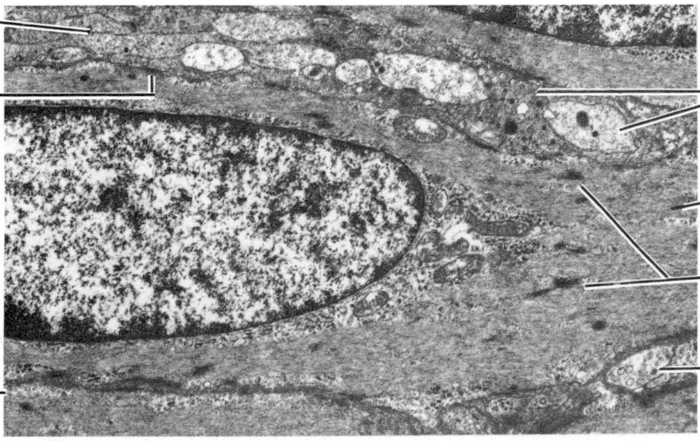

Figure 7-23. Longitudinal section. TEM, ×3000.
Figure 7-24. Cross section. TEM, ×7000.
Figure 7-25. Longitudinal section. TEM, ×15,000.

8

Nervous Tissue

Nervous tissue, one of the four basic tissues, is composed of two types of cells, nerve cells or neurons and supporting cells or neuroglia. Nerve cells are highly specialized to react to stimuli and conduct the excitation from one region of the body to another. Thus, nervous tissue shows both irritability and conductivity, properties which are essential to the functions of nervous tissue, namely, to provide communication and to coordinate body activities. The nervous tissue of the brain and spinal cord makes up the central nervous system. All other nervous tissue comprises the peripheral nervous system. Nervous tissue that is specialized to perceive different exogenous stimuli is called a receptor. The sensory stimulus is transmitted by the peripheral nervous system to the central nervous system, which acts as an integrating and communication center. Other neurons, the effectors, conduct nerve impulses away from the central nervous system to other tissues, where they elicit an effect. Neurons also are able to stimulate or inhibit other neurons that are in contact with them. The specialized contacts between neurons are called synapses. Nerve impulses are transferred between nerve cells either by electrical coupling, or by chemical transmitters. Some neurons of the brain secrete substances (hormones) directly into the blood stream and, therefore, the brain may be considered an endocrine organ.

NEURONS

KEY WORDS: perikaryon, dendrite, axon, neurofibrils, neurofilaments, neurotubules, chromophilic (Nissl) substance, axon hillock, melanin pigment, lipofuscin granules

The nerve cell, or neuron, is the structural and functional unit of nervous tissue. The neuron, usually large and complex in shape, consists of a cell body, the **perikaryon**, and several cytoplasmic processes. Processes that conduct impulses *to* the perikaryon are **dendrites** and usually are multiple; the single process that conducts impulses *away* from the perikaryon is the **axon** or axis cylinder.

The perikarya of different types of neurons vary tremendously in size (4 to 140 μm) and shape and usually contain a large, central spherical nucleus. In most neurons, the nucleus contains a prominent nucleolus. The cytoplasm is rich in organelles and may contain a variety of inclusions. Bundles of

neurofibrils form an anastomosing network around the nucleus and extend into the dendrites and axon. Neurofibrils must be stained selectively (usually with a silver preparation) to be seen with the light microscope. Ultrastructurally, neurofibrils consist of aggregates of slender **neurofilaments** (10 nm in diameter) and microtubules which, although called **neurotubules**, appear to be identical to microtubules found in cells of other tissues. The perikarya of most neurons contain the characteristic **chromophilic** or **Nissl substance**, which is best seen after staining by dyes such as cresyl violet or toluidine blue. The stained Nissl substance appears as basophilic masses within the cytoplasm of the perikaryon and dendrites, but is absent from the axon and the **axon hillock**, which is that region of the perikaryon from which the axon originates. As seen in electron micrographs, Nissl substance consists of several parallel cisternae of granular endoplasmic reticulm.

Small, slender or oval mitochondria are scattered throughout the cytoplasm and contain both the lamellar and tubular cristae. Well-developed Golgi complexes occupy a perinuclear position in the cell. Centrioles are occasionally observed, but neurons of the adult do not engage in mitotic activity.

Inclusions also are found in the perikarya of nerve cells. Dark brown granules of **melanin pigment** occur in neurons from specific regions of the brain such as the substantia nigra, locus ceruleus and dorsal motor nucleus of the vagus nerve and in spinal and sympathetic ganglia. More common inclusions are the **lipofuscin granules**, which increase with age and are thought to be the byproducts of normal lysosomal activity. The lipid droplets observed in neurons represent storage material or may occur as the result of pathological metabolism.

Nerve Processes

KEY WORDS: dendrite, dendritic spines (gemmules), axon (axis cylinder), axon hillock, collateral branches, telodendria, axoplasm, action potential

Nerve processes are cytoplasmic extensions of the perikaryon and are of two types: dendrites and axons (axis cylinder). Each neuron usually has several **dendrites** that extend from the perikaryon, dividing repeatedly to form a vast array, like branches on a tree. Although tremendously diverse in number, size and shape of the dendrites, each variety of neuron has a similar branching pattern. The cytoplasm of dendrites contains elongate mitochondria, Nissl substance, scattered neurofilaments and parallel-running microtubules. The cell membrane of most dendrites forms numerous, minute projections called **dendritic spines** or **gemmules** which serve as areas for synaptic contact between neurons; an important function of dendrites is to receive nerve impulses from other neurons. Dendrites provide most of the surface area for receptive synaptic contact between neurons, although in some neurons the perikaryon and initial segment of the axon also may act as receptor areas. The number of synaptic points on the dendritic tree varies with the type of neurons but may be in the hundreds of thousands. Dendrites play an important role in integrating the many incoming impulses.

In contrast to dendrites, a neuron has only one **axon** (or **axis cylinder**), which conducts impulses away from the parent neuron to other functionally related neurons or to effector organs. The axon arises from the **axon hillock**, an elevation on the surface of the perikaryon that can be identified with the light microscope due to the absence of Nissl substance. In some instances axons may arise from the base of a major dendrite. Axons usually are much longer and more slender than dendrites and may or may not give rise to side branches called **collaterals** which, unlike the branches of the dendritic tree, usually leave the parent axon at right angles. The axon also differs in that the diameter is constant throughout most of its course and the external surface generally is smooth. Axons end in several terminal branches called **telodendria**. The terminal branches vary in number and shape and may form a network or a basket-like arrangement around postsynaptic neurons.

The cytoplasm of the axon, the **axoplasm**, contains long, slender mitochondria, numerous neurofilaments, neurotubules and elongate profiles of smooth endoplasmic reticulum. Since axoplasm does not contain Nissl substance, protein synthesis does not occur in the axon. Protein metabolized by the axon during nerve transmission is replaced by that synthesized in cisternae of rough endoplasmic reticulum in the Nissl substance of the perikaryon. The newly synthesized protein is transported down the length of the axon: neurotubules are thought to play a role in this transport.

Axons transmit a response as an electrical impulse, the **action potential**, which begins in the region of the axon hillock and the initial segment of the axon. The impulse behaves in an "all-or-none" fashion, and only when the threshold of activity is reached is the action potential transmitted along the entire length of the axon to its termination. The axon endings synapse with adjacent neurons or terminate on effector cells. The influence of the axon on muscle or epithelial cells is always to elicit some activity, that is, they are stimulated to contract or to secrete, whereas the impulse directed to another neuron may be excitatory or inhibitory in nature.

Distribution of Neurons

KEY WORDS: gray matter, white matter, nuclei, ganglia

The central nervous system is divided into **gray matter** and **white matter**, according to the concentration of perikarya. Gray matter contains the perikarya of the neurons and their closely related processes, whereas white matter is composed chiefly of bundles or masses of axons and their surrounding sheaths. In the spinal cord, gray matter occupies a central position surrounded by white matter. In the cerebral and cerebellar cortices the gray matter assumes a peripheral position covering the white matter. Aggregates of perikarya occur in the gray matter of the central nervous system and act as distinct, functional units called **nuclei**. Similar aggregates or individual neurons located outside the central nervous system are called **ganglia**.

Types of Neurons

KEY WORDS: Golgi type I neuron, Golgi type II neuron, unipolar neuron, bipolar neuron, pseudounipolar neuron, multipolar neuron

Neurons may be divided into categories according to their location, number of dendrites and length and position of their axons. Most neurons in the vertebrates lie in the gray matter of the central nervous system. Some have numerous, well-developed dendrites and very long axons that leave the gray matter to enter the white matter of the central nervous system. They either ascend or descend in major fiber tracts of the brain or spinal cord, or leave the central nervous system and contribute to the formation of peripheral nerves. Neurons of this type conduct impulses over long distances and are called **Golgi type I neurons**. Other neurons, whose axons are short and do not leave the region where the perikaryon resides, are called **Golgi type II neurons** and are especially numerous in the cerebellar and cerebral cortices and in the retina of the eye. They vary greatly in size and shape and have several, branching dendrites. Golgi type II neurons serve primarily as association neurons, that is, they collect and disseminate nerve impulses to surrounding neurons.

Individual neurons also can be classified according to the number of dendrites. **Unipolar neurons** lack dendrites and have only a single process, the axon. Although common in the developing nervous system, they are rare in the adult. **Bipolar neurons** have a single dendrite and axon, usually located at opposite poles of the perikaryon, and are found in the retina, olfactory epithelium, and cochlear and vestibular ganglia. Neurons of all craniospinal ganglia were originally bipolar in the vertebrate embryo, but during development, the dendrite and axon migrate around the cell body and unite to form a single process. Such neurons of the adult are described as being **pseudounipolar neurons**. The combined process, often called a dendraxon, may course for a short distance and then divide into two processes. One serves as the dendrite and receives stimuli from peripheral regions of the body; the other acts as an axon and enters the gray matter of the central nervous system to synapse with other neurons. Although the process directed toward the periphery acts as a dendrite, morphologically it is unusual in that it resembles an axon. This functional dendrite is smooth, unbranched and usually receives nervous input from a receptor organ. **Multipolar neurons** are the most common type of neuron. They vary considerably in size and shape and are characterized by multiple dendrites.

Ganglia

KEY WORDS: cranial and spinal ganglia, satellite cells, sensory ganglia, pseudounipolar neuron, glomerulus, autonomic ganglia, visceral motor efferents, multipolar neurons

Ganglia are divided into cranial and spinal ganglia, and autonomic ganglia.

Macroscopically, **cranial and spinal ganglia** appear as globular swellings on the sensory roots of their respective nerves. Each ganglion is enveloped by a connective tissue capsule and may contain the perikarya of only a few neurons or as many as 55,000. A delicate network of collagenous and reticular fibers, accompanied by small blood vessels, extends between individual neurons and, together with bundles of nerve processes, often separates the perikarya into groups. The perikarya are surrounded by two distinct capsules. The inner capsule is made up of a single layer of low cuboidal supporting cells called **satellite cells**. The other capsule lies immediately outside the basal lamina of the satellite cells and consists of a vascular connective tissue. Cranial and spinal ganglia are **sensory ganglia** and contain the **pseudounipolar** type of **neuron**. The perikarya appear spherical or pear-shaped and vary from 15 to 100 μm in diameter. They often show a large, central nucleus and a distinct nucleolus. The dendraxon of the pseudounipolar neuron may become convoluted, forming what is termed a **glomerulus**. This nerve process then divides: one branch (the functional dendrite) passes to a receptor organ; the other (the functional axon) passes into the central nervous system. The perikarya of these pseudounipolar neurons do not receive synapses from other neurons.

Autonomic ganglia consist of collections of perikarya of **visceral efferent motor neurons** and are situated in swellings along the sympathetic chain or in the walls of organs supplied by the autonomic nervous system. Like cranial and spinal ganglia, they usually have a connective tissue capsule. The **neurons** are generally **multipolar** with numerous, branched dendrites and assume various shapes and sizes. Perikarya range in size from 15 to 60 μm. The nucleus is large, round and often eccentrically placed in the cell; binucleate cells are not uncommon. Lipofuscin granules are more frequent in neurons of autonomic ganglia than in craniospinal ganglia. The ganglia of the larger sympathetic chains are encapsulated by satellite cells, but a capsule may be absent around the perikarya located in the walls of the viscera. Unlike craniospinal ganglia, neurons of the autonomic ganglia receive numerous synapses and are influenced by other neurons.

Nerve Fiber

KEY WORDS: myelin, myelinated fiber, Schwann cells, neurilemmal sheath (sheath of Schwann), node of Ranvier, internodal segment (internode), neurokeratin, major dense line, intraperiod line, incisures, unmyelinated fiber, mesaxon, action potential, saltatory conduction

A nerve fiber consists of an axon or axis cylinder and a surrounding sheath derived from ectoderm. Large nerve fibers are enclosed by a lipoprotein material called **myelin**: smaller nerve fibers may or may not be surrounded by myelin and therefore nerve fibers may be classed as myelinated or unmyelinated (Fig. 8-1).

Axons of all **myelinated** peripheral **nerves** are enclosed by a sheath of flattened cells called **Schwann cells**. Like neurons, Schwann cells are derived from ectoderm but take origin from neural crest. They invest nerve fibers from near their beginnings almost to their terminations. The resulting **neurilemmal sheath (sheath of Schwann)** is continuous with the capsule of satellite cells that surrounds the perikarya of neurons in craniospinal ganglia. Schwann cells are thin, attenuated cells with flattened, elongate nuclei located near the center of the cells. The cytoplasm contains a small Golgi complex, a few scattered profiles of granular endoplasmic reticulum, scattered mitochondria, microtubules, microfilaments and, at times, numerous lysosomes. The outer cell membrane is covered by a layer of proteoglycan. The Schwann cell is responsible for the production and maintenance of the myelin on nerve fibers of the peripheral nervous system.

Both the neurilemmal and myelin sheaths are interrupted by small gaps at regular intervals along the length of the nerve fiber. These interruptions represent points of discontinuity between individual Schwann cells and are called the **nodes of Ranvier**. Thus,

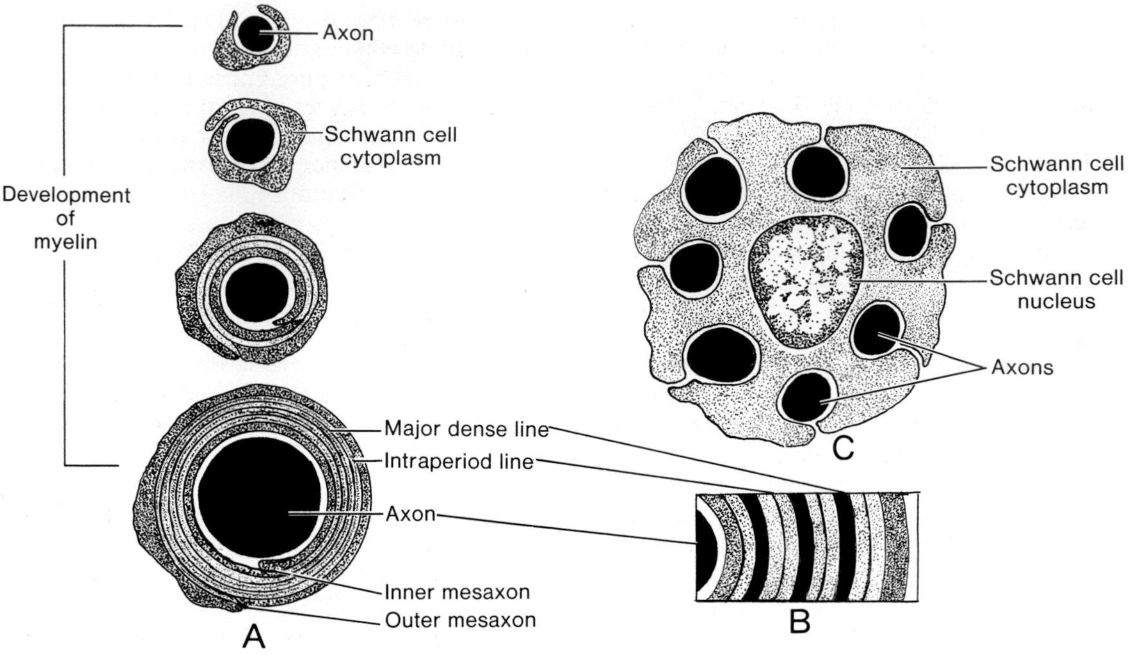

Figure 8-1. Myelinated fiber (*A* and *B*) and nonmyelinated nerve (*C*).

the neurilemmal and myelin sheaths are actually a series of small individual segments. Each segment, (the region between two consecutive nodes of Ranvier) is termed an **internodal segment**, or **internode**, and represents the area occupied by a single Schwann cell and its myelin. Myelin is not a secretory product of the Schwann cell but a mass of lipoprotein that results from successive layering of the Schwann cell plasmalemma as it wraps around the axon. Myelin may appear homogeneous but, after some methods of preparation, may be represented by a network of residual protein called **neurokeratin**. Ultrastructurally, myelin appears as a series of regular, repeating light and dark lines. The dark line, called the **major dense line**, represents apposition of the inner surfaces of the Schwann cell plasmalemma. A less dense **intraperiod line**, which represents the fusion of the outer surfaces of the Schwann cell plasmalemma, lies between the repeating major dense lines. Oblique discontinuities often are observed in the myelin of peripheral nerves and are called **incisures**, or clefts of Schmidt-Lantermann. These clefts represent a local separation of the myelin lamellae.

Unmyelinated fibers (axons) also are surrounded by Schwann cells. In electron micrographs, 15 or more unmyelinated axons often are found in recesses in the plasmalemma of a single Schwann cell. The membrane of the Schwann cell closely surrounds each axon and is intimately associated with it. As the cell membrane of the Schwann cell encircles the axon, it courses back to come in contact with itself; this point of contact is termed the **mesaxon**. In myelinated nerves, the primary infolding of the Schwann cell membrane at the axon-myelin junction is termed the internal mesaxon. The junction between the superficial lamellae of the myelin sheath and the Schwann cell plasmalemma is the external mesaxon.

The speed with which an impulse is transmitted along a nerve fiber is proportional to the diameter of the nerve fiber. The diameter of heavily myelinated nerve fibers is much greater than that of unmyelinated fibers; therefore, impulse conduction is faster in myelinated fibers. Nerve fibers in peripheral nerves can be classed according to the diameter and speed of conduction. Type A nerve fibers are large myelinated motor and sensory fibers 3 to 20 μm in diameter that conduct impulses at 15 to 120 m/second. More finely myelinated fibers with diameters up to 3 μm conduct impulses at 3 to 15 m/second and are type B fibers. They represent many of the visceral sensory fibers. Type C fibers are small unmyelinated nerve fibers that conduct impulses at 0.5 to 2 m/second.

The first event in the development of an **action potential** (Fig. 8-2) along a nerve fiber is a sudden increase in permeability to sodium ion, resulting in depolarization of the axon and development of a negative charge along the axon surface. The local current created between the depolarized and resting surface membranes causes an increased permeability of the resting membrane to sodium ion. A cycle of membrane activation is established that results in the transmission of the depolarization process (nerve impulse) along the nerve fiber. Once depolarization occurs, it will travel along the entire cell membrane of the axon. The nerve impulse lasts for only a short time and repolarization is achieved by means of a sodium pump mechanism in the axon cell membrane. The generation of the nerve impulse is an "all-or-none" phenomenon.

In the faster conducting myelinated nerves, impulses are conducted from node to node, and this method of impulse conduction is known as **saltatory conduction**. Because depolarization occurs only at the nodes of Ranvier, nerve impulses jump from node to node across the intervening internodal segment. This explains, in part, the high velocity of nerve transmission in myelinated nerve fibers.

Peripheral Nerves

KEY WORDS: mixed nerve, epineurium, fascicle, perineurium, endoneurium

Peripheral nerves consist of several nerve fibers (axons) united by surrounding connective tissue. They are **mixed nerves** consisting of sensory (afferent) and motor (efferent) nerve fibers which may by myelinated or unmyelinated. The sheath of connective tissue surrounding a peripheral nerve is called the **epineurium** and unites several bundles (**fascicles**) of nerve fibers into a single unit, the peripheral nerve. The epineurium consists of fibroblasts, longitudinally oriented collagen fibers and scattered fat cells. Each bundle or fascicle of nerve fibers is enclosed by concentric layers of flattened, fibroblast-like cells and collagen fibers that form a dense connective tissue sheath called the **perineurium**. Delicate collagenous fibers, reticular fibers, fibroblasts

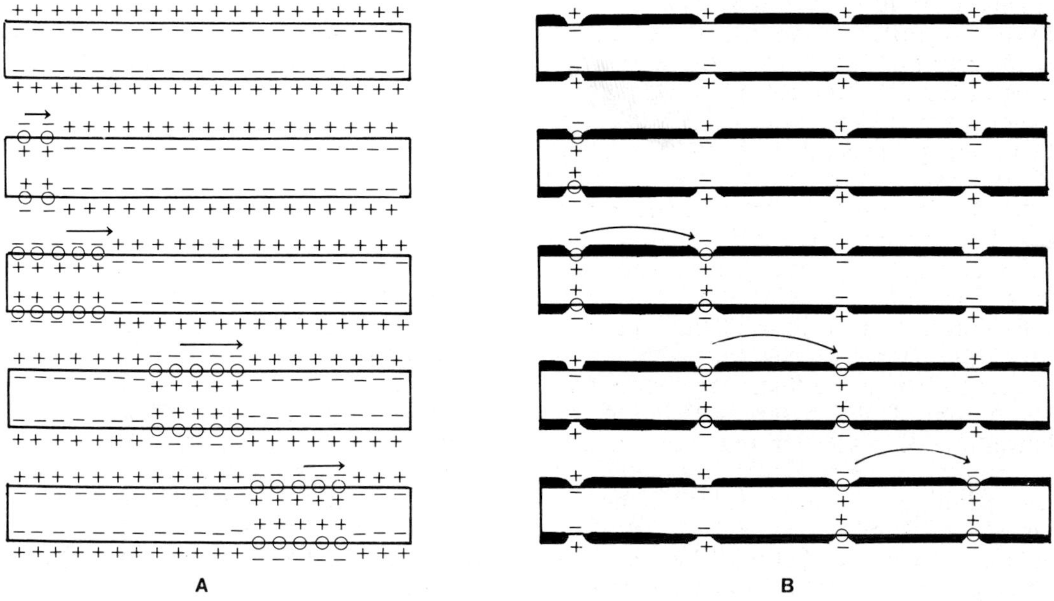

Figure 8-2. Schematic representation of action potential in (*A*) nonmyelinated and (*B*) myelinated fibers.

and macrophages lie between individual nerve fibers within each fascicle and constitute the **endoneurium**. Small blood vessels are found primarily in the epineurium and perineurium but in thicker regions of the endoneurium they may occur as delicate capillary networks.

Peripheral Nerve Endings

KEY WORDS: somatic efferents, motor end plate, motor unit, visceral efferents, receptors, free nerve endings, encapsulated nerve endings

Nerve endings increase the surface area for contact between nervous and nonnervous structures and allow stimuli to be transferred from the nerve ending to muscle, causing them to contract, or to epithelial cells, causing them to secrete. Dendrites at the periphery, when stimulated, generate impulses that are transferred along the nerve fiber to sensory ganglia and ultimately to the central nervous system.

Peripheral efferent (motor) nerve fibers can be divided into two groups. **Somatic efferent** fibers terminate in skeletal muscle as small, oval expansions called **motor end plates**. The number of skeletal muscle cells supplied by a single motor neuron constitute a **motor unit**. Muscles with a large number of motor units are capable of more precise movements than those with fewer units for the same number of muscle cells. **Visceral efferent** nerve fibers stimulate smooth muscle, cardiac muscle and glandular epithelium. Visceral motor endings of smooth muscle terminate as two or more swellings that pass between individual muscle cells. In cardiac muscle, numerous thin nerve fibers end near the surface of individual muscle cells but form no specialized contacts with them. Endings in glands are from unmyelinated nerves and form elaborate, delicate nets along the external surface of the basal lamina of the gland parenchyma; fine branches penetrate the basal lamina and pass between individual epithelial cells.

Terminal peripheral nerve fibers which are excitable to stimuli are **receptors** and are capable of transforming chemical and physical stimuli into nerve impulses. Receptors vary in morphology, may be quite complex and often are grouped into free (naked) or diffuse nerve endings and encapsulated nerve endings.

Free nerve endings are widely distributed and, although most numerous in the skin, also are found in the connective tissue of visceral organs, in deep fascia, in muscle and in serous and mucous membranes. They arise from myelinated and unmyelinated fibers of relatively small diameter. As the myelinated fibers near their terminations, they lose their myelin and form unmyelinated terminal arborizations. The unmyelinated nerve fibers end in numerous fibrils that terminate as small knob-like thickenings. Many naked nerve endings function as pain receptors. A diffuse type of naked receptor encircles the base of hair follicles to form the peritrichal nerve endings which are sensitive to hair movement. They are particularly well developed in the vibrissae of some mammals. In addition to the naked interepithelial nerve endings that terminate among epithelial cells, some form concave neurofibrillar disks applied to a single modified epithelial cell of stratified squamous epithelium. These more specialized nerve endings are known as the tactile disks of Merkel.

In **encapsulated nerve endings** the terminal is enclosed in a capsule of non-nervous tissue (Fig. 8-3). They vary considerably in size, in shape and location and in the stimuli that are perceived. As the nerve fibers near their respective capsules, they generally lose their myelin and neurolemmal sheathes and enter the capsule as a naked ending. A number of encapsulated nerve endings, their location and proposed functions are summarized in Table 8-1.

Synapse

KEY WORDS: terminal bouton, calyces (basket endings), bouton en passage, synaptic vesicles, presynaptic membrane, synaptic cleft, postsynaptic membrane, subsynaptic web, threshold of excitation, gap junction

The site where nerve impulses are transmitted from one neuron to another is called a synapse (Fig. 8-4) and may occur between axon and dendrite (axodendritic), axon and cell body (axosomatic), axon and axon (axoaxonic), dendrite and dendrite (dendrodendritic), dendrite and perikaryon (somatodendritic) or between cell bodies (somatosomatic) of adjacent neurons. The number of synapses associated with a single neuron

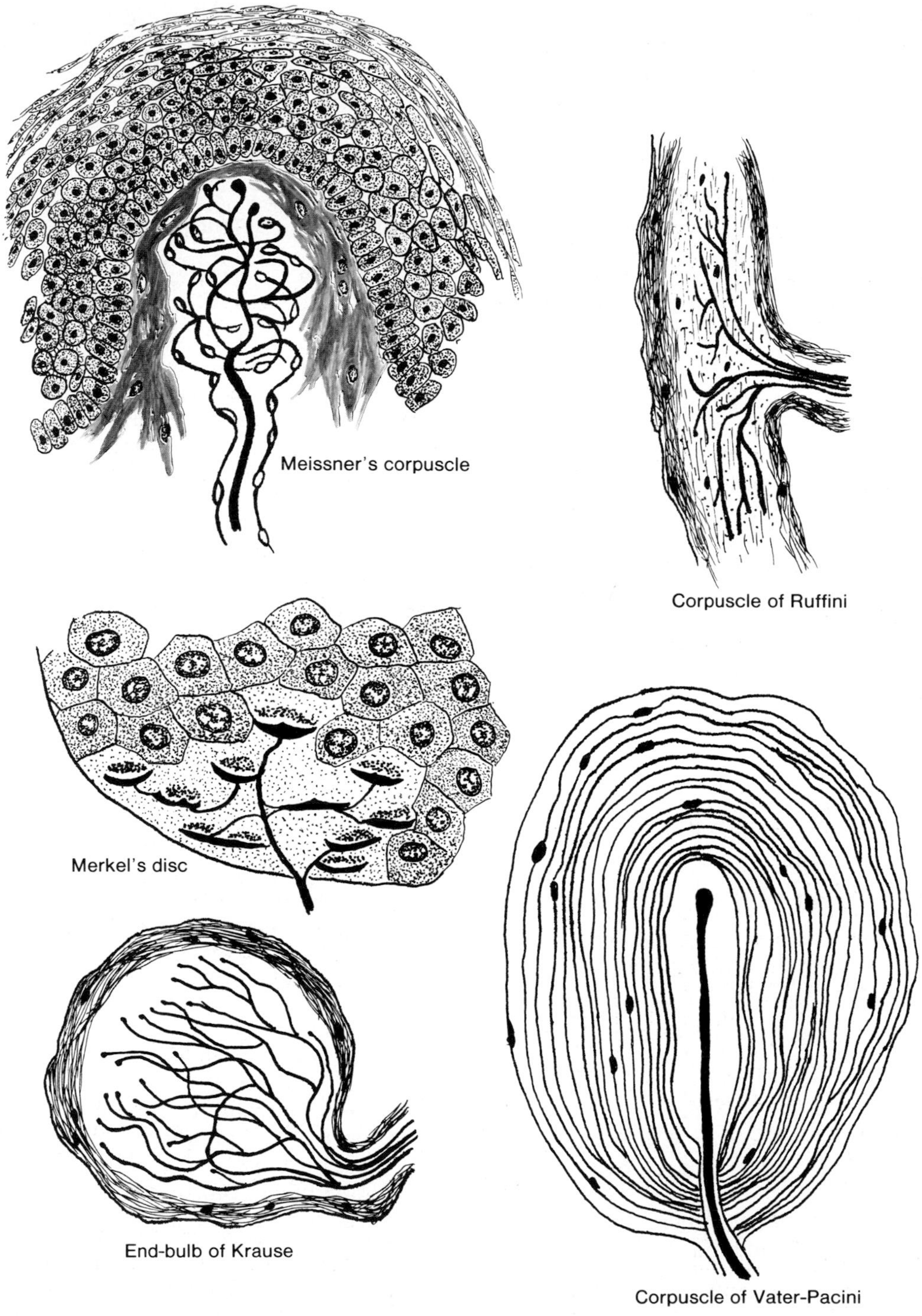

Figure 8-3. Diagram of types of sensory nerve endings.

varies according to the type of neuron. Small Golgi type II neurons (granule cells) of the cerebellum, for example, may have only a few synaptic points, whereas other neurons, such as a Golgi type I neuron (the Purkinje cell of the cerebellum), may have several hundred thousand. Physiologically, both excitatory and inhibitory synapses occur.

Table 8-1.
Encapsulated Sensory Nerve Endings

Name of Receptor	Locations	Functions
Lamellated corpuscles of Vater-Pacini	Dermis of skin, periosteum, mesenteries, pleura, nipple, pancreas, tendons, joint capsules, ligaments, walls of viscera, penis, clitoris	Proprioception, pressure, and vibration
Corpuscles of Meissner	Dermal papillae of digits, lips, genitalia and nipples	Touch
End bulbs of Krause	Dermis, conjunctiva, oral cavity	Cold, pressure
Genital corpuscles	Pernis, clitoris, nipple	Touch, pressure
Corpuscles of Ruffini	Dermis, joint capsules	Heat
Neurotendinous endings (of Golgi)	Tendons	Proprioception
Neuromuscular spindles	Skeletal muscle	Proprioception

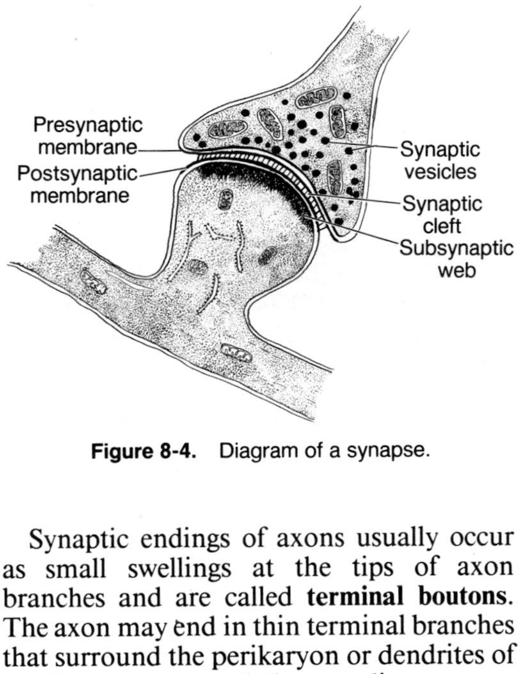

Figure 8-4. Diagram of a synapse.

Synaptic endings of axons usually occur as small swellings at the tips of axon branches and are called **terminal boutons.** The axon may end in thin terminal branches that surround the perikaryon or dendrites of another neuron, and these endings are referred to as **calyces** or **basket endings**. In addition, synaptic contacts may occur at intervals along the terminal segment of an axon, forming the **boutons en passage**.

Synaptic terminations vary considerably in form from one type of neuron to another but generally exhibit some common features. Each neuron is a distinct cellular unit and cytoplasmic continuity between cells does not occur. In some ways synaptic points resemble desmosomes and may aid in maintaining contact between nerve cells. Ultrastructurally, the presynaptic area (terminal bouton) contains clusters of mitochondria and numerous membrane bound, electron lucent vesicles with a diameter of 40 to 60 nm. These **synaptic vesicles** contain neurotransmitter substances and congregate near the **presynaptic membrane**, which is a slightly thickened area of the axon plasmalemma at the synaptic contact. Pre- and postsynaptic membranes are separated by a narrow space, 20 to 30 nm wide, called the **synaptic cleft**, which may contain fine filaments and a glycosaminoglycan. The **postsynaptic membrane** shows increased electron density, is slightly thickened and on its internal surface is associated with a network of dense filamentous material called the **subsynaptic web**. The cytoplasm of the postsynaptic region lacks the synaptic vesicles and the number of mitochondria found in the presynaptic area.

As an action potential reaches the presynaptic area of an axon, the synaptic vesicles fuse at sites along the presynaptic membrane and release transmitter substance into the synaptic cleft. The transmitter substance reacts with special receptors in the postsynaptic membrane, causing an immediate increase in the permeability of the postneuronal membrane, to sodium ion thus changing the resting membrane potential. If the postsynaptic membrane potential rises above a certain level, called the **threshold of excitation**, an action potential is transmitted by the postsynaptic neuron. The first portion of the postsynaptic neuron to initiate an action potential is the axon hillock and the initial segment of the axon.

If transmitter substances decrease the permeability of the postsynaptic membrane, the threshold of excitation rises and the net effect is inhibitory. Inhibition is thought to depend on the receptor sites in the postsynaptic membrane rather than upon specific neurotransmitter substance and transmitter substances that have an excitatory effect at one synapse may have an inhibitory influence at a synapse in a different region.

The initial segment of the axon is a few microns long and lacks a myelin sheath. In most neurons the cell membrane of this region has a lower threshold of excitation than that of the perikaryon or dendrites. Acetylcholine is the transmitter substance most commonly found in the electron-lucent synaptic vesicles of the central nervous system and motor end plates. Synaptic vesicles of most sympathetic postganglionic axons are characterized by an electron-dense core and contain catecholamines. Electrical coupling is another method of transferring impulses in some forms of synapse and occurs at **gap junctions**.

NEUROGLIA

KEY WORDS: astrocytes, protoplasmic and fibrous astrocytes, end feet (foot process), oligodendrocytes, interfascicular and perineuronal oligodendrocytes, microglia, Gitterzellen, ependyma, tela choridea, choroid plexus, cerebrospinal fluid, blood-brain barrier

Neurons form a relatively small percentage of the cells in the central nervous system, and the remainder consist of nonneuronal supporting cells called neuroglia. Depending on the location in the central nervous system, neuroglia may outnumber neurons by as much as 10:1 to 50:1 and account for more than one-half of the total weight of the brain. Neuroglia generally are smaller than neurons and in light microscope preparations can be identified by their small, round nuclei which are scattered among neurons and their processes. The term neuroglia includes the ependyma, astrocytes, oligodendrocytes and microglia. Astrocytes and oligodendrocytes are often collectively referred to as macroglia.

Morphologically the **astrocytes** are divided into protoplasmic and fibrous types. **Protoplasmic astrocytes** are found primarily in the gray matter and are characterized by numerous thick, branched processes. **Fibrous astrocytes** occur mainly in the white matter and are distinguished by long, thin, generally unbranched processes. The two forms of astrocyte may represent a single cell type that varies in its morphology, depending on its location and metabolic state. In electron micrographs, astrocytes generally show an electron-lucent, largely organelle-free cytoplasm and euchromatic nuclei. The cytoplasm of the cell body and its processes contains bundles of microfilaments.

The cell processes vary considerably in appearance. Some are thick and elongate; others are thin and sheet-like. The processes often expand to form **foot processes** or **end feet** that are aligned along the internal surface of the pia mater and around the walls of blood vessels. The largest concentration of foot processes is beneath the pial surface, where they surround the brain and spinal cord to form a membrane-like structure called the glia limitans. Astrocytes may provide a framework to give some structural support to the neurons and contribute to their nutrition and metabolic activity. However, the precise function of astrocytes in the central nervous system is unknown.

Smaller neuroglial cells with fewer processes and more deeply staining nuclei constitute the **oligodendrocytes**, two types of which usually are described. The **interfascicular oligodendrocytes** are found primarily in the fiber tracts forming the white matter of the brain and spinal cord. **Perineuronal** satellite **oligodendroctyes** are restricted to the gray matter and are closely associated with the cell bodies of neurons. The cytoplasm of both types of oligodendroglia contains free ribosomes, short cisternae of rough endoplasmic reticulum, an extensive Golgi complex and numerous mitochondria. Large numbers of microtubules that form parallel arrays course through the cytoplasm of the cell body and into its processes.

Schwann cells are not present in the central nervous system and oligodendrocytes serve as the myelin-forming cells for this region. Myelinated nerve fibers of the central nervous system have nodes of Ranvier but, unlike peripheral myelinated nerve fibers, lack incisures. The myelin sheath begins at the end of the initial segment of the axon, a few microns from the axon hillock, and ensheaths the remainder of the axon to near its termination. Each internodal segment of a nerve fiber in the central nervous system is formed by a single cytoplasmic process from an adjacent oligodendrocyte which wraps around the axon. Unlike Schwann cells of the peripheral nervous system, a single oligodendrocyte provides the internodal segments of the myelin sheath for several separate, but adjacent axons. In some regions, as in the optic nerve, a single oligodendrocyte may be responsible for the internodal segments on 40 to 50 axons. Because perineuronal satellite oligodendrocytes lie close to the perikarya of neurons, it has been proposed that the oligodendrocytes may influence the metabolism or nutrition of the neurons, but this remains to be shown conclusively. Myelination in the central nervous system is shown in Figure 8-5.

In the central nervous system, perineuronal and interfascicular oligodendrocytes have the same relationship to perikarya and their axons as that between the satellite cells of ganglia and the Schwann cells of peripheral nerve fibers. In fact, Schwann cells and satellite cells may be considered as neuroglial elements of the peripheral nervous system.

Small cells called **microglia** also are present in the central nervous system and in areas of damage or disease are thought to proliferate and become phagocytic. As cellular debris is phagocytosed, the cells enlarge and then are known as **Gitterzellen**, or compound granular corpuscles. Labeled cells identical to microglia can be found in the central nervous system after intravenous injection of radiolabeled monocytes. Thus, the monocyte appears to be the precursor of microglial cells, consistent with the concept of a mononuclear system of phagocytes in which, regardless of where the phagocytic cells reside, all are derived from bone marrow monocytes.

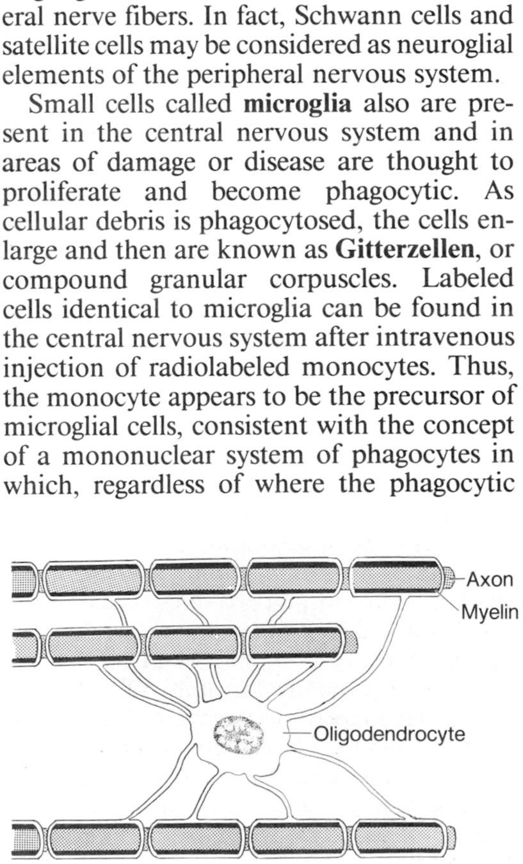

Figure 8-5. Myelination in the central nervous system.

The **ependyma** lines the central canal of the spinal cord and ventricles of the brain. It consists of a simple epithelium in which the closely-packed cells vary from cuboidal to columnar. The luminal surfaces of the cells show large numbers of microvilli and, depending upon the location, may exhibit cilia. Adjacent cells are united by desmosomes and zonulae adherens, but zonulae occludens generally are not seen between ependymal cells. Hence, cerebrospinal fluid in the central canal and ventricles can pass between ependymal cells and enter the parenchyma of the central nervous system. The bases of ependymal cells have long, thread-like processes that branch enter the substance of the brain and spinal cord and may extend to the external surface, where they contribute end feet to the glia limitans.

The ependyma constitutes a secretory epithelium in the ventricles of the brain, where it is in direct contact with a highly vascularized region of pia mater called the **tela choroidea**. The modified ependyma and tela choroidea form the **choroid plexus**, which produces **cerebrospinal fluid**. Ependymal cells of the choroid plexus are columnar, closely-packed and bear numerous microvilli on their luminal surfaces. Unlike other regions of the ependyma, cell apices here are joined by zonulae occludens, which prevent passage of materials between cells. The ependymal cells lie on a continuous basal lamina which separates them from a connective tissue that contains small bundles of collagen fibers, pia-arachnoid cells and numerous blood vessels. Capillary endothelial cells in this region, unlike those elsewhere in the brain, have numerous fenestrations. Fluid readily moves through the capillary walls but is prevented from entering the ventricles by the zonula occludens. Ependymal cells secrete sodium ion into the ventricles and chloride ion, water and other substances follow passively. Protein and glucose concentrations are relatively low. Cerebrospinal fluid is formed continuously, moves slowly through the ventricles of the brain and finally enters the subarachnoid space. It surrounds and protects the central nervous system from mechanical injury and is important in the metabolism of the central nervous system.

Certain substances in the blood are prevented from entering the central nervous system although they readily gain access to other tissues. Capillaries deep in the spinal cord and brain are sheathed by end feet of astrocytes, and the nonfenestrated endothelial cells are united by occluding tight junctions. In addition, the internal plasma membrane of the endothelial cells is thought to have special properties which prevent passage of these substances. Together, the tight junctions and internal plasmalemma of the endothelial cells constitute the **blood-brain barrier**.

Spinal Cord

KEY WORDS: gray matter, internuncial neurons, central canal, ependyma, white matter, funiculus, tracts

The spinal cord is subdivided into a central H-shaped region of gray matter and a surrounding layer of white matter. **Gray matter** consists mainly of perikarya of neurons, their dendrites, and surrounding neuroglial cells. It is arranged into two dorsal horns and two ventral horns. The dorsal horns contain perikarya of multipolar neurons receiving sensory impulses that enter the spinal cord from the peripheral nervous system. Neurons of the dorsal horns transmit the impulses to other neurons in this and other areas of gray matter and are referred to as **internuncial neurons**. The multipolar neurons in the ventral horns are the largest in the spinal cord and transmit motor impulses from the spinal cord to the periphery. In the thoracic and upper lumbar regions of the spinal cord, small multipolar neurons form an intermediolateral horn that provides preganglionic sympathetic fibers for the autonomic nervous system. The **central canal** of the spinal cord lies in the center of the crossbar of the H-shaped gray matter and is lined by **ependyma**.

The surrounding **white matter** consists primarily of myelinated axons and lacks the perikarya and dendrites of the neurons. It is subdivided into anterior, lateral and posterior funiculi by the dorsal and ventral horns of the gray matter. A **funiculus** consists of several **tracts**, each tract in turn containing several bundles of nerve fibers. Nerve fibers in each tract carry similar impulses, motor or sensory, that either ascend or descend along the long axis of the spinal cord.

CEREBELLAR AND CEREBRAL HEMISPHERES

The cerebellar and cerebral hemispheres differ from the spinal cord in that the gray matter is located at the periphery and the white matter lies centrally. Both regions of the brain consist of an outer cortex of gray matter and a subcortical region of white matter.

Cerebral Cortex

KEY WORDS: laminated appearance, pyramidal cells, apical dendrite, cells of Betz, stellate (nonpyramidal) cells

The cerebral cortex ranges from 1.5 to 4.0 mm in thickness and contains about 14 billion neurons in addition to nerve processes and supporting glial elements. In all but a few regions it is characterized by a **laminated appearance**. Perikarya generally are organized into five layers. Starting at the periphery of the cerebral cortex the general organization of neurons is: molecular layer (I), external granular layer (II), external pyramidal layer (III), internal granular layer (IV), internal pyramidal layer (V) and multiform layer (VI). The molecular layer (I) is a largely cell-free zone just beneath the surface of the cortex. Neurons of similar type tend to occupy the same layer in the cerebral cortex, although each cellular layer is composed of several different types. For convenience of description, these neurons are often placed in two major groups: pyramidal cells and stellate or nonpyramidal cells.

The perikarya of **pyramidal cells** are pyramidal in shape and have a large **apical dendrite** that usually is orientated toward the surface of the cerebral cortex and enters into the overlying layers; a single axon enters the subcortical white matter. They are found in layers II, III, V and to a lesser degree in layer VI. Very large pyramidal-shaped neurons (the **cells of Betz**) are present in the internal pyramidal layer (V) of the frontal lobe. **Stellate (nonpyramidal) cells** lack the pyramidal-shaped perikarya and the large apical dendrite. They occur in all layers of the cerebral cortex but are concentrated in the internal granular layer (IV). Impulses entering the cortex are relayed primarily to stellate cells and then are transmitted to pyramidal cells in the various layers by the vertical axons of the nonpyramidal cells. Axons of pyramidal cells generally leave the cortex and extend to other regions of the brain and to the spinal cord.

The cerebral cortex functions in hearing, vision, speech, voluntary motor control and learning.

Cerebellar Cortex

KEY WORDS: molecular layer, stellate cells, basket cells, Purkinje cell layer, granule cell layer, mossy fibers, climbing fibers

The cerebellar cortex is characterized by three layers: an outer molecular layer, a middle Purkinje cell layer and an inner granule cell layer.

The **molecular layer** is largely a synaptic area with relatively few nerve cells. It consists primarily of unmyelinated axons from the granule cells, the axons running parallel to the cortical surface. It also contains large dendrites of the underlying Purkinje cells and, in its superficial portion, contains small scattered neurons called **stellate cells**. Other small neurons located deep in this layer adjacent to Purkinje cells are called **basket cells**.

The **Purkinje cell layer** is formed by the cell bodies of the Purkinje cells—large pear-shaped neurons aligned in a single row and characterized by large, branching dendrites that lie in the molecular layer. They represent Golgi type I neurons and number approximately 15 million. Three-dimensionally, the large dendritic trees occupy a narrow plane, reminiscent of fan coral, so arranged that each dendritic tree is parallel to its neighbor. A single, small axon from the Purkinje cell passes through the granule cell layer and synapses with neurons in the central cerebellar area.

The **granule cell layer** consists of numerous, closely-packed, small neurons the axons of which enter the molecular layer to synapse with dendrites of Purkinje cells. The granule cell represents a Golgi type II neuron. They have small, round nuclei with a coarse chromatin pattern and only scant cytoplasm; dendrites are short and claw-like. The axon enters the molecular layer, bifurcates and runs parallel to the surface but perpendicular to the wide plane of the Purkinje cell dendritic tree. The axon of a granule cell synapses with approximately 450 Purkinje cells in a relationship similar to that of wires coursing along (through) telephone poles. Axons of granule cells also form synapses with stellate and basket neurons in the molecular layer. Another type of small neuron, the Golgi cell, is found in the outer zone of the granule cell layer.

Two types of afferent nerve fibers enter the cerebellar cortex from other regions of the central nervous system. These are the **mossy fibers,** which synapse with granule cells, and the **climbing fibers**, which enter the molecular layer and wind about the dendrites of the Purkinje cells. The cerebellum primarily modulates and coordinates the activity of skeletal muscle.

Meninges

KEY WORDS: dura mater, epidural space, subdural space, arachnoid, trabeculae, subarachnoid space, pia mater

In addition to a covering of bone (skull, vertebral column), the central nervous system is contained within three connective tissue membranes called meninges. The outermost, the **dura mater**, consists primarily of dense collagenous connective tissue. Around the brain it comprises two layers and serves both as a periosteum for the cranium and as the external covering of the brain. The periosteal layer is rich in blood vessels, nerves and cells. The inner layer is less vascular and the interior surface is lined by a simple squamous epithelium. Around the spinal cord, the dura is a single layer of dense collagenous connective tissue that contains scattered elastic fibers. The outer surface is covered by a simple squamous epithelium, separated from the periosteum of surrounding vertebrae by an **epidural space** filled by loose connective tissue rich in fat cells and veins. The inner surface of the spinal dura also is lined by a simple squamous epithelium. Between it and the next meninx, the arachnoid, is a narrow fluid-filled space called the **subdural space.**

The **arachnoid** (Figure 8-6) is a thin, netlike, avascular membrane made up of fine collagenous fibers and scattered elastic fibers. The outer region forms a smooth sheet while the inner surface gives rise to numerous strands or **trabeculae**, which extend into

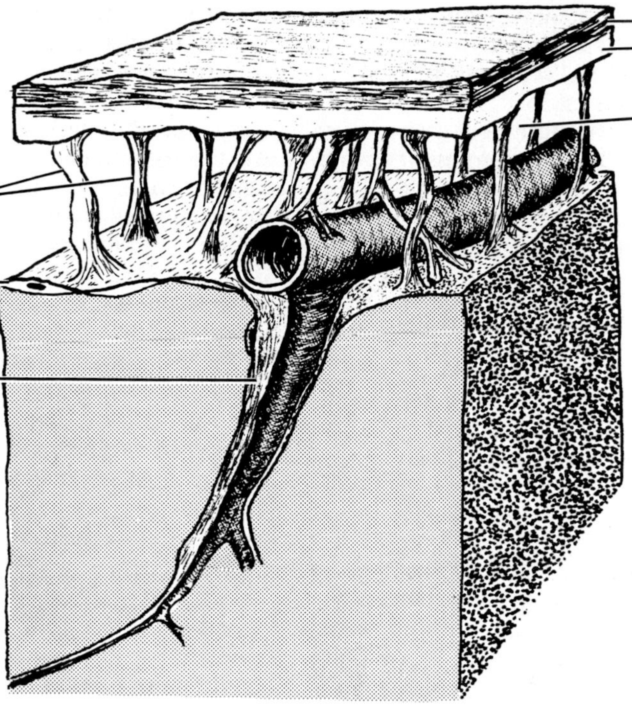

Figure 8-6. Diagram of the pia arachnoid.

and blend with, the underlying pia mater. The inner surface of the arachnoid, the trabeculae, and the external surface of the pia are covered by simple squamous epithelium that also lines a large space, the **subarachnoid space**, which contains cerebral spinal fluid.

The **pia mater** is a thin, vascular membrane that closely invests the brain and spinal cord. Because the pia and arachnoid are closely related, they often are considered together as the pia arachnoid. The pia consists of delicate collagenous and elastic fibers, together with fibroblasts, macrophages and scattered mesenchymal cells. Blood vessels entering and leaving the brain substance are invested by a sheath of pia mater. A perivascular space surrounds the vessels as they extend into the substance of the central nervous system and is continuous with the subarachnoid space.

DEVELOPMENT OF NERVOUS TISSUE

Most of the nervous tissue arises from ectoderm on the dorsal surface of the embryonic disc, in the region called the neural plate. As a result of mitotic activity and cell growth, the lateral edges of the neural plate fold upward to form a neural groove. The edges of the folds converge, fuse, and create a hollow neural tube which separates from the overlying ectoderm. Differential proliferation of ectoderm cells along the internal aspect of the neural tube ultimately gives rise to the brain and spinal cord. Some of the proliferating cells differentiate into neurons; others become the various glial elements.

Three concentric zones become visible in the wall of the neural tube—an internal ependymal layer, a wide intermediate mantle layer and an outer marginal layer. Cells of the ependymal layer divide, migrate to the mantle layer and differentiate into neuroblasts or glioblasts. Neurons differentiate first, followed by astrocytes and, later, by oligodendrocytes.

In the spinal cord, the ependymal zone gives rise to the ependyma; the mantle zone becomes the gray matter, while the white matter develops from the marginal zone. Presumptive neurons in the mantle layer initially are apolar neuroblasts but with development of cytoplasmic processes at opposite sides of the cell body, they become bipolar neurons. As differentiation proceeds, one process (a primitive axon), elongates while the other is replaced by several small processes (primordial dendrites) and multipolar neurons develop. The axons enter into and form the marginal layer. Depending on the region, myelinization follows the differentiation of oligodendrocytes.

The regions of the neural tube that initially form the cerebral and cerebellar cortices show three zones similar to those in the spinal cord. Differentiating neurons in the mantle zone of the cerebral cortex migrate into the marginal zone to establish superficial cortical layers. The stratified appearance of the adult cerebral cortex results from successive waves of migration of neuroblasts into the marginal zone and the differentiation of different types of neurons in the cortex. Sensory areas of the cerebral cortex are typified by numerous granular cells (neurons) whereas motor areas are characterized by large numbers of pyramidal cells.

Initially, the developing cerebellar cortex also is arranged into ependymal, mantle and marginal zones. As development progresses, some neuroblasts from the mantle zone migrate into the marginal zone of the cerebellar cortex to become Golgi and granular cells, while others remain in the mantle zone to form cerebellar nuclei. As this takes place, a second migration occurs and these (the Purkinje cells), together with cells from the first migration, establish the definitive cerebellar cortex.

Simultaneously with development of the neural tube, a second source of neurons, the neural crest, develops and gives rise to neurons and supportive (glial) elements. The neural crest arises at the time the neural tube fuses. Along the crest of each neural fold, ectodermal cells lose their epithelial characteristics, detach and migrate into the mesoderm along either side of the neural tube, where they acquire the characteristics of mesenchymal cells. Neural crest is a major contributor to the peripheral nervous system and gives rise to neurons and supporting cells (glia and satellite cells) of spinal root ganglia; Schwann cells; some neurons in the sensory ganglia of cranial nerves V, VII, IX and X; supporting cells (but not the neurons) of the geniculate, acoustic, petrosal and nodose ganglia. Other cells of the neural crest envelop the neural tube and contribute to the formation of the meninges.

FUNCTIONAL SUMMARY

An essential function of nervous tissue is communication. Nerve tissue is able to fulfill this role because of its ability to react to various stimuli and to transmit the impulses from one region to another. Thus, the organism is able to react to the external environment, to internal events and integrate and coordinate body functions. In cortical regions of the brain, complex interrelationships between different types of neurons provide intellect, memory and conscious experience and for the interpretation of special impulses from the eye and ear into the sensations of sight and sound, respectively. All contribute to the formation of the personality and behavior of the individual.

Neurons are the structural and functional units of nervous tissue. They generally are complex in shape and usually have several cytoplasmic processes. Dendrites conduct impulses to the perikaryon and a single axon conducts impulses from the perikaryon to other neurons or effector organs. Receptor organs of nerve tissue convert mechanical, chemical or other stimuli into nerve impulses which are transmitted along a physiological dendrite to its cell body located in spinal or cranial ganglia. From ganglia the impulses are relayed to other neurons in the central nervous

system. Nerve fibers of most somatic sensory neurons are large and myelinated and impulses are relayed quickly to the central nervous system to elicit a response. Most effector and internuncial neurons are multipolar and their numerous dendrites summate the excitatory and inhibitory impulses that influence a specific neuron. Dendrites of this type of neuron are generally unmyelinated. When the threshold of activity is attained, an action potential is generated in the region of the axon hillock and/or initial segment of the axon. These regions of the neuron have a lower threshold of excitation than the dendrites or perikaryon. The impulse is conducted by the axon to other neurons or an effectory organ to elicit a response. The speed of conduction depends on fiber diameter and usually reflects the degree of myelinization, both in peripheral nerve fibers and in those of the central nervous system. Myelin is formed by consecutive layerings of the plasmalemma of adjacent supporting cells. In the peripheral nervous system it is formed by Schwann cells scattered at intervals along a single axon. Oligodendrocytes are responsible for myelination in the central nervous system and form internodal segments on more than one axon. Myelin is thought to act as an insulating material and to prevent the wave of depolarization (action potential) from traveling along the entire length of the axolemma as occurs in unmyelinated nerve fibers. Depolarization occurs only at the nodes of Ranvier in myelinated nerves because of the insulating effect of myelin, and nerve impulses jump the internodal segment to adjacent nodes. This saltatory conduction explains in part the greater speed of nerve impulses transmitted by myelinated nerve fibers.

Communication between neurons or between neurons and effector organs takes place at specific contact points called synapses. At these points nerve impulses are transferred directly to other cells either by chemical transmitters or electrical coupling. The terminal axons of some neurons, such as those in the hypothalmic and paraventricular regions, may secrete peptides or other substances directly into the blood stream and act as endocrine tissues. These particular neurons influence cells that are not in direct contact with them.

Neurons are surrounded by supporting cells. In the peripheral nervous system neurons are intimately associated with Schwann and satellite cells which, like astrocytes and oligodendrocytes of the central nervous system, provide both structural and metabolic support to their associated neurons. The ependyma represents glial cells that form a simple epithelium lining, for the central canal of the spinal cord and the ventricals of the brain. In regions of the ventricles, ependyma comes in direct contact with vascularized regions of the pia mater (tela choroidea) to form the choroid plexus. The choroid plexus actively and continuously produces cerebrospinal fluid which surrounds and protects the brain and spinal cord and plays an important role in their metabolism.

The meninges provide protective coverings for the brain and spinal cord and also contain numerous blood vessels which supply the structures of the central nervous system.

Atlas for Chapter 8

8-7 Neurons

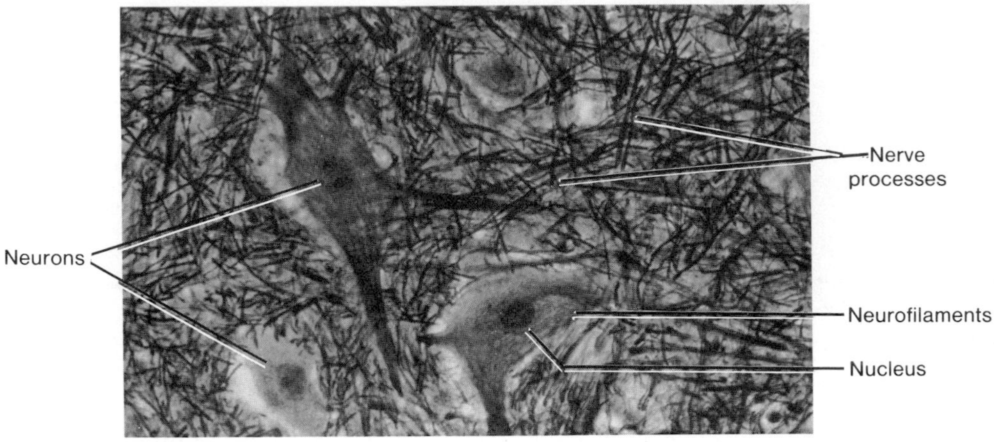

8-8

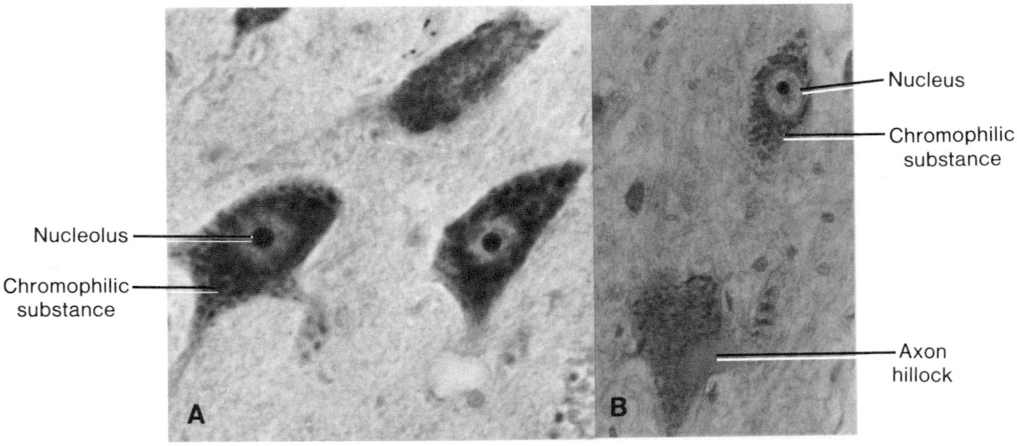

8-9

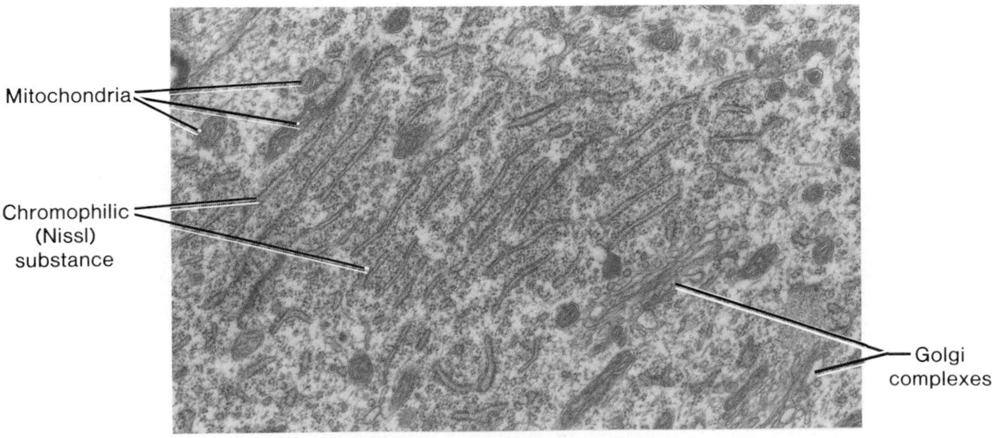

Figure 8-7. Spinal cord. LM, ×400.
Figure 8-8. *A*, spinal cord (human). LM, ×400. *B*, spinal cord. LM, ×400.
Figure 8-9. Nissl body in inferior olivary neuron. TEM, ×20,500.

8-10 Nerve

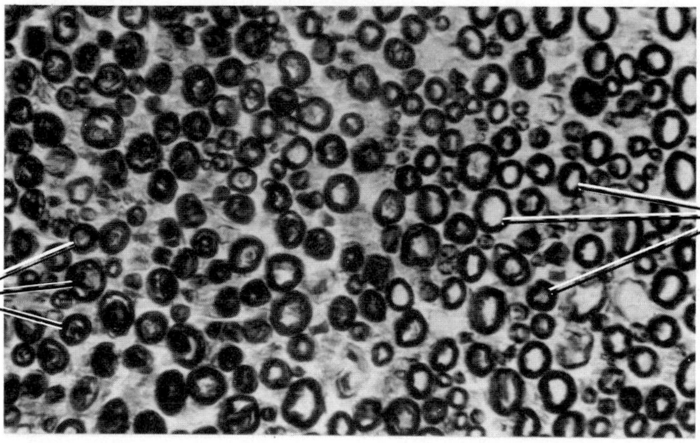

8-11

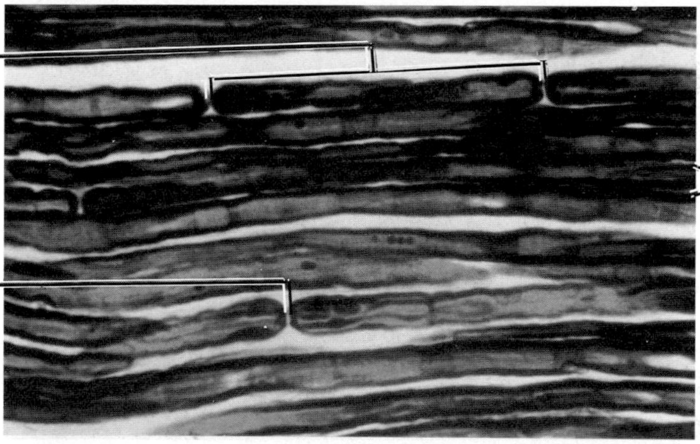

8-12

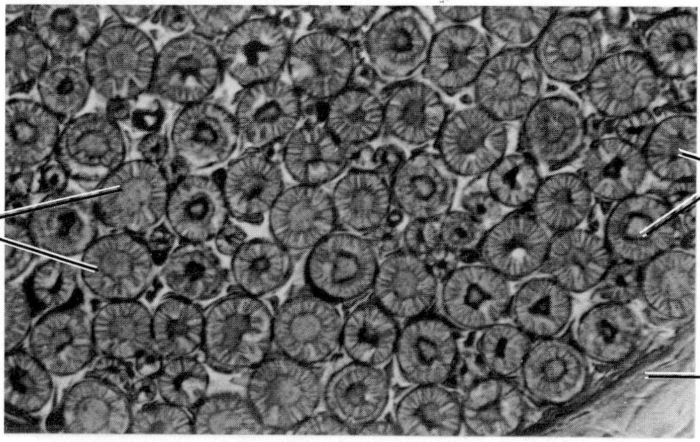

Figure 8-10. Peripheral nerve. LM, ×400.
Figure 8-11. Peripheral nerve. LM, ×400.
Figure 8-12. Peripheral nerve (cross section). LM, ×400.

8-13

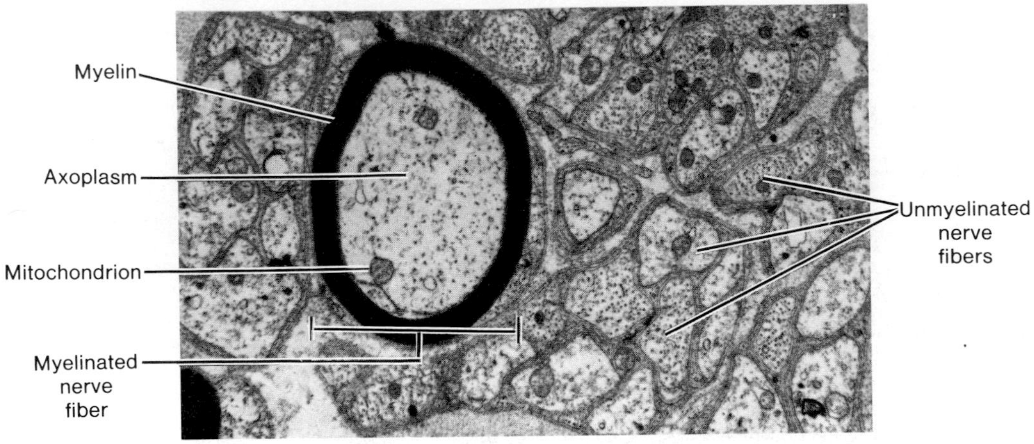

8-14

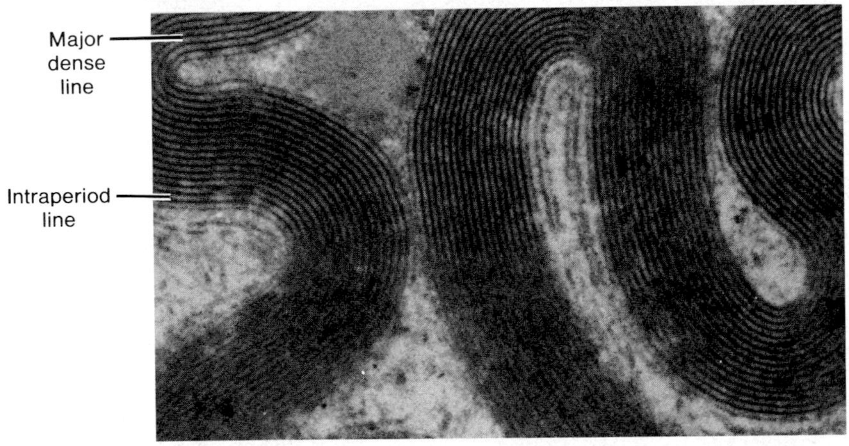

8-15

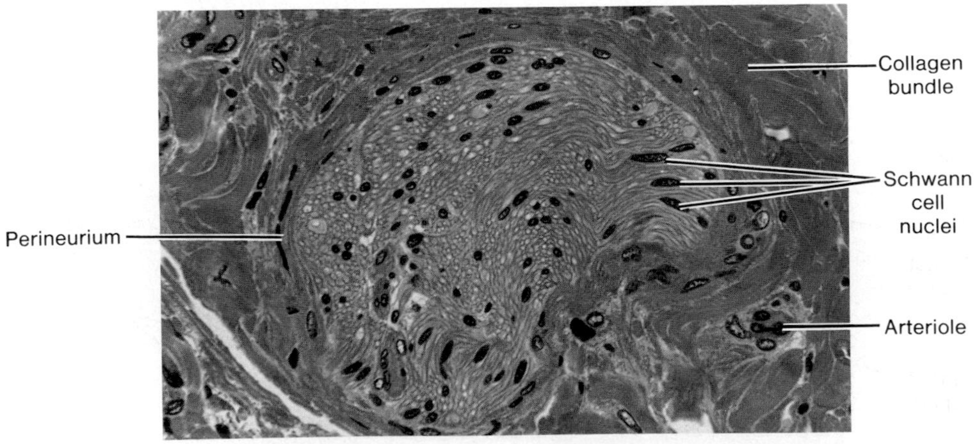

Figure 8-13. Peripheral nerve (mixed). TEM, ×8000.
Figure 8-14. Myelin. TEM, ×54,000.
Figure 8-15. Peripheral nerve. LM, ×250.

8-16

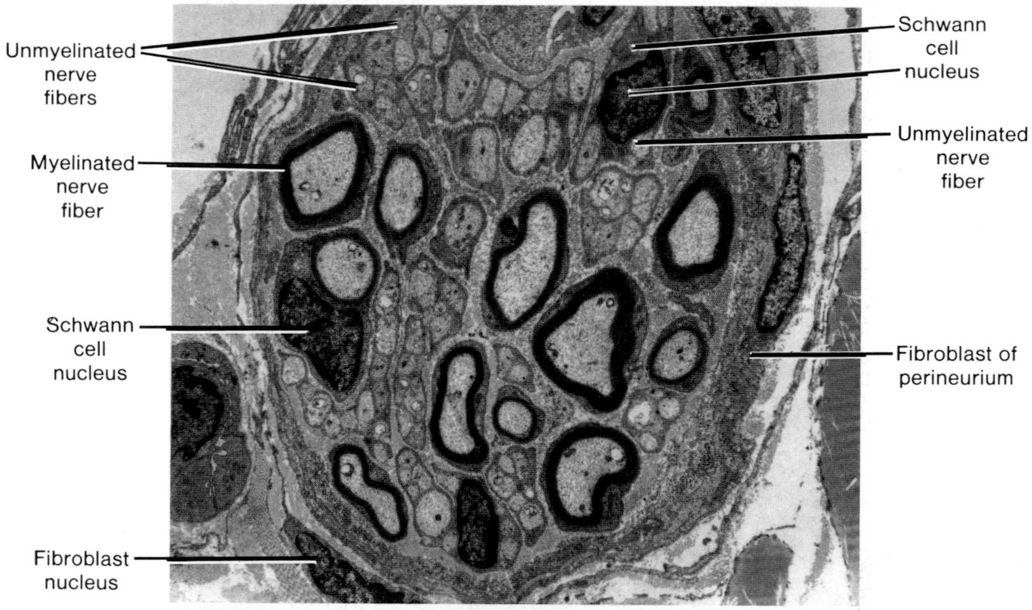

8-17 Synapse

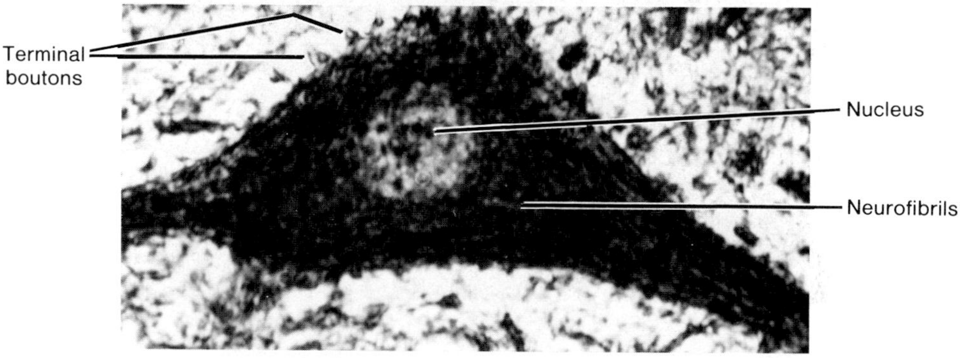

8-18

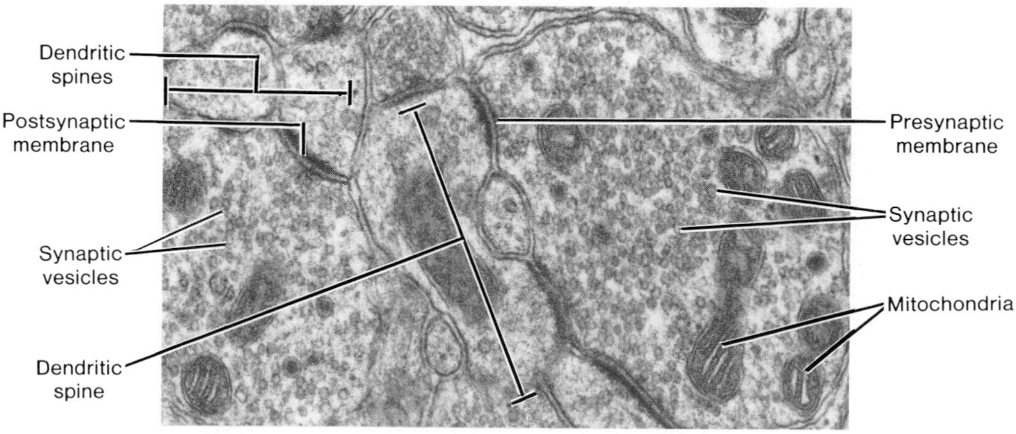

Figure 8-16. Peripheral nerve (mixed). TEM, ×2000.
Figure 8-17. Perikaryon of spinal neuron. LM, ×1000.
Figure 8-18. Synaptic endings of dendritic spines. TEM, ×39,900.

Nerve Endings

8-19

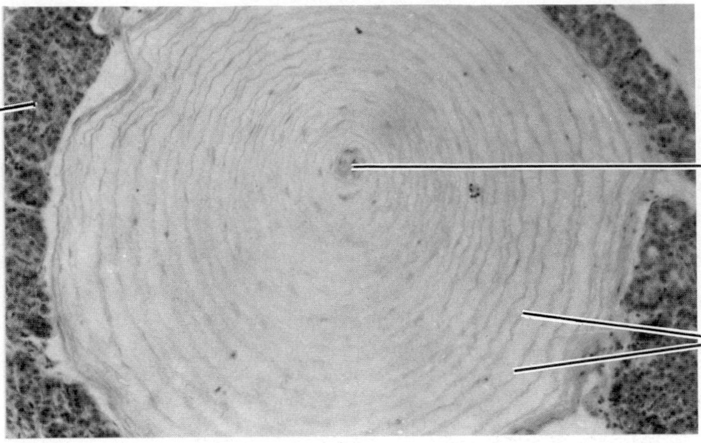

8-20

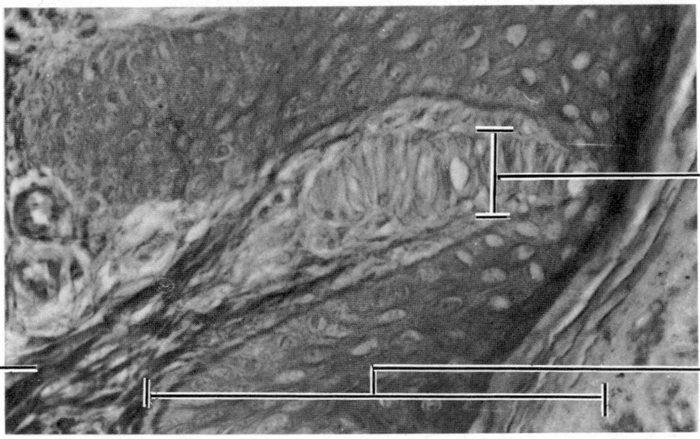

8-21

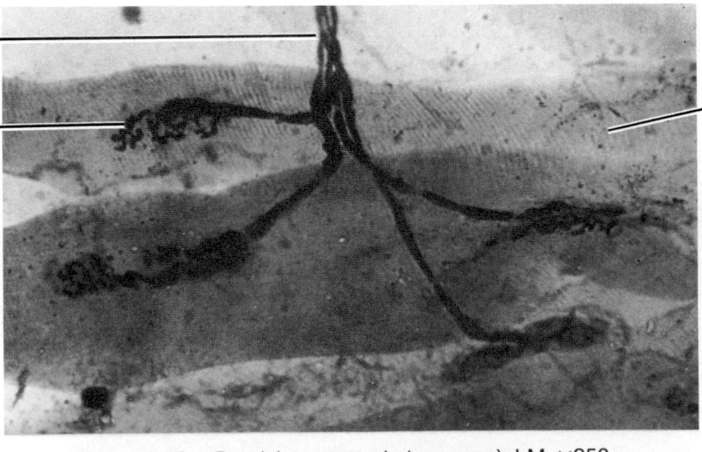

Figure 8-19. Paccinian corpuscle (pancreas). LM, ×250.
Figure 8-20. Meissner's corpuscle (human skin). LM, ×400.
Figure 8-21. Motor end plates (human muscle). LM, ×400.

8-22 Ganglia

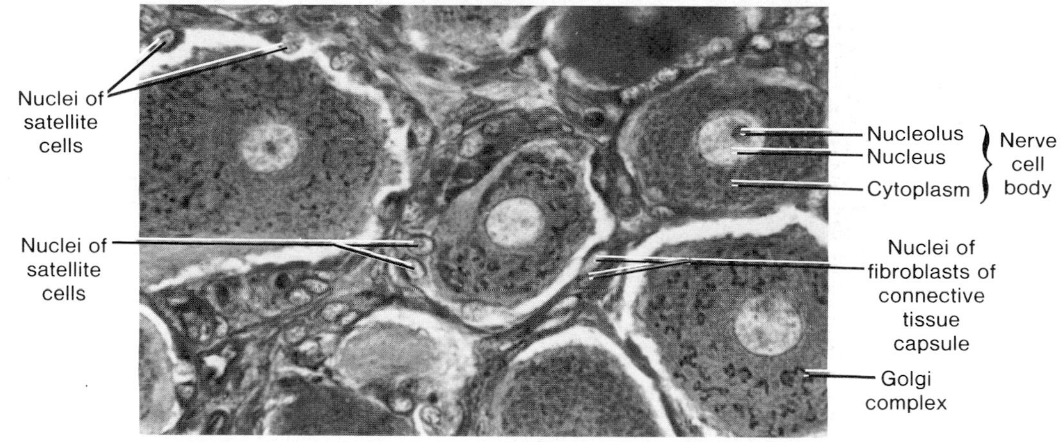

8-23

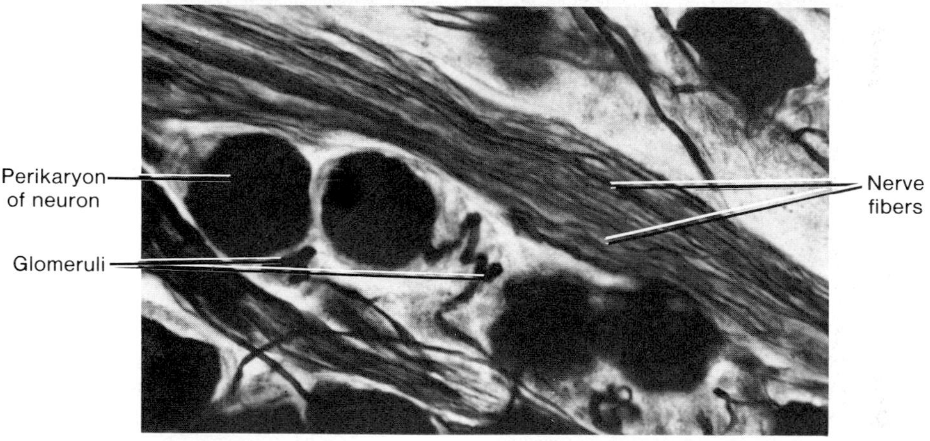

8-24

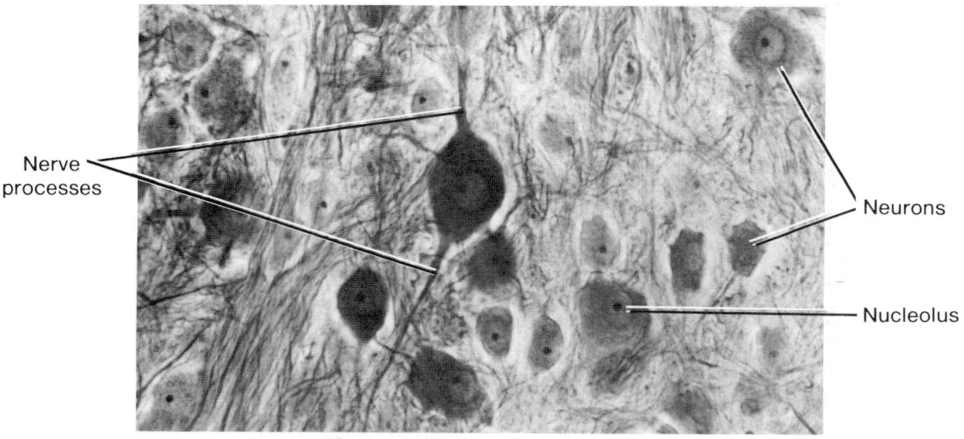

Figure 8-22. Dorsal root ganglion. LM, ×300.
Figure 8-23. Dorsal root ganglion. LM, ×250.
Figure 8-24. Autonomic ganglion. LM, ×250.

8-25

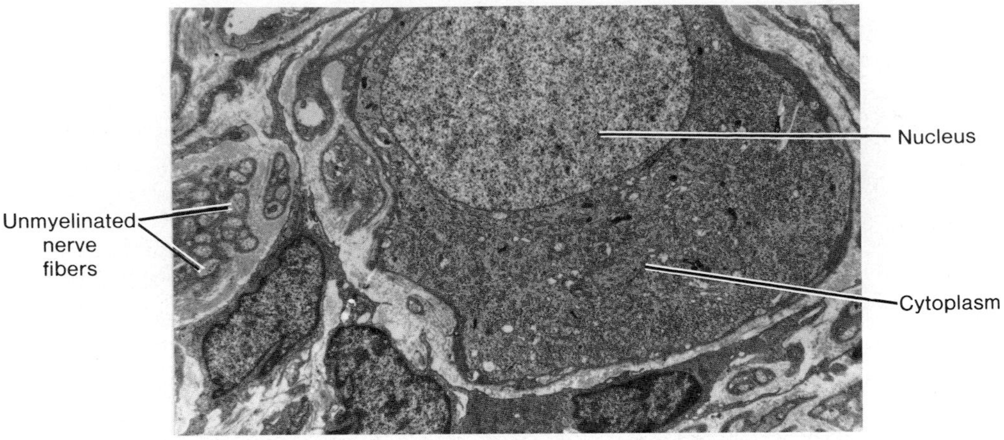

8-26 Central Nervous System

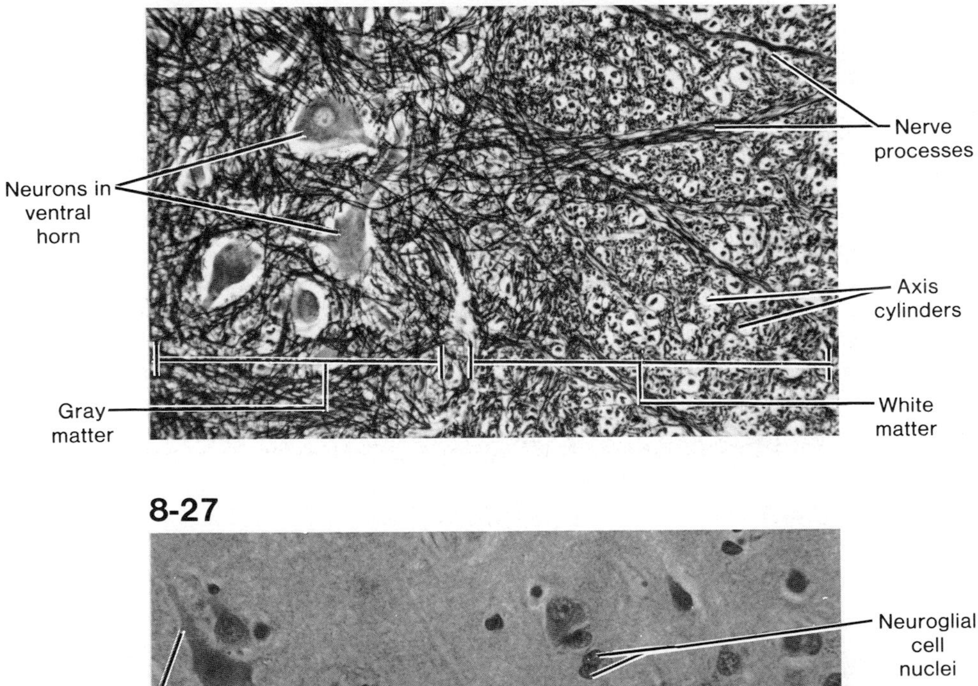

8-27

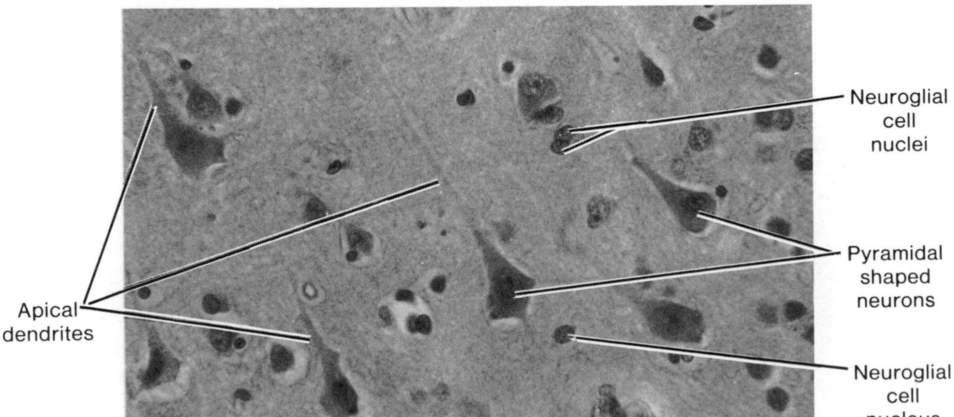

Figure 8-25. Autonomic neuron (salivary gland). TEM, ×2000.
Figure 8-26. Spinal cord (human). LM, ×400.
Figure 8-27. Cerebral cortex (human). LM, ×250.

8-28

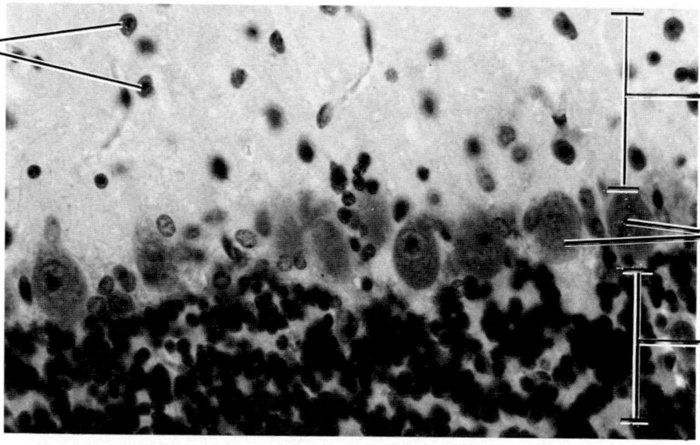

8-29

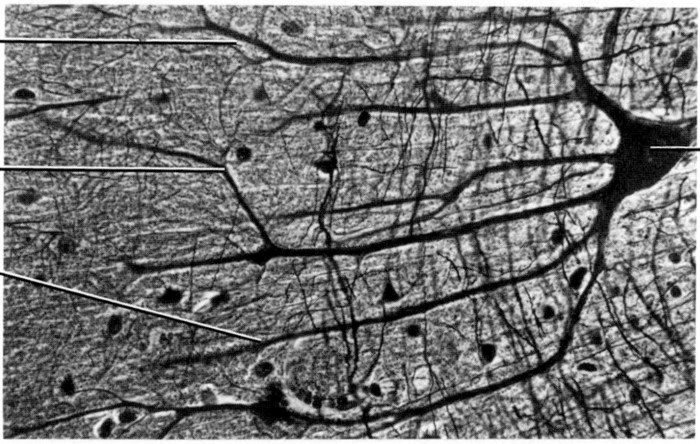

8-30 **Glia**

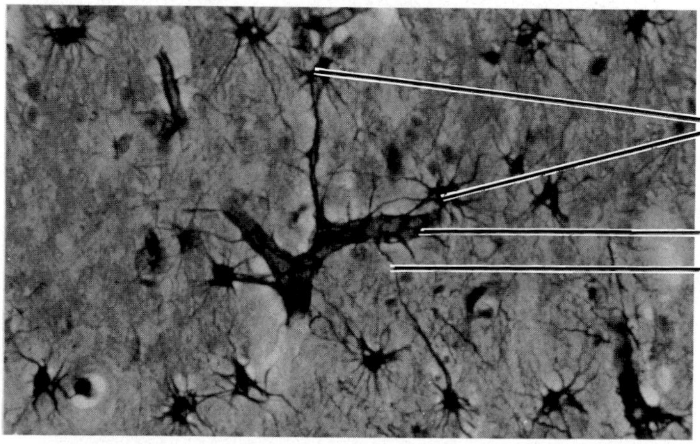

Figure 8-28. Cerebellar cortex. LM, ×250.
Figure 8-29. Cerebellar cortex. LM, ×250.
Figure 8-30. Fibrous astrocytes (white matter). LM, ×300.

8-31 Development

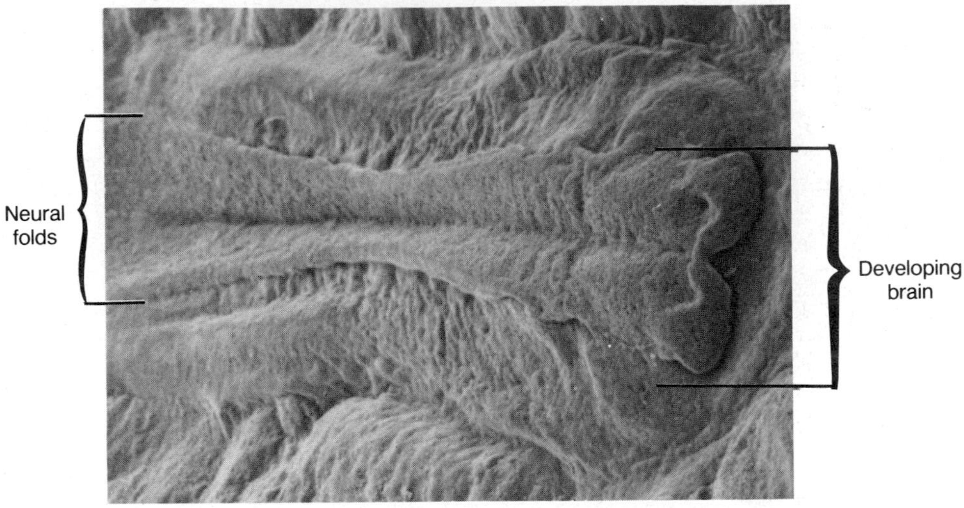

8-32

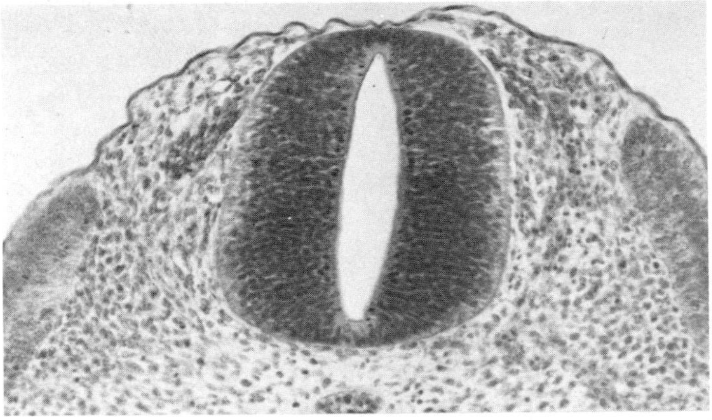

8-33

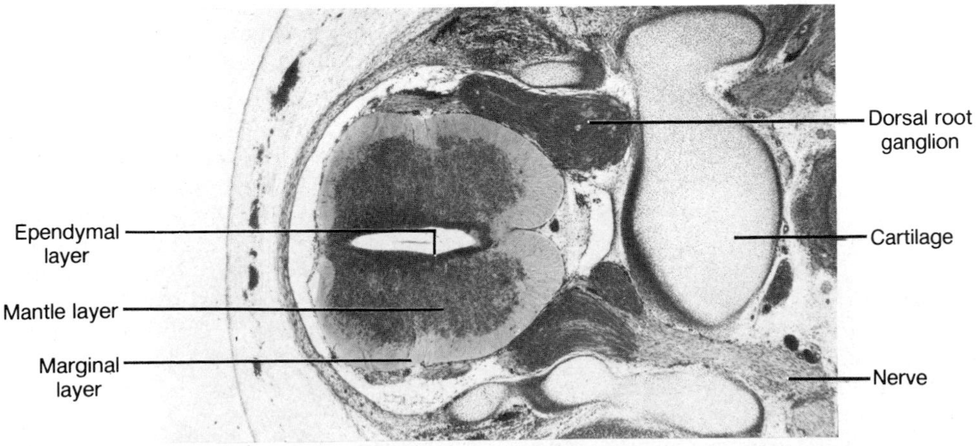

Figure 8-31. Developing nervous system (opossum). SEM, ×40.
Figure 8-32. Neural tube (pig). LM, ×250.
Figure 8-33. Developing spinal cord (human). LM, ×50.

9

The Eye

Eyes are photoreceptors which contain systems of convex surfaces that transmit and focus light on a sensitive surface. Images formed there are transmitted to the brain where they are interpreted, correlated and translated into the sensation of sight. The image-forming surface is sensitive to the intensity of wavelength (color) of light and eyes can regulate the amount of light admitted and change their focal lengths.

In the human, the eyes are almost spherical in shape and are located in and protected by bony sockets provided with a protective padding of fat. Because the eyes are offset from each other, the images formed are correspondingly offset and provide for binocular vision. Integration of the binocular images results in a three-dimensional quality of sight through which depth and spacial orientations are recognized.

GENERAL STRUCTURE

The wall of the eyeball consists of an outer corneoscleral coat, a central coat called the uvea and an inner coat, the retina.

The corneoscleral coat is divided into a smaller, transparent, anterior cornea which allows light to enter the interior of the eye and the sclera, a larger, white-colored segment. The sclera is a tough fibrous layer that protects the delicate internal structures of the eye and aids in maintaining the shape of the eyeball.

The uveal coat consists of the choroid, ciliary body and iris. The choroid is the vascular portion of the uvea immediately subjacent to the retina. It is continuous with the ciliary body, which forms a belt-like structure around the interior of the eyeball just forward of the anterior margin of the retina. The ciliary body controls the diameter and shape of the lens, which focuses light upon the retina. The last portion of the uvea, the iris, is continuous with the ciliary body and has a central opening called the pupil, the diameter of which can be increased or reduced by contractile cells of the iris. It serves as a diaphragm to regulate the amount of light passing into the eyeball.

The retina consists of photoreceptors that contain photopigments which, on exposure to light, produce chemical energy that is then converted into the electric energy of nerve impulses. A chain of conducting neurons in the retina transmits the nerve impulses to the optic nerve. The optic disk is the point where nerve fibers from the retina gather together to form the optic nerve and leave the eyeball.

The interior of the eyeball is subdivided into an anterior chamber, a posterior chamber and a vitreal cavity. Each is filled with a transparent medium which aids in maintaining the shape and turgor of the eye. The anterior and posterior chambers are continuous through the pupil. They contain a watery aqueous humor which provides nutrients for the anterior structures of the eye. The large vitreal cavity is filled with a viscous transparent gel called the vitreous humor or vitreous body.

The general structure of the eye is shown in Figure 9-1.

Corneoscleral Coat

The corneoscleral coat forms the outermost layer of the eyeball and consists of the cornea and sclera.

Sclera

KEY WORDS: fibrous outer tunic, lamina cribrosa

The sclera forms the tough, opaque **fibrous outer tunic** of the posterior five-sixths of the eyeball and varies in thickness in different regions averaging about 0.5 mm. It is composed of flat bundles of collagen that run in various directions but parallel to the scleral surface. Between the collagen bundles are delicate networks of elastic fibers and elongated flattened fibroblasts. Melanocytes occur in the deeper layers. The sclera thins and forms a fenestrated membrane, the **lamina cribosa**, at the point where fibers of the optic nerve penetrate the sclera to exit from the eye. The sclera protects the interior of the eye, aids in maintaining its shape and serves as the site of attachment for the extrinsic muscles of the eye.

Cornea

KEY WORDS: corneal epithelium, Bowman's membrane, substantia propria, keratocytes, Descemet's membrane, corneal endothelium

The transparent cornea is the most anterior portion of the eye and measures about 11 mm in diameter, approximately 0.8 mm in thickness near the center and 1.0 mm at the periphery. Its curvature is considerably greater than that of the posterior sclera. The cornea is uniform in structure and consists of corneal epithelium, Bowman's membrane, substantia propria, Descemet's membrane and corneal endothelium (mesothelium).

The **corneal epithelium** is stratified squamous with a smooth outer surface. It usually consists of five layers of large squamous cells and averages about 50 μm in depth. Individual cells possess few organelles but often contain glycogen. The superficial cells retain their nuclei, and their external surfaces form numerous fine ridges (microplicae) that help retain moisture on the corneal surface. The epithelium lies on a distinct basal lamina and the lateral membranes of adjacent cells are extensively interdigitated and united by numerous desmosomes. The corneal epithelium contains many free nerve endings and is very sensitive to a number of stimuli, especially pain.

The basal lamina of the corneal epithelium lies upon the outer layer of the substantia propria and is called **Bowman's membrane**. It appears homogeneous and measures 6 to 15 μm in thickness. Bowman's membrane ends abruptly at the peripheral margin of the cornea. It consists of a feltwork of small collagen fibrils and lacks elastin. Bowman's membrane is well developed in man but is absent in other primates and in rabbits. The **substantia propria**, or stroma, forms the bulk of the cornea. It consists of numerous bundles of collagen fibers arranged in thin lamellae that run parallel to the corneal surface. The collagen bundles in each successive lamella run in different directions and cross at various angles. Adjacent lamellae are tightly knit together by interchanging collagenous fibers. Sulfated polysaccharides, chondroitin sulfate and keratosulfate form a proteoglycan matrix between collagen fibers, bundles and lamellae. These proteoglycans are not present in the sclera. Between the parallel bundles of collagen fibers are elongated, flattened fibroblast-like cells termed **keratocytes**. Blood vessels and lymphatics normally are absent in the substantia propria, although occasional lymphoid wandering cells are observed.

Descemet's membrane is an homogeneous membrane, 6 to 8 μm thick, lying between

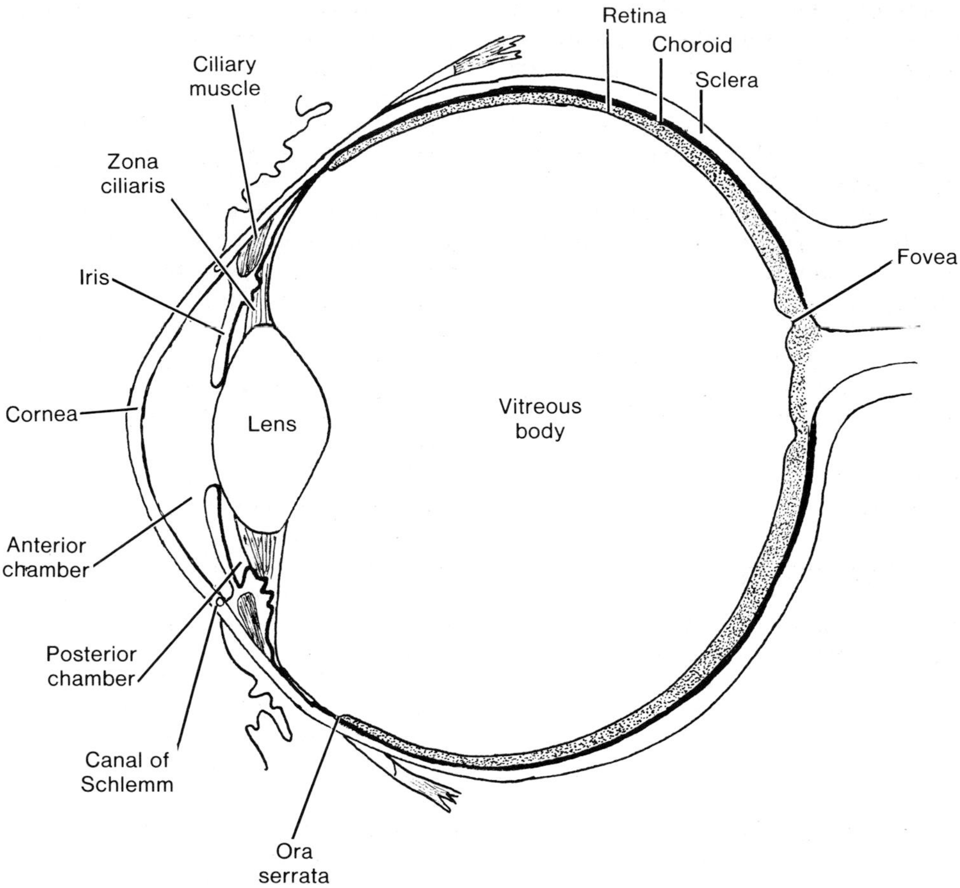

Figure 9-1 General structure of the eye.

the posterior surface of the substantia propria and the corneal endothelium. It may correspond to a thick basal lamina secreted by the corneal endothelium. It is resilient and elastic, although elastic fibers are not present, and appears to consist primarily of an atypical form of collagen.

The **corneal endothelium** (or mesenchymal epithelium) lines the inner surface of the cornea and consists of a layer of large hexagonal squamous cells. The apices of the cells are joined by tight junctions and the cytoplasm contains numerous mitochondria and vesicles. The cells appear active and may be involved in transport of materials from the anterior chamber. The transparency of the cornea is due to the uniform diameter and orderly arrangement of collagen fibers and to the properties of the ground substance. The cornea is avascular and depends upon the aqueous humor and blood vessels of the surrounding limbus to supply its nutritional needs.

Ion pumps of the corneal endothelial cells maintain a critical tissue fluid level within the substantia propria. If excess fluid accumulates, the cornea becomes less transparent.

Corneal endothelium cells do not divide after birth and therefore are not replaced. Each individual is born with his or her complement of corneal endothelial cells.

Limbus

KEY WORDS: external scleral sulcus, internal scleral sulcus, scleral spur, trabecular meshwork, canal of Schlemm

The limbus represents a zone of transition about 1.5 to 2.0 mm wide, between the transparent cornea and the opaque sclera. The outer surface exhibits a shallow groove, the **external scleral sulcus**, where the more convex cornea joins the sclera. A similar structure, the **internal scleral sulcus**, lies on the inner surface of the limbus. The **scleral spur** is a small ridge of tissue that projects from the posterior lip of the internal scleral sulcus and attaches anteriorly to tissue that comprises the outflow system for fluid from the anterior chamber. The limbus is further characterized by the terminations of Bowman's and Descemet's membranes. The collagen fibers and bundles of the cornea become larger and their arrangement more irregular as they blend with those of the sclera. Numerous small blood vessels form arcades in this region and nourish the peripheral portions of the avascular cornea.

Descemet's membrane is replaced by the spongy tissue of **trabecular meshwork,** which is attached to the anterior part of the scleral spur. It contains numerous flattened, anastomosing trabeculae that consist of collagen fibers and ground substance covered by an attenuated endothelium continuous with the corneal endothelium. The trabeculae form a labyrinth of spaces that communicate with the anterior chamber. Between the bulk of the limbal stroma and the trabecular meshwork, a flattened endothelial lined channel (the **canal of Schlemm**) courses around the circumference of the cornea. Aqueous humor enters the trabecular spaces from the anterior chamber and crosses the endothelial lining of the trabeculae, the juxtacanalicular connective tissue, and finally the endothelium of the canal to enter its lumen. Several channels arise from the peripheral wall of the canal to join veins in the limbus and eventually drain to episcleral veins. Obstruction to the drainage of aqueous humor results in a rise in the intraocular pressure which is characteristic of the condition known as glaucoma.

Uveal Layer

The uvea, the middle vascular coat of the eye, is divided into the choroid, ciliary body and iris.

Choroid

KEY WORDS: suprachoroid lamina, perichoroidal space, vessel layer, choriocapillary layer, glassy membrane (Bruch's membrane)

The choroid is a thin, brown, highly vascular membrane that lines the inner surface of the posterior sclera. Its outer surface is connected to the sclera by thin avascular lamellae that form a delicate, pigmented layer called the **suprachoroid lamina**. The lamellae consist primarily of fine elastic fibers between which are numerous large, flat melanocytes and scattered macrophages. The lamellae cross a potential cleft, the **perichoroidal space**, between the sclera and choroid to enter the choroid proper.

The choroid proper consists of three regions. The outer **vessel layer** is composed of loose connective tissue with numerous melanocytes, and contains the larger branches of the ciliary arteries and veins. The central **choriocapillary layer** consists of a net of capillaries lined by a fenestrated endothelium. The vessels of the choriocapillary layer provide for the nutritional needs of the outer layers of the retina. The choriocapillary layer ends near the ora serrata. The innermost layer of the choroid is the **glassy membrane (Bruch's membrane)** that lies between the remainder of the choroid and the pigment epithelium of the retina. With the light microscope it appears as a homogeneous layer 1 to 4 μm thick. Ultrastructurally, it shows five separate strata: the basal laminae of capillaries in the choriocapillary layer, the pigment epithelium of the retina, and between them, two thin layers of collagen fibers separated by a delicate elastic network.

In some teleosts, a layer of cells rich in crystals of guanine lies between the suprachoroid and choroid. It extends to the iris and forms the argenteum layer, which gives a silvery quality to the eyes of these species of fish. A reflecting layer, the tapetum lucidum, lies between the choriocapillary and vessel layers of the choroid of several species. Although not present in man, it is found in most other mammals. It may consist of several layers of fine fibers as in herbivores, or of several layers of flattened cells characteristic of carnivores. This layer reflects light, causing the eyes to "glow" in the dark.

Ciliary Body

KEY WORDS: ciliary epithelium, inner nonpigmented cells, outer pigmented cells, blood-aqueous barrier, aqueous humor, ciliary processes, zonule fibers, ciliaris muscle

The ciliary body is located between the ora serrata of the neural retina and the outer edge of the iris, where it attaches to the posterior aspect of the scleral spur at the corneoscleral junction. It forms a thin triangle when seen with the light microscope, and consists of an inner vascular tunic and a mass of smooth muscle immediately adjacent to the sclera. The internal surface is lined by the **ciliary epithelium**, a continuation of the pigment epithelium of the retina which lacks photosensitive cells.

The ciliary epithelium consists of an **inner layer of nonpigmented cells** and an **outer layer of pigmented cells** and is unusual in that cell apices of both layers closely appose one another, each resting on a separate basal lamina. The outer pigmented layer is separated from the stroma of the ciliary body by a thin basal lamina continuous with that underlying the pigment epithelium in the remainder of the retina. The basal lamina of the nonpigmented layer lies adjacent to the posterior chamber of the eye and is continuous with the inner limiting membrane of the retina. The basal plasmalemma of the nonpigmented cells shows numerous infoldings and is thought to be actively involved in ion transport. The cells contain numerous mitochondria and a well developed supranuclear Golgi complex. The adjacent pigmented cells of the outer layer also show prominent basal infoldings and the cytoplasm is filled with melanin granules. The apices of cells of the inner, nonpigmented epithelium are united by well developed tight junctions and form the anatomic portion of the **blood-aqueous barrier,** which selectively limits passage of materials between the blood and the interior of the eye.

The ciliary epithelium elaborates the **aqueous humor,** which differs from blood plasma both in electrolyte composition and in the lower content of proteins. It fills the posterior chamber, provides nutrients for the lens and, posteriorly, enters the vitreous body. Anteriorly, it flows from the posterior chamber through the pupil into the anterior chamber and aids in nourishing the cornea. It leaves the anterior chamber via the trabecular meshwork and canal of Schlemm to the episcleral veins.

The inner surface of the anterior portion of the ciliary body is formed by 60 to 80 radially arranged, elongated ridges called **ciliary processes**. These are lined by ciliary epithelium and contain a highly vascular stroma and scattered, stellate melanocytes. **Zonule fibers**, which hold the lens in position, are produced primarily by the nonpigmented cell layer of the ciliary epithelium and are attached to its basal lamina. They extend from the ciliary processes to the equator of the lens.

The bulk of the ciliary body consists of smooth muscle, the **ciliaris muscle**, which controls the shape and therefore the focal power of the lens. Muscle cells are organized into regions with circular, radial and meridional orientations. Numerous elastic fibers and melanocytes form a small amount of connective tissue between the muscle bundles. When the ciliaris muscle contracts, it draws the ciliary processes forward, thus relaxing the suspensory ligament (the zonule fibers) of the lens. This allows the lens to become more convex and focus near objects on the retina; hence, the ciliaris muscle is important in eye accommodation.

Iris

KEY WORDS: pupil, anterior chamber, posterior chamber, ciliary margin, pupillary margin, myoepithelial cells, dilator, sphincter muscle

The iris is a thin disk suspended in the aqueous humor between the cornea and lens and has a central, circular aperture known as the **pupil**. The iris is continuous with the ciliary body at the periphery and divides the space between the cornea and lens into anterior and posterior chambers. The **anterior chamber** is bounded anteriorly by the cornea and posteriorly by the iris and central portion of the lens. The **posterior chamber** is a narrow space behind the peripheral portion of the iris and anterior to the peripheral portion of the lens, ciliary zonule and ciliary processes. The two chambers communicate through the pupil. The anterior surface of the iris is irregular due to numerous fissures or crypts. The margin attached to the ciliary body is the **ciliary margin**; that surrounding the pupil is the **pupillary margin**.

The stroma of the iris consists primarily of loose, vascular connective tissue with scattered collagenous fibers, melanocytes and fibroblasts embedded in a homogenous ground substance. Its anterior surface lacks a definite endothelial or mesothelial lining but is lined in part by a discontinuous layer of melanocytes and fibroblasts. Tissue spaces of the stroma often appear to communicate with the anterior chamber. The posterior surface is covered by two rows of pigmented cuboidal cells that are continuous with the ciliary epithelium. Where it passes onto the posterior surface of the iris, the inner nonpigmented layer of the ciliary epithelium becomes heavily pigmented. Cells of the outer layer are less pigmented and in addition, become modified into **myoepithelial cells** to form the **dilator** of the iris. Thus, the dilator of the pupil consists only of a single layer of radially-arranged myoepithelial cells whose contraction increases the diameter of the pupil. In contrast, the **sphincter muscle** consists of a compact bundle of smooth muscle cells arranged in a circular pattern near the pupillary margin. Contraction of the sphincter muscle reduces the diameter of the pupil. The iris acts as a diaphragm to modify the amount of light entering the eye, thus permitting a range of vision under a variety of lighting conditions.

The color of the iris is determined by the amount and distribution of pigment. In the various shades of blue eyes, melanin is restricted to the posterior surface of the iris, whereas in gray, brown and dark eyes, melanin is found in increasing concentration within melanocytes present throughout the stroma of the iris. In albinos, where melanin pigment is absent, the iris assumes a pink hue due to the vasculature of the iridial stroma.

Retina

KEY WORDS: pigment epithelium, neural retina (retina proper), ora serrata, macula leuta, fovea centralis, optic disk

The retina, the innermost of the three tunics, is a delicate sheet of nervous tissue that forms the photoreceptor of the eye. Its outer surface is in contact with the choroid and its inner surface is adjacent to the vitreous body. The posterior retina consists of an outer **pigment epithelium** and an inner **neural retina** or **retina proper**. The retina decreases in thickness anteriorly, and the nervous component ends at a jagged margin called the **ora serrata**. A thin prolongation of the retina (minus the nervous component) extends anteriorly to cover the ciliary processes as the ciliary epithelium, and the posterior aspect of the iris where it forms the iridiae retinae. This forward extension of the retina consists only of the pigmented layer and an inner layer of columnar epithelial cells.

The neural retina is anchored only at the optic disk, where nerve fibers from the retina congregate before passing through the sclera to form the optic nerve, and at the ora serrata. Although the cells of the pigment epithelium interdigitate with photoreceptor cells of the neural retina, there is no anatomical connection between these two components of the retina. Following trauma or disease, the neural retina may detach from the pigment epithelium.

The exact center of the posterior retina corresponds to the axis of the eye and at this point vision is most perfect. This region appears as a small, yellow oval area known as the **macula leuta**. In its center is a depression approximately 0.5 mm in diameter called the **fovea centralis**, where the sensory elements are most numerous and most precisely organized. Nearer the periphery of the retina, neural elements are larger, fewer and less evenly distributed. Approximately 3.0 mm to the nasal side of the macula leuta is the **optic disk**, the site of formation and exit of the optic nerve. Lacking photoreceptor cells, this area is insensitive to light and is often referred to as the "blind spot" of the retina.

Neural Retina

KEY WORDS: three-neuron conducting chain, photoreceptor cells, bipolar neurons, ganglion cells, association neurons, glial cells

Except for the extreme periphery and the fovea centralis, the neural retina consists of the following layers, listed in order from choroid side, as seen with the light microscope: (1) layer of rods and cones, (2) external limiting membrane, (3) outer nuclear layer, (4) outer plexiform layer, (5) inner nuclear layer, (6) inner plexiform layer, (7) ganglion cell layer, (8) layer of nerve fibers, and (9) the internal limiting membrane. The retina consists principally of a **three-neuron conducting chain** (Fig. 9-2) that ultimately forms the nerve fibers in the optic nerve. The neural elements of the conducting chain are the **photoreceptors** (rod and cone cells), **bipolar neurons** and **ganglion cells**.

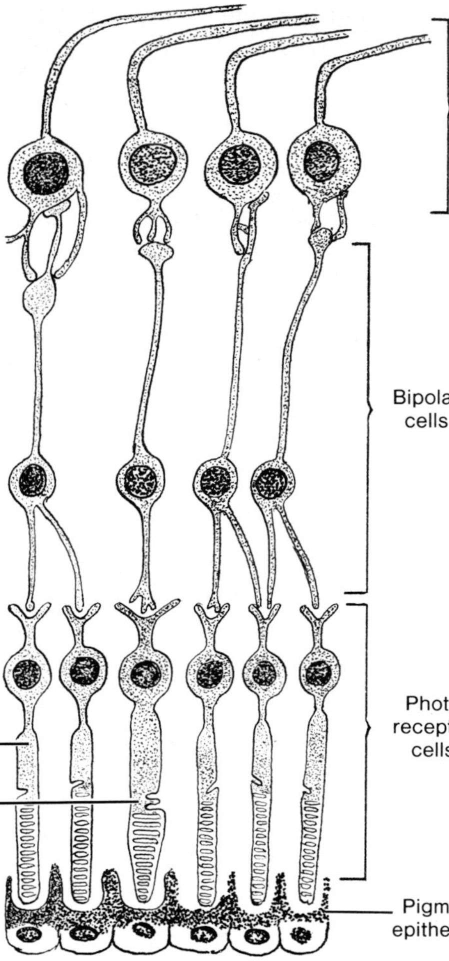

Figure 9-2 Three-neuron chain system.

When stimulated by light, photoreceptor cells transmit an action potential to bipolar neurons, which in turn synapse with ganglion cells. Unmyelinated axons from the ganglion cells enter the layer of retinal nerve fibers and unite at the optic disk to form the optic nerve which transmits the impulse to the brain. Other intraretinal cells are either **association neurons** (horizontal cells, amacrine cells) or **glial cells**.

Glial Cells

KEY WORDS: Muller's cells, inner limiting membrane, outer limiting membrane

The largest and most prominent glial elements in the neural retina are **Muller's cells**, which extend from the outer limiting membrane to the inner limiting membrane of the retina. Cytoplasmic processes run between cell bodies and processes of neurons in the retina and provide physical support for the neural elements. The basal lamina of Muller's cells lies adjacent to the vitreal body and forms the **inner limiting membrane** of the retina. The apices of Muller's cells establish junctional complexes with adjacent photoreceptor cells and form the **outer limiting membrane**. The cytoplasm is rich in smooth endoplasmic reticulum and contains abundant glycogen. In addition to providing structural support, Muller's cells are thought to give nutritional support to other elements of the retina and have been equated with astrocytes of the central nervous system.

A small number of spindle-shaped glial

cells also are present around the ganglion cells and between axons that form the nerve fiber layer of the retina.

Photoreceptor Cells

KEY WORDS: rod cells, rod proper, outer segment, rhodopsin, inner segment, ellipsoid, vitreal portion, myoid, outer fiber, cell body, inner fiber, spherule, synaptic ribbon, cone cells, iodopsin, cone pedicle

The two types of photoreceptors are the rod cells and cone cells (Fig. 9-3). **Rod cells** are long, slender cells that lie perpendicular to the layers of the retina. They measure 40 to 60 μm in length and 1.5 to 3.0 μm in width, depending on their location in the retina, and number between 75 and 170 million in each retina. The scleral (outward) third of each rod, called the rod proper, lies between the pigment epithelium and the outer limiting membrane. The scleral end of rods is surrounded by processes that extend from the subjacent pigment epithelial cells, while the inner or vitreal end extends into the outer plexiform layer.

Each **rod proper** consists of outer and inner segments connected by a slender stalk containing nine peripheral doublets of mi-

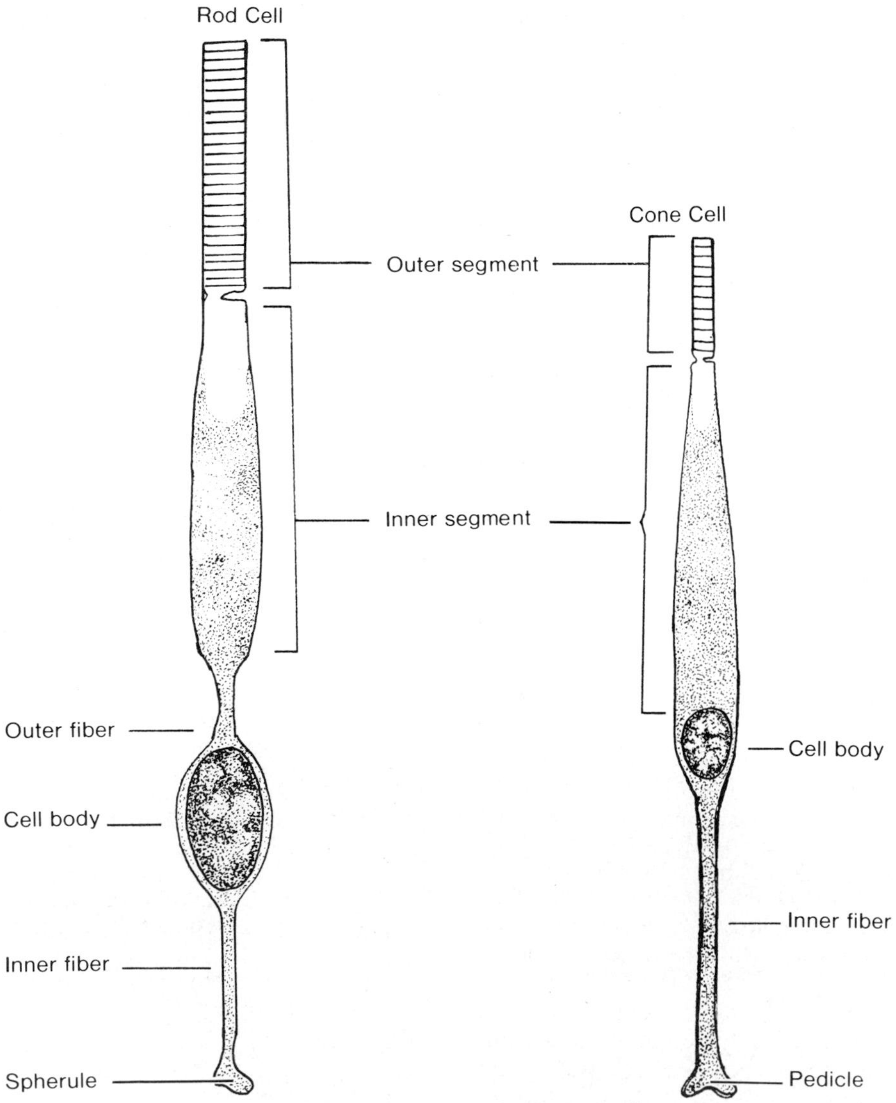

Figure 9-3 Diagram of rod and cone cells.

crotubules. The doublets originate from a basal body in the vitreal end of the inner segment, but the connecting stalk differs from a typical cilium in that it lacks a central pair of microtubules.

The **outer segment** contains hundreds of flattened membranous sacs or disks of uniform diameter. These sacs contain **rhodopsin**, the substance responsible for absorption of light. After exposure to light, rhodopsin changes from *cis* to *trans* and breaks down, resulting in hyperpolarization of the rod cell plasmalemma and the formation of an electrical potential that is transferred to dendrites of associated bipolar cells. After stimulation, rhodopsin is rapidly reconstituted.

The **inner segment** consists of an outer scleral region, the **ellipsoid**, that contains numerous mitrochondria and a **vitreal portion** that houses the Golgi complex, free ribosomes and elements of the granular and smooth endoplasmic reticulum called the **myoid**. Both regions contain numerous microtubules. The myoid region synthesizes and packages new proteins which are transported down the connecting stalk to the vitreal end of the outer rod segment, where they are used in the assembly of new membranous disks. Older sacs are displaced sclerally and eventually are shed during the morning hours from the tips of the rods as new ones are formed. The discarded disks are phagocytized and destroyed by cells of the pigment epithelium.

The remainder of the rod cell consists of the outer fiber, the cell body and the inner fiber. The **outer fiber** is a thin process extending from the inner segment of the rod proper to the **cell body**, which contains the nucleus. The **inner fiber** unites the cell body to the **spherule**, a pear-shaped synaptic ending. The spherule contains numerous synaptic vesicles and the **synaptic ribbon**, a dense proteinaceous plaque which lies perpendicular to the presynaptic surface, often bounded by numerous vesicles. The cell body and nucleus of the rods are located in the outer nuclear layer of the retina, while the spherule lies within the outer plexiform layer.

Cone cells are 75 μm or more in length at the fovea, decreasing to 40 μm at the periphery of the retina: between six and seven million cones are present in the human retina. Cone cells generally resemble rod cells but are flask-shaped with short, conical outer segments and relatively broad inner segments; these are united by a modified ciliary stalk similar to that in the rods. The membranous sacs of the outer cone segments also differ in that they may remain attached to the surrounding cell membrane and decrease in diameter as they approach the tip of the cone.

The inner segment, also called the ellipsoid portion, shows a region with numerous mitochondria and a myoid portion, which contains the Golgi complex and elements of smooth and granular endoplasmic reticulum. As in rods, the cones synthesize proteins, which pass to the outer segments, where they are used in the formation of new membranous sacs. Older sacs appear to be shed during the evening and are phagocytosed by the pigment epithelial cells. Unlike those in rods, each newly formed sac is larger than the one preceding it. In cones, the visual pigment associated with the outer segment is **iodopsin**. Absorption of light and generation of an electrical impulse is similar to that in the rods. Cones function in color perception and visual acuity, responding to light of relatively high intensity. Detection of color is believed to depend on different pigments in the cones, whereas rods are thought to contain only one form of pigment.

Most cones (except for those in the outer fovea) lack an outer fiber and the inner cone segment blends with the cell body. The nuclei of cone cells are larger and paler than those of the rods and form a single row in the outer nuclear layer adjacent to the outer limiting membrane. All cones have a thick inner fiber that runs to the outer plexiform layer to terminate in a club-shaped synaptic ending, the **cone pedicle**, which synapses with processes from bipolar and horizontal neurons.

Bipolar Cells

KEY WORDS: rod bipolar cells, flat cone bipolar cells, invaginating midget bipolar cells, flat midget bipolar cells

Like photoreceptor cells, bipolar cells lie perpendicular to the retinal layers, with their cell bodies and nuclei in the inner nuclear layer of the retina. They give rise to one or more dendrites that extend into the outer plexiform layer, where they synapse with terminals of the photoreceptor cells. A single axon extends into the inner plexiform layer and synapses with processes from ganglion cells. Several types of bipolar neurons have been described. **Rod bipolar cells** make contact with several rod cells; **flat cone bipolar cells** form synapses with several cone pedicles and **invaginating midget** and **flat midget bipolar cells** synapse with a single cone pedicle. Bipolar cells relay impulses from the photoreceptor cells (rod and cones) to the ganglion cells of the next layer.

Ganglion Cells

KEY WORDS: diffuse ganglion cells, midget ganglion cells

Dendrites of ganglion cells synapse with axons of bipolar neurons and represent the third and terminal link in the neuron chain. Axons of the various ganglion cells pass along the vitreal surface in the nerve fiber layer of the retina and join other axons at the optic disk to form the optic nerve. Although several morphological varieties of ganglion cells have been described, two forms have been identified by their synaptic relations with bipolar neurons. **Diffuse ganglion cells** synapse with several types of bipolar cells and **midget ganglion cells**, a monosynaptic type, synapse with a single midget bipolar cell.

Association Neurons

KEY WORDS: horizontal cells, amacrine cells

The cell bodies and nuclei of **horizontal cells** lie in the inner nuclear layer. Their dendrites enter the outer plexiform layer and synapse with a single cone pedicle. The axon also enters the outer plexiform layer and runs parallel to the adjacent retinal layers to end on terminal twigs which synapse with several rod spherules. Although the functional significance of the horizontal cells is poorly understood, because they synapse with cones of one area, rods of another area and bipolar neurons, it has been suggested that they may raise or lower the functional threshold of these cells.

Amacrine cells are pear-shaped neurons that lack an axon but have several dendrites. The cell bodies lie in the inner nuclear layer and their dendrites extend into the inner plexiform layer. Their function is unknown.

The neural retina is composed of photoreceptor cells, conducting neurons forming a neuron chain, association neurons and glial or supportive cells. These elements are organized into the various layers of the retina and can be summarized as shown in Table 9-1.

Table 9-1
Contents of Layers of Retina

Layers of Retina	Principal Contents
1. Layer of rods and cones	Inner and outer segments of rods and cones
2. External limiting membrane	Formed by junctional complexes between the scleral tips of Muller's cells and adjacent photoreceptor cells
3. Outer nuclear layer	Cell bodies and nuclei of rods and cones
4. Outer plexiform layer	Rod spherules, cone pedicles, dendrites of bipolar neurons, processes of horizontal cells
5. Inner nuclear layer	Nuclei of bipolar, horizontal, amacrine and Muller's cells
6. Inner plexiform layer	Axons of bipolar neurons, dendrites of ganglion cells, processes of amacrine cells
7. Ganglion cell layer	Ganglion cells, scattered neuroglial cells
8. Nerve fiber layer	Nonmyelinated nerve fibers from ganglion cells, small neuroglial cells, processes of Muller's cells
9. Internal limiting membrane	Vitreal processes of Muller's cells, and their basal lamina

Fovea Centralis

The fovea centralis is a funnel-shaped depression on the posterior surface of the retina, in direct line with the visual axis. At this point the vitreal layers of the retina that are beyond the outer nuclear layer are displaced laterally, allowing light an almost free pathway to the photoreceptors. The central region of the fovea, approximately 0.5 mm in diameter, consists only of cones, and these are longer and thinner than those elsewhere in the retina. They are closely packed and number approximately 25,000 to 35,000. It is this portion of the retina where vision is most acute.

Pigment Epithelium

KEY WORDS: cylindrical sheaths, elongate microvilli, melanin granules, residual bodies, vitamin A

The pigment epithelium of the retina consists of a simple layer of hexagonal cells that tend to increase in diameter near the ora serrata. The basal cell membranes show numerous infoldings with associated mitochondria and are thought to be actively engaged in transport. The basal lamina contributes to the light microscopic entity of the choroid known as Bruch's membrane. The lateral cell membranes of adjacent cells show some interdigitation and, near the apex, are united by tight junctions. Two types of cytoplasmic processes arise from the apices of the cells. **Cylindrical sheaths** invest the tips of the rod and cone outer segments and **elongated microvilli** extend between photoreceptor cells. In addition to abundant mitochondria near the base of the cell, the cytoplasm is characterized by numerous **melanin granules**. Pigment epithelial cells also show numerous **residual bodies** that may contain remnants of phagocytosed membrane material shed by rod outer segments.

The pigment epithelium absorbs light after it has passed through the neural retina, thereby preventing reflection within the eye, and the apical tight junctions prevent undesirable substances from entering the intercellular spaces of the neural retina. The component cells phagocytose the membranous sacs shed by the outer rod segments. Some products are recycled to the photoreceptor cells. The pigment epithelium also serves for storage of the cyclic supply of **vitamin A** (a precursor for rhodopsin) to the outer rod segment membranes.

Vascular Supply of the Retina

The outer nuclear and plexiform layers and the layer of rod and cone inner segments lack blood vessels. This portion of the retina is nourished by capillaries of the choriocapillary layer of the choroid. The nutrients traverse the pigmented epithelium to enter the intercellular spaces of the outer neural retina. The inner layers of the retina are supplied by retinal vessels arising from the central retinal artery which enters the interior of the eye in the optic nerve. Capillary networks from this source lie in the nerve fiber layer and in the inner plexiform layer.

Lens

KEY WORDS: capsule, anterior lens cells, lens fibers, lens substance, cortex, nucleus, zonule fibers

The lens is a transparent, biconvex epithelial body placed immediately behind the pupil between the iris and the vitreous body. It measures about 10 mm in diameter and 3.7 to 4.5 mm in thickness. The posterior surface is more convex than the anterior surface. The lens consists primarily of a capsule, anterior lens cells and lens substance.

The lens is covered on its anterior and posterior surfaces by a homogenous, carbohydrate-rich **capsule** 10 to 18 μm thick. A simple layer of cuboidal cells, the **anterior lens cells**, forms the epithelium of the lens and is restricted to the anterior surface; the posterior surface lacks an epithelium. The anterior lens cells lie immediately beneath the capsule. Their apices face inward (toward the lens) and attach to a lens fiber; the basal surfaces rest upon a basal lamina. Near the equator, the cells increase in height and gradually differentiate into **lens fibers**, which constitute the bulk of the lens, referred to as the **lens substance**. The lens grows throughout life by addition of new fibers to the periphery of the lens substance. The outer layers of the lens substance form the **cortex**. Nearer the center, the lens substance consists of condensed, concentrically arranged fibers that give it a more homogenous appearance, and is called the **nucleus** of the lens.

At the equator, the anterior lens cells elongate and push into the lens to lie beneath the epithelium anteriorly and the capsule posteriorly. As the cells increase in length they lose their nuclei and basal attachment to the capsule and are called lens fibers. They appear hexagonal in cross section and measure 7 to 10 μm in length. The lateral membranes of lens fibers (cells) from the cortex show large protrusions that interdigitate with concavities in adjacent fibers, in a knob and socket fashion. The knob and socket joints maintain adjacent cells (fibers) in position as the lens changes its shape while focusing. Nexus junctions are common at these points. Lens fibers show few organelles and a homogenous, finely granular cytoplasm. The lens is avascular and derives its nutrition totally from diffusion of nutrients from the aqueous humor and vitreous body. Anterior lens cells are believed to contain ion pumps that maintain the fluid levels of the lens. If the cells fail, fluid levels increase and the lens loses transparency and becomes cloudy.

The lens is held in position by a system of fibers called **zonule fibers** which make up the suspensory ligament of the lens. Zonule fibers arise from the ciliary epithelium covering the ciliary processes and attach to the lens capsule just anterior and posterior to the lens equator. The zonule fibers consist of small bundles of fine filaments, approximately 12 nm in diameter, which may correspond to the microfibril component of elastic fibers.

The thickness and convexity of the lens are under the control of the ciliary muscle. If the ciliary muscle contracts, the ciliary body and choroid are pulled forward and centrally, releasing the tension on the zonule fibers, and the lens becomes thicker and more convex. This action is important when the eye must focus on near objects. When the ciliary muscle relaxes, tension builds on the zonule fibers and the lens becomes thinner and less convex.

Vitreous Body

KEY WORDS: hyaluronic acid, hyalocytes, hyaloid canal

The vitreous body is a colorless, transparent, gelatinous mass filling the vitreal cavity. It is 99% water and contains **hyaluronic acid** and other hydrophilic polysaccharides, as well as thin fibrils of collagen arranged in a random network. The fibrils are most prominent near the periphery. A few cells, called **hyalocytes,** together with occasional macrophages, are present in the outermost portions of the vitreous body. Hyalocytes may be involved in the formation and maintenance of the vitreous body. A thin cylindrical network of fibrils, the **hyaloid canal**, extends from the optic disk to the posterior surface of the lens. It represents the site of the fetal hyaloid artery. The vitreous body provides nutrients to the lens and adjacent structures, and maintains the correct turgor and shape of the eye.

ACCESSORY STRUCTURES

Eyelids

KEY WORDS: conjunctiva, tarsal plate, tarsal (Meibomian) glands, eyelashes, glands of Zeiss, glands of Moll

The eyelids protect the anterior aspects of the eyes. They consist of a connective tissue core covered externally by thin skin. The interior surface of each lid and the anterior aspect of each eye (except for the cornea) are lined by a mucous membrane called the **conjunctiva**. That which lines the interior of the lid is referred to as the palpebral conjunctiva and that which covers the anterior surface of the eyeball is called the bulbar conjunctiva. Both consist of a stratified columnar epithelium interspersed with goblet cells, resting on a dense connective tissue rich in elastic fibers. Goblet cells provide mucus which lubricates and prevents tearing of the corneal epithelium. Numerous lymphocytes may be present. At the margin of the lid, the palpebral conjunctiva is continuous with the keratinized stratified squamous epithelium of the skin. In some lower vertebrates a nictitating membrane is formed by the bulbar conjunctiva. It usually consists of a connective tissue core which contains smooth muscle cells covered by conjunctival epithelium.

The external surface of the eyelid is covered by keratinized stratified squamous epithelium and a subcutaneous layer of loose connective tissue with many elastic fibers. Projecting from these layers are fine hairs associated with small sebaceous glands and sweat glands. Skeletal muscle of the orbicularis oculi and superior levator palpebrae muscles is present in the substance of the lid. A curved plate of dense fibrous connective tissue that conforms to the shape of the eyeball forms a major structure in the lid and constitutes the **tarsal plate**, which maintains the shape of the lid. Large sebaceous glands called the **tarsal** or **Meibomian glands** lie embedded within the tarsal plate and are arranged in a single row, with their ducts opening at the margin of the lid. Each gland consists of a long central duct surrounded by numerous large secretory alveoli. They elaborate a lipid secretion that lubricates the lid margins and prevents them from sticking together.

The **eyelashes** are thick, short curved hairs arranged in two or three irregular rows at the lid margin. Their follicles also extend into the tarsal plate. Sebaceous glands associated with the eyelashes are called the **glands of Zeiss**. Sweat glands located between the eyelash follicles are referred to as the **glands of Moll**.

Lacrimal Gland

KEY WORDS: compound tubuloalveolar, serous, myoepithelial cells, lacrimal ducts, lacrimal sac, nasolacrimal duct

Lacrimal glands are well developed, **compound tubuloalveolar** glands of **serous** type located in the superior temporal region of the orbit. Each gland consists of several separate glandular units that empty into the conjunctival sac via 6 to 12 ducts. The secretory units consist of tall columnar cells with large, pale secretory granules. Numerous **myoepithelial cells** lie between the secretory cells and their limiting basal lamina. Initially the ducts are lined by simple cuboidal epithelium which becomes stratified columnar in the larger ducts. Small accessory lacrimal glands, the tarsal glands, are present in the inner surface of the eyelid.

Secretions of the lacrimal gland moisten, lubricate and flush the anterior surface of the eye and interior of the eyelids. Excess tears collect at a medial expansion of the conjunctival sac which is drained by the **lacrimal duct** to a lacrimal sac at the medial corner of each eye. The lacrimal duct is lined by stratified squamous epithelium. The **lacrimal sac** and the **nasolacrimal duct** which drains it into the inferior meatus of the nasal cavity are lined by pseudostratified columnar epithelium. The remainder of their walls consists of a dense connective tissue.

DEVELOPMENT OF THE EYE

Eyeball. The eyeball arises from neuroectoderm of the embryonic forebrain, surface ectoderm of the head, and the mesenchyme that lies between or around these components.

Eye development begins with the formation of shallow optic grooves on each side of the developing forebrain. As the neural tube closes, the optic grooves expand to form optic vesicles which remain attached to the brain by a hollow optic stalk. Thickenings of the surface ectoderm over the optic vesicles give rise to the lens placodes. These expand along their lateral walls to form the lens pits, from which lens vesicles eventually form. The walls of the vesicles consist of surface ectodermal cells. With loss of the superficial (epitrichial) cells of the surface ectoderm and connecting stalk to the surface, the underlying cuboidal cells of the lens vesicle come to form the definitive cells of the lens.

Simultaneously, the distal wall of the optic vesicle invaginates into itself to form a double-walled optic cup in which the apices of the cuboidal cells in the two layers face each other. As the optic cup forms, the lens vesicle descends into the cavity of the cup, where it continues to develop. The optic cup remains attached to the brain by the optic stalk: The cup forms the retina; the optic stalk becomes the optic nerve.

Meanwhile, mesenchyme of the paraxial area grows in and helps to separate the lens vesicle from the surface ectoderm. Part of the mesenchymal ingrowth differentiates into the corneal endothelium; the remainder contributes to the anterior chamber. A second ingrowth of mesenchyme extends between the surface ectoderm and the corneal endothelium to form the substantia propria of the cornea. The surface ectoderm, previously a simple epithelium, is now two cells thick and forms the corneal epithelium. A third ingrowth of mesenchyme extends into the optic cup from the lateral side near the

Table 9-2
Contributions to the Eye

Embryonic layer	Adult Structures
Neuroectoderm	Neural retina, pigment epithelium, epithelium over the iris, dilator and sphincter pupillary muscles, nervous and neuroglial elements of optic nerve
Surface ectoderm	Epithelium of cornea, lens
Mesenchyme	Substantia propria and endothelium of cornea, sclera, choroid, stroma and vessels of iris, ciliary body and ciliary process, ciliary muscle, sheaths of optic nerve, anterior, posterior and vitreous chambers

lens and forms a loose, acellular matrix between the lens and corneal epithelium. The matrix behind the central cornea liquefies and forms an early anterior chamber which, as it widens, separates the corneoscleral region from the developing iris. Bowman's and Descemet's membranes appear during the 4th month in man and collagen fibrils in the substantia propria reach their full thickness. As the corneal epithelium and substantia propria develop, the cornea thickens, reaching its full dimensions at the end of the first postnatal year.

The outer layer of the double-walled optic cup becomes highly pigmented and forms the pigment epithelium of the retina: endothelial cells in the adjacent undifferentiated mesenchyme form the choriocapillaris. In man, the collagenous portion of Bruch's membrane develops first, followed about 6 weeks later by the elastic part. Melanocytes migrate from the neural crest into the outer layers of the choroid by the 5th month and later appear in its inner layers. The sclera arises as a condensation of mesenchyme around the optic cup, just external to the developing choroid. The condensation begins at the equator of the sclera, and by the 5th month forms a complete layer.

The posterior four-fifths of the inner layer of the optic cup thickens due to cell proliferation and migration and forms the neural retina. The inner layer of the optic cup differentiates into inner and outer neuroblastic layers. Cells of the inner layer develop into the neurons and glial elements of the adult retina; rods and cones arise from ciliated cells in the outer neuroblastic layer. A marginal layer in the forming retina receives axons that extend posteriorly toward the optic stalk. Differentiation of retinal cells begins in the posterior region of the optic cup, gradually extending forward to the area of the (adult) ora serrata. Neuroblastic layers of the macular region develop first so that the more peripheral, later-developing axons must course around this region to reach the optic disk. Some retinal differentiation, especially of the macular region, continues after birth and the density of the retinal pigment also increases postnatally.

Cells in the anterior one-fifth of the inner layer of the optic cup, beyond the region of the ora serrata of the adult eye, remain in a single layer. The cells lie apex-to-apex with cells of the pigment layer that extend to the margin of the optic cup and cover the developing ciliary region and iris.

The ciliary body arises from neuroectoderm of the anterior optic cup and its associated mesoderm. Neuroectoderm forms the outer pigmented and inner nonpigmented epithelia covering the ciliary body and ciliary processes; mesenchyme forms the ciliary muscle, stroma and blood vessels. As the ciliary muscle differentiates, folds appear in the outer layer of neuroectoderm external to the margin of the optic cup. Each fold gives rise to a ciliary process, complete with a core of mesenchyme and blood vessels, covered by the two epithelial layers in which the cells are arranged apex to apex. Zonule fibers develop within the vitreous and extend from the inner surface of the ciliary processes to the lens capsule. In man, they appear during the 3rd month and form the suspensory ligament of the lens.

The iris also is derived from neuroectoderm and mesenchyme. The double layer of epithelium covering the iris develops from the double cell layer of the optic cup. The smooth muscle of the sphincter and dilator muscles of the iris are unusual in that they develop from neuroectoderm. An ingrowth of mesenchyme at the edge of the optic cup provides the stroma and vasculature of the iris.

The optic nerve develops from axons of retinal ganglion cells, neuroectodermal cells and mesoderm associated with the optic stalk. The mesoderm gives rise to the vascular components and connective tissue of the nerve, including its meninges. At first, the optic stalk contains an open ventral groove, the choroid fissure, through which mesenchyme enters the optic cup. Hyaloid vessels that supply the lens and inner surface of the retina during their development, and axons from the brain to the retina, also pass within the groove. As the choroid groove closes, the optic stalk is transformed into the optic nerve with the central retinal (the previous hyaloid) artery at its center. That part of the hyaloid artery which supplied the lens degenerates and is resorbed. The mesenchyme filling the posterior aspect of the optic cup becomes the gelatinous, transparent vitreous.

The lamina cribrosa develops from the neuroectoderm as a condensation of glial cells. It is strengthened by the mesenchymal component that gives rise to fibroblasts and collagenous septae that pass among the neuroglial cells.

Accessory Structures. Folds of integument adjacent to the eyeball differentiate to form the eyelid. Ectoderm on the exterior of the developing eyelid becomes the epidermis; that covering the cornea and anterior part of the sclera forms the conjunctiva. As development proceeds, the folds meet and fuse temporarily. The epidermal union breaks down prior to the opening of the eyes which, in some species, does not occur until well after birth. Eyelashes, sebaceous, sweat and tarsal glands develop along the edge of each eyelid while these still are fused. The follicles of the lashes and their associated glands arise as epidermal ingrowths which develop in a manner identical to the development of hairs elsewhere on the body.

Lacrimal glands develop as a series of solid cords of cells from the conjunctival epithelium. The cords grow, branch and acquire lumina, thus establishing the ductal system. Secretory alveoli are the last components to form. The lacrimal sac and nasolacrimal duct first appear as a solid outgrowth of epithelium from the nasolacrimal groove: a second growth from the epithelium of each eyelid joins it. The distal end of the cord grows toward the nasal cavity and fuses with the nasal epithelium prior to acquiring a lumen.

FUNCTIONAL SUMMARY

The corneoscleral coat, together with the intraocular pressure of the fluid contents within the eye, maintains the proper shape and size of the eyeball. Light entering the eye must traverse several transparent media (cornea, aqueous humor, lens and vitreous body) before reaching neural receptors in the retina. Blood vessels are absent in the transparent elements which rely on the diffusion of substances for their nutrition. Peripheral regions of the cornea receive nutrients from adjacent vessels in the limbus. The remainder of the cornea depends on diffusion of nutrients from the aqueous humor. The lens receives all its nutrition from the aqueous humor, which is thought to be secreted continuously into the posterior chamber by the ciliary epithelium. Aqueous humor then enters the anterior chamber through the pupil or diffuses posteriorly into the vitreous chamber of the eye. From the anterior chamber it passes through the trabecular network into the

canal of Schlemm and then into adjacent episcleral veins. The aqueous humor supplies nutrients to the transparent media of the eye; it also is responsible for maintaining the correct intraocular pressure.

Stationary refraction occurs through the transparent cornea, in contrast to variable refraction, which occurs in the lens as it changes shape to focus near and far objects on the retina during eye accommodation. The other media have negligible refraction. The lens is held in position by zonule fibers which extend from surrounding ciliary processes. It focuses an inverted, real image on the retina. The convexity and thickness of the lens are controlled by the ciliary muscle acting through the ciliary process and zonule fibers. If the ciliary muscle contracts, the ciliary body and choroid are pulled centrally and forward, releasing tension on the zonule fibers, and the lens becomes thicker and more convex to enable the eye to focus on near objects. When the ciliary muscle relaxes, the ciliary body slides posteriorly and peripherally, resulting in increased tension. As this occurs, tension builds on the zonule fibers and the lens becomes thinner and less convex to focus on far objects.

The iris is continuous with the ciliary body at the periphery and divides the space between the cornea and lens into anterior and posterior chambers which communicate through an aperture in the iris, the pupil. Light passes through the pupil to enter the lens and then the vitreous chamber of the eye. The dilator of the pupil consists of a single layer of radially arranged myoepithelial cells along the posterior surface of the iris. Contraction of the myoepithelial cells increases the diameter of the pupil. The sphincter of the iris consists of smooth muscle arranged around the pupillary margin of the iris. It acts as a diaphragm to modify the amount of light entering the eye, permitting vision under a variety of light conditions.

The rods and cones of the retina act as photoreceptor cells that collect visual impressions (light patterns) and translate them into nerve impulses. The membranous sacs of the outer rod segments contain rhodopsin, a substance responsible for absorption of light. Following exposure to light, rhodopsin undergoes a change from *cis* to *trans* and breaks down, resulting in hyperpolarization of the rod plasmalemma and the formation of an electrical potential that is transferred to dendrites of associated bipolar cells. Rods have a lower threshold to light intensity than cones and are important in dark and light discrimination and in night vision.

The visual pigment associated with the cone outer segment is iodopsin. Light absorption and generation of an electrical impulse in cones follows a sequence similar to that which occurs in rod cells. Cones function in color perception and visual acuity, responding to light of relatively high intensity. Detection of color depends on different pigments present in the cones. The central region of the fovea centralis consists only of cones and is in direct line with the visual axis of the eye. Here the inner layers of the retina that are beyond the outer nuclear layer are displaced laterally, allowing light rays almost a free pathway to the photoreceptors, and in this portion of the retina vision is most acute.

The pigment epithelium of the retina absorbs light after it has passed through the neural retina and prevents reflection within the eye. Melanocytes in the choroid, iris and other regions of the eye interior also absorb light and prevent it from reflecting in the eye interior. The cells of the pigment epithelium actively phagocytize and break down the membranous sacs as they are shed at the tips of the outer rod segments. Some components of the digested membranes are transported back to the photoreceptor cells to be reused. The pigment epithelium serves as a storage site for vitamin A, a precursor for rhodopsin, which is recycled to the membranes of the outer rod segments. Apical tight junctions between cells of the pigment epithelium form a barrier to prevent undesirable substances from entering the neural retina, which is nourished by diffusion from capillaries in the choriocapillary layer of the choroid.

The retina basically represents a three-neuron chain of photoreceptors (rods and cones), bipolar neurons and ganglion cells equivalent to three-neuron sensory chains in the peripheral nervous system. Rods and cones can be equated with other sensory receptors, bipolar neurons with craniospinal ganglia and retinal ganglion cells with internuncial neurons of the spinal cord and brain stem. Thus, the arrangement of nervous elements in the sensory chain of the retina is identical to that in other sensory pathways. Indeed, the retina represents an extension of the nervous system (brain) modified to form a special receptor. Other neurons, horizontal cells and amacrine cells in the retina serve as association neurons.

The eyelids are mobile folds of skin that protect the anterior of the eye from physical injury, desiccation and excessive light. The lacrimal glands secrete tears which moisten and lubricate the anterior surface of the eyeball. Together with the eyelids, tears prevent the cornea from drying out and also flush the anterior surface of the eye and the interior surface of the eyelid, washing away potentially dangerous debris.

Atlas for Chapter 9

9-4

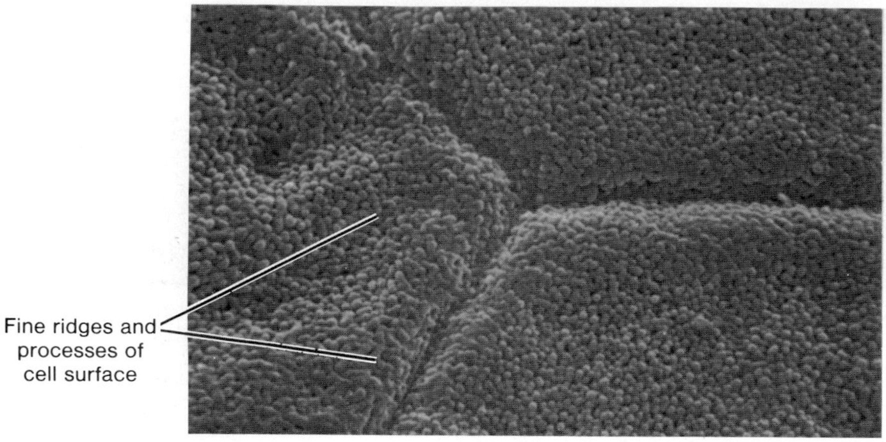

9-5

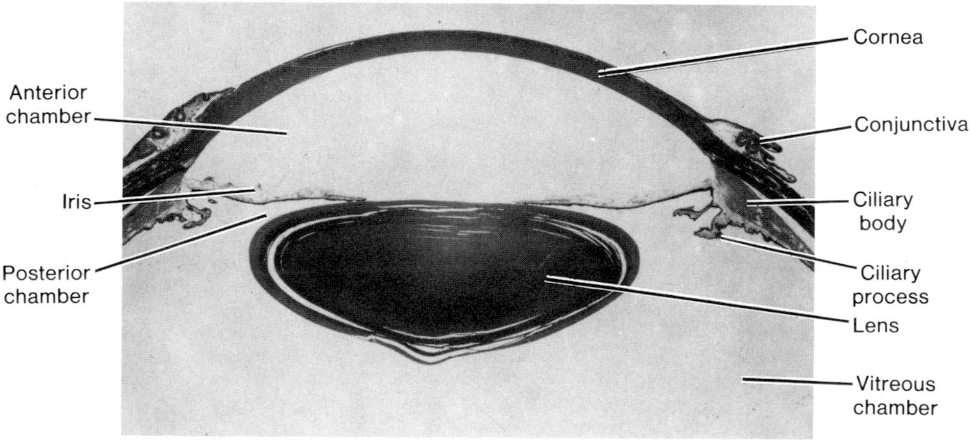

9-6

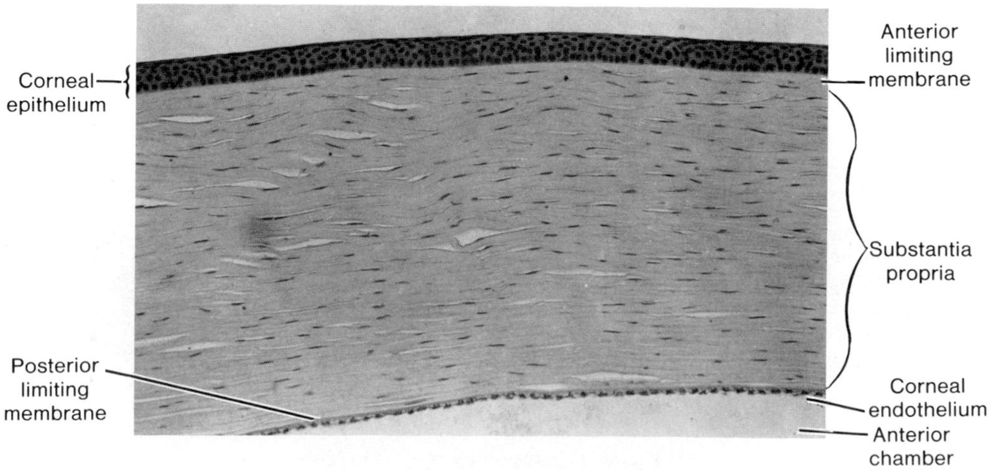

Figure 9-4 Cornea: junction of three superficial cells. SEM, ×5000.
Figure 9-5 Anterior portion of eye. LM, ×6.
Figure 9-6 Cornea. LM, ×100.

9-7

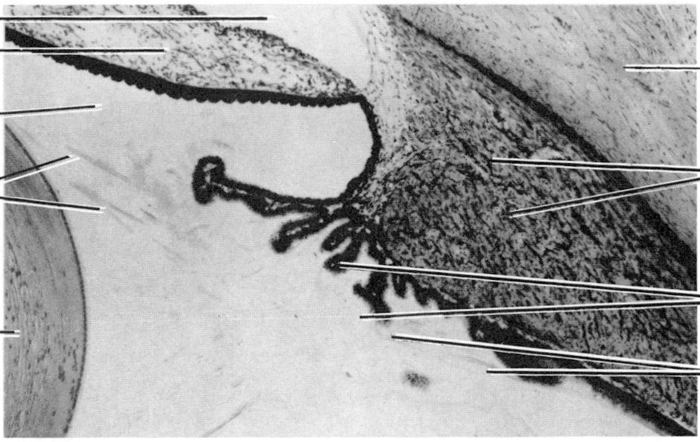

9-8

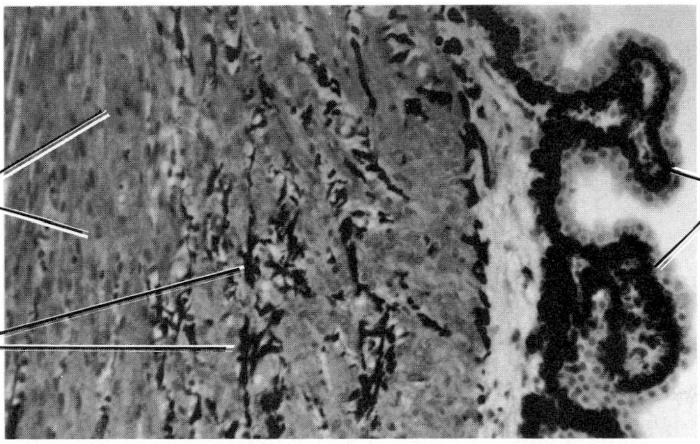

9-9

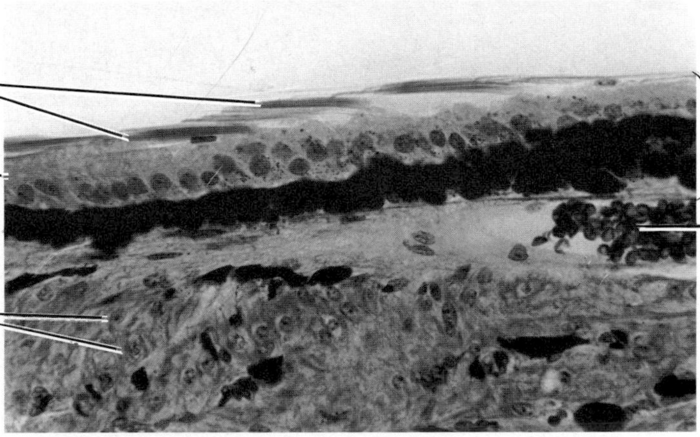

Figure 9-7 Ciliary body. LM, ×100.
Figure 9-8 Ciliary body. LM, ×250.
Figure 9-9 Ciliary epithelium. LM, ×250.

9-10

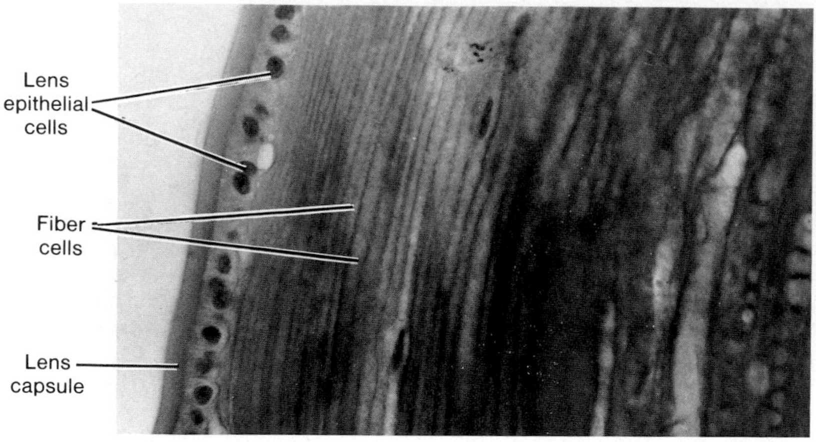

9-11

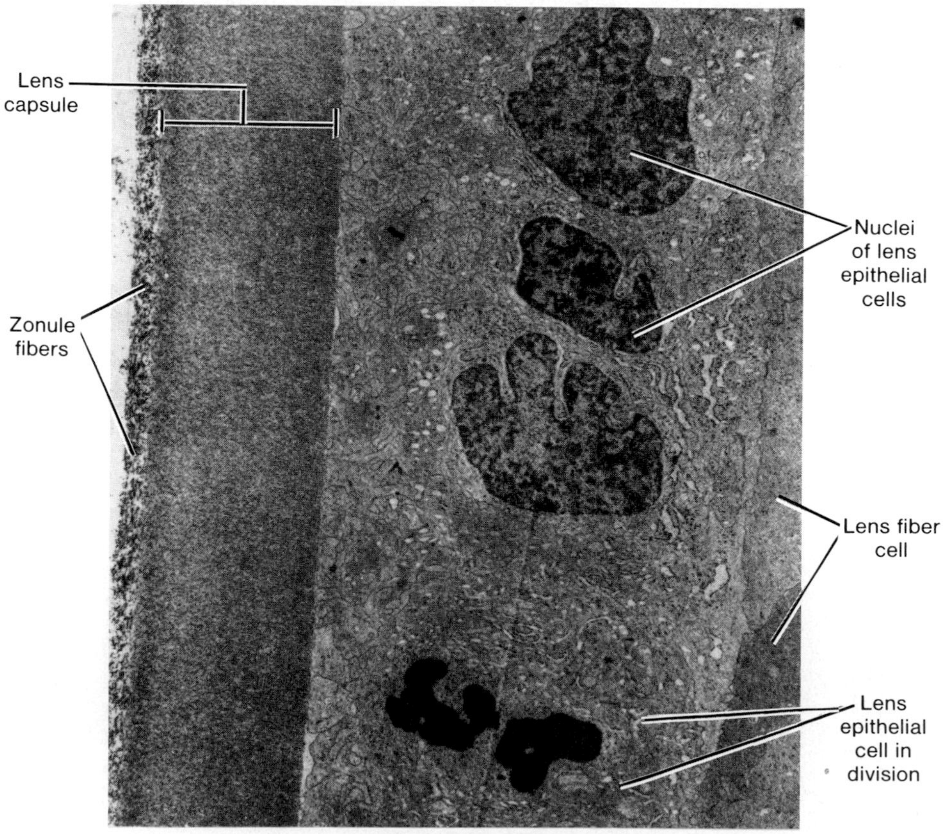

Figure 9-10 Lens. LM, ×250.
Figure 9-11 Lens epithelial cells. TEM, ×4500.

9-12

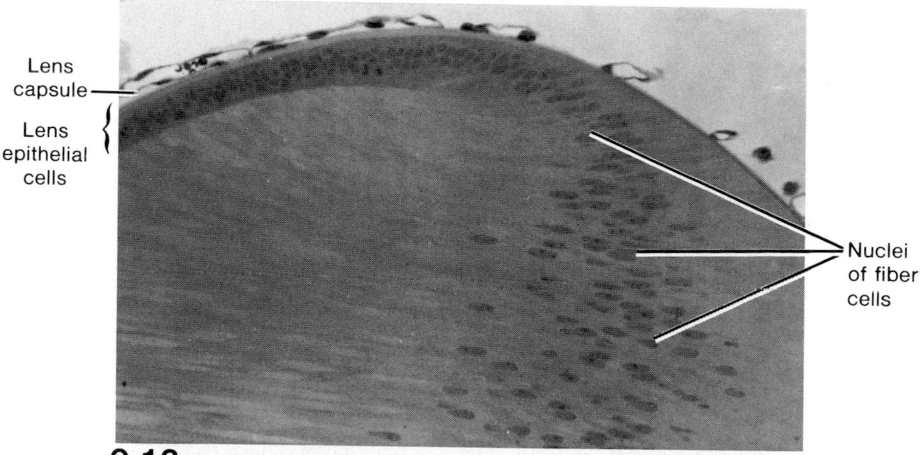

9-13

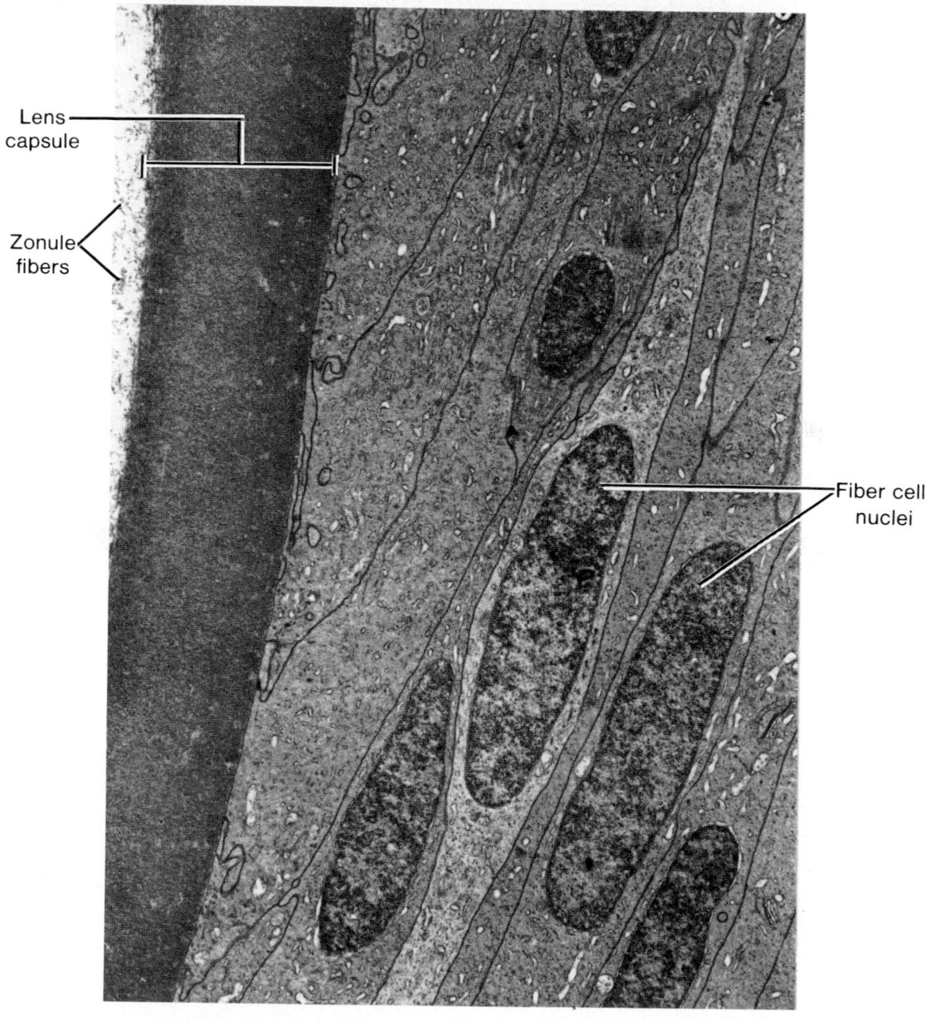

Figure 9-12 Lens. LM, ×125.
Figure 9-13 Fiber cells from lens equator. TEM, ×4500.

9-14

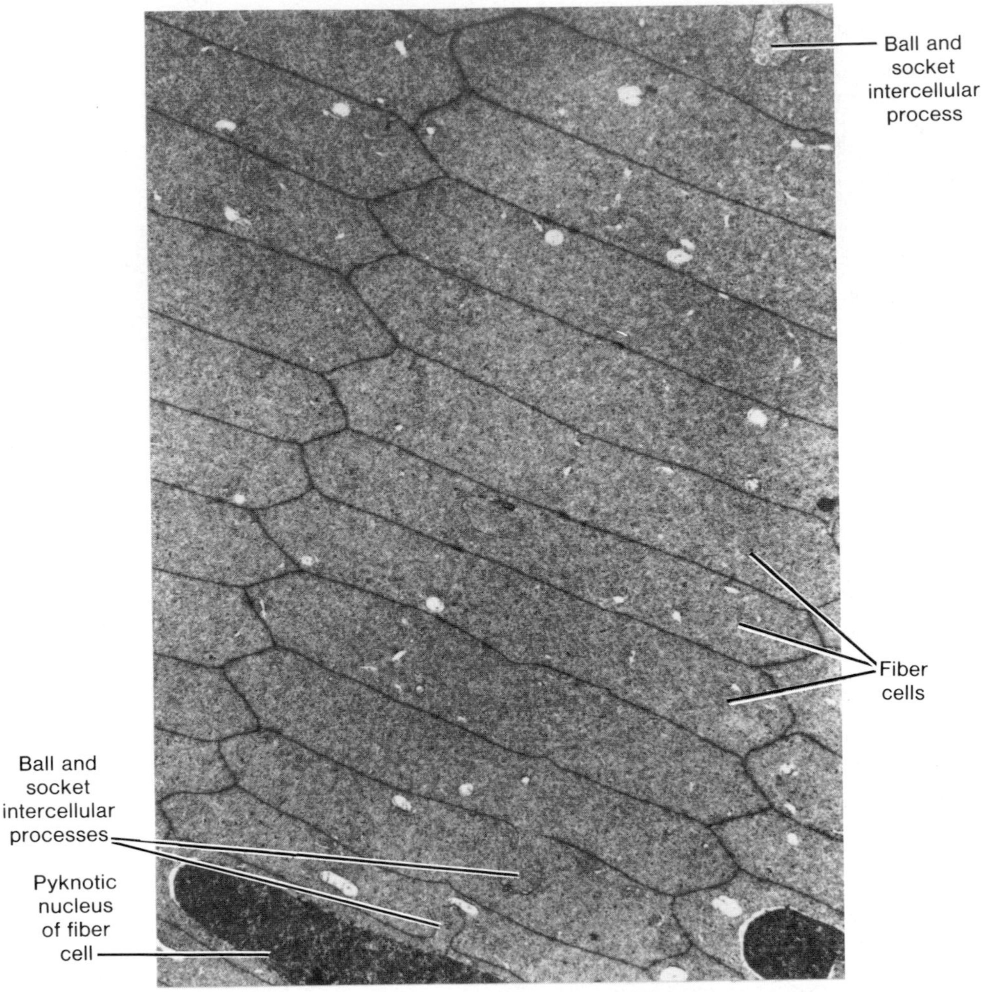

9-15

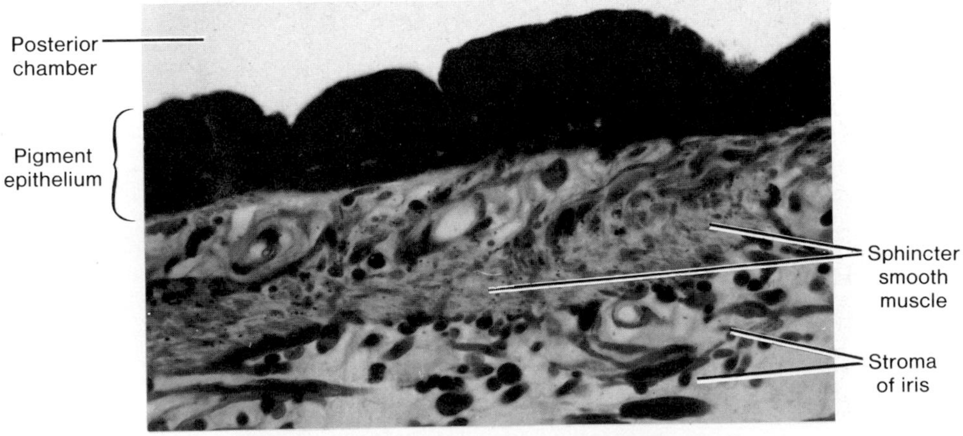

Figure 9-14 Fiber cells of lens cortex. TEM, ×6000.
Figure 9-15 Iris. LM, ×250.

9-16

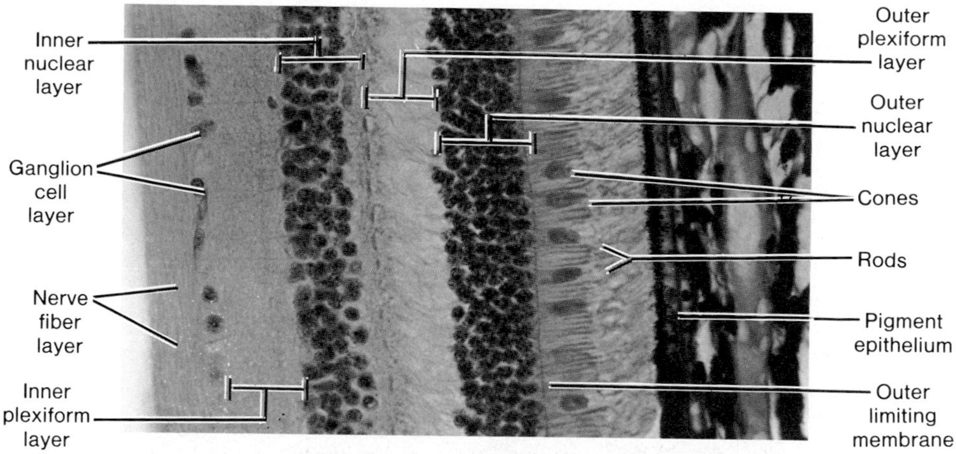

9-17

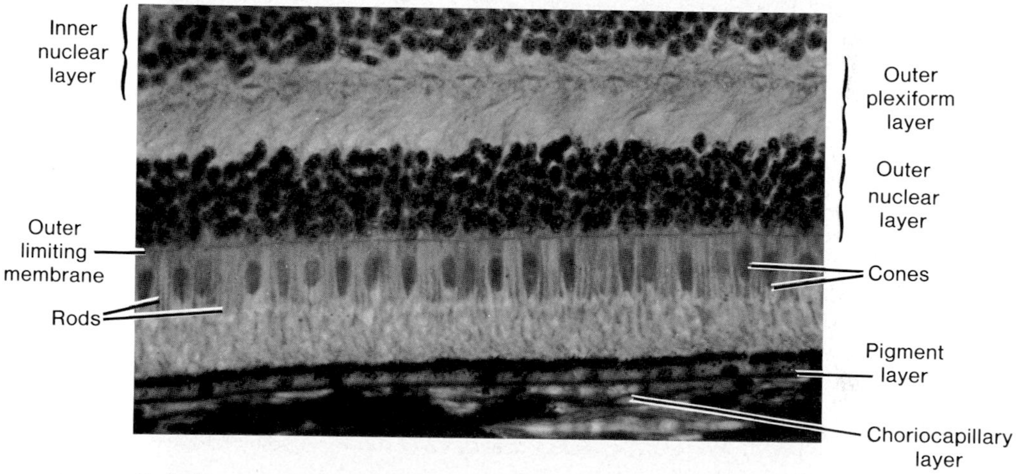

9-18

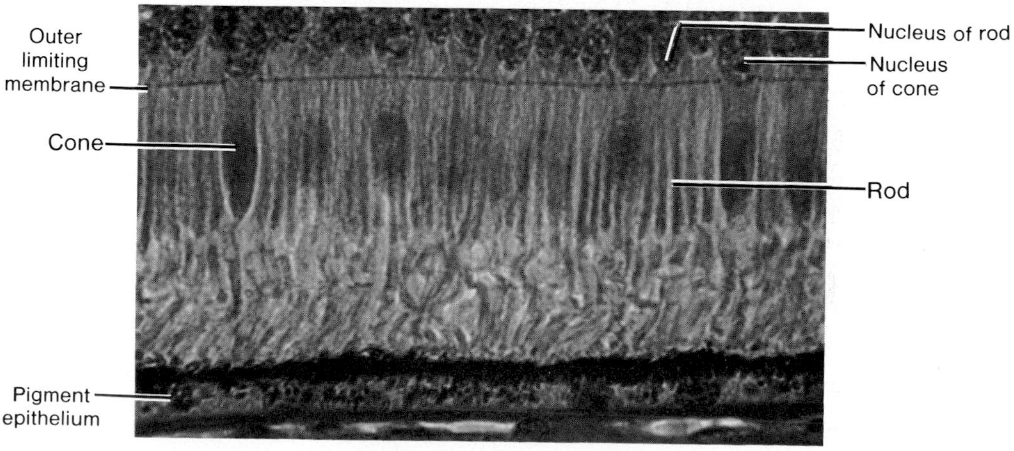

Figure 9-16 Retina. LM, ×250.
Figure 9-17 Retina. LM, ×250.
Figure 9-18 Retina. LM, ×1000.

9-19

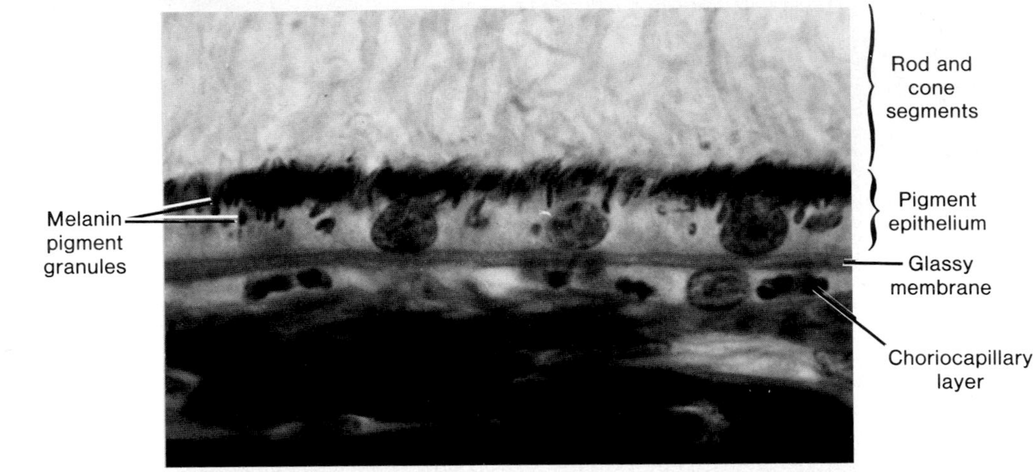

9-20

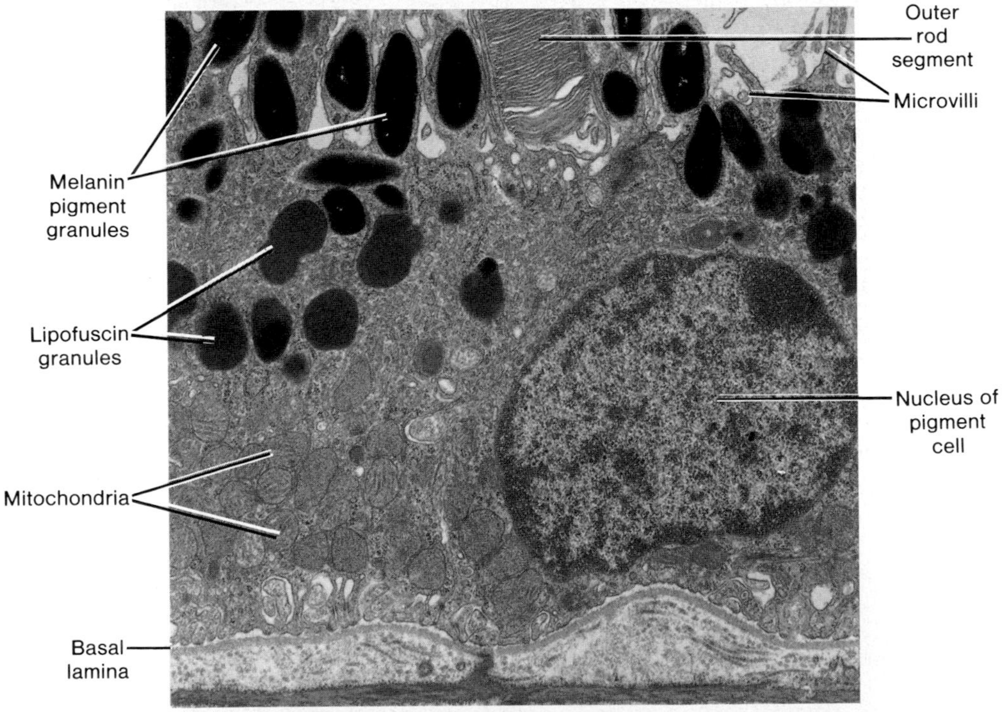

Figure 9-19 Pigment epithelium. LM, ×1000.
Figure 9-20 Pigment epithelium (human). TEM, ×6000.

9-21

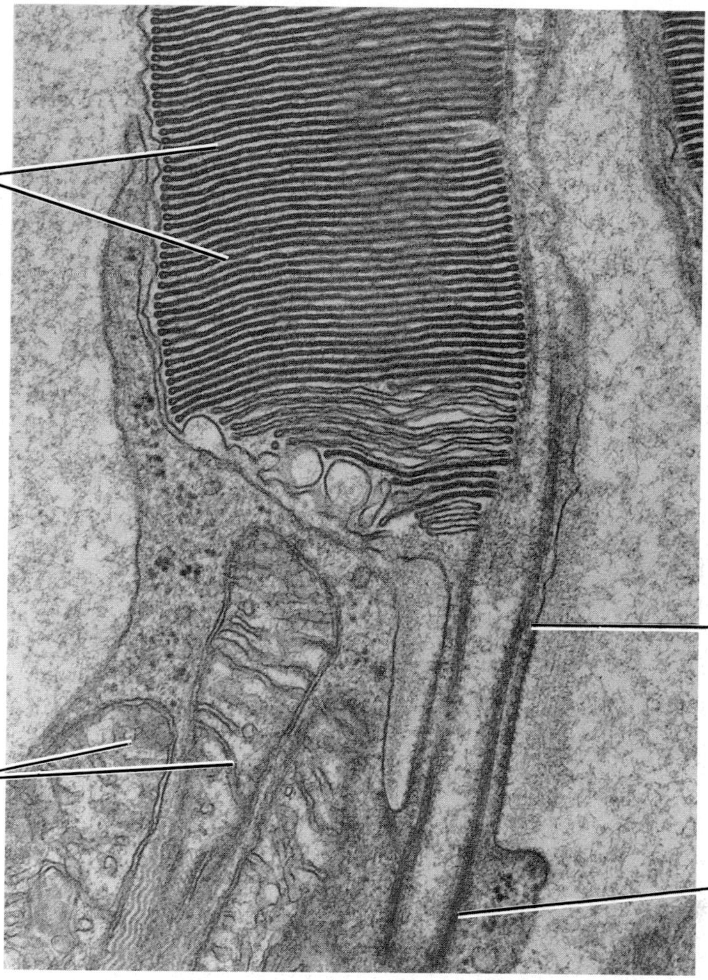

9-22

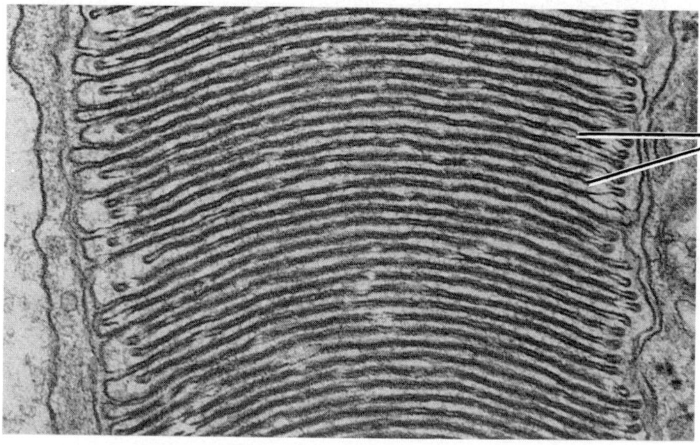

Figure 9-21 Junction of outer and inner segment of rod. TEM, ×45,000.
Figure 9-22 Cone outer segment. TEM, ×56,000.

9-23

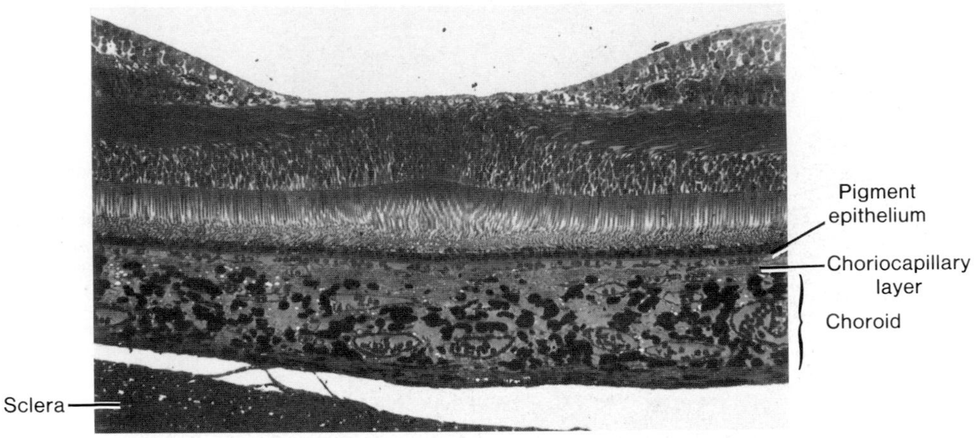
Pigment epithelium
Choriocapillary layer
Choroid
Sclera

9-24

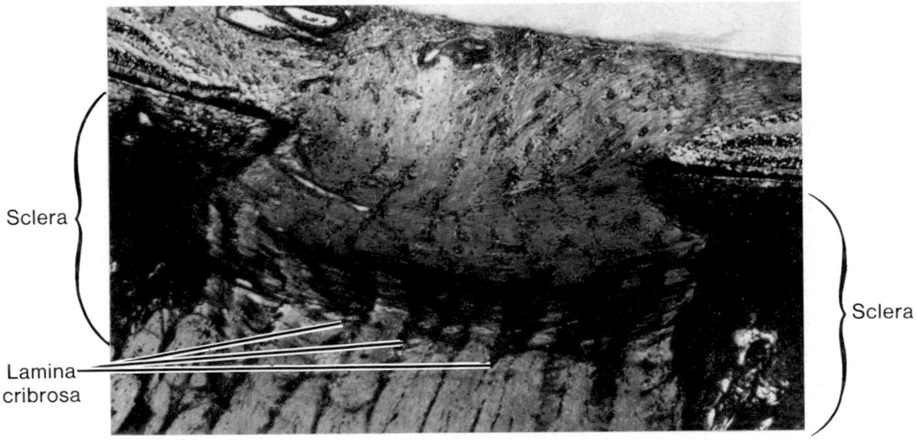
Sclera
Sclera
Lamina cribrosa

9-25

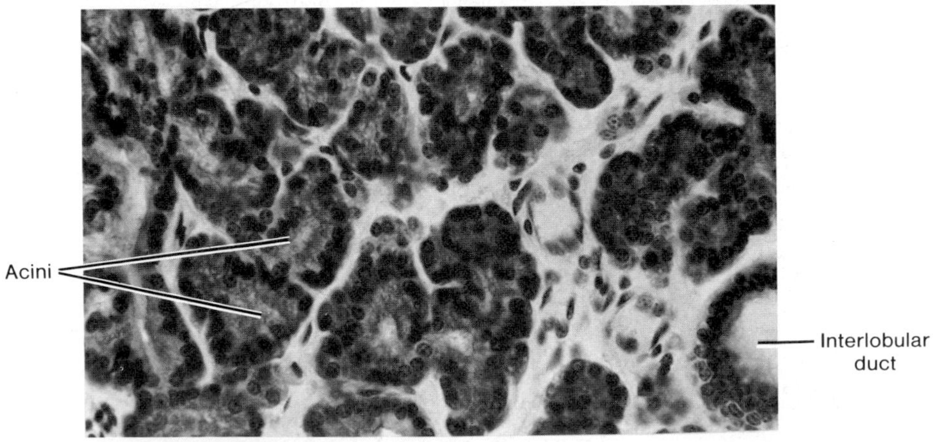
Acini
Interlobular duct

Figure 9-23 Fovea centralis of retina. LM, ×100.
Figure 9-24 Optic disk. LM, ×100.
Figure 9-25 Lacrimal gland. LM, ×250.

Development

9-26

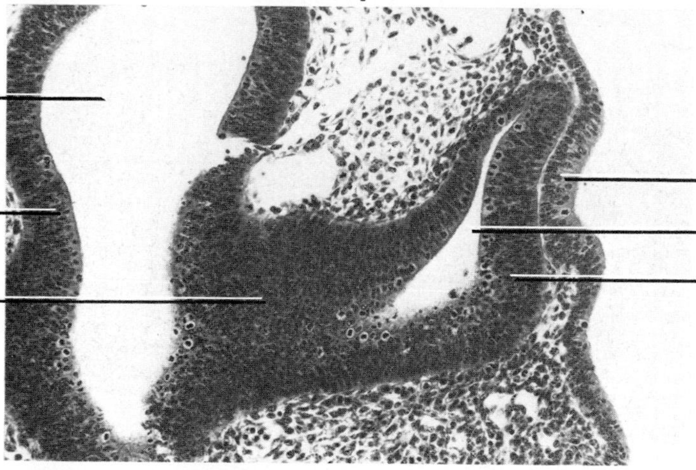

9-27

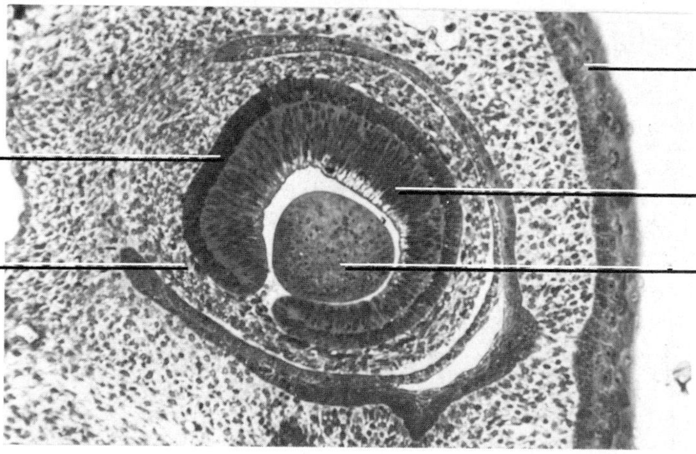

9-28

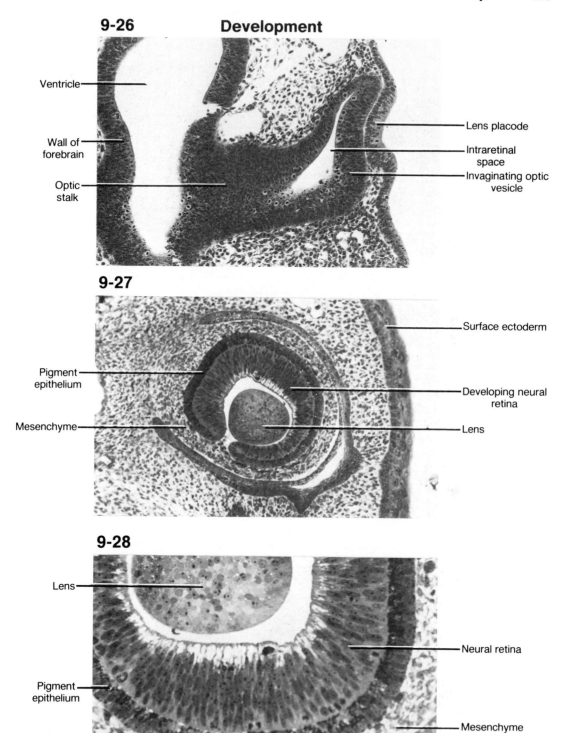

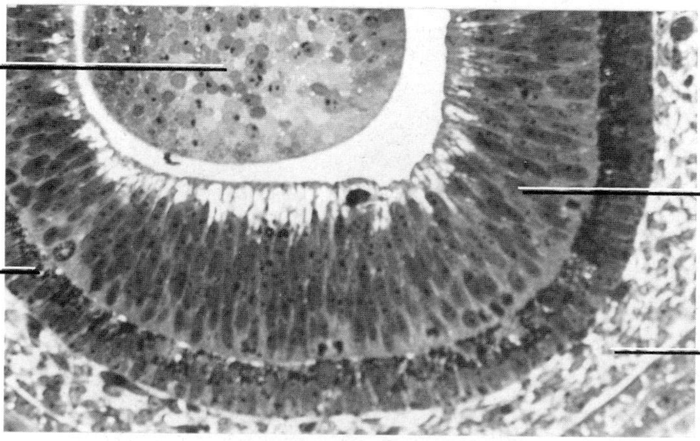

Figure 9-26 Eye. LM, ×100.
Figure 9-27 Eye. LM, ×100.
Figure 9-28 Eye. LM, ×250.

9-29

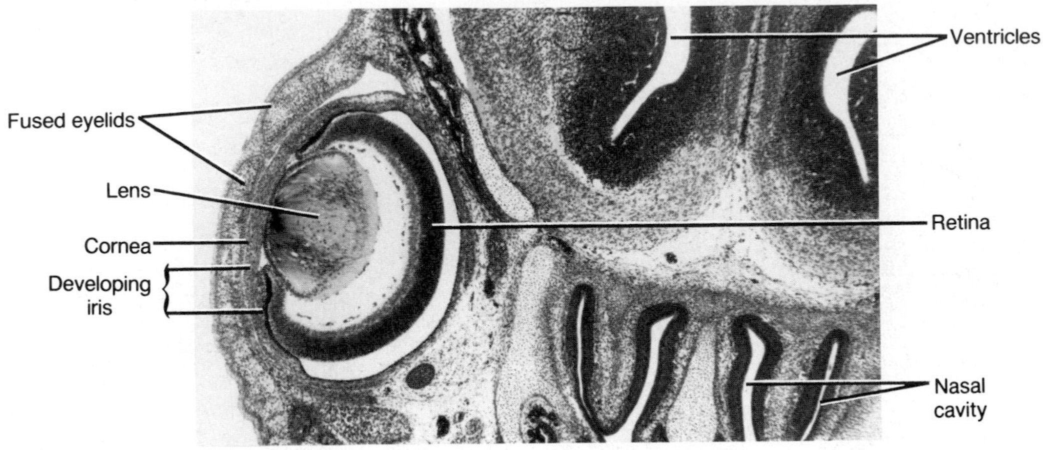

9-30

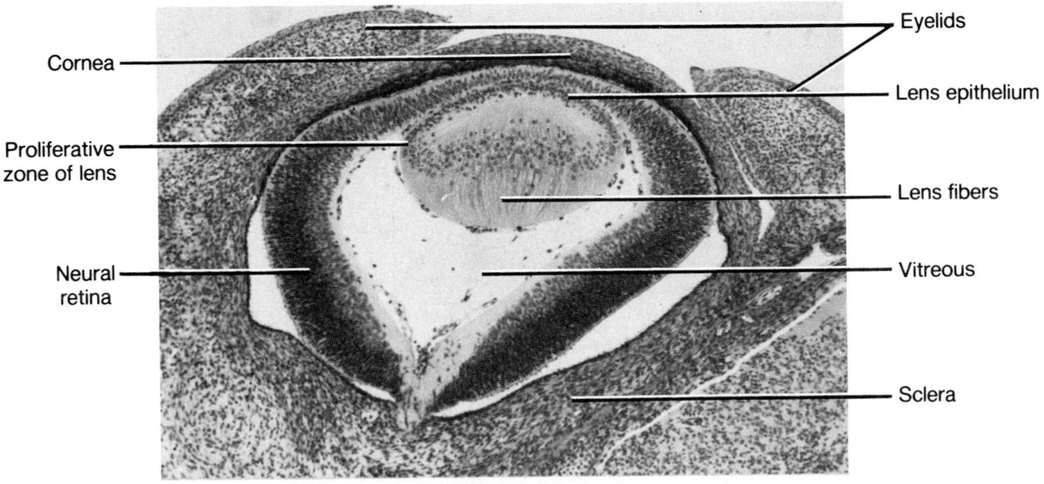

9-31

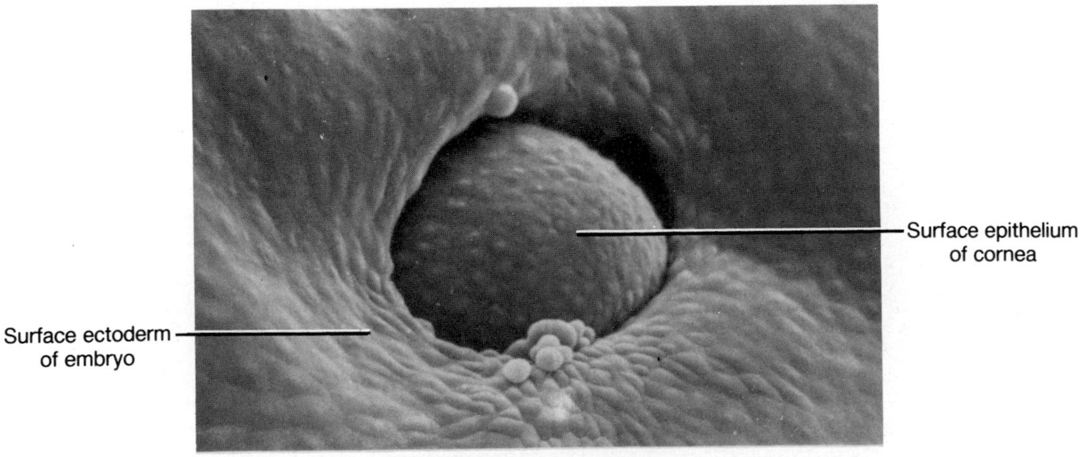

Figure 9-29 Eye. LM, ×50.
Figure 9-30 Eye. LM, ×100.
Figure 9-31 Eye. SEM, ×250.

10

The Ear

The ear (Fig. 10-1) contains receptors that are specialized for hearing and for the awareness of head position and movement. It is usual to subdivide the ear into the external ear, which receives and directs sound waves from the surrounding environment; the middle ear, which transforms sound waves into mechanical vibrations; and the inner ear, where the mechanical vibrations from the middle ear generate nerve impulses that are relayed to the brain to be interpreted as sound. The inner ear also contains the vestibular organs which function in balance.

EXTERNAL EAR

KEY WORDS: auricle (pinna), elastic cartilage, external auditory meatus, ceruminous glands, cerumen

The **auricle**, or **pinna**, of the external ear consists of an irregular piece of **elastic cartilage** surrounded by a thick perichondrium that is rich in elastic fibers. In man, the covering skin contains a few small hairs, their associated sebaceous glands and occasional sweat glands. The skin adheres tightly to the perichondrium, except on the posterior surface, where a subcutaneous layer is present. In most mammals the auricle is associated with sheets of skeletal muscle and in many species is mobile to aid in collecting and directing sound waves into the external auditory meatus.

The **external auditory meatus** is about 2.5 cm in length and follows an open S-shaped course. It consists of an outer portion, the cartilaginous walls of which are continuous with the auricular cartilage, and an inner portion whose walls are formed by temporal bone. The external auditory meatus is lined by keratinized stratified squamous epithelium continuous with the surrounding epidermis of the auricle. The epithelium of the external auditory meatus is firmly anchored to the surrounding perichondrium or periosteum by underlying connective tissue. Small hairs are abundant in the epithelium of the outer portion of the meatus and are associated with large sebaceous glands in the subjacent connective tissue. A special form of coiled apocrine sweat gland, the **ceruminous gland**, is found in the skin that lines the meatus. Depending on their state of activity, the secretory cells of this gland may vary from cuboidal to columnar in shape. Each secretory tubule is surrounded by a network

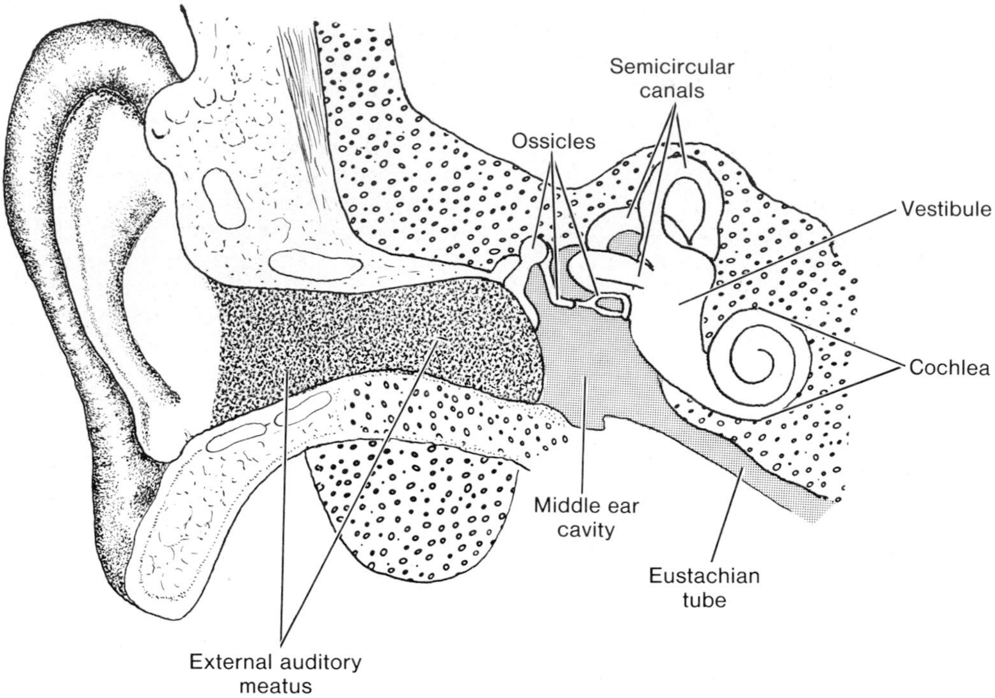

Figure 10-1. Diagram of the structure of the ear.

of myoepithelial cells that lies within the limiting basal lamina of the gland. Ducts of the ceruminous glands may open directly onto the free surface or together with adjacent sebaceous glands, they may open into hair follicles. Their secretory product is a brown, waxy material called **cerumen** that prevents drying of the skin that lines the external auditory meatus. Hair and glands occur only along the roof of the inner (bony) portion of the external auditory meatus.

MIDDLE EAR

KEY WORDS: tympanic cavity, auditory ossicles (malleus, incus, stapes), tensor tympani, stapedius, auditory tube, tympanic membrane

The **tympanic cavity** is an irregularly shaped space in the petrous portion of the temporal bone. It is continuous anteriorly with the auditory or Eustachian tube and posteriorly with mastoid air cells (cavities) in the temporal bone. The lateral wall consists primarily of the tympanic membrane (eardrum), which forms a partition separating the tympanic cavity from the external auditory meatus. The inner, bony wall of the middle ear makes contact with the inner ear via two small, membrane-covered apertures called the oval and round windows. The membrane of the oval window contains the base of an auditory ossicle, the stapes. The membrane covering the round window is often referred to as the secondary tympanic membrane.

The tympanic cavity contains a chain of three small bones, the **auditory ossicles (malleus, incus, stapes)**, which are composed of compact bone. They unite the tympanic membrane of the middle ear with the oval window of the inner ear. Small synovial joints occur between the malleus and incus and incus and stapes. The auditory ossicles are suspended in the air-filled tympanic cavity by thin strands of connective tissue called ligaments. Two small skeletal muscles, the **tensor tympani** and **stapedius**, also are found in the tympanic cavity associated with two of the auditory ossicles. The tendon of the tensor tympani attaches to the malleus and that of the stapedius to the stapes. The bulk of the muscles themselves are contained within small canals in the temporal bone.

The auditory ossicles, their suspending ligaments and the interior walls of the tympanic cavity are covered by a thin mucous membrane consisting of a simple squamous epithelium and a thin underlying layer of connective tissue. The mucous membrane is firmly attached to the adjacent periosteum of the temporal bone, lines the interior of the mastoid air cells and covers the inner surface of the tympanic membrane. Where the tympanic cavity joins the auditory tube, the lining epithelium may become ciliated columnar interspersed with secretory cells.

The **auditory tube** (Eustachian tube) is about 4 cm in length and connects the anterior portion of the tympanic cavity with the nasopharynx. The auditory tube serves as a passageway to ventilate the tympanic cavity and allow pressure equilibration between the middle ear and throat. The supporting wall adjacent to the tympanic cavity is compact bone, whereas the framework for the medial two-thirds of the auditory tube consists of a J-shaped elastic cartilage. The epithelium lining the bony portion of the auditory tube generally is ciliated simple columnar, whereas that of the cartilaginous portion is ciliated pseudostratified columnar. Cilia beat toward the pharyngeal orifice. Near the pharyngeal orifice, goblet cells are found in the lining epithelium and mixed compound tubuloalveolar glands are often encountered in the subjacent connective tissue. A mass of lymphoid tissue, the tubal tonsil, fills the adjacent connective tissues and infiltrates the lining epithelium.

The **tympanic membrane**, which forms most of the lateral wall of the tympanic cavity, is made up of three layers. The outer layer consists of stratified squamous epithelium which reflects onto the tympanic membrane from the external auditory meatus. Two layers of collagenous fibers and fibroblasts form the middle layer. In the external layer, the fibers have a radial arrangement, whereas those of the inner layer form a circular pattern. A simple squamous epithelium and its supporting connective tissue form the third layer and are continuous with the lining of the tympanic cavity. The fibrous layers of the tympanic membrane enter a surrounding ring of fibrocartilage that unites the eardrum to the surrounding bone. The inner surface of the tympanic membrane is attached to the malleus.

The tympanic membrane receives sound waves which cause it to vibrate slightly. The resulting vibrations are transmitted to the fluid-filled chambers of the inner ear via the auditory ossicles. The tympanic membrane is about 18 times as large as the oval window of the inner ear, which contains the foot plate of the stapes. Because of this arrangement, the eardrum and auditory ossicles act as a hydraulic piston that exerts pressure on the confined fluid in the chambers of the inner ear. Thus, the tympanic membrane and the auditory ossicles serve not only to transmit the vibrations but also because of their unique arrangement, also to amplify the weak forces of the sound waves without an expenditure of energy.

The tensor tympani and stapedius muscles protect delicate structures in the inner ear by dampening ossicle movement that results from loud or sudden noise. They also are thought to regulate the degree of tension in the tympanic membrane, so that sounds of moderate intensity can be transmitted in a noisy environment.

INNER EAR

KEY WORDS: bony labyrinth, perilymph, membranous labyrinth, endolymph

The inner ear consists of a system of canals and cavities within the petrous portion of the temporal bone. The compact bone immediately surrounding the canals and cavities forms the **bony labyrinth** and is filled with a fluid called **perilymph.** A series of fluid-filled membranous structures, collectively known as the **membranous labyrinth**, lie suspended in the perilymph. The membranous labyrinth is filled with **endolymph**, a fluid with an ionic composition similar to that of intracellular fluid, being rich in potassium ions and low in sodium ions. Perilymph resembles extracellular fluid, having a high sodium ion and low potassium ion concentration. Endolymph is produced by an area of the cochlear duct known as the stria vascularis. The exact site of perilymph formation is unknown.

The bony and membranous labryinths consist of two major components: the vestibular labyrinth which contains sensory elements for equilibrium (Fig. 10-2) and the cochlea which contains sensory structures for hearing.

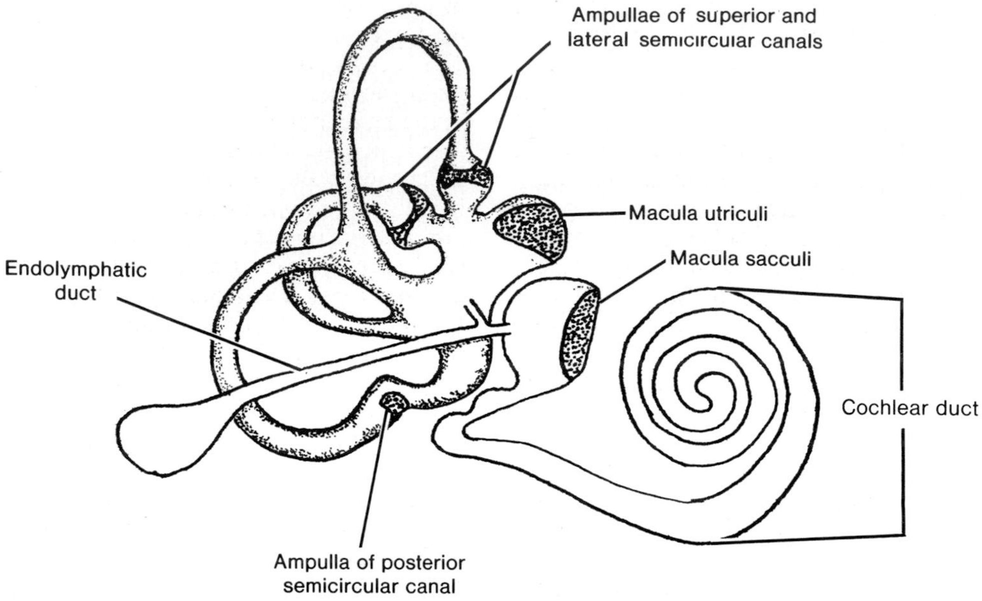

Figure 10-2. Location of sensory regions in membranous labyrinth. The sensory regions are **stippled**.

Vestibular Labyrinth

KEY WORDS: semicircular canals, utricle, saccule, cristae ampullaris, maculae utriculi and sacculi, type I hair cells, kinocilium, type II hair cells, supporting (sustentacular) cells, planum semilunatum, cupula, otolithic membrane, otoliths (otoconia)

The vestibular labyrinth consists of three **semicircular canals** that are continuous with an elliptical structure called the **utricle**. The utricle unites in turn with an anteromedial spherical portion of the vestibular system called the **saccule** by a thin duct that joins a similar duct extending from the saccule. The two ducts unite to form a slender endolymphatic duct which terminates as a small expansion called the endolymphatic sac.

Most of the membranous labyrinth forming the vestibular portion of the inner ear is lined by a simple squamous epithelium. The remainder of its thin wall consists of fine connective tissue fibers and stellate-shaped fibroblasts. Thin connective tissue trabeculae extend from the wall of the membranous labyrinth and cross the perilymphatic spaces to blend with the periosteum of the surrounding bone. The trabeculae suspend the membranous component of the semicircular canals, utricle and saccule in the perilymph that is contained within the osseous labyrinth. The perilymphatic connective tissue is rich in blood capillaries which supply the various segments of the the membranous labyrinth.

In specific regions of each subdivision of the membranous labyrinth, the epithelium assumes a stratified appearance and functions in sensory reception. The sensory epithelium of each semicircular canal is restricted to the dilated ampullary portion, and, together with an underlying core of connective tissue, forms a transverse ridge that projects into the lumen of the ampulla. The connective tissue is rich in nerve fibers. These sensory neuroepithelial regions of the semicircular canals form the **cristae ampullaris**. Similar raised regions of sensory epithelium are found both in the utricle and saccule and form the **macula utriculi** and **macula sacculi**, respectively. The macula of the utricle covers an area approximately 2-mm square along the superior-anterior wall. It lies on a plane perpendicular to the macula of the saccule which occupies an area measuring 2×3 mm on the anterior wall of the saccule. The sensory epithelium of both the cristae and maculae consists of type I and type II sensory hair cells (Fig. 10-3) and supporting (sustentacular) cells.

Type I hair cells are flask-shaped with a narrow apical region and rounded base that contains the nucleus. A large portion of the cell is enveloped by a cup-like afferent nerve ending or calyx. Nearby efferent nerve endings may synapse with the surrounding nerve calyx but are not in direct contact with the type I hair cell; a narrow intercellular space, 30-nm in width, separates the type I hair cell from the nerve ending. The space narrows to approximately 5 nm at gap junctions, which are scattered between the two components. Synaptic ribbons often are found in the cytoplasm of the type I hair cell, immediately adjacent to the limiting cell membrane. Mitochondria are concentrated around the nucleus and at the cell apex. The cytoplasm also contains numerous microtubules concentrated primarily in the apical region. The cytoplasm of the nerve calyx shows scattered mitochondria and numerous vesicles ranging from 50 to 200 nm in diameter.

The apical cell membrane of the type I hair cell is characterized by 50 to 100 large specialized microvilli referred to as "hairs." They are nonmotile, limited by a plasmalemma, have a cytoplasmic core that is rich in fine filaments and are constricted at their bases just before they join the rest of the cell. The longitudinally arranged filaments pass from the microvilli and enter into a thick mat of filaments which forms a terminal web in the apical cytoplasm of the cell. The microvilli show a progressive increase in height from about 1 μm on one side to about 100 μm on the opposite side of the cell. A single eccentric cilium is present on the apical surface and is peculiar in that the two central microtubules terminate shortly after originating from the basal body. It is thought to be nonmotile and is often referred to as a **kinocilium.**

Type II hair cells are simple columnar and are not enveloped by a single afferent nerve ending, but are surrounded by numerous separate afferent and efferent nerve endings. Type II hair cell also bears a single, eccentric, nonmotile cilium and 50 to 100 large microvilli arranged identically to those of type I hair cells. The cytoplasm shows scattered profiles of granular endoplasmic reticulum, abundant mitochondria, smooth-

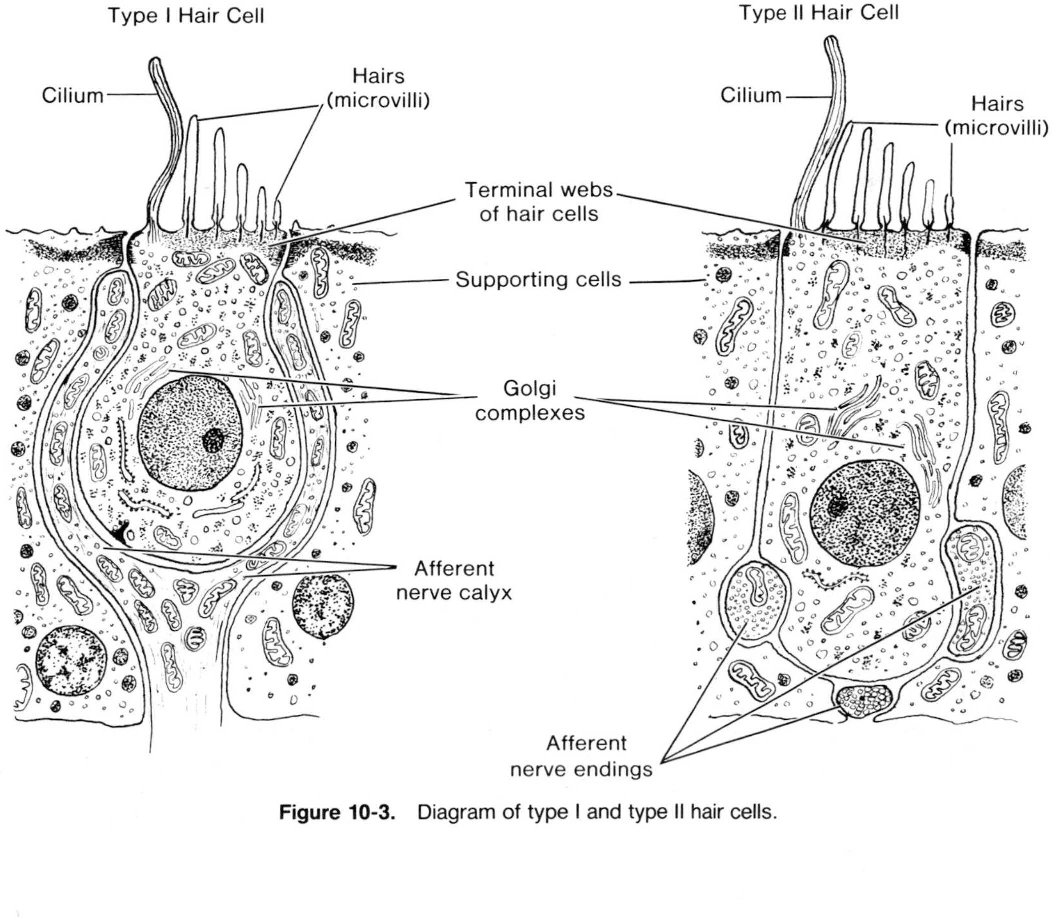

Figure 10-3. Diagram of type I and type II hair cells.

surfaced tubules, and contains numerous vesicles 20 nm in diameter. A well developed Golgi complex occupies a supranuclear position. Synaptic ribbons also are found in the cytoplasm of type II hair cells, immediately opposite the surrounding nerve terminals.

The adjacent **supporting** or **sustentacular cells** are columnar in shape and extend from the basal lamina to the free surface of the sensory epithelium. They follow a very irregular course through the sensory epithelium and in electron micrographs show a well developed terminal web at the cell apex, a prominent Golgi complex, numerous secretory granules and bundles of microtubules extending from the basal cytoplasm to the terminal web. The microtubules form an integral part of the cytoskeleton and provide the rigidity of the supporting cells. Although the function of the supporting cells is controversial, it has been suggested that they may be concerned with the metabolism of endolymph or may contribute to the nutrition of hair cells. At the periphery of the sensory epithelium the supporting cells form a simple columnar layer, the **planum semilunatum**, which is devoid of hair cells.

The microvilli of the hair cells in the cristae are embedded in an overlying gelatinous structure known as the **cupula**, which is composed of viscous proteoglycans that project from the surface of the cristae into the ampullary lumen of each semicircular canal. Supporting cells in the sensory epithelium also may contribute to the cupula. The sulfated proteoglycan is thought to be secreted by the planum semilunatum. Microvilli of hair cells from the maculae of the utricle and saccule also are embedded within a viscous proteoglycan that forms the **otolithic membrane**. In addition, numerous crystalline bodies called **otoliths** or **otoconia** are suspended within this layer of proteoglycan. These bodies consist of protein and calcium carbonate.

The gelatinous cupula of the cristae projects across the lumen of the ampullary region of the semicircular canal in the manner of a "swinging door" and during angular movement of the head is displaced by the motion of endolymph contained within this portion of the membranous labyrinth. The displacement of the cupula excites the sensory hair cells, which in turn generate an action potential received by surrounding nerve terminals. Similarly, gravitational forces on the gelatinous otolithic membrane and the otoconia embedded within it cause a shearing motion on the microvilli of the underlying hair cells in the maculae. Linear acceleration also results in the stimulation of hair cells in the maculae.

Although the exact mechanism is unknown, the sensory epithelium in the vestibular organs transforms the mechanical energy of endolymph movement into the electrical energy of a nerve impulse. The bending or displacement of microvilli is thought to result in the depolarization of hair cells, the impulse being transferred to surrounding nerve endings to result in the generation of a nerve impulse. Efferent nerve endings probably have an inhibitory function and may control the threshold of activity of hair cells.

Cochlea

KEY WORDS: modiolus, spiral ganglion, spiral lamina, basilar membrane, spiral ligament, vestibular membrane, scala vestibuli, cochlear duct, scala tympani, ductus reuniens, cecum cupulare, helicotrema

Like the vestibular portion of the inner ear, the cochlea consists of an outer portion of compact bone and a central membranous portion contained in perilymph. The osseous part of the cochlea spirals for 2¾ turns around a central axis of spongy bone called the **modiolus**, which is shaped like a cone. Blood vessels, nerve fibers and the perikarya of afferent bipolar neurons, called the **spiral ganglion**, lie within the bony substance of the modiolus. Extending from the modiolus into the lumen of the cochlear canal along its entire course is a bony projection called the **spiral lamina**. A fibrous structure, the **basilar membrane**, extends from the spiral lamina to the **spiral ligament**, a thickening of the periosteum on the outer bony wall of the cochlear canal. The thin **vestibular membrane** extends obliquely across the cochlear canal from the spiral lamina to the outer wall of the cochlea.

The basilar and vestibular membranes subdivide the cochlear canal into an upper **scala vestibuli**, an intermediate **cochlear duct**, and a lower **scala tympani**. A cross section of the cochlea is shown in Figure 10-4.

The cochlear duct is part of the endolymphatic system and is connected to the saccule of the membranous labyrinth by the small **ductus reuniens**. The opposite end of the cochlear duct terminates at the apex of the cochlea as the blindly ending **cecum cupulare**. Both the scala vestibuli and the scala tympani contain perilymph and communicate at the apex of the cochlea through a small opening known as the **helicotrema**. At the base of the cochlea the scala tympani is closed by the secondary tympanic membrane which fills the fenestra rotundum (round window). This membrane separates the perilymph of the scala tympani from the air-filled cavity of the middle ear. The scala vestibuli extends through the perilymphatic channels of the vestibule to end at the fenestra ovalis (oval window), which is closed by the foot of the stapes. Movement of the stapes in the fenestra ovalis exerts pressure on the perilymph in the scala vestibuli. Because the fluid cannot be compressed, waves of pressure either pass through the cochlear duct, displacing it to enter the scala tympani, or enter the scala tympani directly through the helicotrema. The pressure is released from the confined perilymphatic spaces of the cochlea by the elasticity of the secondary tympanic membrane which bulges into the tympanic cavity of the middle ear. Figure 10-5 shows the mechanics of hearing.

Cochlear Duct

KEY WORDS: basilar membrane, spiral crest, vestibular membrane, stria vascularis, marginal cells, basal cells, intraepithelial capillaries, spiral prominence

The cochlear duct is a triangular space which follows the spiral course of the cochlea. Its floor is formed by the basilar membrane and its roof by the vestibular membrane. The **basilar membrane** consists of a layer of collagen-like fibers embedded in an amorphous matrix and extends from the osseous spiral lamina of the modiolus to the **spiral crest**, a well vascularized periosteal

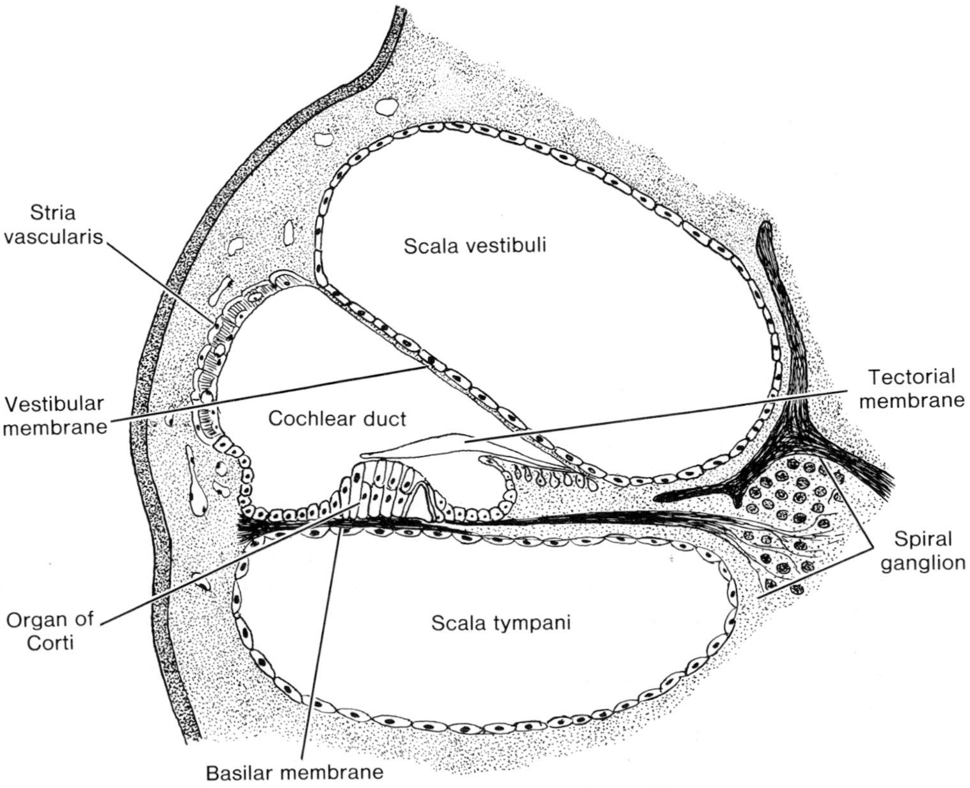

Figure 10-4. Cross section of the cochlea.

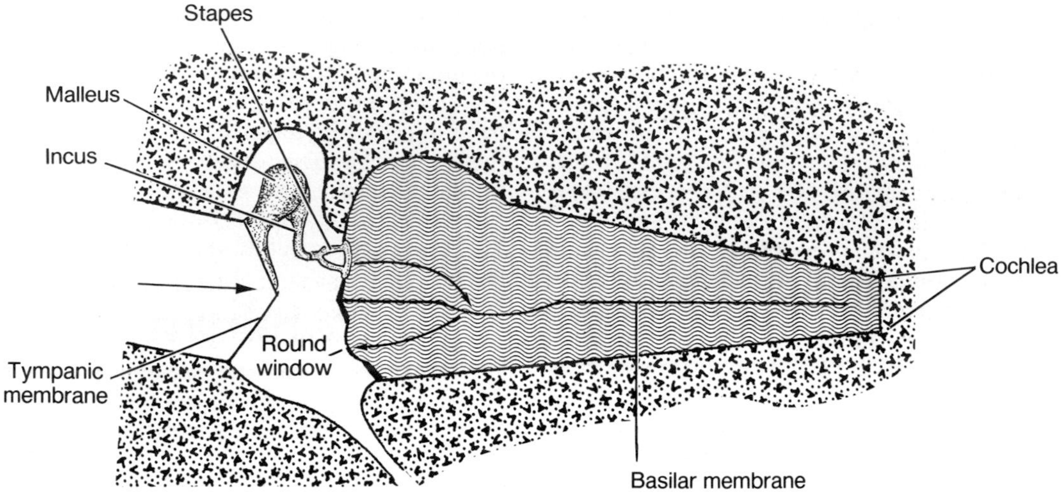

Figure 10-5. Mechanics of hearing.

region along the outer wall of the cochlea. The **vestibular membrane** consists of two layers of simple squamous cells separated primarily by their associated basal laminae.

The outer wall of the cochlear duct is formed by a vascular area called the **stria vascularis**. It occurs along the entire length of the cochlear duct and consists of a pseudostratified columnar epithelium and an underlying vascular connective tissue. The lining epithelium is continuous with the simple squamous epithelium that lines the interior of the vestibular membrane. The epithelium of the stria vascularis consists of basal cells and marginal cells.

The **marginal cells** show deep infoldings of the basal and lateral cell membranes associated with numerous mitochondria, suggesting that these cells are involved in ion transport; they may participate in the elaboration of endolymph. The **basal cells** show few mitochondria or basal infoldings. The epithelium of the stria vascularis differs from that found elsewhere in the body in that it contains **intraepithelial capillaries**.

The epithelium of the stria vascularis is continuous below with a simple layer of attenuated cells which overlies the **spiral prominence**, a highly vascularized thickening of the periosteum. The spiral prominence lies below the stria vascularis and extends along the entire length of the cochlear duct. The cells assume a cuboidal appearance at the point where the epithelium reflects from the outer wall of the cochlear duct onto the basilar membrane.

Organ of Corti

KEY WORDS: inner pillar cells, outer pillar cells, inner phalangeal cells, outer phalangeal cells, border cells, inner spiral tunnel, spiral limbus, interdental cells, tectorial membrane, cells of Hensen, cells of Claudius, inner hair cells, outer hair cells

The cochlear duct contains a region of specialized cells, the organ of Corti (Fig. 10-6), that transforms vibrations of the basilar membrane into nerve impulses. The avascular organ of Corti extends along the entire length of the cochlear duct, lying on the basilar membrane. It consists principally of supporting cells and hair cells. The supporting cells are tall and columnar and consist of inner and outer pillar cells, inner and outer phalangeal cells, border cells, Hensen's cells and cells of Claudius.

The **inner** and **outer pillar cells** form the boundaries of a space known as the inner tunnel that lies within and extends throughout, the length of the organ of Corti. In both types of pillar cells, the nucleus is located in the broad base. The elongated cell bodies contain numerous microtubules which form a cytoskeleton. Inner pillar cells are slightly expanded at the apex and extend over the outer pillar cells. The apices of the outer pillar cells also expand slightly and fit into the concave apical undersurface of the inner pillar cells. The inner and outer pillar cells not only form the boundaries of the inner tunnel but also provide structural support for adjacent cells.

Inner and outer phalangeal cells act as direct supporting elements for the sensory hair cells. The **inner phalangeal cells** form a single row immediately adjacent to the inner pillar cells and completely surround the sensory inner hair cells, except at their apical regions. In contrast, the columnar **outer phalangeal cells** form three to four rows and support outer hair cells which also are arranged in rows. The apex of each outer phalangeal cell forms a cup-like structure which surrounds the basal one-third of an outer hair cell. Afferent and efferent nerves are situated at its base.

Each outer phalangeal cell gives off a slender cytoplasmic process filled with microtubules and extends to the surface of the organ of Corti, where it expands into a flat plate. The plate attaches to the apical edges of the outer hair cell and is supported laterally by outer phalangeal cells and the outer hair cells in the adjacent row. The apical plates of the outer phalangeal cells provide additional support for the outer hair cells, the upper two-thirds of which are not supported by adjacent cells but are surrounded by large fluid-filled intercellular spaces. The fluid that occupies these spaces is said to be similar to that contained within the inner tunnel.

Another supporting cell associated with the inner edge of the organ of Corti is the **border cell**. These slender cells undergo a transition to the squamous cells that line a small space called the **inner spiral tunnel**. This space is formed by the **spiral limbus**, which consists of periosteal connective tissue that extends from the osseous spiral lamina and bulges into the cochlear duct. Within the substance of the limbus are vertically arranged collagenous fibers often referred to as the auditory teeth. **Interdental** cells are specialized cells along the upper surface of the spiral limbus. These cells extend between the collagen fibers to reach the lumen of the cochlear duct. On the upper surface of the limbus they form a continuous cellular sheet in which the cells are united by tight junctions.

The interdental cells secrete a sheet of material known as the **tectorial membrane**,

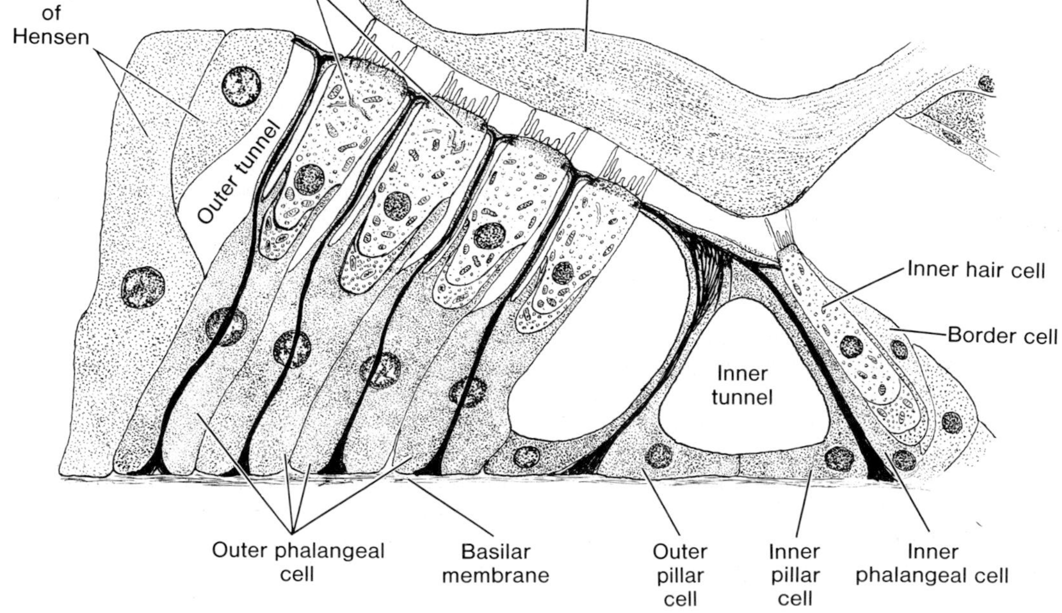

Figure 10-6. Diagram of the organ of Corti.

which consists of a protein thought to be similar to epidermal keratin. The tectorial membrane extends over the interdental cells and beyond the substance of the spiral limbus, to overlie the hair cells of the organ of Corti. Tips of microvilli that extend from the sensory hair cells are firmly embedded in the undersurface of the tectorial membrane.

Near the outer edge of the organ of Corti, immediately adjacent to the outer phalangeal cells, is another group of columnar supporting cells called the **cells of Hensen**. They decrease in height and transform into the adjacent **cells of Claudius**, which form the outer edge of the organ of Corti.

The sensory hair cells are divided into inner and outer hair cells. The **inner hair cells** form a single row along the inner aspect of the organ of Corti and extend along the entire length of the cochlea. Like the type I hair cells of the vestibular labyrinth, the inner hair cells of the cochlea are short, flask-shaped cells with narrow necks. Well developed microvilli extend from the apical surface of the inner hair cells, but unlike the type I hair cells, they lack a kinocilium. The microvilli are arranged in a U at the apical surface and contain numerous filaments which extend into a dense terminal web in the apical cytoplasm. Mitochondria aggregate just beneath the terminal web and are scattered throughout the remainder of the cytoplasm, which also contains scattered ribosomes and profiles of smooth endoplasmic reticulum. Numerous nerve endings form synapses with the bases of the inner hair cells on a plane below the level of the nucleus.

The columnar **outer hair cells** generally are arranged in three or four rows and are supported by the apices of the outer phalangeal cells. Microvilli are arranged in the shape of a "W" and are shorter near the center of the apical cell surface. A cilium is absent. Mitochondria are aggregated at the base of the outer hair cell, which makes contact with afferent and efferent nerve fibers. In all other respects, the outer hair cells are similar to the inner hair cells and both serve as receptors for sound in the organ of Corti.

DEVELOPMENT OF THE EAR

External Ear. Mesenchymal proliferations around the edges of the first and second pharyngeal arches, together with the surface ectoderm, give rise to the auricle. The proliferations occur around the opening of the developing external auditory meatus, and gradually fuse to form the definitive auricle.

The external auditory meatus develops from the first pharyngeal groove and the bounding arches. As the pharyngeal cleft grows centrally, it forms a funnel-shaped, ectodermally-lined pit surrounded by cartilage. A thick epithelial plate forms in the ectoderm, growing from the base of the pit toward the developing tympanic cavity. After making contact, the ectodermal plate degenerates and the epithelium over the floor of the meatus becomes the outer (ectodermal) epithelium of the eardrum. The inner epithelial surface arises from the endodermally-derived lining of the adjacent tympanic cavity. Connective tissue between the two epithelial layers develops from mesenchyme. Initially, the eardrum lies horizontally, almost parallel to the floor of the meatus, but as the meatus continues to grow and lengthen, the eardrum gradually becomes more erect.

Middle Ear. The tympanic cavity is derived from the first pharyngeal pouch and is lined by epithelium of endodermal origin. The distal part of the pouch, the tubotympanic recess, widens to form a provisional tympanic cavity. The narrow proximal connection to the region of the developing nasopharynx becomes the auditory tube. Mesenchyme from the first and second pharyngeal arches above the provisional cavity becomes cartilaginous and forms the first models of the ossicles. These remain embedded in a spongy mesenchyme until the tympanic cavity widens and the mesenchyme degenerates. As this occurs, the epithelium expands to line the newly-formed cavity and inner surface of the eardrum, and to cover the ossicles in a mesentery-like manner. The ossicles thus are suspended in the tympanic cavity, but actually lie outside the epithelium of the cavity. Each cartilaginous ossicle undergoes endochondral ossification.

The tensor tympani and stapedius muscles arise from mesenchyme of the first and second pharyngeal arches, respectively, and lie beyond the lining of the tympanic cavity. Ligaments supporting the ossicles develop from mesenchyme that lies between the mesentery-like folds of the covering epithelium. The lining of the tympanic cavity continues to expand and eventually lines the mastoid air cells of the temporal bone.

Inner Ear. The epithelium of the inner ear is ectodermal in origin. Thickenings of the ectoderm, the auditory placodes, occur midway along both sides of the midbrain and invaginate to form cup-shaped auditory pits. These expand, lose their connections with the surface ectoderm and become detached ovoid sacs—the auditory vesicles or otocysts. A narrow tubular recess, the endolymphatic duct, develops from the region last in contact with ectoderm, eventually expanding into a blind endolymphatic sac. The otocyst elongates and a tubular outgrowth at the ventral pole grows, spiral fashion, for 2¾ turns into the surrounding mesenchyme. This is the cochlear duct which remains connected to the saccule by a narrow ductus reuniens. The dorsal part of the otocyst expands and develops into the semicircular canals; the intermediate region forms the utricle and saccule.

The epithelial lining of the various segments of the membranous labyrinth is, at first, simple low columnar. As nerve fibers grow among the cells of the cristae ampullaris, macula of the utricle, saccule and organ of Corti, the epithelium thickens and differentiates into special sensory and supporting cells. Supporting cells are believed to secrete and maintain the cupula and otolithic membranes in the cristae and maculae, respectively. Differentiation of the organ of Corti progresses slowly, beginning as a thickening of the epithelium in the basal turn and progressing to the apex. Large inner and small outer ridges of epithelium form, both associated with a covering tectorial membrane. The small ridge gives rise to the supporting and inner and outer hair cells of the organ of Corti; the inner ridge involutes to form the lining of the spiral sulcus.

At first, the structures of the developing membranous labyrinth are embedded in mesenchyme which later undergoes chondrification and in turn is replaced by bone to form the bony labyrinth. Cartilage adjacent to the membranous labyrinth degenerates to form a syncytial reticulum, which becomes the perilymphatic spaces filled with perilymph. In the region of the forming cochlear duct, the cartilage is resorbed in such a manner that two perilymphatic spaces (scala vestibuli and scala tympani) are formed on either side of the cochlear duct. The modiolus of the cochlea develops directly from mesenchyme as membranous bone.

FUNCTIONAL SUMMARY

The pinna of the external ear collects external sound and directs it into the external auditory meatus. Sound waves cause the tympanic membrane to vibrate slightly at the same frequency as the sound waves. Auditory ossicles, suspended in the tympanic cavity of the middle ear, conduct the vibrations to the perilymphatic channels of the inner ear. The force of the vibrations created by the sound waves is amplified without expenditure of energy because the tympanic membrane is much larger than the foot plate of the stapes. Together the intervening ossicles act as an hydraulic piston. With each movement, the foot plate of the stapes exerts pressure on the perilymph, which is confined to the scala vestibuli and scala tympani of the inner ear. The pressure waves pass through the perilymph from the scala vestibuli to the scala tympani to be released

from the perilymphatic spaces by the bulging of the secondary tympanic membrane into the air-filled tympanic cavity. As the pressure waves move from the scala vestibuli to the scala tympani, they must first pass through the intervening cochlear duct or travel to the helicotrema at the apex of the cochlea. When a pressure wave passes through the cochlear duct, both the vestibular and basilar membranes are displaced slightly. Such displacement of the basilar membrane and organ of Corti creates a strong shearing force between the microvilli at the apex of the inner and outer hair cells and the overlying tectorial membrane. The shearing action is thought to stimulate the hair cells, which in turn elicit a nerve impulse in the surrounding afferent nerve endings. Supporting cells, particularly the pillar and phalangeal cells, provide strong structural support to the cell bodies of the hair cells, so they are not displaced by this shearing action.

Large areas of the basilar membrane vibrate at several frequencies. However, sound waves of a given frequency produce a maximum displacement along specific regions of the basilar membrane. With sound waves of lower frequency, maximum displacement occurs further away from the oval window. Because both efferent and afferent nerve endings terminate on hair cells in the organ of Corti, both sensory reception and inhibition are said to occur. The inhibitory mechanisms stem from the central nervous system and may aid in the discrimination of both loudness and pitch.

The two skeletal muscles of the middle ear, the tensor tympani and stapedius, act to dampen ear ossicle movement and protect the delicate structures of the inner ear from loud and sudden noises. Contraction of these muscles also may play an important role in regulating the degree of tension placed on the tympanic membrane, so that sounds of moderate intensity can be transmitted in a noisy environment.

Nerve impulses from the organ of Corti are transmitted via the bipolar neurons of the spiral ganglion to the cochlear division of the eighth cranial nerve. From here impulses are relayed to appropriate regions of the brain to be interpreted as sound.

The vestibular portion of the inner ear is important for coordinating and regulating the movements of locomotion and equilibrium. Types I and II hair cells of the cristae in the ampullary region of each semicircular canal are stimulated during angular movement of the head. Sensory stimulation of these receptors results from the movement of endolymph that displaces a gelatinous cupula overlying the cristae. Displacement of the cupula, in which microvilli of underlying hair cells are embedded, causes a shearing force at the apices of the hair cells. Similarly, forces created during linear acceleration act upon the otolithic membrane and the contained otoconia, again resulting in a shearing force on the apices of hair cells in the maculae. Hence, linear acceleration results in the stimulation of hair cells in the maculae, while angular motion results in stimulation of hair cells in the cristae.

Hair cells of the vestibular organs, as well as those in the cochlea, transform mechanical movements of the endolymph (produced by displacement of the cupula, otolithic membrane or basilar membrane) into the electrical energy of a nerve impulse. The bending or displacement of microvilli on the various types of hair cells is thought to result in depolarization of the hair cell, the stimulus then being transferred to surrounding afferent nerve endings to generate a nerve impulse. Associated efferent nerve endings are thought to have an inhibitory function and may elevate the threshold of activity of the hair cells.

Atlas for Chapter 10

10-7 Ear

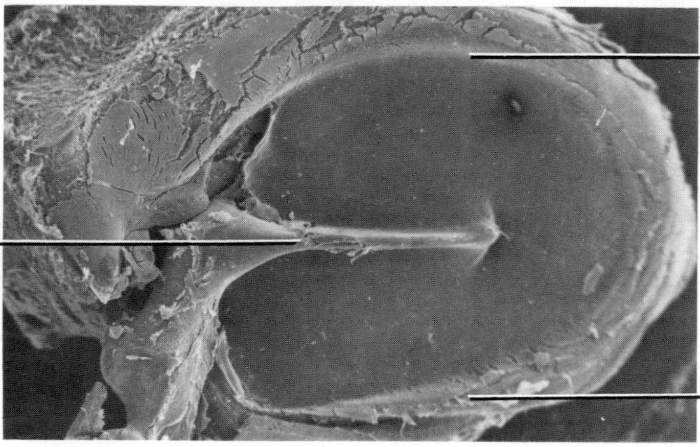

10-8

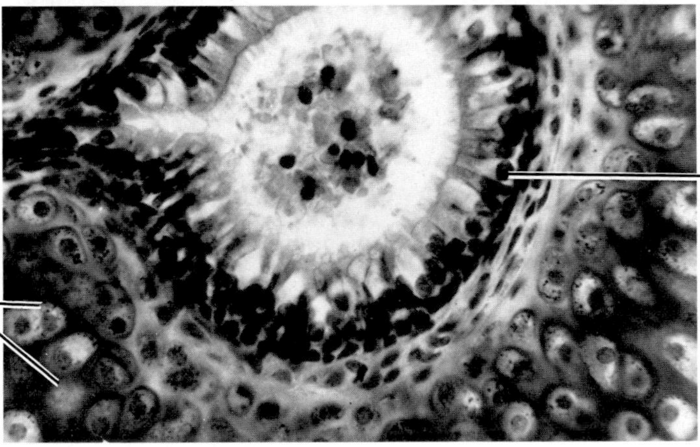

10-9

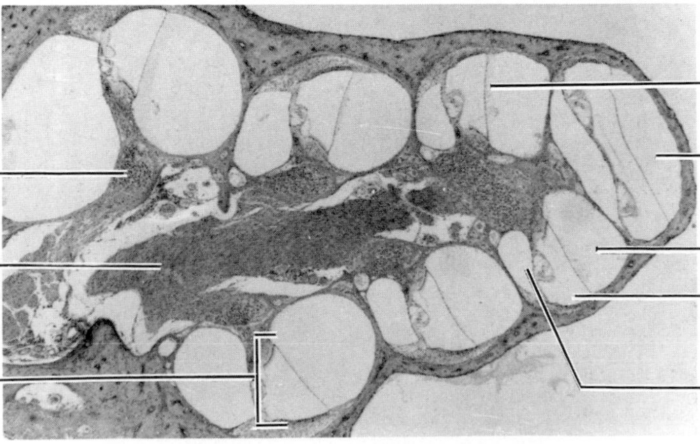

Figure 10-7. Eardrum. SEM, ×20.
Figure 10-8. Eustachian tube. LM, ×350.
Figure 10-9. Cochlea. LM, ×25.

10-10

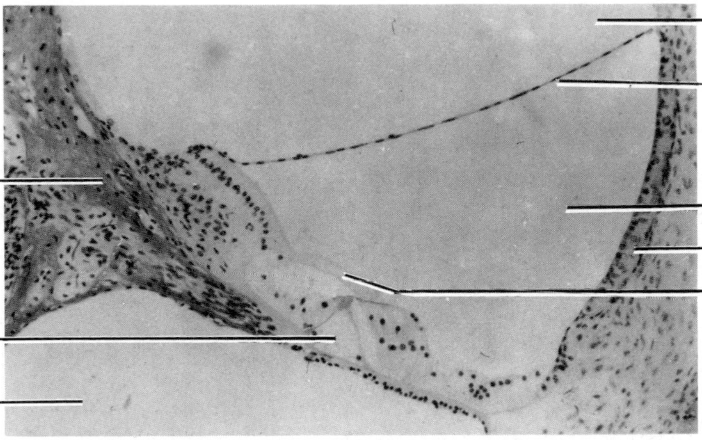

10-11

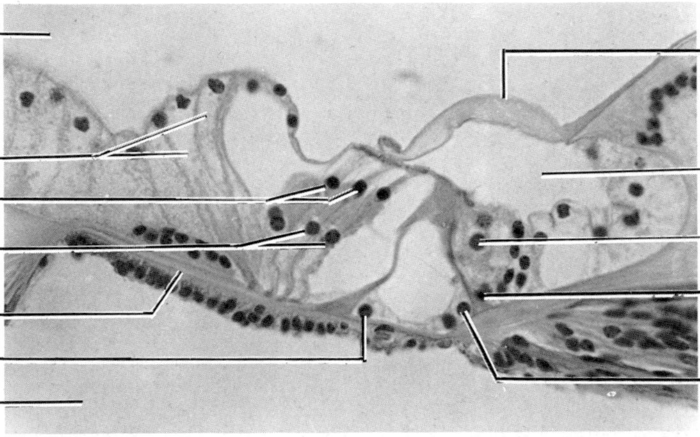

10-12

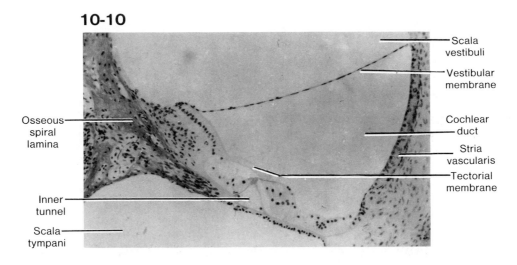

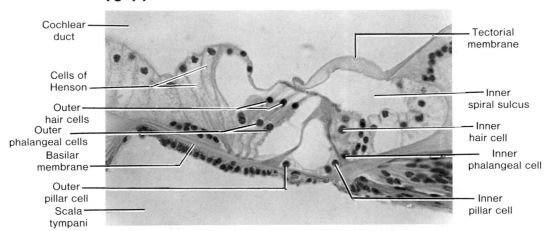

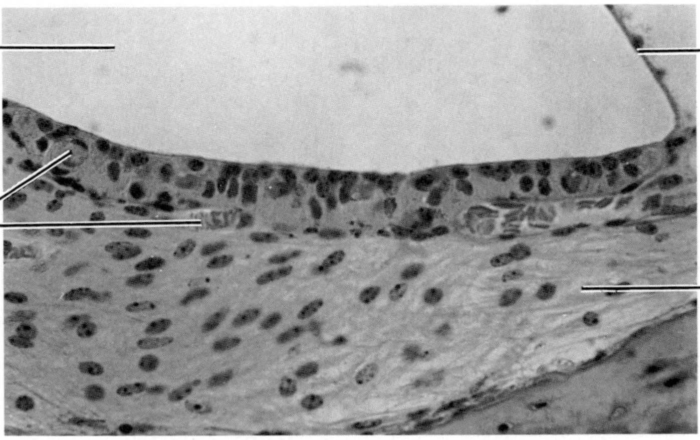

Figure 10-10. Organ of Corti. LM, ×100.
Figure 10-11. Organ of Corti. LM, ×250.
Figure 10-12. Stria vascularis. LM, ×250.

10-13

10-14

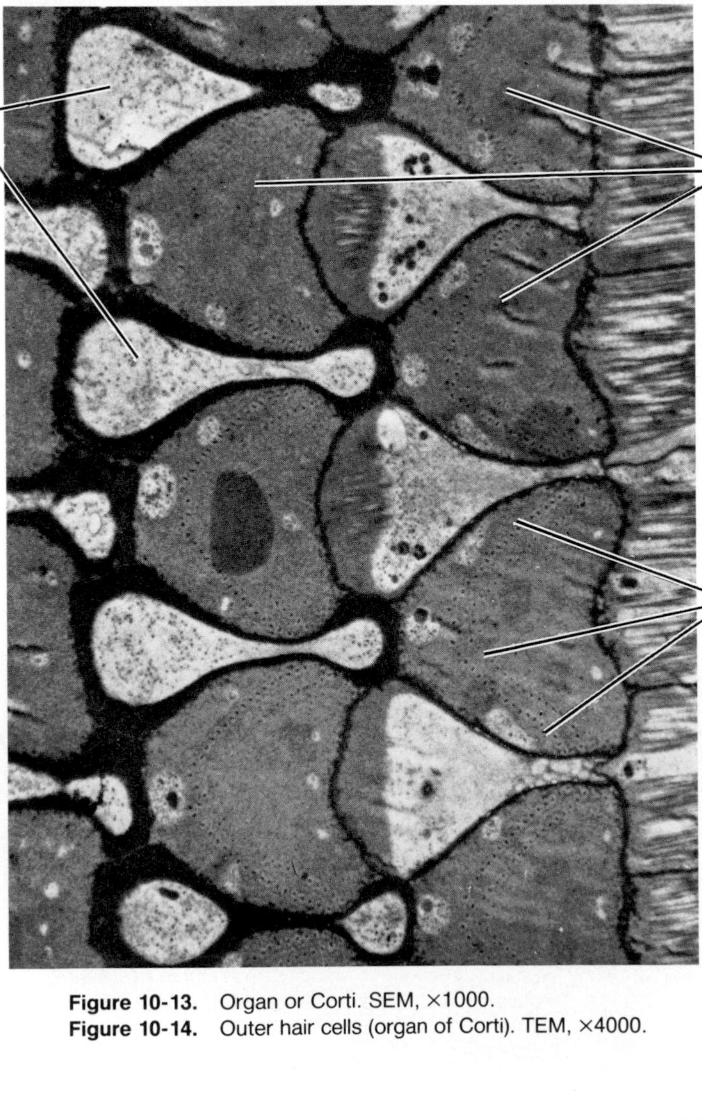

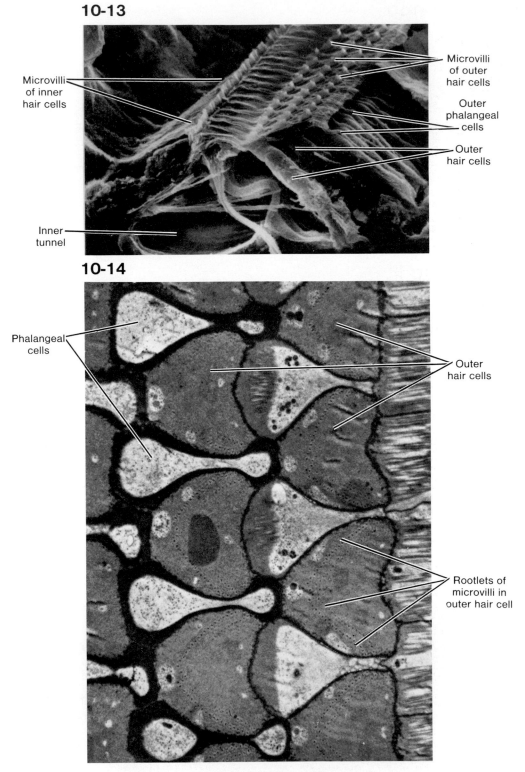

Figure 10-13. Organ or Corti. SEM, ×1000.
Figure 10-14. Outer hair cells (organ of Corti). TEM, ×4000.

10-15

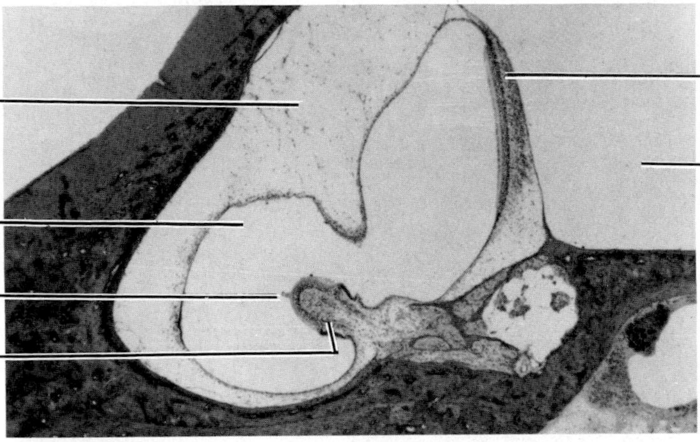

10-16

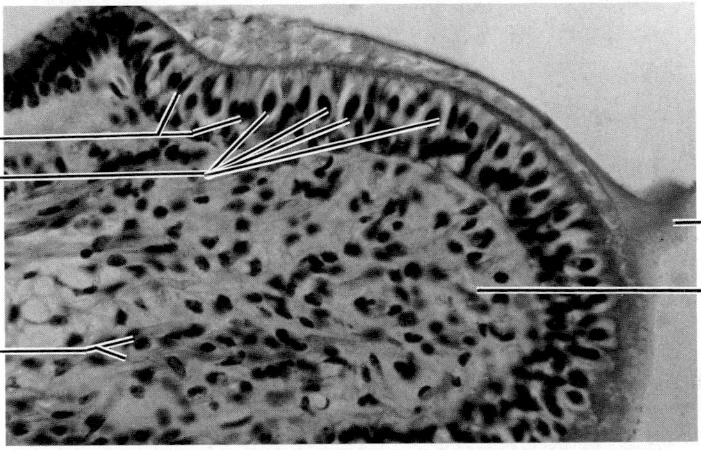

10-17

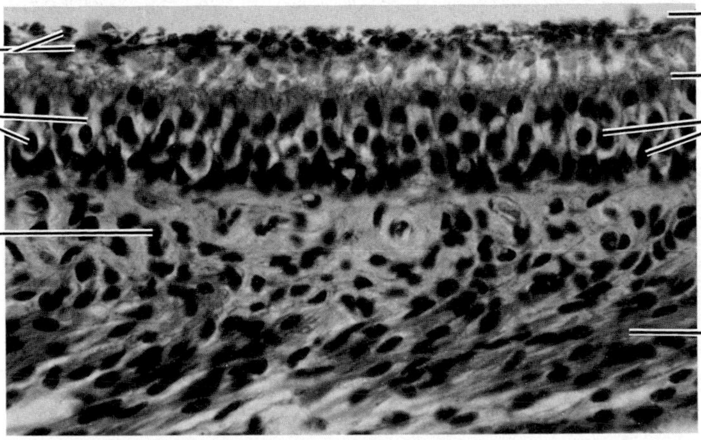

Figure 10-15. Crista ampullaris and macula utriculi. LM, ×40.
Figure 10-16. Crista ampullaris. LM, ×250.
Figure 10-17. Macula utriculi. LM, ×250.

10-18

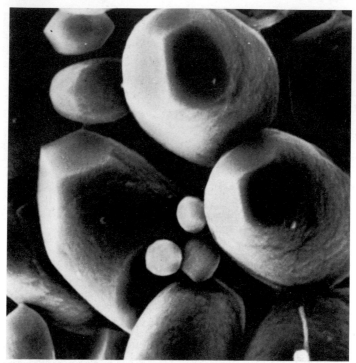

10-19

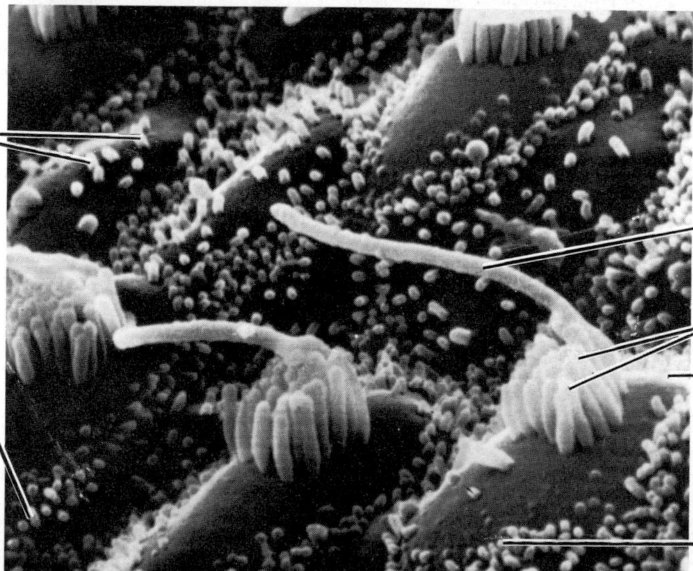

Figure 10-18. Otoconia. SEM, ×4000.
Figure 10-19. Vestibular hair cells. SEM, ×6000.

10-20 Development

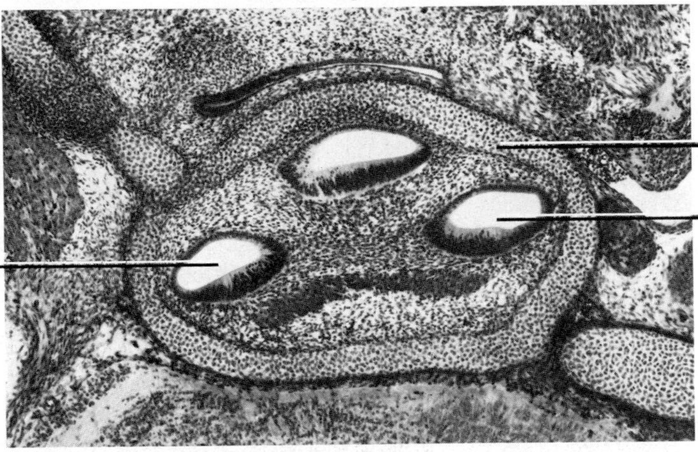

10-21

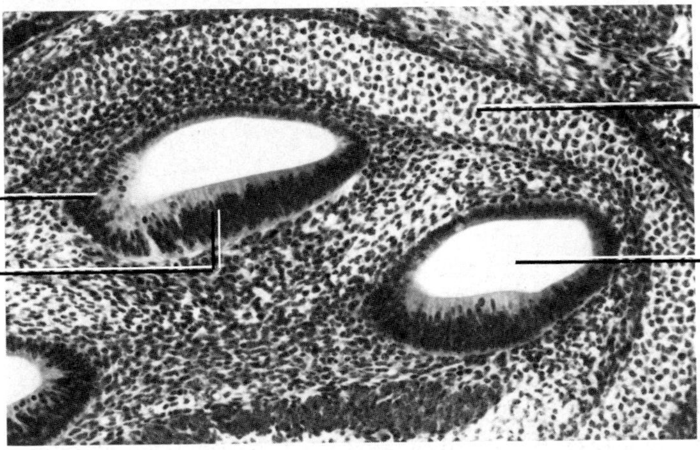

10-22

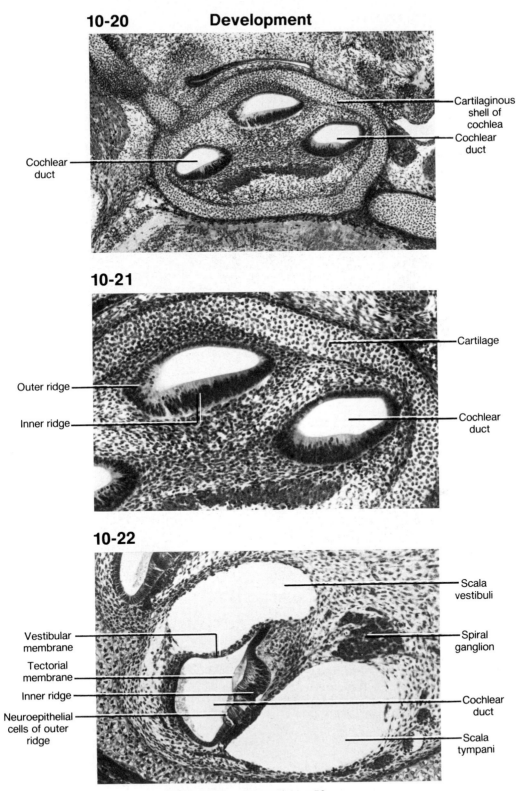

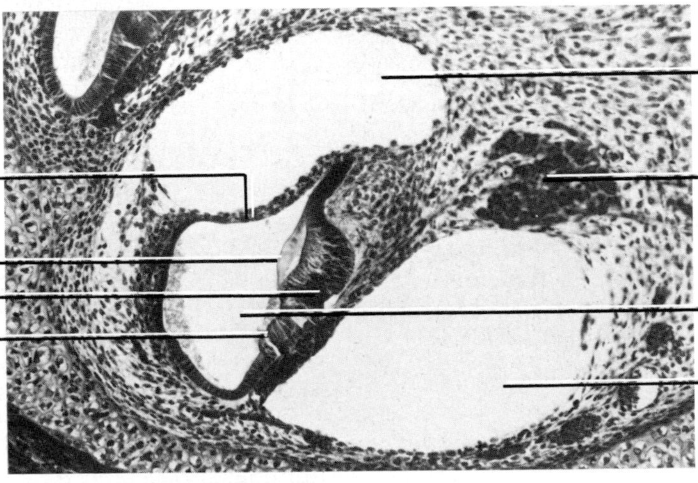

Figure 10-20. Cochlea. LM, ×50.
Figure 10-21. Cochlea. LM, ×100.
Figure 10-22. Cochlear duct. LM, ×100.

11

Cardiovascular and Lymph Vascular Systems

Unicellular animals acquire their nutriments and oxygen directly from the external environment by simple diffusion and other activities of the cell membrane. However, in multicellular animals most of the cells lie deep in the body with no access to the external environment and materials are transported to them through a closed system of branching tubes. Together with a muscular pump, the system of tubes makes up the cardiovascular or blood vascular system. The entire system consists of a heart that serves as the pumping unit, arteries that carry blood to the organs and tissue, capillaries where exchange of material occurs and veins which return blood to the heart.

A second system of vessels, the lymph vascular system, drains interstitial fluid from organs and tissues and returns it to the blood vascular system. It lacks a pumping unit and is unidirectional, carrying lymph toward the heart only. There is no lymphatic equivalent of blood arteries.

HEART

The heart is a modified blood vessel which serves as a double pump and consists of four chambers. On the right side, the atrium receives blood from the body and the ventricle propels it to the lungs. The left atrium receives blood from the lungs and passes it to the left ventricle, from which it is distributed throughout the body. The wall of the heart consists of an inner lining layer, a middle muscular layer and an external layer of connective tissue.

Endocardium

KEY WORDS: squamous cells, tight (occluding) junctions, gap junctions, subendothelial layer, subendocardial layer

The endocardium forms the inner lining of the atria and ventricles and is continuous with and comparable to, the inner lining of the blood vessels. It consists of a single layer of polygonal **squamous cells** with oval or rounded nuclei. The cells are closely apposed and joined by **tight (occluding) junctions**. **Gap junctions** are present also and permit communication between the cells. Electron micrographs reveal a few short microvilli, a thin proteoglycan layer over the luminal surface and the usual organelles in the cytoplasm. The endothelial cells rest on a continuous layer of fine collagen fibers. This layer has been called the **subendothelial layer**. Deep to it is a thick layer of denser connective tissue which forms the bulk of the endocardium and contains elastic fibers and some smooth muscle. Loose connective tissue, the **subendocardial layer**, binds the endocardium to the underlying heart muscle and contains collagen fibers, elastic fibers and blood vessels. In the ventricles it also contains the specialized cardiac muscle fibers of the conducting system.

Myocardium

KEY WORDS: striated cardiac muscle

The myocardium is the middle layer of the heart wall and consists mainly of **striated cardiac muscle**. It is thinnest in the atria and thickest in the left ventricle. The myocardium is arranged in layers that form complex spirals about the atria and ventricles. In the atria, bundles of cardiac muscle form a latticework and are locally prominent as the pectinate muscles. In the ventricles, isolated bundles of muscle form the trabeculae carnae.

Elastic fibers are scarce in the ventricular myocardium, but are plentiful in the atria, where they form an interlacing network between the muscle fibers. The elastic fibers of the myocardium become continuous with those of the endocardium and outer coat of the heart (epicardium).

Epicardium

KEY WORDS: visceral layer of pericardium, subepicardial layer

The epicardium is the **visceral layer of the pericardium**, the fibrous sac that encloses the heart. The free surface of the epicardium is covered by a single layer of flat to cuboidal mesothelial cells below which is a layer of connective tissue that contains numerous elastic fibers. In the layer adjacent to the cardiac muscle, the epicardium contains blood vessels, nerves and a variable amount of fat. This part frequently is called the **subepicardial layer**.

The parietal layer of the pericardium consists of connective tissue lined by mesothelial cells. The mesothelial surface of the parietal layer faces that of the epicardium, separated only by a thin film of fluid which allows the layers to slide over each other during contraction and relaxation of the heart.

Cardiac Skeleton

KEY WORDS: dense connective tissue, anuli fibrosi, trigona fibrosa, septum membranaceum

The so-called cardiac skeleton consists of several **dense connective tissue** structures to which the cardiac muscle is attached. The main part of the skeleton is formed by the **anuli fibrosi**, rings of fibrous tissue that surround the openings of the aorta and pulmonary artery. Also contributing to the skeleton are masses of fibrous tissue, the **trigona fibrosa** that occur between the atrioventricular and arterial openings, and the **septum membranaceum**, which is the upper fibrous part of the interventricular septum. The fibrous rings contain elastic fibers and some fat cells and, with aging, may become calcified. In dogs the rings contain hyaline cartilage, and bone normally occurs in the anuli fibrosi in cattle.

Valves

Valves are present between the atria and ventricles and at the openings of the aorta and pulmonary vessels. Regardless of location, the valves are similar in structure. The atrioventricular valves are attached to the anuli fibrosi, the connective tissue of which extends into each valve to form its core. The valves are covered on both sides by endocardium which is thicker on the ventricular side, where it contains more elastic fibers. Scattered smooth muscle fibers are present in the endocardium on the atrial surface of the valves. On the ventricular side, the valves are connected to the papillary muscles by thin tendinous cords called the chordae tendinae. Valves of the pulmonary arteries and aorta are thinner, but show the same general structure as the atrioventricular valves.

Conducting System

KEY WORDS: sinoatrial node, atrioventricular node, atrioventricular bundle, Purkinje fibers (cells), nodal cells

The conducting system of the heart consists of specialized cardiac muscle fibers and is responsible for initiating and maintaining cardiac rhythm, and for ensuring coordination of the atrial and ventricular contractions. The system consists of the sinoatrial node and atrioventricular bundle.

The **sinoatrial node** is located in the epicardium at the junction of the superior vena cava and right atrium. Impulses initiated in this node spread through the ordinary cardiac muscle of the atria to reach the **atrioventricular node**, which is located on the right side of the interatrial septum. From here the impulse travels rapidly along the **atrioventricular bundle** in the membranous part of the interventricular septum. The bundle divides into two trunks that pass into the ventricles, where they break up into numerous branches that connect with the ordinary cardiac muscle fibers. Thus, the impulse is conducted to all parts of the ventricular myocardium.

The specialized fibers of the atrioventricular bundle and its branches are called the **Purkinje fibers (cells)** and differ in several respects from ordinary cardiac muscle fibers. The Purkinje fibers are larger, contain more sarcoplasm and myofibrils are less numerous and usually have a peripheral location. The fibers are rich in glycogen and mitochondria and often have two (or more) nuclei. Intercalated discs are uncommon, but numerous desmosomes are scattered along the cell boundaries. **Nodal cells** are smaller than ordinary muscle cells but otherwise are similar in structure to the Purkinje cells.

BLOOD VESSELS

The blood vessels consist of variously sized tubes arranged in a circuit, through which blood is delivered from the heart to the tissues, then back to the heart from all parts of the body. By means of this circulatory system, oxygen from the lungs, nutrients from the intestines and liver and regulatory agents such as hormones are distributed to all of the organs and tissues. Waste products also are emptied into the circulation and carried to various organs for elimination.

Structural Organization

KEY WORDS: tunica intima, tunica media, tunica adventitia

Although blood vessels differ in size, distribution and function, their structural organization shows many common features. Like the heart, the walls of blood vessels consist of three major coats or tunics. Differences in the function and appearance of the various segments of the circulatory system are reflected by structural changes in these layers, or by reduction or even omission of some features of the basic structural pattern. From the lumen outward, the wall of a blood vessel consists of a tunica intima, tunica media and tunica adventitia.

Tunica intima corresponds to, and is continuous with, the endocardium of the heart. It consists of an endothelium of flattened squamous cells, resting on a basal lamina and supported by a subendothelial connective tissue.

Tunica media is the most variable layer, in size and in structure. Depending on the function of the vessel, this layer contains variable amounts of smooth muscle and elastic tissue. In the heart the tunica media is represented by the myocardium.

Tunica adventitia also varies in thickness in different parts of the vascular circuit. It consists mainly of connective tissue and corresponds to the epicardium of the heart.

ARTERIES

As the arteries course away from the heart they undergo successive divisions to provide numerous branches whose calibers progressively decrease. The changes in size and corresponding structure of the vessel wall are continuous, but three classes of arteries can be distinguished and are designated as: large elastic or conducting arteries, medium-sized muscular or distributing arteries and small arteries and arterioles.

Elastic or Conducting Arteries

KEY WORDS: tunica intima, endoendothelial coat, caveolae, subendothelial layer, tunica media, elastic laminae, tunica adventitia, vasa vasorum

The aorta is the main conducting artery, but also in this class are the common iliac, pulmonary, brachiocephalic, subclavian and common carotid arteries. A major feature of this type of artery is the width of the lumen, compared to which the wall of the vessel appears thin.

The **tunica intima** is relatively thick and is lined by a single layer of flattened, polygonal cells that rest upon a complete basal lamina.

Adjacent endothelial cells may be interdigitated or overlap and are extensively linked by occluding and communicating junctions. The cells contain the usual organelles but these are few in number. Peculiar membrane-bound, rod-shaped granules, consisting of several tubules embedded in an amorphous matrix, are present but their significance is unknown. At the luminal surface, the cell membrane is coated with a proteoglycan and this layer has been called the **endoendothelial coat**. On the basal surface, the endothelial cells are separated from the basal lamina by an amorphous matrix. Numerous invaginations or **caveolae** are present at the luminal and basal surfaces of the plasmalemma, and the underlying cytoplasm contains many small vesicles 50 to 70 nm diameter. These are believed to form at one surface, detach and cross to the opposite wall, where they fuse and discharge their contents. In man, about one-quarter of the total thickness of the intima is formed by the **subendothelial layer**, which consists of loose connective tissue that contains elastic fibers and a few smooth muscle cells.

The **tunica media** is the thickest layer and consists largely of elastic tissue which forms 50 to 70 concentric fenestrated sheets, or **laminae**, each about 2 to 3 μm thick and 5 to 20 μm apart. The successive laminae are interconnected by elastic fibers or bands. In the spaces between these elastic sheets are thin layers of connective tissue that contain collagen fibers and smooth muscle cells arranged circumferentially. The smooth muscle cells are flattened, irregular and branched, and are bound to the adjoining elastic laminae by elastic microfibrils and collagen. These structures lie in an appreciable amount of amorphous ground substance. Smooth muscle cells are the only cell elements present in the media of elastic arteries and they are able to synthesize and maintain the elastic fibers.

Elastic arteries are those nearest the heart and, because of the large content of elastic tissue, are expansible. As blood is pumped from the heart during its contraction, the walls of the elastic arteries expand; when the heart relaxes, the elastic recoil of these vessels serves as an auxiliary pumping mechanism to force the blood onward at the time when no pumping force is exerted by the heart.

The **tunica adventitia** is relatively thin and contains bundles of collagen fibers and a few elastic fibers, both of which have a loose helical arrangement. Also present are fibroblasts, mast cells and rare, longitudinally oriented smooth muscle cells. The walls of these large arteries are too thick to be nourished by diffusion from the lumen and consequently their walls are provided with their own small arteries, the **vasa vasorum**. These may be branches of the main vessel or may be derived from neighboring vessels; they form a plexus in the tunica adventitia and generally do not penetrate deeply into the media. The tunica adventitia gradually blends into the surrounding loose connective tissue.

Muscular or Distributing Arteries

KEY WORDS: tunica intima, endothelium, subendothelial layer, internal elastic lamina, tunica media, smooth muscle, external elastic lamina, adventitia

This forms the largest class of arteries and, except for the elastic arteries, contains all of the named arteries of gross anatomy. They vary from 0.3 to 1.0 cm in diameter. As compared to the luminal diameter, the walls of these arteries are thick and make up about one-quarter of the total cross-sectional diameter. The thickness of the wall is due mainly to the large amount of smooth muscle present in the media which, by contraction and relaxation, aids in regulating the supply of blood to organs and tissues. The general organization of these vessels is similar to that of elastic arteries, but the proportion of cells and fibers differs.

The **tunica intima** consists of the lining endothelium, a subendothelial layer and an internal elastic lamina. The **endothelium** and **subendothelial layers** are similar to those of the elastic arteries. With decreasing size of the vessel, the subendothelial layer decreases in thickness. It contains fine collagen fibers, a few elastic fibers and scattered smooth muscle cells which have a longitudinal orientation. The **internal elastic lamina** is a fenestrated band of closely interwoven elastic fibers which forms a prominent, scalloped boundary between the tunica media and tunica intima. The basal surfaces of the endothelial cells send slender processes through the discontinuities in the elastic lamina to make contact with the cells of the underlying tunica media.

Tunica media is the thickest coat and consists almost entirely of **smooth muscle** cells arranged in concentric, helical layers. The number of layers varies from 3 to 4 in the smaller arteries to 10 to 40 in the larger muscular arteries. The muscle cells are surrounded by basal laminae and communicate with each other by means of gap junctions. Reticular fibers and small bundles of collagen fibers are present between the layers of smooth muscle, interspersed with elastic fibers. The amount and distribution of elastic fibers correlate with the caliber of the artery; in small vessels the elastic fibers are scattered between the muscle cells, whereas in larger arteries the elastic tissue forms circularly oriented loose networks. At the junction of the tunica media and tunica adventitia, the elastic tissue forms a prominent, fenestrated membrane called the **external elastic lamina**.

The **tunica adventitia** of the muscular arteries is prominent and in some vessels may be as thick as the tunica media. It consists of collagen and elastic fibers which have a longitudinal orientation. This coat continues into the surrounding loose connective tissue with no clear demarcation.

Small Arteries and Arterioles

These vessels have the general structure of the larger muscular arteries and differ only in size and in the thickness of the layers that comprise their walls. The distinction between small arteries and arterioles is mainly one of definition. Arterioles can be regarded as those small arteries with a diameter less than 250 to 300 μm and which have only one or two layers of muscle cells in the tunica media.

In the progresion from distributing arteries to arterioles, the subendothelial tissue progressively decreases in amount. In arterioles the subendothelial layer is lacking and the tunica intima consists of the endothelium and a fenestrated internal elastic lamina. The endothelial cells are joined by occluding junctions and basally are in contact with the smooth muscle cells by processes that penetrate the internal elastic membrane. The basal lamina is thin and becomes less distinct in the smallest arterioles. The layers of smooth muscle progressively decrease in number, and at a diameter of about 30 μm, the muscle coat of the arteriole consists of a single layer of circumferentially oriented smooth muscle cells. No definite external elastic lamina is present and the internal membrane is thin and disappears in the terminal portions of the arteriole. The adventitia is correspondingly thin.

As compared to the size of the lumen, the walls of the arterioles are thick. Because of their smooth muscle content, arterioles control the blood to the capillary bed, which they feed, and are the main controllers of systemic blood pressure. Precapillary sphincters are simply the small terminal arterioles that give rise to capillaries.

CAPILLARIES

Capillaries are the functional units of the blood vascular system and are interposed between arterial and venous limbs of the blood circulatory system. They branch extensively and form elaborate networks, the extent of which reflects the activity of an organ or tissue. Elaborately branched, closely-packed networks of capillaries are present in the lungs, liver, kidneys, glands and mucous membranes. According to the appearance of the endothelium and basal lamina in electron micrographs, capillaries can be classed as continuous, fenestrated and discontinuous (sinusoids). Regardless of the type, the basic structure of capillaries is the same and represents an extreme simplification of the layers of the wall. The tunica intima consists of an endothelium and a basal lamina; a tunica media is absent; and tunica adventitia is greatly reduced.

Continuous Capillaries

KEY WORDS: continuous endothelium, continuous basal lamina, tunica adventitia, pericytes

These form the common type of capillary, found throughout the connective tissues, muscle and central nervous system. The wall consists of a **continuous endothelium** and a thin tunica adventitia. The lumen ranges from 5 to 10 μm in diameter and in smaller vessels may be encompassed by a single endothelial cell. In the larger capillaries, the lumen may be enclosed by three or four cells. The endothelial cells rest on a **continuous basal lamina** and show the same features as endothelial cells elsewhere in the vascular tree. They possess the usual organelles, caveolae and vesicles, a glycoprotein layer, a few short microvilli on their luminal surfaces, and a variable number of membrane-bound granules whose function is unknown. Adjacent cells may abut each other end to end or overlap each other obliquely or in sinuous interdigitations. At intervals, the adjacent cell membranes unite in occluding junctions, but it is not certain that they form complete belts as in other epithelia. The **tunica adventitia** is thin and contains some collagen and elastic fibers embedded in a small amount of ground substance. Fibroblasts, macrophages and mast cells also are present.

Pericytes are irregular, branched, isolated cells that occur at intervals along capillaries, enclosed by the basal lamina of the endothelium. Generally, the cells resemble fibroblasts and characteristically contain a few dense bodies and numerous cytoplasmic filaments. Their function is unknown.

Fenestrated Capillaries

KEY WORDS: fenestrae (pores), diaphragm, continuous basal lamina

Fenestrated capillaries have the same structure as the continuous type, but differ in that the endothelial cells contain numerous **fenestrae (pores)** which appear as circular openings, 70 to 100 nm in diameter. The fenestrae usually are closed by thin **diaphragms** that show central, knob-like thickenings. The diaphragm is a single-layered structure, thinner than a single unit membrane, so it would appear unlikely that the diaphragm is formed by apposition of two cell membranes. The pores may be distributed at random, or occur in groups. The **basal lamina** is continuous across the fenestrae, on the basal side of the endothelium.

Fenestrated capillaries occur in the intestinal villi, choroid plexus, ciliary processes of the eye, endocrine glands and glomeruli and peritubular capillaries of the kidneys. In glomeruli, the fenestrae are not closed by diaphragms and the capillaries also differ in the greater thickness of their basal laminae.

Discontinuous Capillaries (Sinusoids)

KEY WORDS: gaps, discontinuous basal lamina, phagocytes

These thin-walled vessels have much wider bores and their lumina are more irregular in outline than those of other capillaries. The endothelial cells do not form a continuous lining, large **gaps** are present between adjacent cells and the **basal lamina** is **discontinuous**. Phagocytes usually are associated with the wall of the sinusoid, either as a component of the lining as in the liver, or closely applied to the exterior as in the spleen. The endothelial cells themselves show no greater phagocytic properties in sinusoids than do endothelial cells of other blood vessels.

Exchange of nutrients and cell wastes between tissues and blood occurs across the attenuated endothelium of capillaries. It has been estimated that no active cell is more than 30 to 40 μm away from a capillary and the total capillary surface available for exchange has been calculated to be over 100 sq m. The most important means by which materials cross the endothelium is diffusion. Lipid-soluble materials diffuse directly through the endothelial cells, whereas water and water-soluble materials are transmitted through water-filled, physiological "pores." The fenestrae of discontinuous capillaries have been considered the equivalent of these pores. In continuous capillaries micropinocytotic cytoplasmic vesicles have been implicated in transendothelial passage of water-soluble materials. Pinocytosis also takes place and may contribute to the transfer of substances of high molecular weight. Fluid exchange occurs through intercellular clefts between endothelial cells.

Metarterioles

KEY WORDS: capillary sphincter areas, precapillary arterioles, scattered smooth muscle

These vessels are intermediate between capillaries and arterioles and control the flow of blood through the capillary bed. They also are called **capillary sphincter areas** and **precapillary arterioles** (sphincters). Although these vessels are poorly defined morphologically, the lumen generally is wider than that of the capillaries they serve, and circularly-arranged **smooth muscle** cells are scattered in their walls.

VEINS

The venous side of the circulatory system carries blood from the capillary beds to the heart and in their progress, the veins gradually increase in size and their walls thicken. Their structure basically is that of arteries and the three coats—tunica intima, media and adventitia—can be distinguished but are not as clearly defined. Generally, veins are more numerous and larger than the arteries they accompany, but their walls are thinner because of a reduction of muscular and elastic elements. Since their walls are less sturdy, veins tend to collapse when not filled, and in sections may appear flattened with irregular, slit-like lumina.

Veins show much greater variation in structure than do arteries. The thickness of the wall does not always correlate with the size of the vein and the same vein may show structural differences in different parts. Histological classification of veins is less satisfactory than for arteries, but several subdivisions usually are made, namely, venules and small, medium and large veins.

Venules

KEY WORDS: continuous endothelium, pericytes, thin adventitia, incomplete tunica media

Venules arise by union of several capillaries to form vessels that range from 10 to 50 μm in diameter. The tunica intima consists of a thin, **continuous endothelium**, the cells of which are loosely joined by poorly-developed intercellular junctions. The thin basal lamina is penetrated by **pericytes** which appear to make contact with the endothelial cells.

A tunica media is missing in the smallest venules and the relatively **thin adventitia** contains a few collagen fibers, scattered fibroblasts, mast cells, macrophages and plasma cells. The junctions between venules and capillaries are important sites for fluid exchange between tissues and blood.

As the vessels increase in size to reach diameters of about 50 μm, circularly oriented, scattered smooth muscle cells begin to appear and form a somewhat discontinuous and **incomplete tunica media**. The adventitia increases in thickness and consists of longitudinally oriented collagen fibers that form an open spiral around the vessel. Fibroblasts frequently are irregular in shape and bear thin processes.

Small Veins

KEY WORDS: continuous endothelium, complete tunica media, adventitia

Small veins vary from about 0.2 to 1.0 mm in diameter. The tunica intima consists only of a **continuous endothelium** resting on a thin basal lamina. Circular smooth muscle fibers form a **complete tunica media**, which consists of from one to four layers of cells. Between the smooth muscle cells is a thin network of elastic and collagen fibers. The **adventitia** forms a relatively thick coat and contains longitudinally oriented collagen fibers and some thin elastic fibers.

Medium Veins

KEY WORDS: thin tunica intima, inconspicuous subendothelial layer, tunica intima, thick tunica adventitia, vasa vasorum, valves

This class of veins contains most of the named veins of gross anatomy, except for major trunks. They vary in size from 1 to 10 mm in diameter. The **thin tunica intima** consists of endothelial cells resting on a basal lamina. An **inconspicuous subendothelial layer** may be present and contains delicate collagen fibers and scattered, fine elastic fibers. An external elastic lamina is poorly defined. In most medium veins the **tunica media**, although well developed, is thinner than that of corresponding arteries. The **tunica adventitia** is **thicker** than the media and forms the bulk of the wall. It consists of collagen and elastic fibers and frequently contains longitudinal smooth muscle cells. **Vasa vasorum** are present in the larger vessels of this class.

Most medium veins are provided with **valves**, pocket-like flaps of the tunica intima that project into the lumen, their free edges oriented in the direction of blood flow. They consist of a core of connective tissue covered on both surfaces by endothelium. A rich network of elastic fibers is present in the connective tissue beneath the endothelium on the downstream side of the valves. As blood flow towards the heart, the valves are pressed against the vessel wall but with backflow, the valves are forced outward, against each other, to occlude the vessels and prevent reversal of blood flow.

Large Veins

KEY WORDS: tunica adventitia, vasa vasorum, thin tunica media, tunica adventitia

In large venous trunks such as the venae cavae, renal, external iliac, splenic, portal and mesenteric veins, the **thick tunica adventitia** forms the greater part of the wall. It consists of loose connective tissue with thick, longitudinally oriented bundles of collagen and elastic fibers. Smooth muscle layers, also longitudinally arranged, are present and are especially well-developed in the inferior vena cava. **Vasa vasorum** are present and may extend into the tunica media. The **tunica media** is **thin**, poorly developed and may even be absent; otherwise, it shows the same organization as that in medium veins. The **tunica intima** is similar in composition to that of medium veins, except that the subendothelial connective tissue may be prominent.

Veins with Special Features

Some veins, such as the trabecular veins of the spleen, veins of the retina, bone, maternal placenta, most of the meningeal and cerebral veins and those of the nail bed, lack a tunica media. Veins in the pregnant uterus contain smooth muscle in all three coats. In the intima, the fibers are longitudinally arranged, as they are in the tunica intima of the saphenous, popliteal, femoral, umbilical and internal jugular veins. At their junctions with the heart, the adventitia of the pulmonary veins and the venae cavae are provided with a coat of cardiac muscle: the fibers are run longitudinally and circularly about the vessels for a short distance.

Arteriovenous Anastomoses

In addition to their capillary connections, arteries and veins may unite by shunts called arteriovenous anastomoses. Generally, these arise as side branches of arterioles and pass directly to venules. They are thick-walled, muscular vessels of small caliber which usually are coiled and surrounded by a connective tissue sheath. They are plentiful in the sole of the foot, palm of the hand, skin of the fingertips, toes, lips and nose, and also occur in the thyroid. When open, the anastomoses shunt blood around the capillary bed and thus regulate the blood supply of many tissues.

Carotid and Aortic Bodies

KEY WORDS: epithelioid (glomus) cells, type II glomus cell, chemoreceptors

The carotid bodies are encapsulated structures, one on each side of the neck at the bifurcations of the common carotid arteries. They consist of masses of large, polyhedral **epithelioid (glomus) cells** that are closely related to a rich network of sinusoidal vessels. The cells have large, pale nuclei and light, finely granular cytoplasm. In electron micrographs, the granules show a dense core and contain catecholamines and 5-hydroxytryptamine. A second cell type, the **type II glomus cell**, lacks granules. Many nerves ramify through the structures. Carotid bodies act as **chemoreceptors** and monitor blood for change in oxygen and carbon dioxide content, and also are sensitive to changes in the pH and pressure of blood.

Aortic bodies are similar structures that lie close to the aorta between the angle of the subclavian and carotid arteries on the right, and near the origin of the subclavian artery on the left. They are believed to have functions similar to those of carotid bodies. The carotid and aortic bodies are derived from neural crest.

LYMPH VASCULAR SYSTEM

The lymph vascular system consists of endothelial-lined tubes that recover intercellular fluids not picked up by the blood vascular system, and return them to the blood. The fluid carried by the vessels, lymph, essentially is a blood filtrate formed as fluid crosses the blood capillaries into the tissues. Unlike the blood vascular system, lymph flow is unidirectional— from tissue to the union of lymph and blood vascular systems at the base of the neck.

The lymph vascular system begins in the tissues as blind capillaries which drain into larger collecting lymphatics and, thence, into two main trunks. Lymph nodes occur along the course of the lymphatic vessels and serve to filter the lymph. Lymphatic vessels are present in most tissues but are absent from bone marrow, the central nervous system, coats of the eye, internal ear and fetal placenta.

Lymph Capillaries

KEY WORDS: thin continuous endothelium, discontinuous basal lamina, anchoring filaments

The lymphatic capillaries are thin-walled, blind tubes that branch and anastomose freely, forming a rich network in organs and tissues. They are wider and have a more irregular outline than blood capillaries. The wall consists only of a **thin continuous endothelium.** A **basal lamina** is lacking or is present only in **discontinuous** patches. Adjacent endothelial cells may overlap, but junctional complexes are rare, so intercellular clefts are present. Externally, the endothelial tube is surrounded by a small amount of collagenous connective tissue. Fine filaments run perpendicularly from the collagen bundles and attach to the outer surfaces of the endothelium as **anchoring filaments** that maintain the patency of the capillary.

Collecting Lymph Vessels

KEY WORDS: tunica intima, tunica media, tunica adventitia, valves

These vessels differ from lymph capillaries in size and in the thickness of their walls. Although three coats—intima, media and adventitia—are describes as for blood vessels, they are not as clearly delineated.

The **tunica intima** consists of an endothelium supported by a thin network of longitudinally arranged elastic fibers. The **tunica media** is composed of smooth muscle with a predominantly circular arrangement, but some fibers are longitudinally oriented. Between the muscle fibers are a few fine elastic fibers. **Tunica adventitia** forms the thickest coat and consists of bundles of collagen fibers, elastic fibers and some smooth muscle cells, all of which have a longitudinal orientation.

Valves are numerous along the course of lymphatic vessels, and occur at closer intervals than in veins. They arise in pairs and represent folds of the intima, as in veins.

Lymphatic Trunks

KEY WORDS: thoracic duct, right lymphatic duct, tunica intima, subendothelial layer, tunica media, tunica adventitia

The collecting lymphatic ducts ultimately gather into two main trunks, the thoracic duct and the right lymphatic duct. The **thoracic duct** is the longer and has a greater field of drainage. It begins in the abdomen, passes along the vertebral column and opens into the venous system at the junction of the left jugular and subclavian veins. It receives lymph from the lower limbs, abdomen and left side of the thorax, head, neck and upper limb. The **right lymphatic duct** receives lymph only from the upper right portion of the body and empties into the right brachiocephalic vein.

The structure of the trunks is the same, and generally resembles that of a large vein. The **tunica intima** consists of a continuous endothelium, beneath which is a subendothelial layer of fibroelastic tissue with some smooth muscle. Near the junction with the tunica media, the elastic fibers condense into a thin internal elastic lamina. The **tunica media** is the thickest layer in the wall of lymphatic trunks and contains more smooth muscle than does the media of large veins. The fibers have a predominantly circular arrangement and are separated by abundant collagenous connective tissue and some elastic fibers. **Tunica adventitia** is poorly defined and merges with the surrounding connective tissue. It contains bundles of longitudinal collagen fibers, elastic fibers and occasional smooth muscle fibers. The wall of the thoracic duct contains nutrient blood vessels similar to the vasa vasorum of large blood vessels.

DEVELOPMENT OF CARDIOVASCULAR SYSTEM

Initially the developing embryo is nourished by simple diffusion of nutrients, at first from the uterine lumen then, after implantation, from maternal blood lakes. With growth, diffusion is unable to meet the nutritional demands of the embryo, and a vascular system arises early in development.

The Heart. The earliest cardiac structure

appears as an aggregation of the splanchnic mesoderm into two longitudinal strands. Each acquires a lumen and becomes a simple endothelial-lined tube lying in a fold of mesoderm. The tubes fuse to form a single, saccular cardiac primordium, and the mesodermal folds merge into a single surrounding coat. Thus, the primitive heart appears as a simple endothelial tube with a thick mesodermal coat that acquires a rhythmic contractility. The endothelial tube will give rise to the endocardium while the myocardium and epicardium develop from the outer mesodermal layer. At first the endothelial tube is separated from the myocardial layer by a jelly-like fluid which, after being invaded by mesenchyme, is transformed into the connective tissue of the subendocardial layer. The cells at the external surface of the myocardial coat flatten into a mesothelium that, together with a sublayer of connective tissue, becomes the epicardium. The remainder of the myocardial coat forms an outer, compact layer of cardiac muscle and an inner layer of loosely-arranged trabeculae. In mammals, the entire muscle wall becomes compact, except for the trabeculae carnae of the ventricles, which remains as remnants of the spongy inner layer.

The atrioventricular node, according to some investigators, is the first part of the conducting system to develop, arising from cardiac muscle cells around the atrioventricular canal. From this, the atrioventricular bundle arises. An alternative view suggests that the bundle arises first, from muscle on the dorsal wall of the atrioventricular canal, then spreads to form the atrioventricular node and the right and left limbs of the bundle. The sinoatrial node is the last to appear, from a narrow muscular band in the lateral surface of the superior vena cava. Later in fetal life, the node is incorporated into the wall of the atrium.

Vessels. The earliest blood vessels arise from extraembryonic mesenchyme, appearing first in blood islands of the yolk sac and body stalk. Initially the islands and cords are solid, but the outermost cells flatten to become the first endothelial cells, while the innermost become primitive blood cells. This process occurs in several places and by growth and union, the isolated vascular spaces unite to form a plexus of vessels. The first vessels of the embryo proper are formed in similar fashion. After a circulation is established, further development of blood vessels occurs by budding and extension of preexisting vessels. The formation of capillary-like vessels precedes development of definite arteries and veins. Smooth muscle and connective tissue coats are acquired by differentiation of surrounding mesenchyme.

Lymphatic vessels arise quite separately, originating as isolated spaces in mesenchyme. Cells bordering the spaces flatten to become endothelial cells lining the spaces. By progressive unions, the spaces link up to form continuous, branching channels that ultimately lead to a complete set of lymphatic vessels. In the larger lymphatics, the outer tunics are derived from the surrounding mesenchyme.

FUNCTIONAL SUMMARY

The heart provides the propelling force that moves blood through the systemic and pulmonary circulations, this function being carried out by the myocardium. Cardiac muscle is characterized by its ability to contract spontaneously, without external stimulus. However, the heart is provided with a system of specialized fibers which regulate the contractions into rhythmical beats, coordinated throughout the chambers of the heart. The contraction impulse is initiated in the sinoatrial node, the pacemaker of the heart, whose fibers contract with inherent rhythm due to their ability to depolarize spontaneously. From the sinoatrial node, impulses pass through ordinary cardiac muscle fibers of the atria. Conduction along atrial fibers is relatively slow and by the time the impulse has reached the atrioventricular node, the atrium has completed its contraction. The

impulse then is conducted rapidly along the atrioventricular bundle and by its branches is distributed throughout the ventricular myocardium.

Flow of the blood from the heart is intermittent and the arteries immediately joining the heart are subjected to pulses of high pressure. Because of the large amounts of elastic tissue in their walls, these large conducting vessels are expansible and able to absorb the forces without damage. During the intervals in which the heart is resting, the elastic recoil of the arterial wall serves as an additional propelling mechanism and helps to smooth out the blood flow, protecting delicate venules and capillaries from severe changes in pressure.

The distribution of blood to organs is controlled largely by the muscular distributing arteries. The caliber of these vessels is regulated by the degree of contraction of the tunica media, in response to changes in blood pressure and demands of organs. Pressure within the capillary bed is controlled by the arterioles and by the opening or closing of shunts formed by the arteriovenous anastomoses.

Exchange of material between blood and tissue occurs at the level of capillaries and venules. Passage of fluid across capillary walls depends partly on the blood pressure and partly on the colloidal osmotic pressure in the capillaries. Blood pressure promotes passage of fluid into tissues; osmotic pressure promotes resorption. At the arterial end of capillary beds, the blood pressure is greater and fluid is driven outward; at the venous end, osmotic pressure is greater and fluid is resorbed. Venules, with their thin walls and loosely joined endothelial cells, also are important sites of fluid exchange. Lipid-soluble materials readily diffuse through endothelial cells, whereas water-soluble materials are carried through intercellular clefts and pores. These may correspond to fenestrae of fenestrated capillaries, or to caveoli and cytoplasmic vesicles of continuous capillaries. Materials, including whole cells, readily cross the rather leaky walls of sinusoids.

Blood returns to the heart via venous blood vessels. They are able to constrict or enlarge, and store large quantities of blood. From 70 to 75% of the circulating blood is contained in veins and much of it can be made available to organs as needed. Blood moves along the veins by the massaging action of muscles and fascial tissues. As the veins are compressed, blood flows away from the area of compression and valves prevent any backflow. A similar mechanism propels lymph along the lymphatic vasculature.

Although most of the fluid filtered from the blood capillaries is resorbed by them, about 10% is not recovered by the blood vascular system, and it is this fluid that is recovered by the lymph capillaries. Substances of high molecular weight such as proteins, pass into the blood capillaries with difficulty but are recovered by lymphatic capillaries almost unhindered. Lymphatic channels are one of the main routes by which nutrients, especially fats, are absorbed from the gastrointestinal tract.

The endothelium of blood vessels plays an important role in hemostasis. It provides a surface to which platelets do not normally stick, and so prevents their aggregation. However, it contains thromboplastic substances and the antihemophilic factor VIII of the blood coagulation system. The luminal surface bears a negative charge, as do blood cells, thus preventing aggregation of these elements.

Atlas and Table of Key Features for Chapter 11

Table 11.1.
Key Features of Arteries and Veins

	Tunica Intima	Tunica Media	Tunica Adventitia	Other
Arteries				
Large	Thick subendothelial layer with elastic fibers and smooth muscle; internal elastic lamina prominent	Major coat, 40–60 elastic laminae; smooth muscle, fibrous connective tissue between laminae	Thin; no external elastic lamina	Compared to lumen, wall is thin; vasa vasorum extend through aventitia and about one-third of the way through media
Small and medium	A thin subendothelial layer present; prominent internal elastic lamina	Major coat; up to 40 layers of smooth muscle, some elastic tissue	May equal thickness of media; external elastic lamina present	Muscular (distributing) arteries, includes most of named arteries
Arteriole	Thin, no recognizable subendothelial layer: internal elastic lamina	Forms the main coat; 1–5 layers of smooth muscle	Thin; No external elastic lamina, fibroelastic	Wall (relative to lumen), is thicker than in any other vessel
Capillaries				
(a) Continuous	Endothelium plus basement membranes: pericytes, tight junctions, desmosomes	Absent	Scant reticular fibers	5–8 μm in diameter
(b) Fenestrated	Endothelial cells bear openings in cytoplasm, usually closed by diaphragm	Absent	Scant reticular fibers	In glomeruli, fenestrae not closed by diaphragm
(c) Discontinuous	Spaces between adjacent endothelial cells	Absent	Scant reticular fibers	Large diameter, tortuous (sinusoids); basal lamina missing or discontinuous
Veins				
Venule	Endothelium only; no internal elastic lamina	Very thin: 1–3 layers of smooth muscle cells	Thick compared to total wall, wholly collagenous	
Small and medium	Thin; subendothelial layer lacking in smaller veins	Thin; layer of smooth muscle, elastic fibers and collagen fibers	Well developed; thick fibroelastic layer; no elastic lamina	
Large	Thicker than in small veins; a delicate internal elastic lamina may be present	Thin or even lacking	Thickest coat, fibromuscular; no elastic lamina	

11-1 Heart

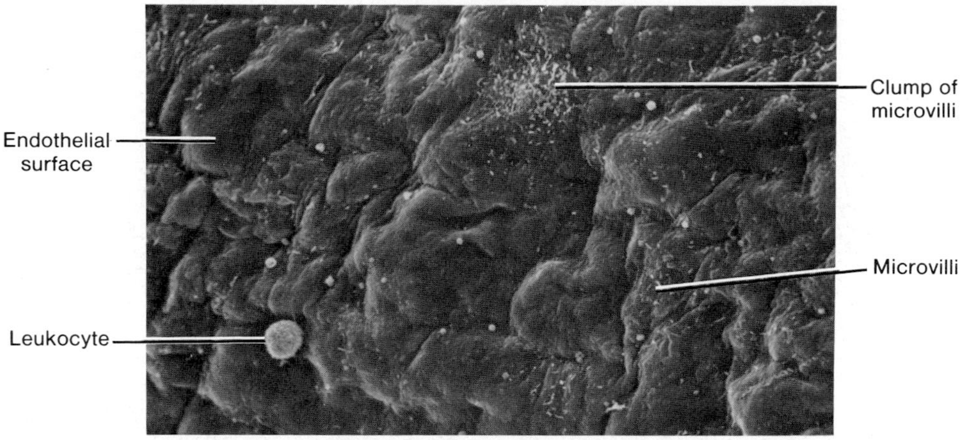

11-2

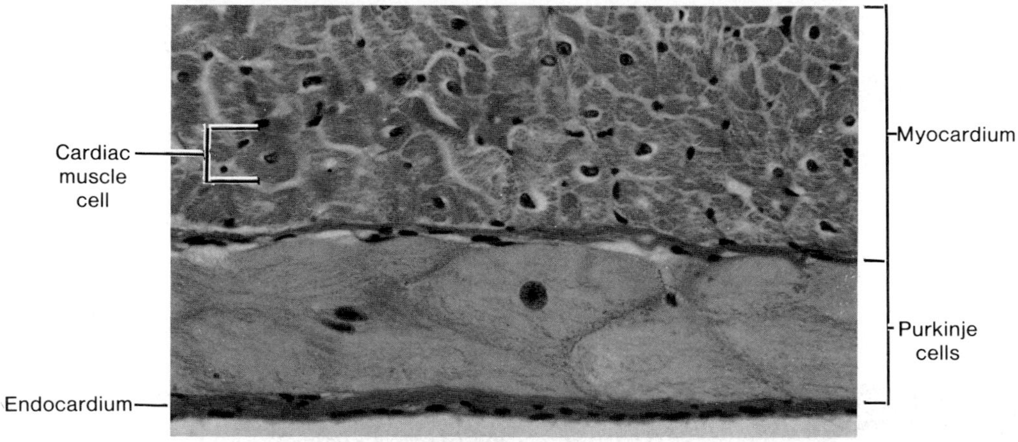

11-3 Arteries

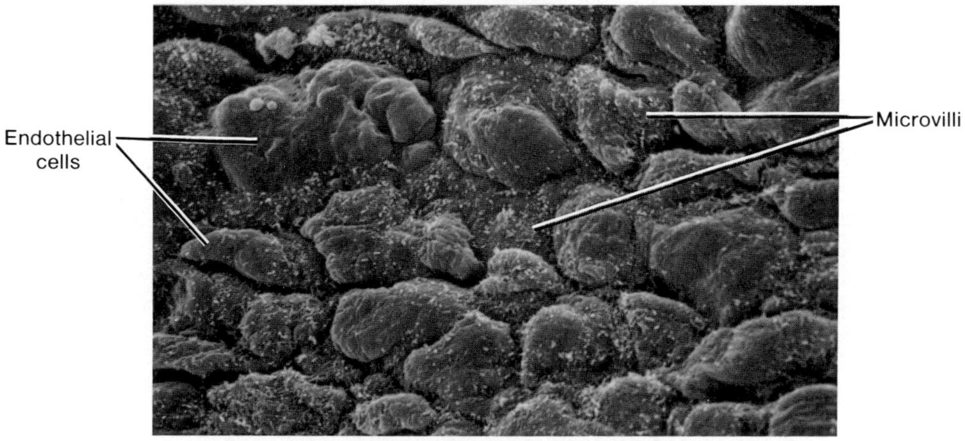

Figure 11-1. Endocardium. SEM, ×1000.
Figure 11-2. Purkinje cells. LM, ×250.
Figure 11-3. Aorta. SEM, ×1000.

11-4

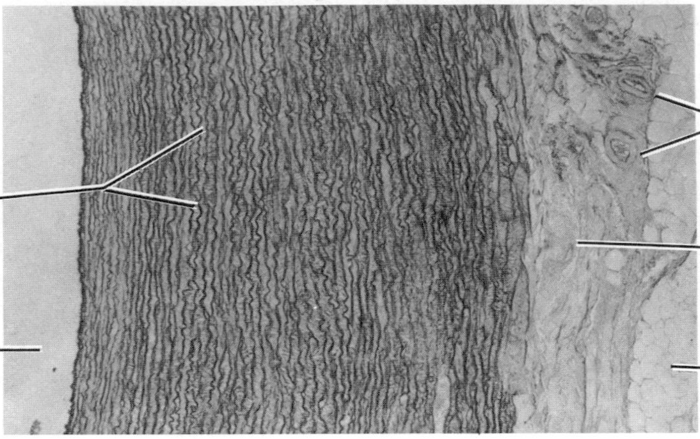

11-5

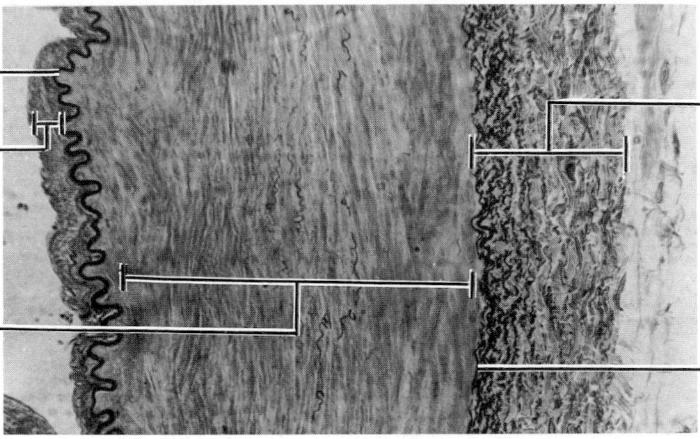

11-6

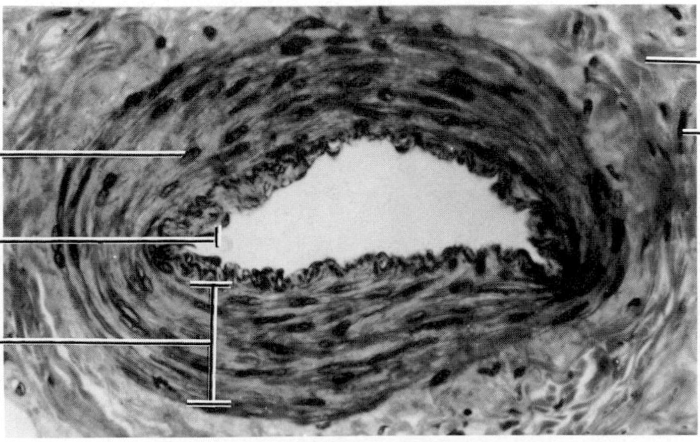

Figure 11-4. Wall of aorta. LM, ×40.
Figure 11-5. Muscular artery. LM, ×200.
Figure 11-6. Small artery. LM, ×250.

11-7

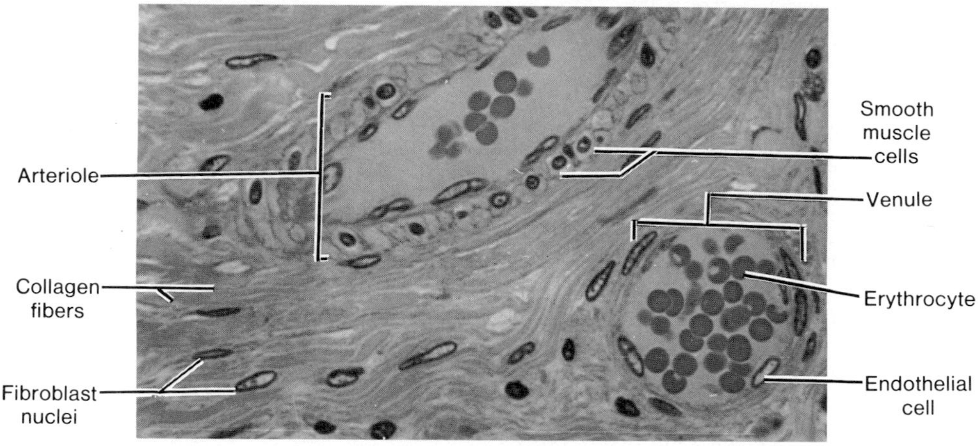

11-8

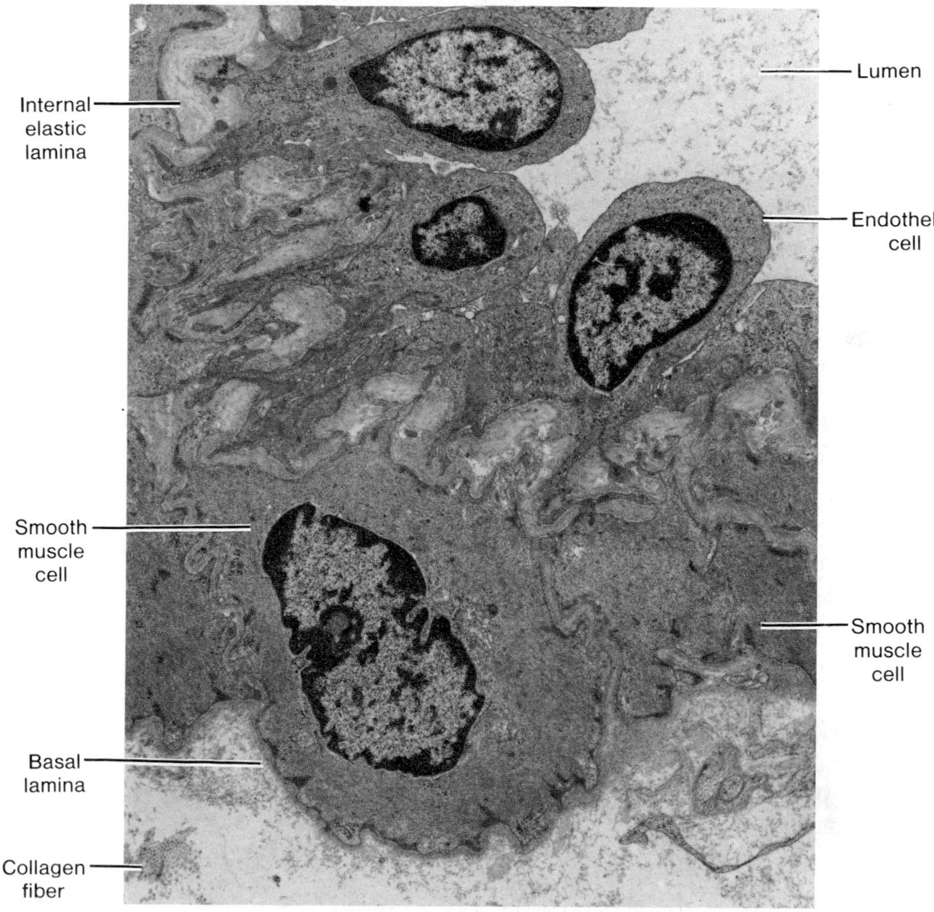

Figure 11-7. Arteriole. LM, ×250.
Figure 11-8. Arteriole. TEM, ×6000.

11-9

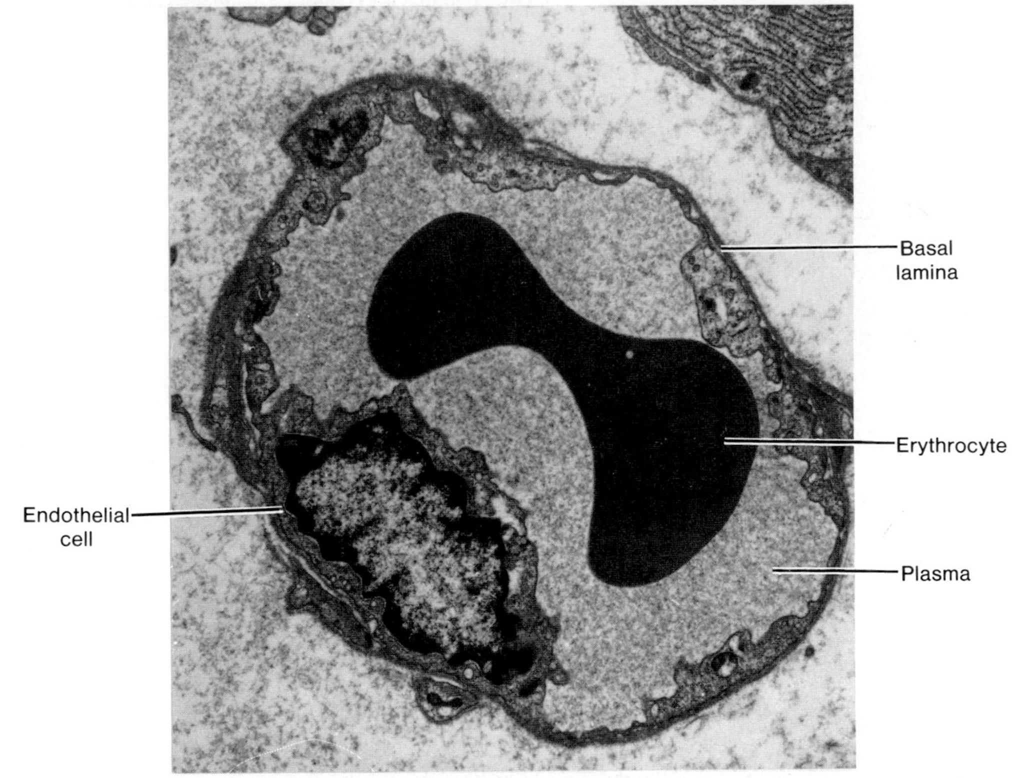

11-10

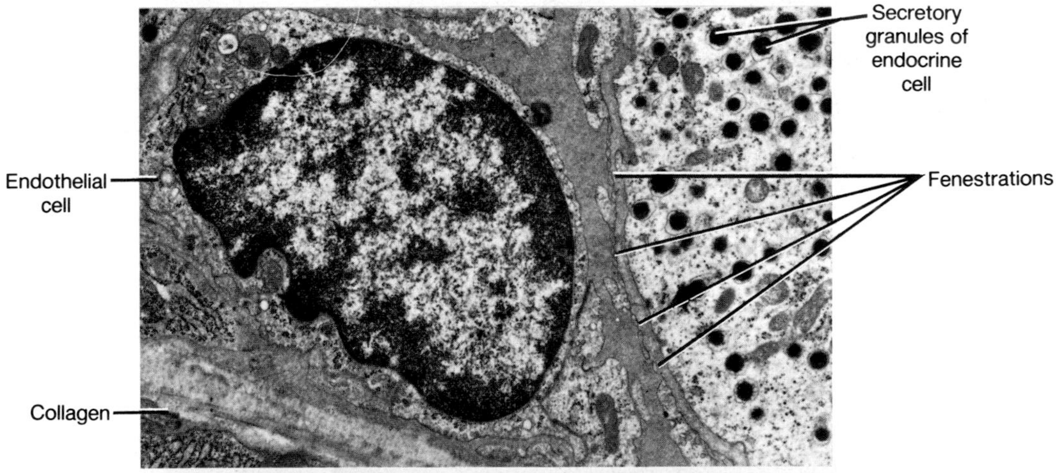

11-11

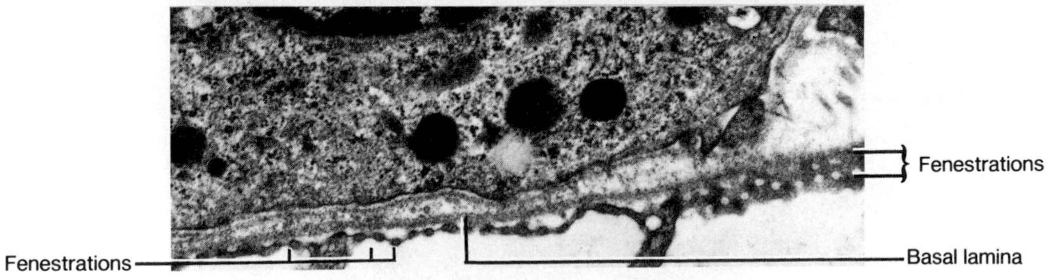

Figure 11-9. Capillary (human). TEM, ×5000.
Figure 11-10. Capillary (fenestrated endothelium). TEM, ×6000.
Figure 11-11. Capillary (fenestrated endothelium). TEM, ×15,000.

11-12 Veins

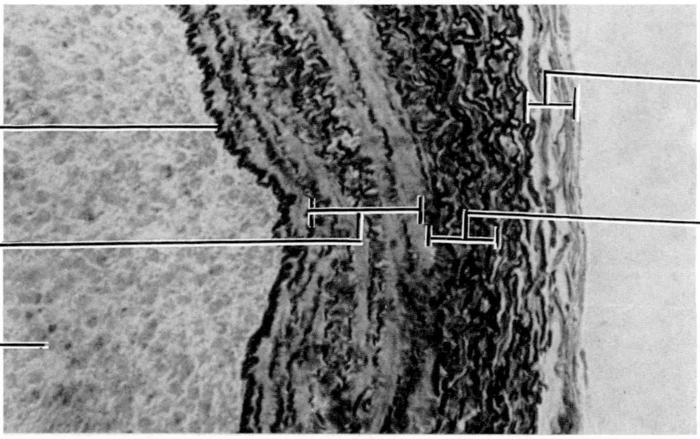

11-13

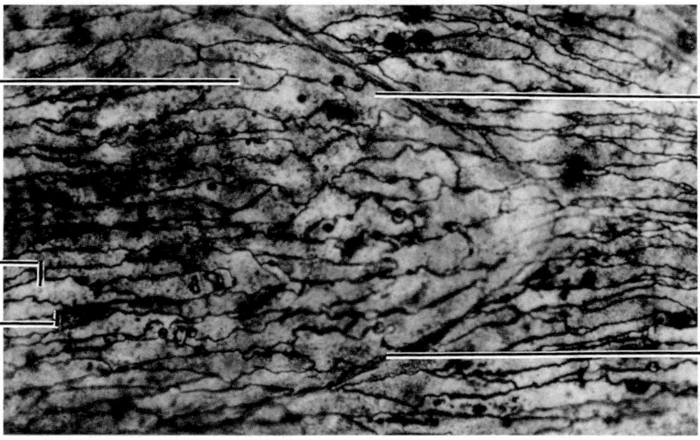

11-14

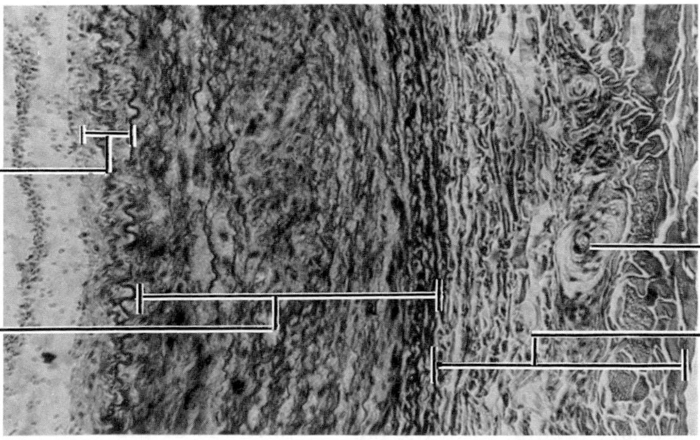

Figure 11-12. Medium-sized vein. LM, ×100.
Figure 11-13. Valve of vein. LM, ×250.
Figure 11-14. Inferior vena cava. LM, ×40.

they possess an internal system of lymphatic sinuses for the filtering of lymph. However, at the outer surfaces of the tonsils, plexuses of blindly ending lymph capillaries form the beginnings of efferent lymphatic vessels.

The tonsils contribute to the formation of lymphocytes, many of which migrate through the covering epithelium and appear in the sputum as the salivary corpuscles. Bacteria that penetrate the lymphoid tissue of the tonsil act as antigens to stimulate the production of antibodies.

LYMPH NODES

Lymph nodes are small encapsulated lymphatic organs set into the course of lymphatic vessels. They are absent in fishes, amphibia and reptiles, although nodular collections of lymphatic tissue about blood vessels have been described in the toad, and rudimentary, lymph-node-like structures have been reported in the crocodile. In aves, simple aggregates of lymphatic tissue occur beside the terminal part of the cervical duct and in the abdomen superior to the genital gland. Lymph nodes are more characteristic of mammals, in which they have reached their fullest development. They are prominent in certain regions of the body such as the neck, axilla, groin, mesenteries and along the course of large blood vessels in the thorax and abdomen. In some mammals, the lymph nodes of the mesentery are aggregated to form a single large organ, the pancreas of Aselli. This appears to be a general feature of rodents and carnivores but no such organ is found in man.

Structure

KEY WORDS: hilus, afferent lymphatics, efferent lymphatics, diffuse lymphatic tissue, nodular lymphatic tissue, capsule, trabeculae, reticular network, cortex, outer cortex, inner (deep) cortex (paracortical area), thymus-dependent area, medulla, medullary cords

Grossly, lymph nodes appear as flattened, ovoid or bean-shaped structures with a slight indentation at one side, the **hilus**, through which blood vessels enter and leave the organ. Lymph nodes are the only lymphatic structures to be interposed into the lymphatic drainage and thus, unlike the other lymphatic organs, have both **afferent** and **efferent lymphatics.** The afferent lymphatic vessels enter the node at multiple sites anywhere over the convex surface; the efferent vessels leave the node at the hilus. Both sets of vessels have valves that are arranged to provide undirectional flow of lymph through the node. The valves of the afferent vessels open toward the node while those of the efferent vessels open away from the node.

Essentially, lymph nodes consist of accumulations of **diffuse** and **nodular lymphatic tissue** enclosed in a capsule which is greatly thickened at the hilus. The **capsule** consists of closely packed collagenous fibers, scattered elastic fibers and a few smooth muscle cells that are concentrated around the entrance and exit of the lymphatic vessels. From the inner surface of the capsule, branching connective tissue **trabeculae** extend into the node and provide a kind of skeleton for the lymph node. The space enclosed by the capsule and trabeculae is filled by an intricate, three-dimensional **reticular network** of reticular fibers and their associated reticular cells. The meshes of the network are crowded with the cells of lymphatic tissue and these are so disposed as to form the outer cortex and the inner medulla.

The **cortex** forms a layer beneath the capsule and extends for a variable distance toward the center of the node. It consists of lymphatic nodules, many with germinal centers, set in a bed of diffuse lymphatic tissue. Trabeculae are fairly regularly arranged and run perpendicular to the capsule, subdividing the cortex into a number of irregular compartments. However, the trabeculae do not form complete walls but represent bars or cylinders of connective tissue, and compartmentation of the cortex is incomplete. The cortical areas communicate laterally with each other where trabeculae are deficient.

The cortex customarily is divided into the **outer cortex**, which lies immediately beneath the capsule and contains nodular and diffuse lymphatic tissues, and the **deep cortex (inner cortex, paracortical area),** which consists of diffuse lymphatic tissue only. The deep cortex becomes depleted of cells after thymectomy and has been called the **thymus-dependent area.** There is no sharp boundary between the two zones and their proportions differ from node to node and with the functional status of the node. The deep cortex continues without interruption or clear demarcation into the medulla. In general, B lymphocytes are concentrated in the nodular lymphatic tissue, while T cells are present in the diffuse tissue.

The **medulla** appears as a paler staining area of variable width, more or less surrounding the hilus of the node. It consists of diffuse lymphatic tissue arranged in irregular cords, the **medullary cords,** which branch and anastomose. The medullary cords contain abundant plasma cells, macrophages and lymphocytes. The trabeculae of the medulla are more irregularly arranged than are those of the cortex, and also branch and anastomose freely.

The general structure of a lymph node is shown in Figure 12-2.

Lymph Sinuses

KEY WORDS: subcapsular (marginal) sinus, cortical (trabecular, intermediate) sinus, medullary sinus

Within the lymph node is a system of channel-like spaces, the lymph sinuses, through which the lymph percolates. Lymph enters the node through the afferent lymphatic vessels that pierce the capsule and empty into the **subcapsular (marginal) sinus** which separates the cortex from the capsule. The sinus does not form a tubular structure but is present as a wide space extending beneath the capsule, interrupted at intervals by the trabeculae. The subcapsular sinus is continuous with the **cortical (trabecular, intermediate) sinuses** which extend radially into the cortex, usually along the trabeculae. These in turn become continuous with the **medullary sinuses** that run between the medullary cords and the trabeculae of the medulla. At the hilus, the medullary and subcapsular sinuses unite, penetrate the capsule and become continuous with the efferent lymphatics.

In sections, the sinuses appear as regions in which the reticular net is coarser and more open. Stellate cells, supported by reticular fibers, crisscross the lumen, and are joined to each other and to the cells bordering the lumen, by slender processes. Numerous macrophages are present in the luminal network and also project from the boundaries of the sinus. The cells that form the boundaries of the sinuses and extend through the sinus space, generally are regarded as flattened reticular cells. However, they also have been considered to be attenuated endothelial cells akin to those of the lymphatic vessels, with which they become continuous.

Sinuses are less numerous in the cortex than in the medulla and the cortical sinuses are relatively narrow. Those in the medulla are large, irregular and show repeated branchings and anastomoses. They pursue a tortuous course in the medullary parenchyma and account for the irregular, cord-like arrangement of the lymphatic tissue in this area.

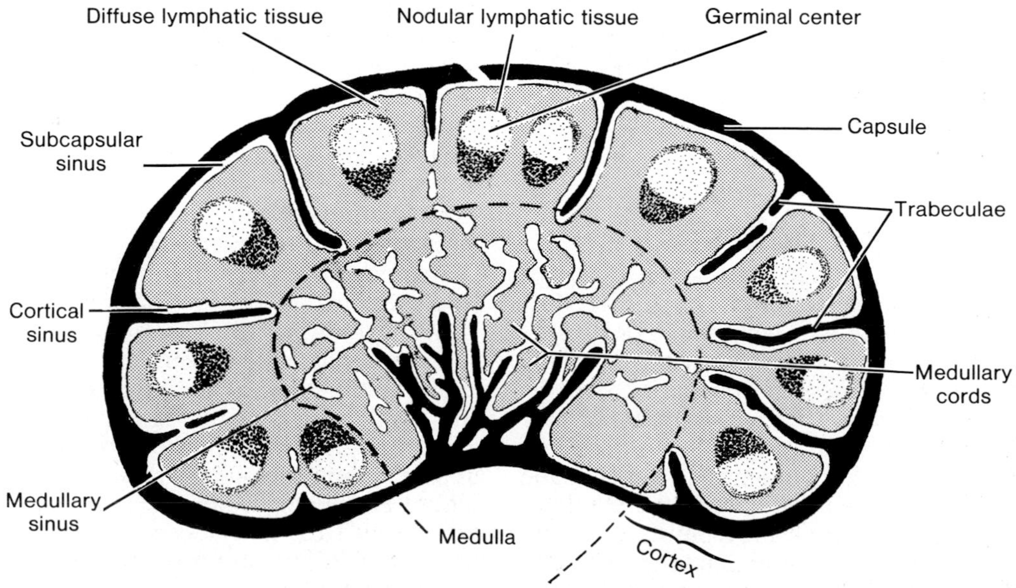

Figure 12-2. General structure of a lymph node.

Blood Vessels

KEY WORDS: postcapillary venules, high endothelium

The major blood supply reaches the node through the hilus and only occasionally do smaller vessels enter from the convex surface of the capsule. The arteries (arterioles) at first run within the trabeculae of the medulla but soon leave these and enter the medullary cords to pass to the cortex. Here they break up into a rich capillary network that distributes to the diffuse lymphatic tissue and forms a network around the lymphatic nodules of the cortex.

The capillaries regroup to form venules which run from the cortex and enter the medullary cords as small veins. These in turn are tributaries of the larger veins that pass out of the node at the hilus. In the deep cortex, the venules take on a special appearance and have been given the name **postcapillary venules.** These vessels are characterized by the presence of a **high endothelium** which varies from cuboidal to columnar and at times may appear to occlude the lumen. The walls of these vessels are often infiltrated with small lymphocytes that generally are presumed to be passing into the lymph node. The lymphocytes pass between the adjacent endothelial cells, indenting their lateral walls as they cross through the endothelium. The significance of the high endothelium is not known. It has been suggested that, as the lymphocytes sink deeper between them, the adjacent endothelial cells resume their original relationship to each other and seal off the interendothelial cleft above the lymphocyte, thereby limiting the loss of plasma from the venule.

Functions

Lymph nodes contribute to the production of lymphocytes (lymphocytopoieses) as indicated by the mitotic activity, especially in germinal centers. It is assumed that the maturational sequence proceeds from large to small, i.e., from lymphoblast to prolymphocyte to small lymphocyte. However, the progression is complicated by the ability of the small lymphocyte to respond to external stimuli, revert to blast-like state and produce more small lymphocytes. The lymphocytopoietic activity of the quiescent node does not appear to be great, and the bulk of the cells of an unstimulated node are recirculating lymphocytes. The lymph nodes receive both B cells and T cells from the blood stream, the cells entering the node via the postcapillary venules. Some also may enter through the afferent lymphatics. Once within the parenchyma, B cells "home-in" on the lymphatic nodules of the outer cortex. The T cells occupy the deep cortex, and because this region becomes depleted of cells after thymectomy, it is referred to as the thymus-dependent area. The cells remain in the lymph node for variable periods of time, then leave through the efferent lymphatics to again reach the blood stream in which they circulate. Eventually the lymphocytes again encounter a lymph node and the process is repeated. Only small lymphocytes recirculate.

Lymph nodes form an extensive filtration system that removes foreign particles from the lymph and prevents their dissemination throughout the body. A single lymph node is capable of removing 99% of particulate matter presented to it. Lymph usually passes through several successive nodes before entering the blood stream. The sinuses form a settling chamber in which the flow of lymph is slow, while baffles of the crisscrossing reticular meshwork serve as a mechanical filter and produce an eddying of the lymph. The bulk of the lymph that enters a node flows centrally through the sinuses, where it comes into progressively greater contact with phagocytic cells. Filtration by a lymph node may be impaired if the number of particles is excessive or if an organism is exceptionally virulent. Agents not destroyed by the lymph node may disseminate throughout the body and the node itself can become a focus of infection.

Lymph nodes are immunological organs and participate both in the humoral and cellular immune responses. Administered antigen accumulates about and within primary nodules and at the junctions of deep and outer cortex. Some of the antigen appears to be retained on the surface of macrophages and possibly on reticular cells. Thus, the retained antigen is available for reaction with B and T cells as these move into and sort out within the parenchyma of the lymph node.

Antigens that evoke antibody production react with uncommitted B cells to elicit their activation and proliferation. The first antibody-producing cells appear in the cortex and then migrate into the medullary cords where, as plasma cells, they accumulate. Following this response in the cortex, intense antibody formation then occurs in newly formed germinal centers. This primary response is elicited on the first exposure to an antigen. The response takes several days to develop; relatively few cells respond to the stimulus, and a low titer of antibody results. On second exposure to the same antigen, a rapid and greatly increased production of antibody occurs. This represents the secondary response, marked by an explosive development of germinal centers which expand rapidly. During the primary response, the reaction to the antigen results not only in the production of antibody but also of conditioned cells which do not form antigen in response to the stimulus. These cells persist for long periods as memory cells which participate in the rapidly evolving response to a second challenge by the antigen.

Cell-mediated immune responses, as in the rejection of a foreign graft, involve the T cells, and the deep cortex of the draining node becomes very thick. Lymphoblasts in this area divide and rapidly increase in number. Following a short time lag, small lymphocytes leave the node, infiltrate the region of the graft and destroy it. Antigen from the graft may reach the lymph node via the afferent lymphatics and react with the T cells of the deep cortex, inducing them to assume a blast-like state and produce committed small T cells. These then leave the node and by recirculation are disseminated throughout the body. The T cells also form memory cells. Since there also is an associated humoral response, newly formed germinal centers appear in the cortex and antibody is present in the blood.

SPLEEN

The spleen embodies the basic structure of a lymph node and can be regarded as a modified, enlarged lymph node inserted into the blood stream. Unlike lymph nodes, the spleen has no afferent lymphatics and no lymphatic sinus system. It does have a distinctive pattern of blood circulation and specialized vascular channels which facilitate the filtering of blood. Also unlike the lymph node, the lymphatic tissue of the spleen is not arranged into a cortex and medulla.

Structure

KEY WORDS: capsule, hilus, trabeculae, reticular network, splenic pulp, white pulp, red pulp, splenic sinusoids

The spleen is enclosed in a well developed **capsule** of dense connective tissue. Elastic fibers are present between bundles of collagenous fibers and are most abundant in the deeper layers of the capsule. Smooth muscle fibers also may be present in small groups or cords, but the amount varies with the species. It is prominent in the capsule of horses, carnivores and ruminants, but little muscle is found in the splenic capsule in man and laboratory animals. On the medial surface of the spleen, the capsule is indented to form the cleft-like **hilus**, through which blood vessels, nerves and lymphatic vessels enter or leave the spleen. Broad bands of connective tissue, the **trabeculae**, extend from the inner surface of the capsule and pass deeply into the substance of the spleen forming a rich, branching and anastomosing framework. As in the lymph node, the trabeculae subdivide the organ into communicating compartments.

The spaces between the trabeculae are filled with a **reticular network** of fibers and associated reticular cells. The meshes of this network vary in size and there is a tendency for the reticular fibers to condense somewhat about blood vessels and the aggregates of lymphatic tissue.

The substance of the spleen is referred to as the **splenic pulp**, and sections from a fresh spleen show a clear separation of the splenic tissue into rounded or elongated grayish areas set within a greater mass of dark red tissue. Collectively, the gray areas compose the **white pulp** and consist of diffuse and nodular lymphatic tissue. The dark red tissue is termed the **red pulp** and consists of a reticular network that is suffused with blood. The large number of erythrocytes present imparts the red color. In many species, including man, the red pulp contains large, branching, thin-walled blood vessels, the **splenic sinusoids** (sinuses). Such spleens are said to be sinusal. In animals such as the cat and opossum the spleen lacks sinusoids and are called asinusal.

The general structure of the spleen is shown in Figure 12-3.

White Pulp

KEY WORDS: periarterial lymphatic sheaths, lymphatic nodules, splenic follicle (Malpighian corpuscle), marginal zone

The white pulp generally is associated with the arterial supply to the spleen and forms the **periarterial lymphatic sheaths** that extend about the arteries where these leave the trabeculae to enter the splenic pulp. The sheaths have the structure of diffuse lymphatic tissue and contain the usual cellular elements of lymphatic tissue. Small lymphocytes make up the bulk of the cells in the sheath, and most of these are T cells. Here and there along the course of the sheath, the lymphatic tissue expands to incorporate **nodular lymphatic** tissue which resembles the cortical nodules of lymph nodes and represents accumulations of B cells. Many of the nodules contain germinal centers. The lymphatic nodules of the spleen have been called **splenic follicles** or **Malpighian corpuscles.** At the periphery of the lymphatic sheath, the reticular net is more closely meshed than

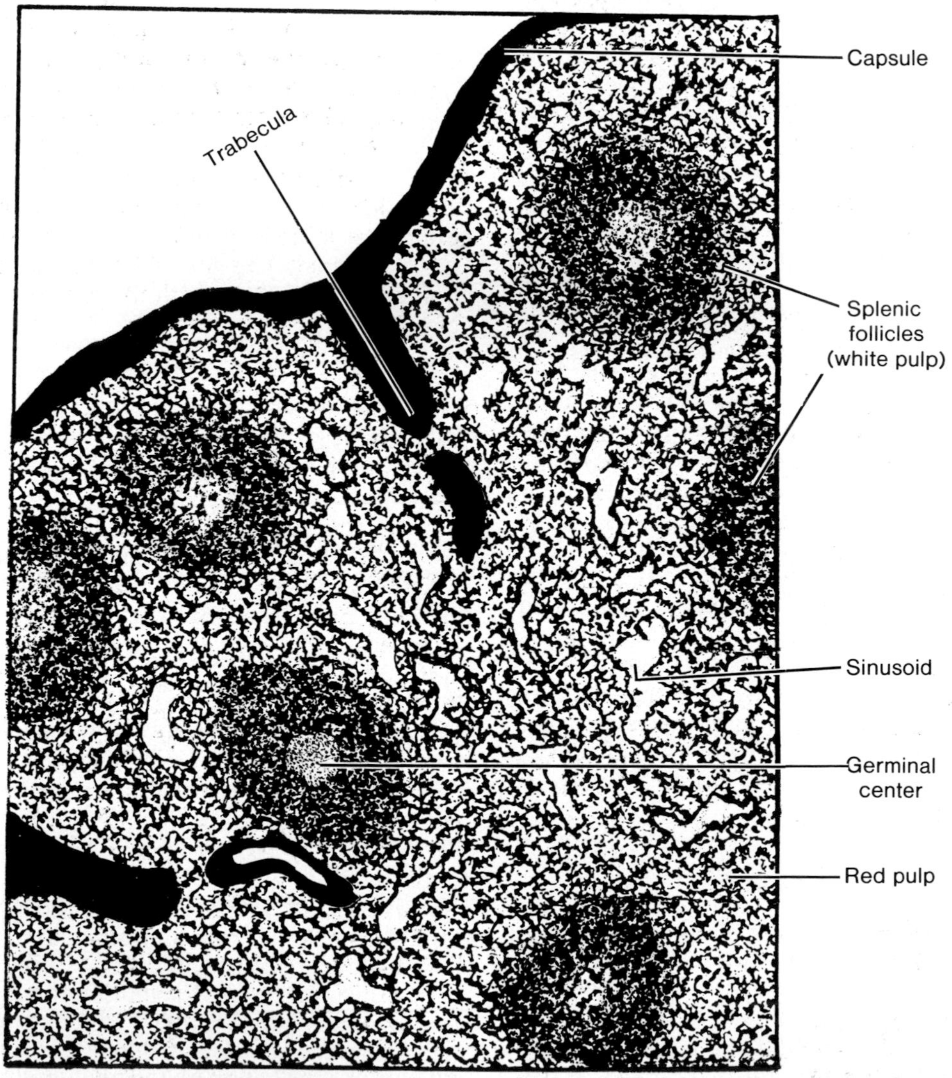

Figure 12-3. General structure of the spleen.

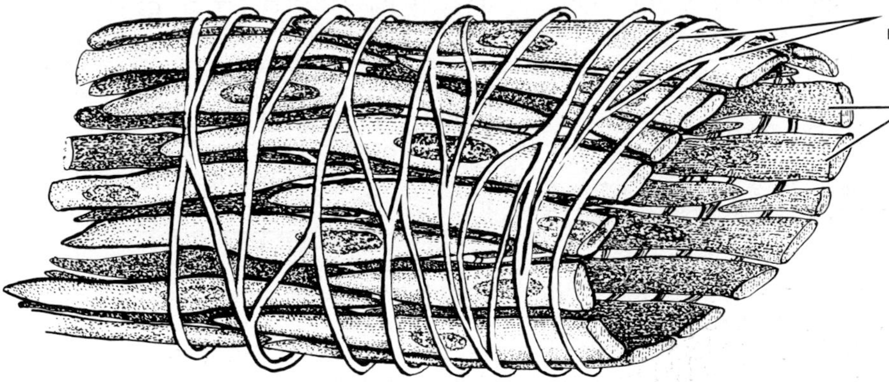

Figure 12-4. Structure of a splenic sinusoid.

elsewhere and the reticular cells and fibers form concentric layers that tend to delimit the lymphatic tissue from the red pulp. This has been called the **marginal zone.**

In the rat and rabbit the periarterial lymphatic sheaths are well developed and the lymphatic nodules are small and not numerous. In the dog and cat, however, the sheaths are poorly developed while the lymphatic nodules are large.

Red Pulp

KEY WORDS: venous sinusoids, (splenic cords)

The red pulp is associated with the venous system of the spleen. The reticular meshwork is continuous throughout the red pulp and is filled with large numbers of free cells, including all of those ordinarily found in blood. Thus, the red pulp is suffused with red cells, granular leukocytes, platelets, lymphocytes, macrophages and a few plasma cells. Occasionally, macrophages can be found that contain ingested red cells or granulocytes or are laden with a yellowish-brown pigment, hemosiderin, that is derived from the breakdown of hemoglobin.

The red pulp is riddled throughout by large, irregular, tortuous blood vessels, the **venous sinusoids** (Fig. 12-4). Between the sinusoids, the red pulp assumes a branching cord-like arrangement, forming the **splenic cords.** The sinusoids have a wide lumen (20 to 40 μm in diameter) and show a unique arrangement of their walls. A muscular supporting coat is lacking and the endothelial cells are elongated, fusiform elements that lie parallel to the long axis of the vessel. The cells lie side by side around the vessel but are not in contact and are separated by a slit-like space. Outside the endothelium, the wall is supported by a basement membrane which is not continuous but which forms widely spaced, thick bars that encircle the sinusoid. The bars or ribs of basement membrane are joined by thinner strands of the same material. The ribs of basement membrane are continuous with the reticular cells of the splenic cords.

Blood Supply

KEY WORDS: trabecular arteries, central arteries, penicillar arteries, sheathed capillaries, open circulation, closed circulation, pulp veins, trabecular veins

The architecture of the spleen is perhaps best understood in relationship to the blood circulation, which shows some special and characteristic features (Fig. 12-5). The branches of the splenic artery enter the spleen at the hilus, where they provide branches that pass within the trabeculae into the interior of the organ. These **trabecular arteries** continue to branch repeatedly and ultimately emerge from the trabeculae as the **central arteries**, which immediately become surrounded by the lymphatic tissue of the periarterial lymphatic sheath. Where the sheath expands to form nodules, the central artery (now better called a follicular artery) is displaced to one side and assumes an eccentric position in the nodule and only rarely does the vessel retain a central position in the nodular lymphatic tissue. Throughout its course in the white pulp, the

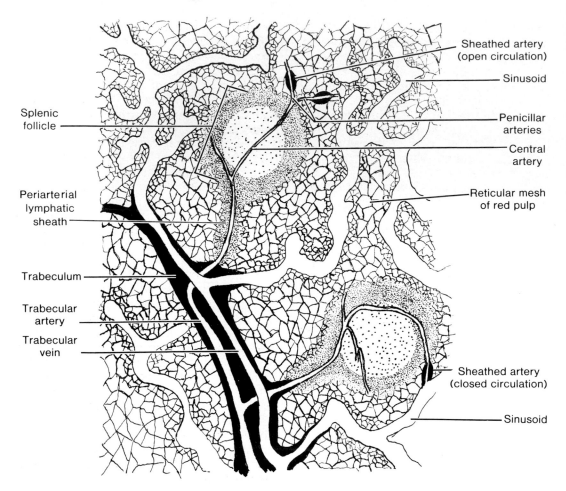

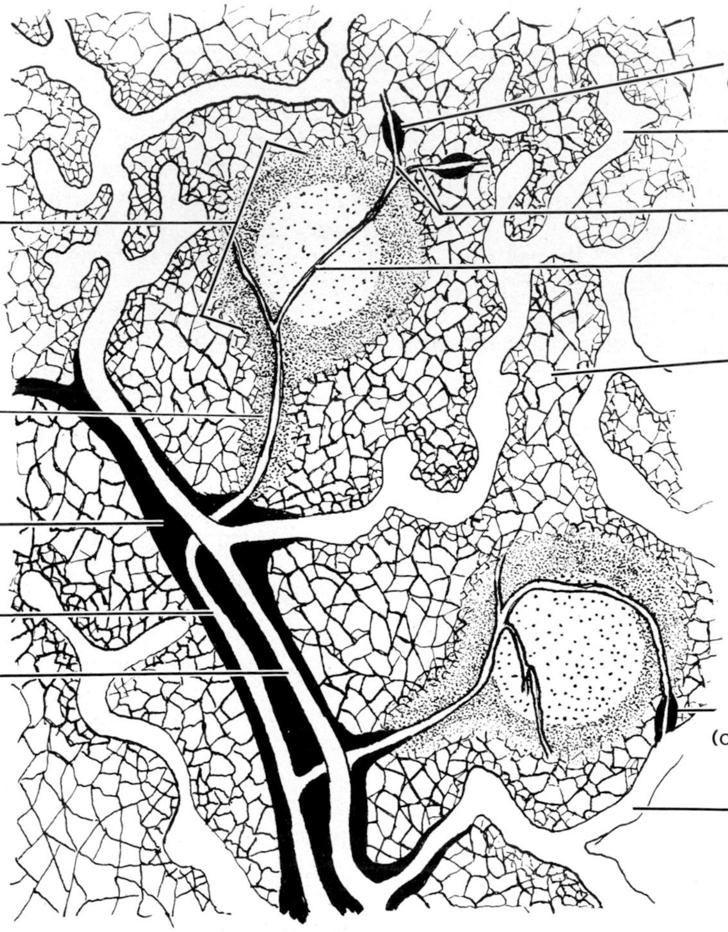

Figure 12-5. Blood supply of the spleen.

central artery provides numerous capillaries which supply the lymphoid tissue of the sheath. The capillaries then pass into the marginal zone surrounding the white pulp. How these capillaries terminate is unknown. Many arterial branches appear to open into the marginal zone, often with a funnel-shaped terminal part. There is no direct venous return and thus the white pulp is associated only with the arterial supply to the spleen.

The central artery continues to branch and its attenuated stem passes into the splenic cords of the red pulp, where it divides into several short, straight, **penicillar arteries**, some of which show a thickening of their walls and now are termed **sheathed capillaries**. The sheath consists of compact masses of concentrically arranged cells and fibers that become continuous with the reticular network of the red pulp. Close to the capillary, the cells of the sheath are rounded, while in the periphery of the sheath the cells assume a stellate shape. The cells of the sheath show a marked capacity for phagocytosis. Not all of the capillaries are sheathed and occasionally a single sheath may enclose more than one capillary. Sheathed capillaries are prominent in dogs, pigs, reptiles and birds, are less well developed in man and are lacking in laboratory animals. The sheathed capillaries either continue as simple capillaries, or they may divide once to provide two terminal capillaries. The manner in which these capillaries terminate is still a matter of debate and has led to the "**open**" and "**closed**" theories of **circulation**.

According to the open circulation theory, the capillaries empty into the meshwork of spaces in the red pulp of the splenic cords.

The blood slowly percolates through the red pulp and finds its way into the venous system through the wall of the splenic sinusoids. The closed theory holds that the capillaries open directly into the lumina of the venous sinusoids; blood leaves the sinusoid at the capillary end and returns at the venous end because of a decreasing pressure gradient between these two ends of the sinusoid. A compromise between these divergent views suggests that both types of circulation exist and that a closed circulation in a contracted spleen becomes open when the spleen is distended.

The splenic sinusoids drain into the **veins of the pulp**, which are supported by a thin muscle coat and, more externally, are surrounded by reticular and elastic fibers. A sphincter-like activity of the smooth muscle has been described at the junction of the pulp veins and sinusoids. The pulp veins enter the trabeculae where, as the trabecular veins, they pass in company with the artery. The **trabecular veins** unite and leave at the hilus as the splenic vein.

The spleen has no afferent lymphatics, but efferents arise deep in the white pulp and converge on the central artery. The lymphatics enter trabeculae and form large vessels that leave at the hilus. Areas of the spleen supplied by sinusoids, i.e., the red pulp, lack lymphatics.

Functions

A reservoir or storage function is highly developed in those species in which the splenic capsule is muscular, and in these species, the spleen can store large numbers of red cells which can be given up to the circulation as needed. In the dog, the spleen can accommodate up to one-third of the circulating mass of erythrocytes and in the horse it has been estimated that the spleen can deliver to the circulation a volume of blood equal to 40% of the resting circulating volume. Normal man has no significant splenic reserve of erythrocytes (only 30 to 40 ml), but there are indications that even this small reserve can be mobilized from the spleen. About one-third of the platelets of the body are sequestered in the spleen where they form a reserve pool, available on demand.

The spleen serves as a filter for the blood, removing particulate matter which is taken up and phagocytized by macrophages in the marginal zone, the splenic cords and the sheathed capillaries. The sinusoidal endothelial cells and the reticular cells of the reticular network have no special phagocytic capacities and contribute little to the clearing of foreign materials from the blood.

In addition to filtering particulate matter, the spleen constitutes the graveyard for worn out red cells and platelets and possibly for granular leukocytes as well. As the blood percolates through the splenic cords it comes under constant scrutiny and monitoring by macrophages. Viable cells are allowed to pass through the spleen but damaged or aged cells are retained and phagocytized. How the spleen recognizes the cells to be removed is not known, but several factors may be involved. Changes in the cell surface with aging may permit antigenic reaction with antibodies that enhance phagocytosis (opsonizing antibodies). Red cells do not undergo lysis or fragmentation within the splenic cords but appear to be phagocytized intact. The sinusoidal walls also serve as a barrier for the re-entrance of cells into circulation, since the cells must insinuate themselves through the narrow slits between the sinusoidal endothelial cells. Normal red cells are pliant and are able to squeeze through these interendothelial clefts, whereas cells such as spherocytes and those of sickle cell anemia are rigid and unable to pass through the endothelial barrier. As red cells age, their cell membranes become more permeable to water. The relatively slow passage through the red pulp may allow the aged cells to imbibe fluid, swell and thereby become too rigid to pass into the sinusoids. Components of erythrocytes that can be reutilized in the production of new blood cells are recovered by the spleen and this organ is highly efficient in conserving the iron freed from hemoglobin and returning it to accessible stores.

Another role of the spleen is that described as the "pitting" function. Red cells that contain rigid inclusions, such as malarial parasites and the iron-containing granules of siderocytes, but which are otherwise normal are not destroyed by the spleen, but the inclusion is removed at the wall of the sinusoid. The flexible portion of the erythrocyte passes through the sinusoidal wall, but the rigid inclusion becomes held back by the narrow interendothelial clefts and is stripped from the cell, which then passes into the lumen of the sinusoid. The rigid portion remains behind in the splenic pulp.

The spleen has great importance in the immune response, mounting a large scale production of antibody against blood-borne antigen. However, antigen introduced by other routes will also evoke a response in the spleen, since the antigen soon finds its way into the blood stream. The reactions in the spleen are the same as those that occur in the lymph node and include both primary and secondary responses. In the primary response, clusters of antibody-forming cells appear at first within the periarterial lymphatic sheath. The cells increase in number and become concentrated at the periphery of the sheath. Immature and mature plasma cells appear and germinal centers develop in the nodules. Ultimately, plasma cells become numerous in the marginal zone between white and red pulp and in the cords of red pulp, either as a result of direct emigration from the white pulp, or indirectly via the circulation. During the secondary response, as in lymph nodes, the germinal center response dominates, occurs almost immediately and is of large scale.

The spleen has important hemopoietic functions in all vertebrates and serves as a primary hemopoietic tissue in lower forms, where all types of blood cells are produced. In most mammals the spleen is active in the production of red cells, platelets and granulocytes only during embryonic and fetal life but production of lymphoid cells continues throughout life. In some conditions in man such as some anemias or in leukemia, the red pulp of the spleen contains islands of hemopoietic tissue. This is referred to as myeloid metaplasia and probably occurs as the result of the sequestration of stem cells by the spleen and not by reactivation of an indigenous population of potential hemopoietic cells. In some animals production of red cells and platelets continues in the spleen even during adult life. In the bat, production of red cells and granulocytes by the spleen continues throughout life and is conspicuous during winter hibernation when there is little such activity in the bone marrow. In rodents such as rats and mice and in the opossum, both granulocytes and erythrocytes are formed in small numbers in the spleen, and megakaryocytes are commonly found.

THYMUS

Thymic tissue is present in all vertebrates except the cyclostomes (lampreys and hagfishes). In man, the thymus forms a bilobed, encapsulated lymphatic organ situated in the superior mediastinum dorsal to the sternum and anterior to the great vessels that emerge from the heart. It is the first organ of the embryo to become lymphoid and, unlike the spleen and lymph nodes, is well developed and relatively large at birth. The greatest weight (30 to 40 g) is achieved at puberty, after which the organ undergoes progressive involution and is partially replaced by fat and connective tissue.

Structure

KEY WORDS: lobes, capsule, septa, lobules, cortex, medulla, reticular network, endoderm, epithelial reticular cells, cytoreticulum

In man the thymus consists of two **lobes** closely applied and joined by connective tissue. Each lobe arises from a separate primordium and there is no continuity of thymic tissue from one lobe to the other. A thin **capsule** of loose connective tissue surrounds each lobe and provides **septa** that extend into the thymus, subdividing each lobe into a number of irregular compartments, or **lobules**. Each lobule consists of a **cortex** and **medulla** and, in the usual sections, the medulla appears as isolated, palely staining areas surrounded by the denser cortical tissue. Serial sections, however, reveal that the lobules are not completely isolated by the septa and that the medullary areas are continuous with each other throughout each lobe.

The free cells of the thymus are contained within the meshes of a **reticular network** which, however, differs from that of lymph nodes and the spleen. In the thymus the reticular cells are of **endodermal** rather than mesenchymal origin and are not associated with reticular fibers. These **epithelial reticular cells** are stellate in shape, with greatly branched cytoplasm. The cytoplasmic processes are in contact with the processes of other reticular cells and at their points of contact are united by desmosomes. Thus, the stroma of the thymus consists of a **cytoreticulum** and is composed of epithelial cells. Reticular fibers are found only in relation to the blood vessels of the thymus.

Cortex

KEY WORDS: lymphocytes, large, medium and small lymphocytes, macrophages

The cortex consists of a thick, deeply stained layer extending beneath the capsule and along the septa. The majority of the cells of the cortex are **lymphocytes** which are closely packed and in contact and there is little intervening material. Because of the mutual compression the cells appear polyhedral in shape. **Large, medium** and **small lymphocytes** are present, the latter being the most abundant and indistinguishable from other small lymphocytes found elsewhere. Large lymphocytes tend to concentrate at the periphery of the cortex beneath the capsule, and mitotic figures are frequent in this region. They represent stem cells that have newly emigrated from the bone marrow. Small lymphocytes become increasingly more numerous toward the deeper cortex, where degenerating cells with pyknotic nuclei are found. Unlike the lymph node, nodular lymphatic tissue is not present in the cortex of the thymus, and there is no internal sinus system.

The reticular cells in the cortex are highly branched but their processes are obscured by the mass of lymphocytes. They form a continuous layer at the periphery of the cortex, separating it from the connective tissue of the capsule and septa. These epithelial reticular cells contain tonofilaments and membrane-bound structures that appear to be secretion granules.

Macrophages are consistently present but in small numbers scattered throughout the cortex. They are difficult to distinguish from reticular cells by light microscopy, unless phagocytosed material can be demonstrated in their cytoplasm. Macrophages that have engulfed degenerating cells can be found scattered throughout the thymus. In electron micrographs they are distinguished from the epithelial reticular cells by the lack of desmosomes. Macrophages tend to be increased in number toward the junction of the cortex and medulla.

Medulla

KEY WORDS: pleomorphism of reticular cells, thymic corpuscles

The medulla occupies the central region of the thymus, where it forms a paler-staining, broad band of tissue that is continuous throughout each lobe. Frequently, however, it appears to be isolated within a lobule, surrounded by a complete layer of cortex. Lymphocytes are less numerous than in the cortex and the epithelial reticular cells are not as widely dispersed, or as markedly branched. There is some degree of **pleomorphism**, however, and the reticular cells vary from stellate to rounded or flattened cells. The free cells of the medulla are predominantly small lymphocytes but a small and variable number of macrophages are present, and plasma cells, mast cells and eosinophil granulocytes can be found, usually in relation to blood vessels. Collagenous and reticular fibers extend from the blood vessels and wind between the epithelial cells.

Rounded or ovoid epithelial structures, the **thymic corpuscles**, are a prominent feature of the medulla. These bodies vary in size from 20 to 100 μm or more in diameter and consist of flattened epithelial reticular cells, wrapped about one another in concentric lamellations. The cells are joined by numerous desmosomes and contain granules of keratohyalin. The cells at the center of the structure undergo hyalinization or necrosis and may become lysed to leave a cystic structure. Some of the cells at the periphery retain their connections with the surrounding cytoreticulum. The function of the thymic corpuscles is unknown and they have been regarded as degenerated structures. Although considered characteristic of the thymus, similar structures occur in the palatine tonsils in the dog and horse. Thymic corpuscles are only poorly developed in mice but are prominent in the thymi of humans, guinea pigs, and rats.

The general structure of the thymus is shown in Figure 12-6.

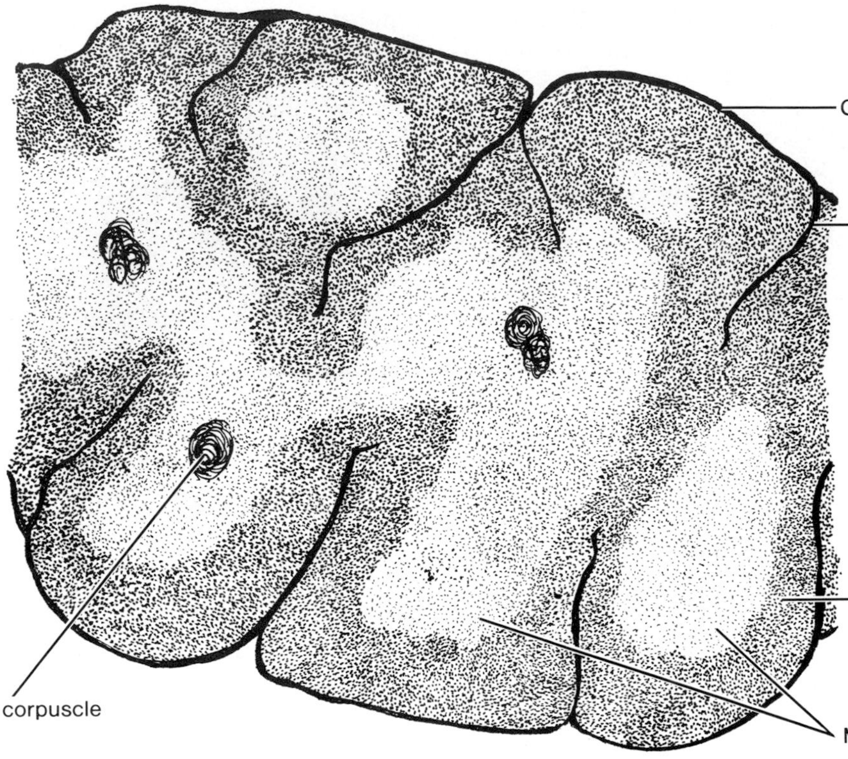

Figure 12-6. General structure of the thymus.

Blood Supply

KEY WORDS: corticomedullary junction, cortical capillaries, blood-thymic barrier

The arteries to the thymus penetrate the organ within the connective tissue septa. Arteriolar branches from these vessels course along the **corticomedullary junction** and provide arterioles and capillaries to the medulla and capillaries to the cortex. Thus, the cortex is provided with capillaries only and larger vessels do not pass through the cortex. Within the cortex, the capillaries run toward the capsule, then form branching arcades and return back through the cortex to drain into venules and thence into veins that accompany the arterioles in the corticomedullary region and medulla. The veins leave the parenchyma by way of the septa and ultimately unite to form a single thymic vein.

The **cortical capillaries** are enveloped by a collar of connective tissue which forms part of the **blood-thymic barrier**. This envelope in turn is surrounded by a continuous layer of epithelial reticular cells. The perivascular connective tissue space varies in width and is traversed by reticular fibers that accompany the vessel. Contained within the space are granular leukocytes, plasma cells, macrophages and lymphocytes. The blood-thymic barrier in the cortex consists then of the capillary endothelium and its basal lamina, the perivascular connective tissue sheath, and the layer of epithelial reticular cells and their associated basal laminae. There is little movement of macromolecules across this barrier, and cortical lymphocytes develop in relative isolation from antigens. On the other hand, vessels of the medulla and corticomedullary junction are permeable to circulating macromolecules.

Involution

Growth of the thymus during fetal life is very rapid and the organ attains its greatest relative size by the time of birth. It continues to grow, but at a reduced rate, until the onset of sexual maturity, after which it undergoes progressive involution. The organ decreases in weight, shows a loss of cortical lymphocytes and an increase in the size and number of thymic corpuscles. The cortical areas become infiltrated by fat cells and the replacement may become extensive. Increased width of the connective tissue septa also has been reported in the involuting thymus. However, the thymic parenchyma does not entirely disappear, even in old age, and the thymus maintains functional activity in the adult.

Functions

The thymus is essential for the production of those lymphocytes (T lymphocytes) that are involved in cell-mediated immune responses such as the rejection of foreign grafts and the immunological responses to fungi and certain bacteria and viruses. Although not directly involved in elaboration of the conventional type of antibodies, the T cells do cooperate with B cells for the production of antibody against antigens such as foreign red cells. All of these responses are impaired in animals that have been thymectomized at birth. There also is a marked decrease in the number of circulating small lymphocytes and the deep cortex of lymph nodes and the periarterial lymphatic sheath of the spleen fail to develop. The hagfish, which has no thymus, appears to be immunologically incompetent.

Most of the lymphocytes within the thymus seem to be inert and acquire immunological capabilities in the blood stream or after migrating to their preferred sites in other lymphatic organs. The T cells have a long life span and, with the exception of the thymus, recirculate between lymphatic organs, lymph and blood. Thymic lymphocytes show a high rate of mitotic activity, but many die within the thymus or emigrate from the thymus to other organs.

Thymic tissue contained in diffusion chambers and transplanted into thymectomized newborn animals partially prevents the effects of thymectomy. Permeable molecules, but not cells, diffuse from the chambers, indicating the presence of a thymic-produced humoral factor. This agent has been called thymosin and is regarded as a hormone that induces T cell differentation. Thymosin may be a product of the reticular epithelial cells.

Other Constituents

The thymuses of birds, reptiles and amphibians frequently show a number of peculiar structural elements, the significance of which is not known. Among these structures are cyst-like spaces lined by cells with brush borders, cilia or mucus-producing cells and reticular cells that contain microvillus-lined vacuoles. Most peculiar are the so-called "myoid" cells which have an imperfect resemblance to striated muscle. These may resemble embryonal muscle fiber or structures similar to adult muscle and in which typical banding with Z lines and A, I and M bands have been described. It is not known whether these various inclusions have functional implications or whether they represent aberrant differentiation of embryonal elements.

DEVELOPMENT OF LYMPHATIC ORGANS

Lymphatic organs have been divided into primary (central) and secondary (peripheral). Primary lymphatic organs, which are the first to develop, include the thymus and in aves, the bursa of Fabricius. The mammalian equivalent of the bursa is unknown but probably is the bone marrow, although the spleen and gut-associated lymphatic tissues, or GALT (Peyer's patches, lamina propria of small intestine, appendix), have been considered also. The secondary lymphatic organs are the lymph nodes, spleen, tonsils and the GALT.

Thymus. The thymus arises as paired endodermal outgrowths from the third pharyngeal pouches. Each outgrowth extends caudally to lie in the midline, beneath the upper part of the sternum and initially contains a slit-like lumen which disappears as the epithelial cells proliferate. Centrally the cells assume a stellate shape and become loosely arranged but still retain cytoplasmic connections with each other. These cells form the epithelial reticular cells that make up the cytoreticulum of the thymus. Lymphoid precursor cells enter the developing thymus from the bone marrow and give rise to the lymphocyte population. Simultaneously, the surrounding mesenchyme condenses to form the capsule and also invades the cellular mass to provide the septae.

Lymph Nodes. Lymph nodes develop locally in vascular mesenchyme at the sites normally occupied by lymph nodes. Their formation is related closely to the development of the lymph vascular system. Aggregates of mesenchymal cells occur about loops of lymphatic capillaries, in close association with lymphatic sacs. At the periphery of the aggregates, the lymphatic vessels form isolated spaces separated by slender bridges of connective tissue. As the lymph spaces gradually fuse to form the marginal (subcapsular) sinus, the connective tissue outside the sinus and in the bridges condenses to form the capsule and its trabeculae. As they fuse, the sinuses follow the course of the developing trabeculae, subdivide, and develop into trabecular and medullary sinuses. The mesenchymal aggregates give rise to the reticular cells and network of the cortex and medulla. The entire mass is seeded by lymphocytes from the bone marrow and thymus, and the cells take up their characteristic locations in the node.

The Spleen. The spleen first appears as several thickenings in the cranial end of the greater omentum. With continued growth, the primordia fuse to form a lobulated spleen which extends into the body cavity. As the organ expands, it loses the lobulated appearance. Mesenchymal cells in the body of the cellular mass differentiate into reticular cells, which provide the splenic reticular stroma. The outermost connective tissue gradually condenses to form the capsule from which mesenchymal projections also condense to form the trabeculae. Early in development, the spleen rudiment is invaded by lymphocytes by seeding of cells from the bone marrow and thymus. Enlargement of the white pulp to form nodules occurs late, and during much of the development the lymphatic tissue is mainly in the form of periarterial lymphatic sheaths. Germinal centers do not appear until after birth. The fetal spleen is hemopoietic, producing erythrocytes and granular leukocytes, but this function ceases just before birth in man but may continue throughout life in rodents.

FUNCTIONAL SUMMARY

The assembly of lymphatic tissue, both the lymphatic organs and that spread throughout the connective tissue as lymphatic tissue, constitutes the immune system. This system serves to protect the body against invading foreign macromolecules and also constantly scrutinizes the circulating body fluids (lymph and blood) for the presence of abnormal components. Antigenic materials evoke a specific defense reaction, the immune response, that gives rise either to cells (plasma cells) that produce specific antibodies or to a population of cells (cytotoxic lymphocytes) that attack foreign cells directly or release nonspecific toxic agents. Antibodies may act by binding the antigen and neutralizing it, or they may inhibit entrance of antigen into a cell, enhance its phagocytosis or initiate its lysis.

Stimulation by antigen results in the proliferation and differentiation of lymphocytes, some of which go on to react against the antigen, while others remain as committed memory cells. On second exposure to the same antigen, the memory cells react swiftly and with great efficiency. Germinal centers are associated with production of humoral antibody, especially during a secondary response, and may represent clones of cells geared to the production of a single antibody.

Tonsils may be valuable sources of interferon, an antiviral factor, and tonsillar tissue may be more important in fighting infection than previously was recognized.

The lymph nodes also serve as filters of the lymph, straining out particulate matter which is then phagocytized by macrophages. The spleen serves a similar function for the blood but has additional functions. It is the site of the destruction of aged red cells and platelets, and possibly for granular leukocytes, and conserves material for reuse in hemopoiesis. In some animals it has a reservoir function for red cells, which can be mobilized on demand. In man, platelets are sequestered there, and these form a reserve pool. The spleen has hemopoietic functions in embryonic and fetal life and retains this function in the adults of many species. The thymus is the source of T cells which are conditioned to respond in the cell-mediated immune responses and which may elaborate a hormone affecting T cell differentiation. Cells from the thymus are seeded to other lymphatic tissues.

Atlas and Table of Key Features for Chapter 12

Table 12-1
Key Histological Features of Lymphatic Organs

	Tonsil	Lymph Node	Spleen	Thymus
Capsule	Partial, at base	Yes	Yes	Thin
Trabeculae	No	Yes	Yes	Forms thin septae
Lymphatic tissue arranged as cortex and medulla	No	Yes	No	Yes
Nodular lymphatic tissue	Yes	Yes	Yes	No
Special features	Crypts: closely associated with overlying epithelium (a) Palatine and lingual—stratified squamous, nonkeratinized (b)Pharyngeal—pseudostratified, ciliated columnar	Subcapsular, trabecular, and medullary sinuses; only lymphatic organ with afferent and efferent lymphatics	Lymphatic tissue arranged as red and white pulp; splenic follicles (nodules) associated with central arteries; sinusoids in red pulp	Thymic corpuscles in medulla; stroma is a cytoreticulum of endododermal origin

12-7 Lymphatic Organs — Tonsils

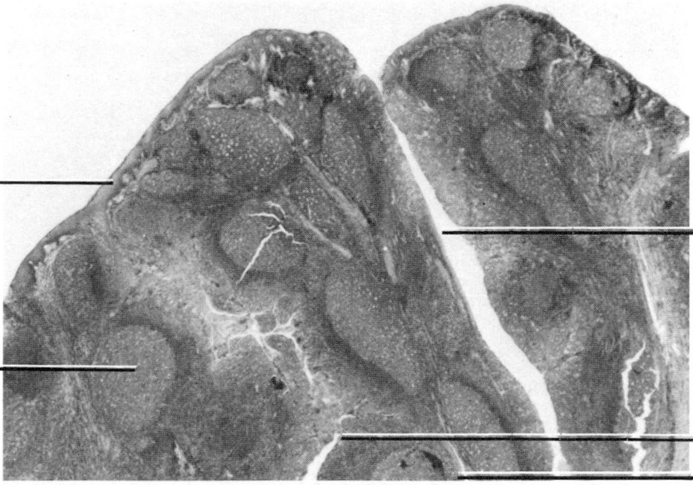

12-8

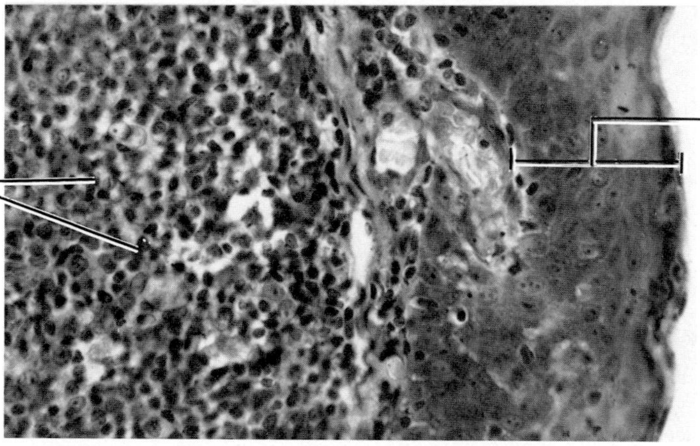

12-9

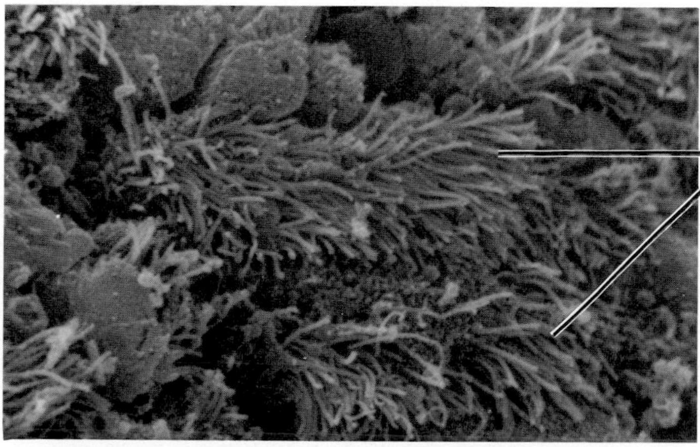

Figure 12-7. Palatine tonsil (human). LM, ×20.
Figure 12-8. Palatine tonsil (human). LM, ×250.
Figure 12-9. Surface of pharyngeal tonsil (human). SEM, ×2000.

12-10

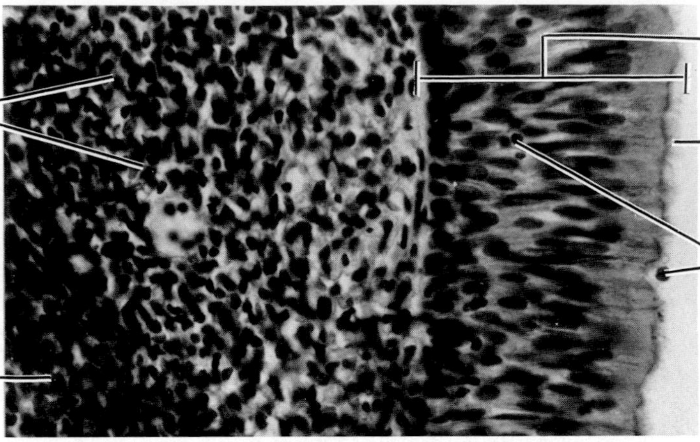

12-11 Lymph Node

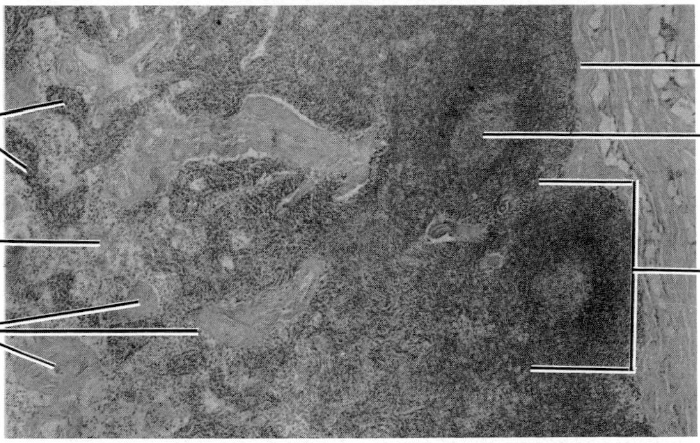

12-12

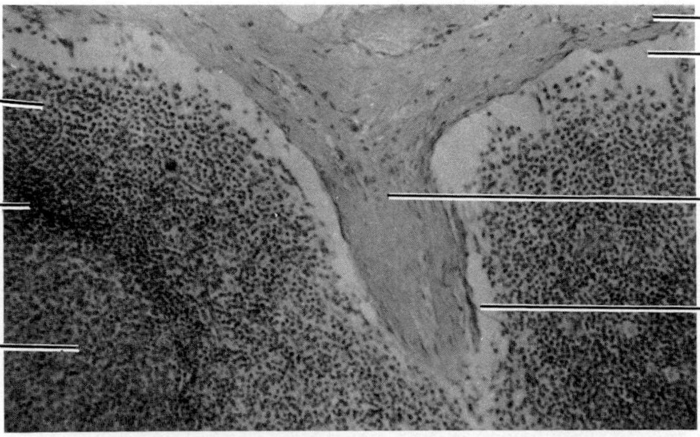

Figure 12-10. Pharyngeal tonsil (human). LM, ×250.
Figure 12-11. Lymph node. LM, ×40.
Figure 12-12. Lymph node. LM, ×250.

12-13

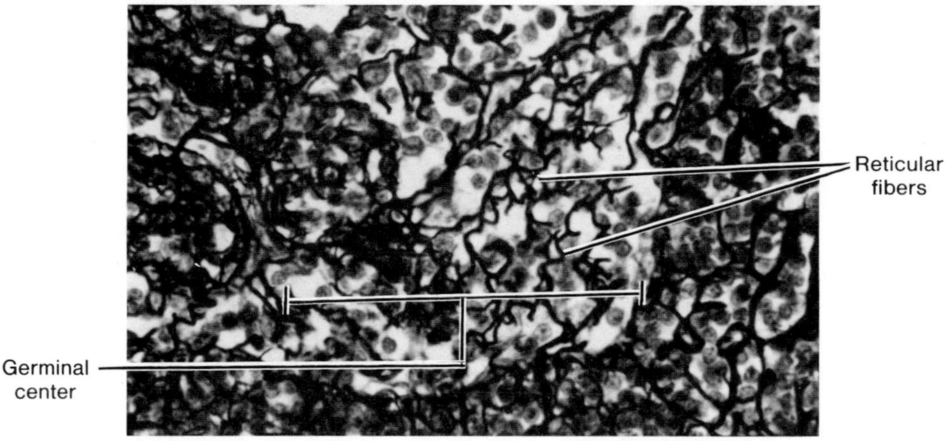

12-14

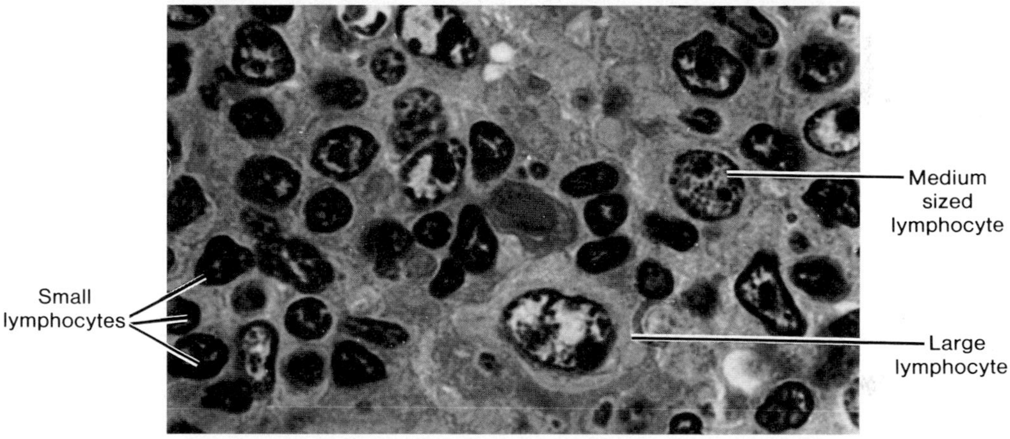

12-15

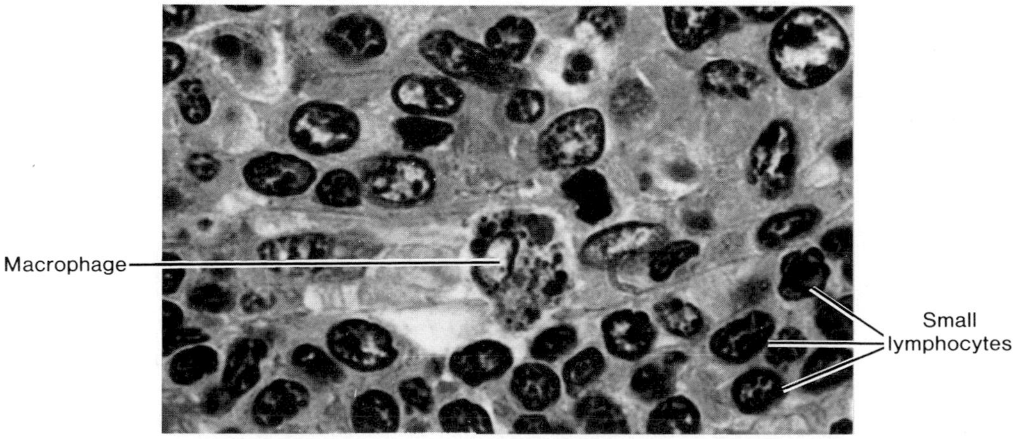

Figure 12-13. Lymph node (lymphatic nodule). LM, ×250.
Figure 12-14. Lymph node. LM, ×400.
Figure 12-15. Lymph node. LM, ×400.

12-16

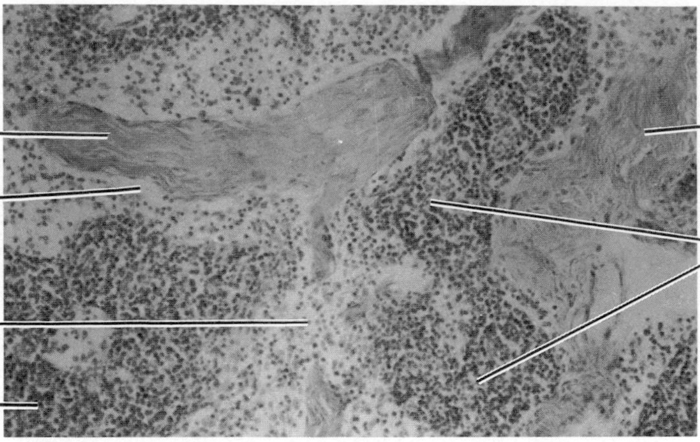

12-17 Spleen

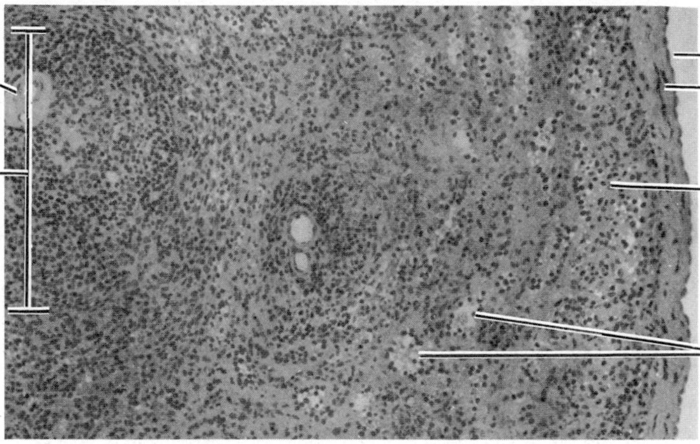

12-18

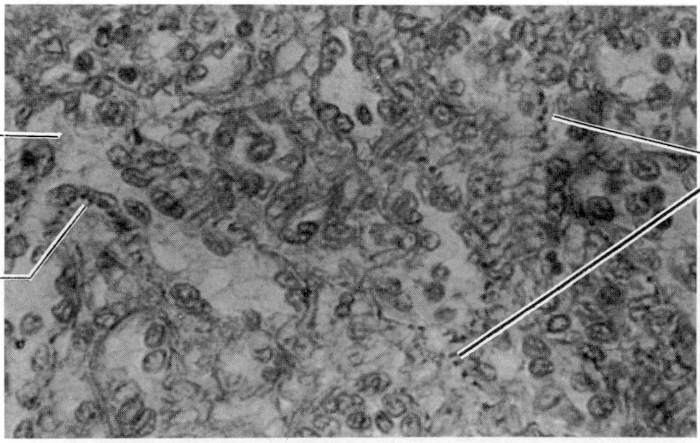

Figure 12-16. Medulla of lymph node. LM, ×100.
Figure 12-17. Spleen. LM, ×100.
Figure 12-18. Red pulp of spleen. LM, ×300.

12–19

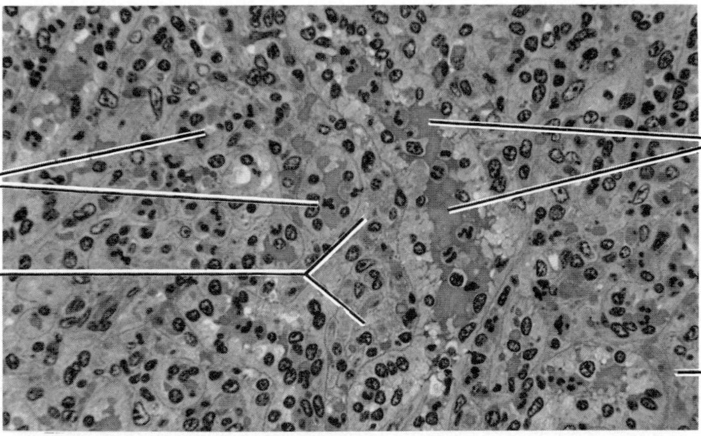
Sinusoids
Billroth's cord
Sinusoid
Basement membrane

12–20

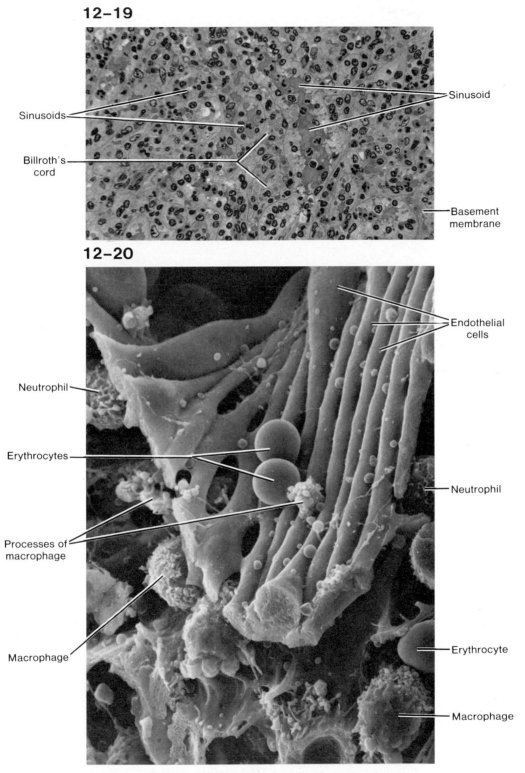

Endothelial cells
Neutrophil
Erythrocytes
Neutrophil
Processes of macrophage
Macrophage
Erythrocyte
Macrophage

Figure 12-19. Red pulp (spleen). LM, ×250.
Figure 12-20. Sinusoidal wall. SEM, ×3000.

12–21

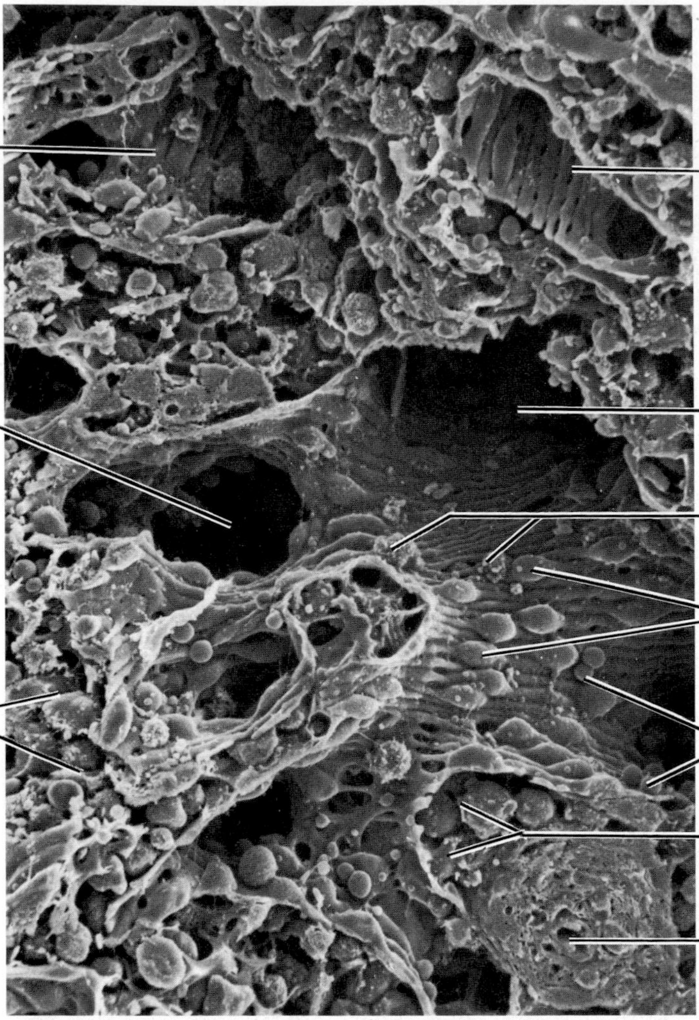

12–22

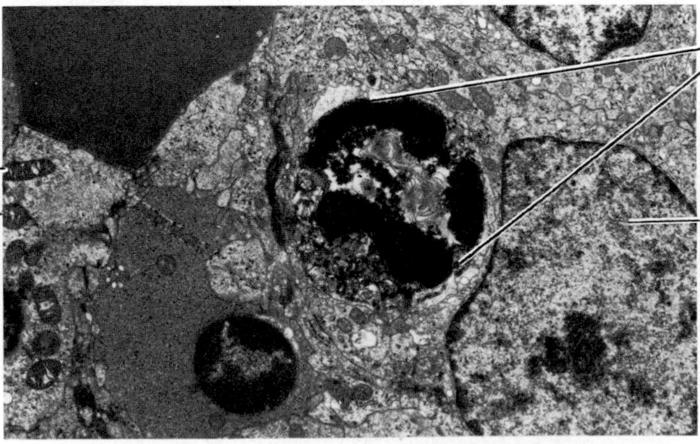

Figure 12-21. Sinusoid (spleen). SEM, ×700.
Figure 12-22. Macrophage (spleen). TEM, ×2500.

12–23

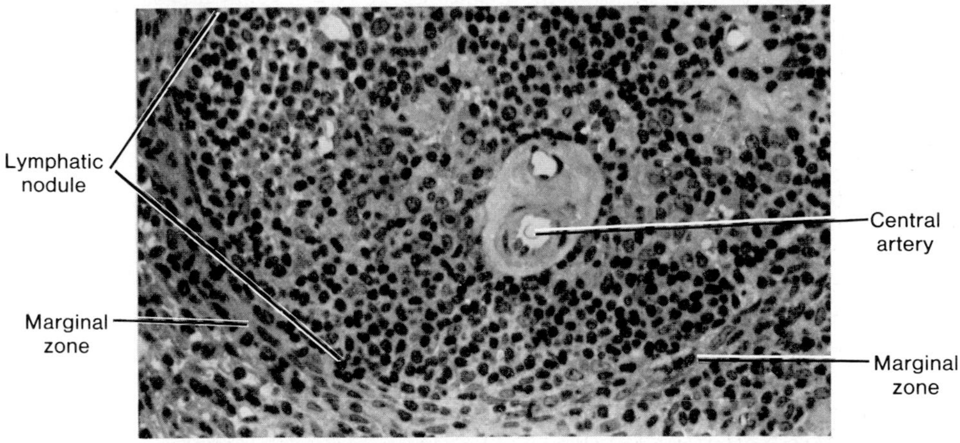

12–24

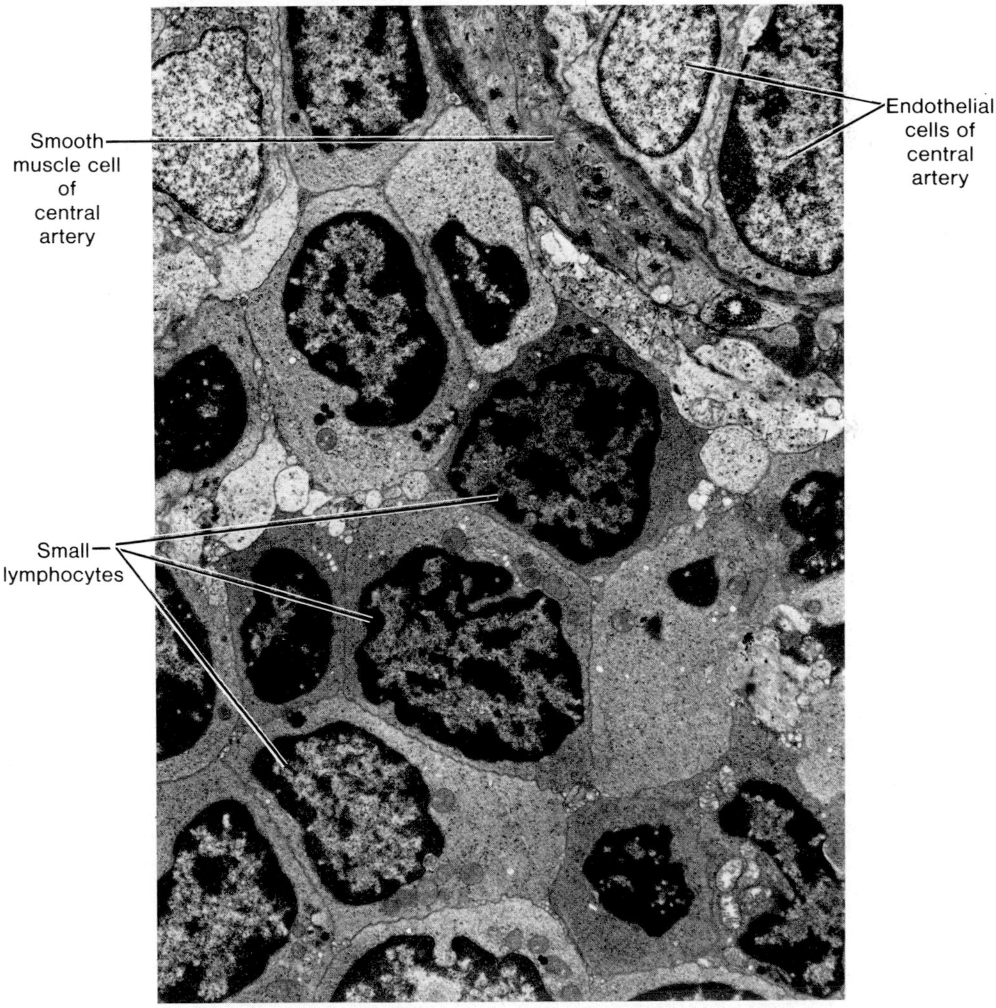

Figure 12-23. White pulp (spleen). LM, ×250.
Figure 12-24. White pulp (spleen). TEM, ×1500.

12–25 Thymus

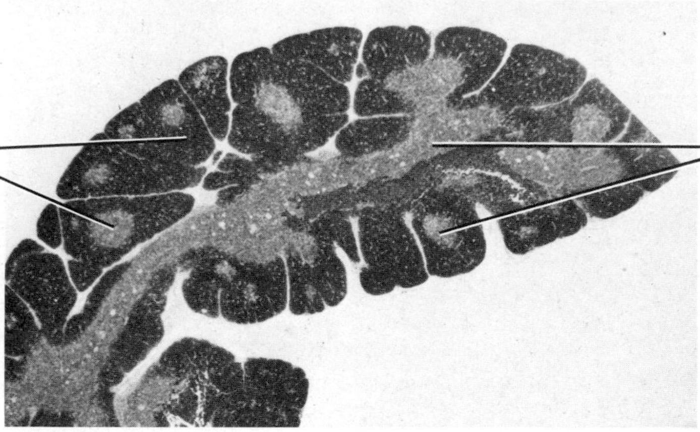

12–26

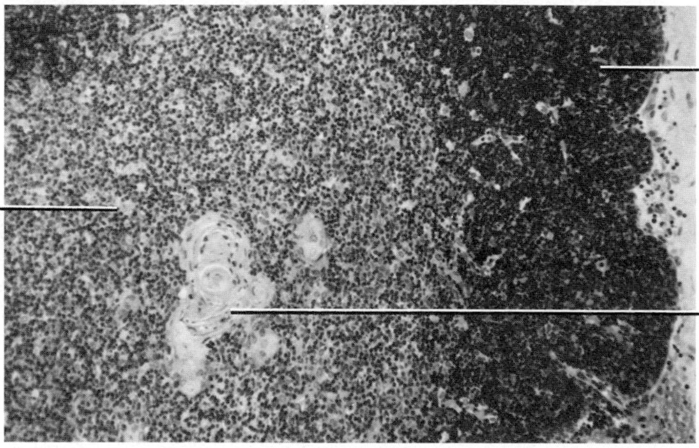

12–27

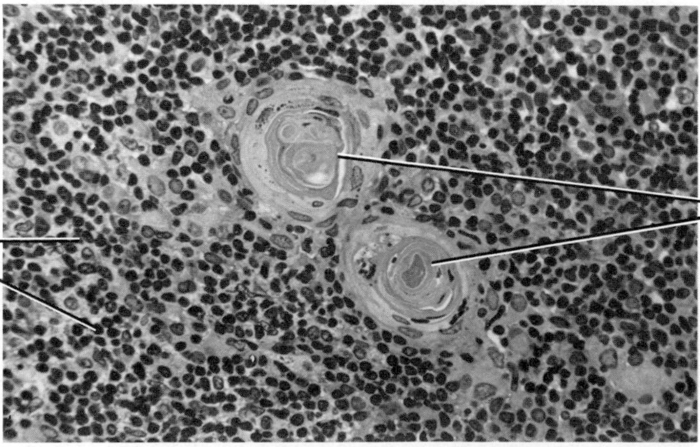

Figure 12-25. Thymus (human). LM, ×10.
Figure 12-26. Thymus (human). LM, ×50.
Figure 12-27. Thymic corpuscles. LM, ×250.

13

Skin

The skin forms the external covering of the body and constitutes a large organ with several functions. It protects the body from mechanical injury and loss of fluid, acts as a barrier against noxious agents, aids in temperature regulation, excretes various waste products and, through its receptors for sensations of heat, cold, touch and pain, provides information about the external environment.

STRUCTURE

KEY WORDS: epidermis, dermis (corium), appendages, integument, thick skin, thin skin, epidermal ridges, dermal papillae

The skin consists of a surface layer of epithelium called the **epidermis** and an underlying layer of connective tissue, the **dermis** or **corium.** A looser layer of connective tissue, the hypodermis, attaches the skin to underlying structures but is not considered a component of skin. The **appendages** of the skin—hair, nails, sweat and sebaceous glands—are local specializations of the epidermis. Together the skin and its appendages form the **integument.**

The skin varies in thickness in different parts of the body, and the proportions of dermis and epidermis also differ. Between the scapula, the dermis is especially thick, whereas on the palms of the hands and soles of the feet the epidermis is thickened. The terms **thick skin** and **thin skin** refer to the thickness of the *epidermis* and not to the thickness of the skin as a whole. In thick skin the epidermis is especially well developed, whereas in thin skin it forms a relatively narrow layer.

At its junction with the dermis, the epidermis forms numerous ridge-like extensions, the **epidermal ridges,** that project into the underlying dermis. Complementary projections of the dermis fit between the epidermal ridges and form the **dermal papillae.** The surface patterns of the skin, such as those associated with fingerprints, reflect the pattern of the dermal papillae.

Epidermis

KEY WORDS: stratified squamous epithelium, keratinization, melanocytes, pigmentation, stratum basale, stratum spinosum, stratum granulosum, stratum lucidum, stratum corneum

The epidermis forms the surface layer of the skin and consists of a **stratified squamous epithelium.** The cells undergo an orderly progression of maturation and **keratinization** to produce a superficial layer of dense, flattened, dead cells at the surface. A smaller population of cells, the **melanocytes,** is associated with **pigmentation** of the skin. The epidermis completely lacks blood vessels and is nourished by diffusion of materials from the vessels in the underlying dermis.

The epidermis can be divided into several layers, reflecting the sequential differentiation of the cells as they progress from the base of the epidermis to the surface, where they are sloughed off. In thick skin these layers are: **stratum basale, stratum spinosum, stratum granulosum, stratum lucidum** and **stratum corneum.** In thin skin these layers are less well defined and the stratum lucidum is absent.

Stratum Basale

KEY WORDS: columnar epithelium, growing layer, stratum germinativum

The stratum basale abuts the underlying dermis and is separated from it only by a basement membrane. It consists of a single row of **columnar epithelial** cells that follows the contours of the ridges and papillae. The stratum basale constitutes the **growing layer** of the epidermis, and most, but not all, of the mitotic activity occurs in this layer; for this reason the stratum basale is often called the **stratum germinativum.**

The cells are limited by a typical trilaminar membrane and are attached to adjacent cells along their lateral surfaces by numerous desmosomes. At the basal surfaces, hemidesmosomes attach the cells to the underlying basement membrane, which in turn is anchored to the dermis by short filaments. The cytoplasm of the basal keratinocytes is fairly dense and contains many tonofilaments scattered throughout the cell. Clusters of ribosomes are prominent and the cells contain a moderate number of mitochondria, some profiles of rough endoplasmic reticulum and a few Golgi saccules.

Stratum Spinosum

KEY WORDS: prickle cells, membrane coating granules, stratum Malpighii

This layer consists of several strata of irregular, polyhedral cells which become somewhat flattened in the outermost layers. The cells normally are closely applied to each other and joined at all surfaces by desmosomes. However, during tissue preparation the cells tend to shrink and pull apart except at their points of attachment. Thus, the cells appear to have numerous, short, spiny projections that extend between adjacent cells, and because of this, the cells commonly are called **prickle cells.** The projections are not areas of cytoplasmic continuity between cells but are the sites of typical desmosomes.

In addition to the organelles seen in basal cells, the cytoplasm of prickle cells in the upper layers of stratum spinosum contains ovoid granules, 0.1 to 0.5 μm in diameter, called **membrane coating granules.** These structures consist of parallel laminae bounded by a double membrane. Their function is unknown, but they may contribute material to the inner and/or outer aspects of the cell membrane. Tonofilaments are numerous and may form dense bundles. The stratum spinosum and stratum basale frequently are grouped together and are referred to as the **stratum Malpighii.**

Stratum Granulosum

KEY WORDS: keratohyalin granules

The stratum granulosum consists of three to five layers of flattened cells whose long axes are oriented parallel to the surface of the skin. The distinguishing feature of the cells is the presence of **keratohyalin granules,** which vary in size and shape and consist of amorphous, densely packed particles. The granules are not limited by membranes and are closely associated with bundles of filaments. Chemically, they possess large quantities of sulphur-containing amino acids. The keratohyalin granules increase in number and size in the outermost layers of the stratum granulosum and these cells show evidence of degenerative changes. The nuclei stain more palely and the contacts between adjacent cells become less distinct.

Stratum Lucidum

KEY WORDS: loss of nuclei, thickened cell membranes, thick skin

The stratum lucidum appears as a narrow, undulating, lightly stained zone at the surface of the stratum granulosum. It is formed by several layers of cells so compacted together that outlines of individual cells cannot be made out. Traces of flattened nuclei may be seen but generally **nuclei are lacking.** Only a few remnants of organelles are present and the main constituents of the cytoplasm are aggregates of tonofilaments which show a more regular arrangement, generally parallel to the skin surface. The **cell membrane** is **thickened** and more convoluted, and the amount of intercellular material is increased.

The stratum lucidum is prominent in the **thick skin** of the palms and soles but is absent from the epidermis in other parts of the body.

Stratum Corneum

KEY WORDS: squames, keratin, soft keratin, desquamation, stratum disjunctum

The stratum corneum (see Fig. 13-1) forms the outermost layer of the epidermis and is composed of scale-like cells, frequently called **squames**, that become increasingly flattened toward the surface. The squames represent the remnants of cells that have lost all of the organelles and their nuclei. The cells are completely filled with **keratin**, which consists of tightly packed filaments embedded in an opaque, structureless material. Keratin is thought to be derived from tonofibrils, and in the cornified layer of the epidermis is said to be **"soft" keratin,** in distinction from that of the "hard" keratin of the nails and hair. Soft keratin has a

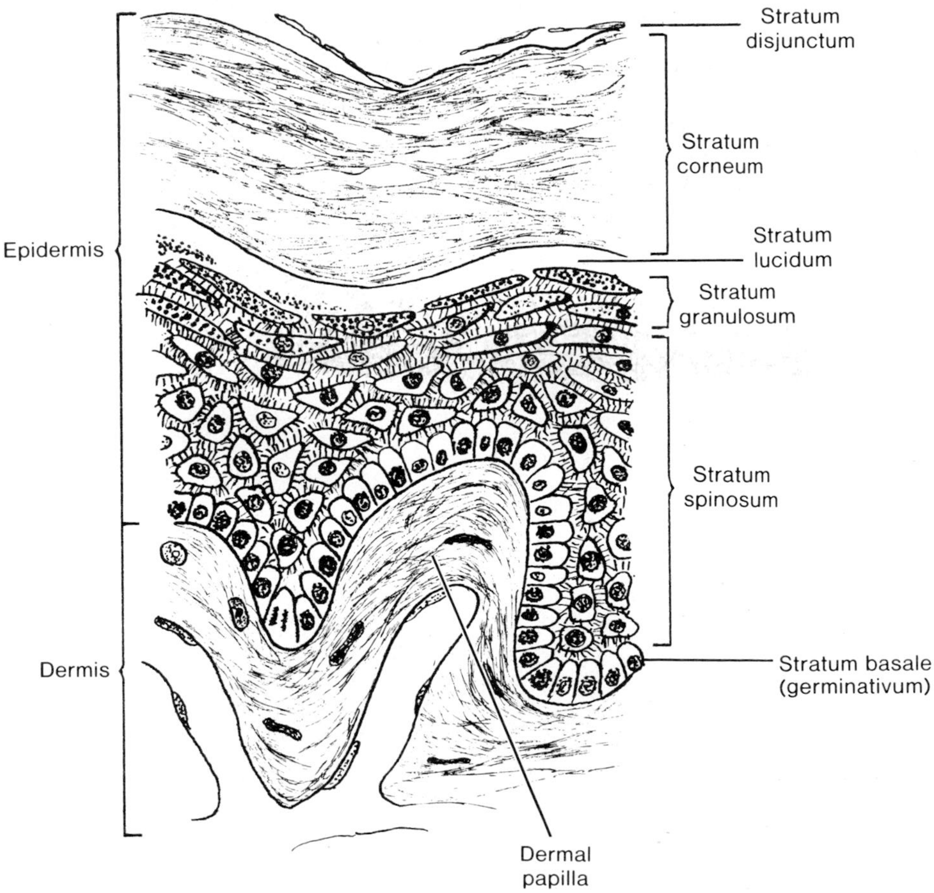

Figure 13-1. Structure of thick skin.

lower sulphur content and is somewhat more elastic than hard keratin. The squames are enclosed by a thickened, modified cell envelope. The outermost cells of the stratum corneum are constantly being sloughed off or **desquamated**, and this region often is referred to as the **stratum disjunctum.**

Pigmentation

KEY WORDS: carotene, melanin, melanocytes, melanosomes

The color of the skin is determined by the pigments carotene and melanin and also by the blood in the capillaries of the dermis. **Carotene** is a yellowish pigment present in the stratum corneum and in the fat cells of the dermis and hypodermis. **Melanin**, a brown pigment, is present mainly in the cells of the stratum basale and deeper layers of the stratum spinosum.

Melanin is formed in specialized cells of the epidermis, the **melanocytes,** that originate from cells that emigrated from the neural crest during embryonic development. Melanocytes are scattered throughout the basal layer of the epidermis and give off numerous cytoplasmic processes that extend between the cells of the stratum spinosum. In electron micrographs, the epidermal melanocytes can be distinguished from surrounding cells because they lack tonofilaments and contain melanin granules, or **melanosomes**, in various stages of development. Melanocytes also contain the usual array of cytoplasmic organelles. While the melanocyte lacks desmosomal junctions with neighboring cells, it is affixed to the dermis by hemidesmosome-like junctions.

Mature melanosomes are transferred from the melanocytes via their processes to the cells of the basal layer and stratum spinosum. In the human, the melanosomes frequently aggregate above the nuclei of the basal cells, but in the superficial layers of the epidermis, the granules are more evenly distributed and become progressively more dust-like. Since epidermal cells are constantly shed from the surface, the melanocyte must provide for continual renewal of melanin. Although melanocytes may die and be replaced by division of neighboring cells, this is a random event, and there does not appear to be a regular cycle of replacement of melanocytes.

The number of melanocytes and the size of the melanosomes is somewhat greater in Negroid and Mongoloid races than in the Caucasian race, but difference in skin color is due mainly to the distribution of pigment. In the Caucasian race, melanin is concentrated in the lower regions of the Malpighian layer, whereas in the Negroid race it is distributed throughout all the layers of the epidermis. The degree of pigmentation also varies in different regions of the body. The axilla, circumanal region, scrotum, penis, labia majora, nipples and areola are areas of increased pigmentation. In contrast, the palms of the hands and soles of the feet contain little or no pigment. Freckles represent local areas of increased pigmentation but paradoxically contain fewer melanocytes than adjacent paler skin. Pigmentation of freckles and of the areola and nipples may be intensified with pregnancy. A general increase in pigmentation by melanin occurs from exposure to sunlight, at first by darkening of existing melanin and later by an increased formation of new melanin.

A deficiency of melanin also may occur. The white spotted patterns of piebald animals and of piebaldism in humans result from abnormalities in the morphology of melanocytes in which the length and number of the cell processes is deficient. Complete albinism results from an inability of the melanocytes to synthesize melanin and not from an absence of melanocytes.

Other Cell Types

KEY WORDS: Langerhans cells, Merkel cells

Two other cell types are present in the epidermis, the Langerhans cells and the Merkel cells. The **Langerhans cells** are present throughout the epidermis but are especially prominent in the upper layers of the stratum Malpighii. In routine sections, these cells have darkly staining nuclei surrounded by a clear cytoplasm. With special stains they are seen to be stellate cells which extend cytoplasmic processes into the stratum spinosum. In electron micrographs, the nucleus is highly irregular in outline and the cytoplasm lacks tonofilaments, desmosomes and melanosomes but is characterized by the presence of membrane-bound, rod-shaped granules with a regular, granular interior. Some of these granules appear to be in continuity with the cell membrane. Langerhans cells apparently are able to trap antigen that penetrates the skin, and to transport it to regional lymph nodes. They may have their origin in bone marrow.

Merkel cells tend to lie in close association with sensory nerve endings in the basal layer of the epidermis. Morphologically they resemble the cells of the stratum spinosum but are distinguished, in electron micrographs, by the indented nucleus, prominent Golgi complex and numerous dense-cored vesicles. The vesicles tend to concentrate basally, at the site where nerve cells approach the cell. The function of these cells is unknown but they may play a role in sensory processes. They have been compared to polypeptide and hormone-containing cells, but a definite relationship with these has not been developed.

Dermis

KEY WORDS: Reticular layer, papillary layer, dermal papillae, arrectores pilorum muscles, panniculus carnosus

The dermis, or corium, varies in thickness in different regions of the body. It is especially thin and delicate in the eyelids, scrotum and prepuce, very thick in the palms and soles, thicker on the posterior than the anterior aspect of the body and also thicker in men than in women. The dermis is tough, flexible, highly elastic and consists of a felt work of collagenous fibers and abundant elastic fibers. The connective tissue is arranged in two layers: a deep or reticular layer and a superficial papillary layer.

The **reticular layer** is the thicker, denser part of the dermis and consists of dense bundles of collagenous fibers that for the most part run parallel with the surface. Below, the reticular layer merges indistinctly into the subcutaneous tissue which generally contains abundant fat cells. Collagen in the reticular layer is mostly type I with a smaller amount of type III. The **papillary layer** lies immediately beneath the epidermis and extends into it in the form of the **dermal papillae**. The papillary layer is not clearly demarcated from the reticular layer, but the collagenous fibers tend to be thinner and more loosely arranged, and this layer also has a more cellular appearance. Most of the collagen is type III.

The papillae are small, conical projections with round or blunted apices that fit into corresponding pits on the undersurface of the epidermis. They are particularly prominent on the palmar surfaces of the hands and fingers, where they are closely aggregated and arranged in parallel lines which correspond to the surface ridges of the epidermis. Capillary loops are present within the papillae and in some, especially in the palms and fingers, nerve endings and tactile corpuscles are present.

Smooth muscle cells are present in the deeper parts of the reticular layer in the penis, scrotum, perineum and areola. In these areas, the skin becomes wrinkled as the muscles contract. The **arrectores pilorum muscles** are small bundles of smooth cells associated with hairs. Many animals contain an extensive subcutaneous layer of skeletal muscle, the **panniculus carnosus,** which permits the voluntary movement of large areas of the skin.

APPENDAGES OF THE SKIN

The appendages of the skin are derived from the epidermis and in man include the hair, nails, sebaceous and sweat glands. In other animals, the epidermis gives rise to such structures as claws, hooves, beaks, feathers and scales, to the salt glands of certain marine reptiles and birds and to the shells of turtles.

Nails

KEY WORDS: body (nail plate), root, proximal nail fold, lateral nail fold (nail wall), eponychium, hyponychium, lunule, nail bed, nail matrix, hard keratin

The nails (Fig. 13-2) are hard, elastic, keratin structures that cover the tips of the fingers and toes on their dorsal surfaces. Each nail consists of two parts: a visible portion, the **body** (nail plate), and the proximal part called the **root** which is implanted into a groove in the skin. The root of the nail is overlapped by the **proximal nail fold**, a fold of skin that also continues along the lateral borders of the nail, where it forms the

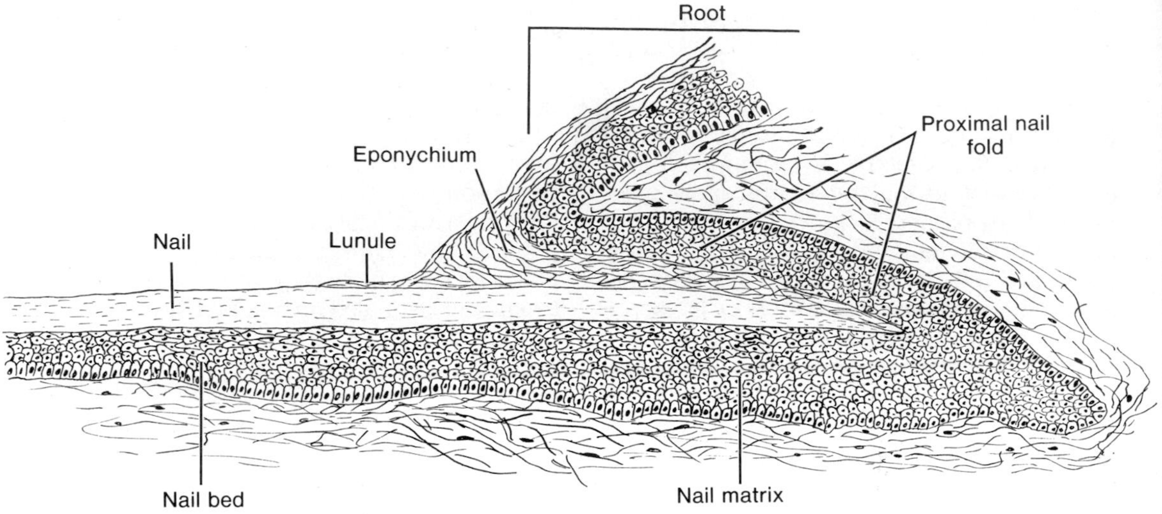

Figure 13-2. Longitudinal section of a nail.

lateral nail fold, or **nail wall**. The stratum corneum of the proximal nail fold extends over the upper surface of the nail root and for a short distance onto the surface of the body of the nail as a thin cuticular fold called the **eponychium.** At the free border of the nail, the skin is attached to the undersurface of the nail, forming the **hyponychium**.

The nail itself is analogous to the cornified zone of the epidermis and consists of several layers of flattened cells with shrunken and degenerated nuclei. The cells are hard, tightly coherent and throughout most of the body of the nail are clear and translucent. The pink color of the nails is due to the transmission of color from the underlying capillary bed. Near the root, the nail is more opaque and forms a crescentic area, the **lunule**, which is most visible in the thumbnail, becoming smaller and more hidden by the proximal nail fold towards the little finger.

Beneath the nail lies the **nail bed**, which corresponds to the stratum Malpighii of the skin. It consists of prickle cells and a stratum basale resting upon a basement membrane. The underlying dermis is thrown into numerous longitudinal ridges which are very vascular, but near the root the ridges become more irregular, smaller and less vascular. The nail bed beneath the root and lunule is thicker, actively proliferative and is concerned with the growth of the nail; it is called the **nail matrix**. The nail bed beneath the rest of the nail is thinner and is not involved with nail growth. Cells in the deepest layer of the matrix are cylindrical and show frequent mitoses while above them are several layers of polyhedral cells and flattened squames that represent the differentiating cells of the nail. These cells are enclosed by a thickened plasma membrane and are filled with keratin. Nail keratin has a higher sulphur content than the keratin of the epidermal cells of the skin and is termed **hard keratin**.

Claws are similar to nails in their development and structure; they differ mainly in their final form. Whereas nails are flat and cover the upper surface of the digit, claws are compressed laterally and arch over the top, sides and tip of the digit. The hyponychium is thicker and shows a greater degree of cornification in clawed animals.

Hair

KEY WORDS: lanugo, vellus hairs, terminal hairs

Hairs are present on almost all surfaces of the skin, except for the palmar surfaces of the hands, plantar surfaces of the feet, margin of the lips, prepuce, glans penis, clitoris, labia minora and inner surfaces of the labia majora. They consist of elastic, keratinized threads that vary in length and thickness in different regions of the body and in different races. From the middle of fetal life the skin of the human is covered by a fine hair called

lanugo; this mostly has been shed by birth and replaced by downy hair, the **vellus hairs**. Vellus hairs are retained in most regions, where they are present as short, soft colorless hair such as that of the forehead. In the scalp and eyebrows, vellus hairs are replaced by coarser **terminal hair** which also forms the axillary and pubic hair, and in the male, the hair of the beard and chest. Modified hairs form the spines or quills of porcupines, hedgehogs and echidna, and a closely packed bundle of hair forms the "horn" in the rhinoceros.

Structure

KEY WORDS: shaft, medulla, cortex, cuticle, root, hair bulb, papilla

Each hair consists of a root embedded in the skin and a hair shaft projecting for a variable distance above the surface of the epidermis. In cross section, the **shaft** appears round or oval and is made up of three concentric layers. The core or **medulla** is composed of flattened, cornified, polyhedral cells in which the nuclei are shrunken or absent. Air spaces are present between the cells. A medulla is lacking in thin fine hairs (lanugo) and may be absent in some hairs of the scalp or extend only part way along the shaft. The bulk of the hair consists of the **cortex**, composed of several layers of intensely cornified, elongated cells tightly compacted together. Most of the pigment of colored hair is found in the cortex and is present in the cells and in the intercellular spaces. Variable accumulations of air spaces occur between and within the cells and, together with fading of pigment, result in graying of the hair. The outermost layer is thin and forms the **cuticle.** It contains a single layer of clear keratinized cells that overlap each other, shingle-fashion, from below upwards.

The **root** of the hair is that portion which is embedded in the skin. At the lower end, the root expands to form the **hair bulb,** which is indented at its deep surface by a conical projection of the dermis called a **papilla**. Papillae contain blood vessels that provide nourishment for the growing and differentiating cells of the hair bulb.

The structure of the hair at the root differs somewhat from that of the shaft. In the lower part of the root, the cells both of the medulla and cortex tend to be cuboidal in shape and contain nuclei of normal appearance. At higher levels in the root, the nuclei become indistinct and finally are lost. The cells of the cortex become progressively flattened toward the surface of the skin.

Hair Follicle

KEY WORDS: inner epithelial root sheath, cuticle of root sheath, Huxley's layer, trichohyalin granules, Henley's layer, outer epithelial root sheath, stratum Malpighii, glassy (vitreous) membrane

The root of each hair is enclosed within a tubular sheath called the hair follicle, which consists of an inner epithelial component and an outer connective tissue portion. The epithelial component is derived from the epidermis and consists of the inner epithelial root sheath and the outer epithelial root sheath. The connective tissue sheath is derived from the dermis.

The **inner epithelial root sheath** corresponds to the superficial layers of the epidermis that have undergone specializations to produce three layers. The innermost layer is the **cuticle of the root sheath,** which abuts the cuticle of the hair. The cells are thin, scale-like and are overlapped from above downward; the free edges of the cells interlock with the free edges of the cells of the hair cuticle. Immediately surrounding the cuticle of the root sheath are several layers of elongated cells which form **Huxley's layer**. The cells contain granules which are similar to keratohyalin granules but differ chemically and are called **trichohyalin granules**. Huxley's layer in turn is surrounded by **Henley's layer**, a row of clear, flattened cells that contain keratin fibrils. The cells of these three layers are nucleated in the deeper parts of the sheath, but as the sheath approaches the surface, the nuclei are lost.

The **outer epithelial root sheath** is a direct continuation of the **stratum Malpighii**. The outermost layer of cells are columnar, arranged in a single row and at the surface become continuous with the stratum basale of the epidermis. The inner layers of cells are identical to and continuous with the prickle cells of the stratum spinosum.

The connective tissue portion of the follicle consists of three layers. A narrow clear band, the **glassy** or **vitreous membrane,** is closely applied to the columnar cells of the outer epithelial root sheath and equates with the basement membrane. The middle layer consists of fine circular connective tissue fibers; the outermost layer is poorly defined and contains collagenous fibers arranged in loose, longitudinal bundles, interspersed with some elastic fibers.

In summary, the hair follicle consists of an outer component derived from the dermis, separated from an inner epithelial layer by the glassy membrane. The epithelial layer is a continuation of the epidermis and itself contains two layers. The outer layer of the epithelial root sheath consists of an extension of the stratum basale and stratum spinosum of the epidermis, while the inner root sheath represents a modification of the stratum granulosum and stratum corneum. The cuticle of the root sheath might be likened to the stratum disjunctum.

The bulbous expansion of the hair root surrounds the papilla and the cells of the hair bulb are not arranged in layers but form a matrix of growing cells. Matrix cells at the tip of the papilla differentiate into the medulla of the hair; those on the slopes develop into the cortex and medulla and laterally the cells of the bulb form the inner epithelial root sheath. Pigmentation of the hair results from the activity of melanocytes present in the matrix.

The structure of a hair and a hair follicle are shown in Figure 13-3.

Sebaceous Glands

KEY WORDS: alveoli, holocrine secretion, sebum

Sebaceous glands occur in most parts of the skin, are especially numerous in the scalp and face and around the mouth, nose and anus and are absent in the palms of the hand and soles of the feet. Generally the sebaceous glands are associated with hairs and drain into the upper part of the hair follicle, but in the lip, glans penis, inner surface of the prepuce and on the labia minora, the glands open directly onto the surface of the skin without relationship to hairs. The glands vary in size and consist of a cluster of two to five oval **alveoli** drained by a single duct.

The secretory portion (alveolus) lies within the dermis and is composed of epi-

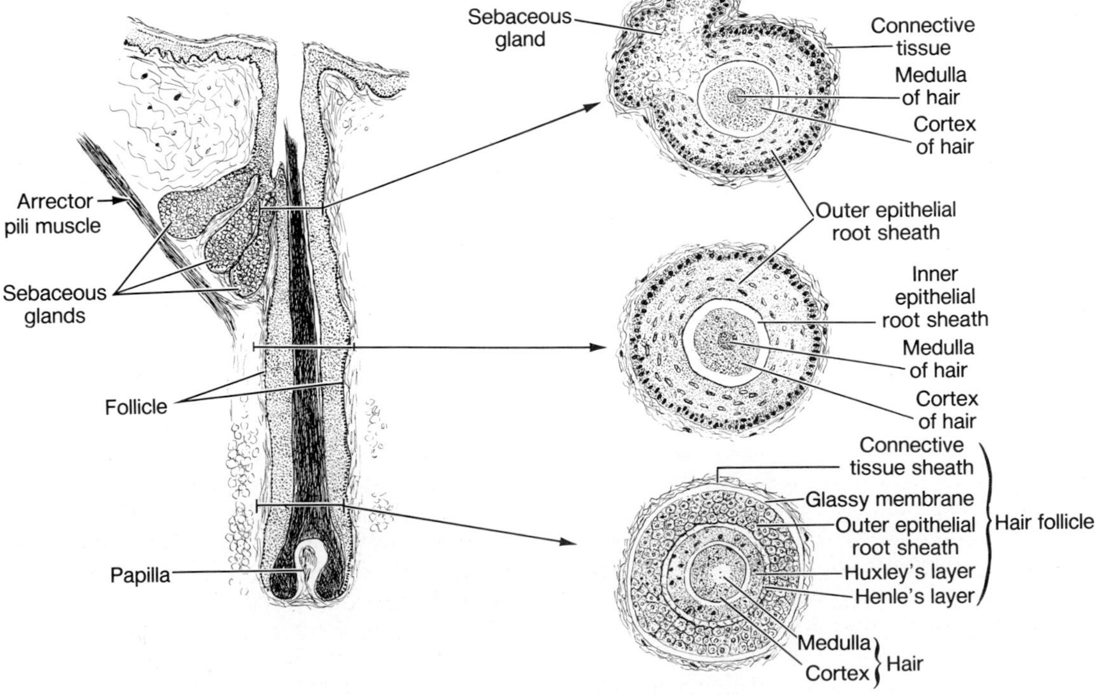

Figure 13-3. Structure of a hair and hair follicle.

thelial cells enclosed in a basement membrane and supported by a thin connective tissue capsule. The cells abutting the basement membrane are small, cuboidal and contain rounded nuclei. The entire alveolus is filled with cells which centrally become larger and polyhedral and gradually accumulate a fatty material. The nuclei become compressed, shrunken and finally disappear. **Secretion** is of the **holocrine** type, in which the entire cell breaks down and the cell debris, along with the secretion product, is released as the **sebum**.

The duct is lined by stratified squamous epithelium that is a continuation of the outer epithelial root sheath of the hair follicle. Replacement of the secretory cells of the alveolus is by division of cells close to the walls of ducts near their junctions with the alveoli and from cells at the periphery of the alveoli.

Sweat Glands

KEY WORDS: eccrine sweat glands, simple tubular, coiled, dark cells, clear cells, myoepithelial cells, apocrine sweat glands, ceruminous glands

Two classes of sweat glands are distinguished; ordinary sweat or eccrine glands and apocrine glands such as those of the axilla and circumanal region.

Eccrine sweat glands are distributed throughout the skin, except at the lip margins, glans penis, inner surface of the prepuce, clitoris and labia minor. Elsewhere the numbers vary, being plentiful in the palms and soles and least numerous in the neck and back. Each gland is a **simple tubular** structure, the deep part of which is tightly **coiled** and forms the secretory part located in the dermis. The secretory portion consists of a simple epithelium resting on a thick basement membrane. Two types of cells, the clear cells and the dark cells, are present. The **dark cells** are narrow at their bases and broad at the luminal surface; in electron micrographs they contain numerous ribosomes, secretory vacuoles and few mitochondria. These cells secrete protein-polysaccharides which have been identified in the secretory vacuoles.

The **clear cells** are broad at their bases and narrow at the apex. Intercellular canaliculi are present and extend between adjacent clear cells. They contain abundant glycogen, considerable smooth endoplasmic reticulum, numerous mitochondria, but few ribosomes. The plasmalemma at the base of the cell shows extensive, complex infoldings. The clear cells appear to secrete sodium chloride, urea, uric acid, ammonia and water.

Myoepithelial cells are present in the secretory portion, located between the basal lamina and the bases of the secretory cells. These stellate cells are contractile and are believed to aid in the discharge of secretion.

The secretory portion of the gland empties into a narrowed duct which at first is coiled, then straightens as it passes through the dermis to reach the epidermis. The lining consists of two layers of cuboidal cells. At their luminal surfaces, the cells of the inner layer show an aggregation of filaments that are organized into a terminal web. The epithelium lies on a basal lamina, but myoepithelial cells are lacking. In the epidermis, the duct consists of a spiral channel which is simply a cleft between the epidermal cells; those cells immediately adjacent to the duct are concentrically arranged.

The **apocrine glands** of the axilla, circumanal regions, areola of the nipple, labia majora and eyelids are enlarged, specialized sweat glands. Their secretions are thicker than those of the ordinary sweat glands and their histological appearance also differs in several respects. The apocrine glands also are coiled tubes but are wider, the myoepithelial cells are larger and more numerous and there is only a single type of secreting cell, which resembles the dark cells of the eccrine sweat glands. The ducts are similar in structure to those of the ordinary sweat glands but empty into a hair follicle rather than through the epidermis. The **ceruminous** (wax) **glands** of the external auditory canal are of the apocrine type: the secretory portions branch, as may the ducts. Glands in the margin of the eyelid (Moll's glands) also are apocrine glands and differ in that the terminal portions show less coiling and wider lumina. Secretion by the apocrine glands is of the merocrine type and involves no loss of cell structure; although retained, the term apocrine is misapplied.

DEVELOPMENT OF SKIN

The skin has a dual origin, the epidermis and its appendages arising from ectoderm, while the dermis is formed from mesoderm. Initially, the epidermis consists of a single layer of cuboidal cells resting on a basal lamina. Only a few desmosomes unite the loosely-arranged cells. With proliferation, the cells become organized into two layers—an outer periderm of flattened cells and a basal layer of cuboidal to columnar cells. The basal layer forms the stratum germinativum from which all the epidermis will develop. As the cells of stratum germinativum multiply, successive layers of cells come to lie between the periderm and the basal layer. The periderm forms a temporary protective layer and is lost just before birth, by which time the epidermis presents all the layers seen in adult skin. Meanwhile, cells have migrated from the neural crest and have taken residence in the basal layer of the epidermis as melanocytes. The Langerhans cells of the epidermis are of mesenchymal origin, possibly arising in the bone marrow.

Dermis develops from a condensation of adjacent mesenchyme. The cells differentiate and fibroblasts appear which begin to lay down collagen and elastic fibers. The dermis soon is well-defined and organized into reticular and papillary layers. Initially, the dermoepidermal junction is smooth but dermal ridges soon appear and in the human, can be identified by the 4th month of gestation.

All of the epidermal appendages (hairs, nails, feathers, quills, sweat glands, sebaceous glands, etc.) arise as outgrowths of the primitive epidermis. Hairs arise from solid cords or cylinders of epidermis (hair buds) that grow into the dermis at an angle. Each hair bud has an outer layer of columnar cells and an inner core of polygonal cells. The deepest part of the hair bud swells to form the hair bulb, which comes to sit, cup-like, over a small mound of mesenchyme that forms the papilla of the hair. The primitive dermal connective tissue along the length of the hair bud condenses to form the connective tissue component of the hair follicle. The cells at the periphery of the hair bud give rise to the epidermal portions of the outer root sheath, while the inner cell mass forms the substance of the hair.

Sebaceous glands are derived from thickenings of the outer root sheath. Solid buds of cells grow down into the surrounding mesenchyme, branching into several flask-shaped alveoli. The lining cells (derived from stratum germinativum) proliferate, pushing older cells towards the center, where they degenerate to form the sebum. A cellular bulge on the root sheath, below the origin of the sebaceous glands, provides for the attachment of the arrectores pilorum, which arise independently from mesenchyme.

Sweat glands also begin as solid downgrowths of the epidermis. As these elongate, their deeper parts become coiled to form the secretory portions of the glands. A lumen develops in each epithelial cord, which now form tubes opening onto the surface and lined by a double layer of epithelium. Myoepithelial cells associated with the secretory portions of the glands arise locally from the same epidermal bud. Some sweat glands develop from superficial epidermal swellings on hair follicles; their ducts empty into the uppermost part of the follicle.

FUNCTIONAL SUMMARY

The outer horny layers of the epidermis are highly impermeable to water and are rather inert chemically. It is this portion of the epidermis which acts as the chief barrier to mechanical damage, dessication and invasion by bacteria. Membrane-coating granules may contribute to or constitute the primary, intercellular barrier to water. The epidermis has a high capacity for self-renewal, the

new cells being derived mainly from the stratum basale. The main function of melanin is to protect the germinal layer from the effects of ultraviolet irradiation. It has been suggested that melanin may capture harmful free radicals generated in the epidermis by ultraviolet light. Accumulation of melanin above the nuclei of the basal cells affords maximum protection from incoming irradiation. Poorly melanized skin is more subject to sunburn, skin cancer and degenerative changes following chronic exposure to sunlight than is darker skin.

The dermis provides considerable mechanical strength due to the high content of collagen and elastic fibers. The vascular supply of the skin is contained wholly within the dermis and the epidermis is nourished by diffusion from the underlying vascular bed. The area of contact between dermis and epidermis is increased by the dermal papillae, which facilitate the exchange of nutrients from the capillaries in the papillary layer of the dermis.

In furred animals, hairs serve as insulating material and function in temperature regulation by minimizing heat loss. The erection of hair by the arrectores pilorum muscles contributes to thermal insulation by permitting the incorporation of an air blanket in the fur. In man, hair contributes little to this function, which is served mainly by the subcutaneous fat and the greater thickness of the epidermis, which is a relatively poor conductor of heat. Hairs in man are largely concerned with cutaneous sensations of touch. Each hair follicle is elaborately innervated and some of the nerve endings are associated with tactile disks of the Merkel type. In some mammals tylotrich hairs (the so-called "feelers") are present in specialized patches of epithelium of the face. The nerve endings associated with these hairs show especially rapid conduction of impulses.

Man, equine species and some Bovidae regulate their body temperature by the evaporation of sweat, which contains about 98% water. Dogs cannot sweat; eccrine sweat glands are restricted to the pads of the paw, and the temperature regulation is brought about by panting. Some lizards have a highly developed panting mechanism and their extremely vascular tongues can be extended well outside the body to act as an effective heat exchange mechanism. Birds also lack sweat glands and have the most effective panting mechanism of all animals. Regulation of temperature by panting depends upon respiratory heat loss and the evaporation of salivary secretions. The copious saliva produced by the opossum has been implicated in thermoregulation.

The sebum from sebaceous glands acts as a lubricant for the skin, protects it from drying and aids in "waterproofing" the skin. It also has some slight antibacterial activity, but the effect appears to be insignificant. The preen glands of aquatic birds provides an oily secretion which, when spread over the feathers, makes them impervious to water.

Nails not only have a protective function but also serve as rigid bases for the support of the pads at the ends of the digits and, thus, may have a role in tactile mechanisms.

Atlas and Table of Key Features for Chapter 13

Table 13.1
Key Histological Features of Thick and Thin Skin

	Epidermis	Dermis	Other
Thick skin	Shows five layers: stratum corneum, stratum lucidum, stratum granulosum, stratum spinosum and stratum germinativum	Papillary and reticular layers very thick	Only on palms of hand, soles of feet; contains eccrine sweat glands, the only glands present in thick skin.
Thin skin	Lacks stratum lucidum; stratum corneum, stratum granulosum and stratum spinosum are more thin	As for thick skin, depth varies with area; thick dermis in skin between scapulae; delicate dermis over eyelids, scrotum, penis; thinner on anterior surface of body than on posterior surface	Contains hair follicles, eccrine sweat and sebaceous gland; apocrine sweat glands in axilla and groin

13-4 Integument—Epidermis

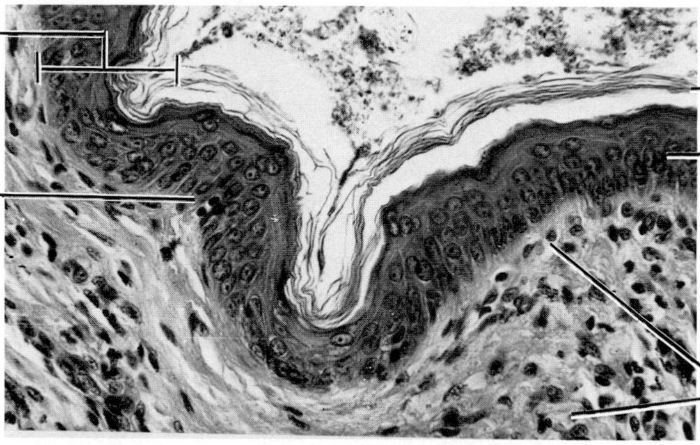

13-5

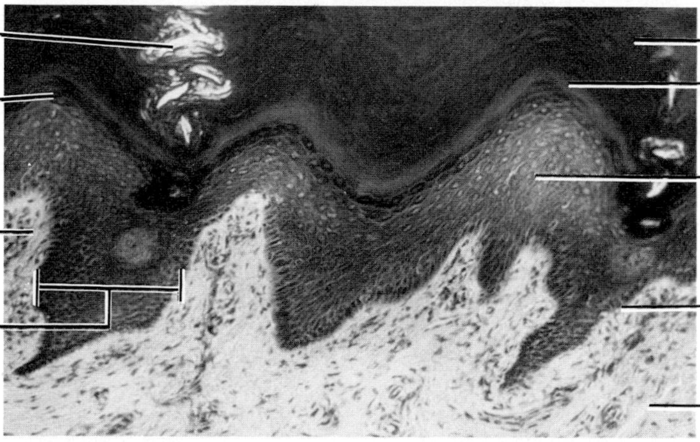

13-6

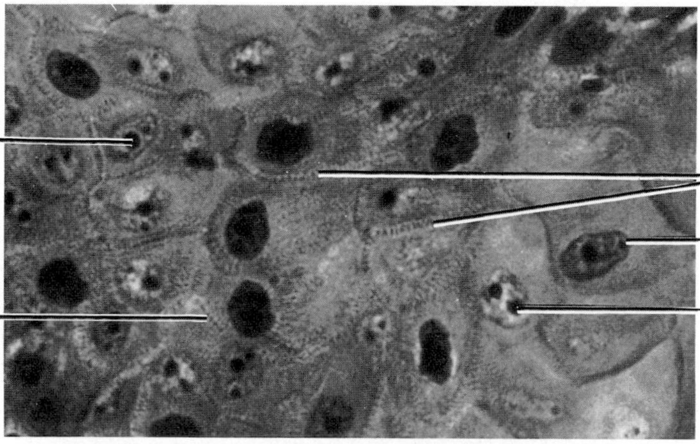

Figure 13-4. Thin skin (human). LM, ×250.
Figure 13-5. Thick skin (human). LM, ×100.
Figure 13-6. Cells of stratum spinosum. LM, ×1000.

13-7

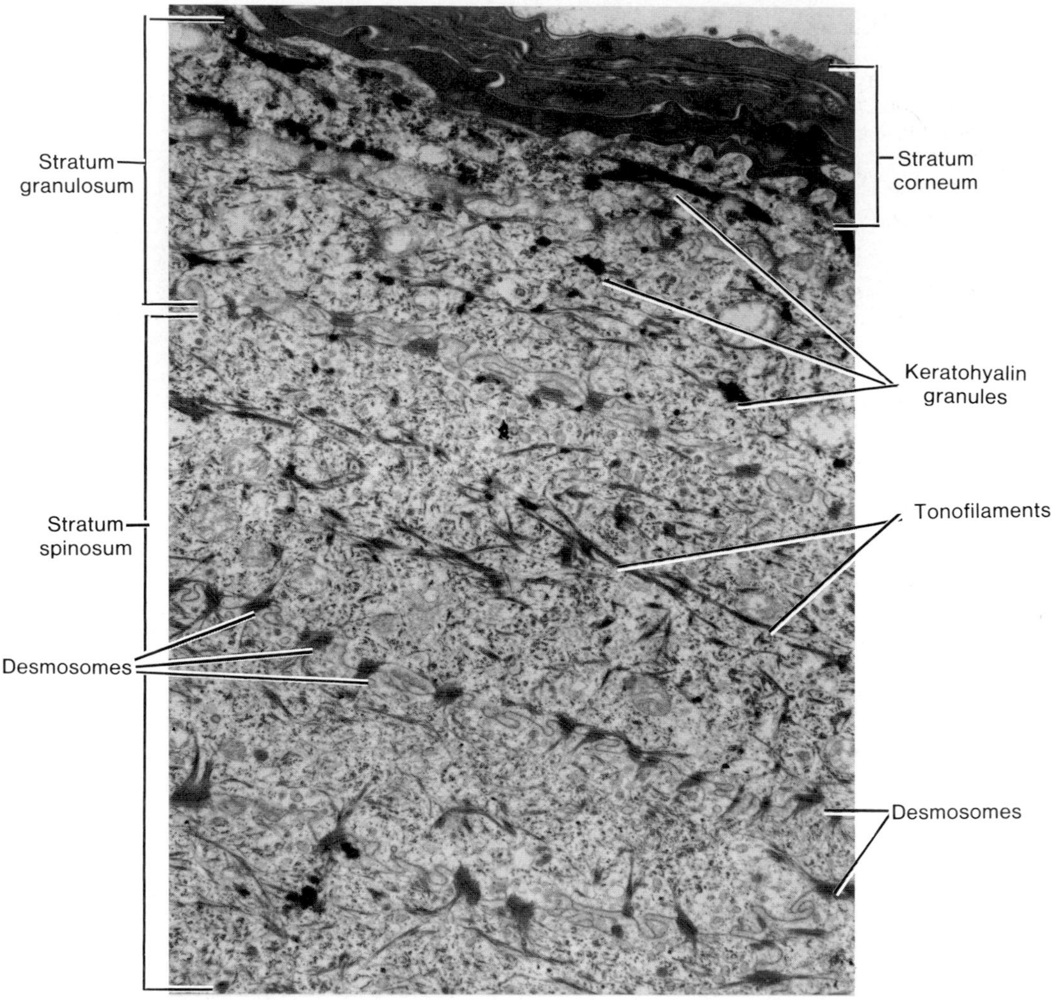

13-8

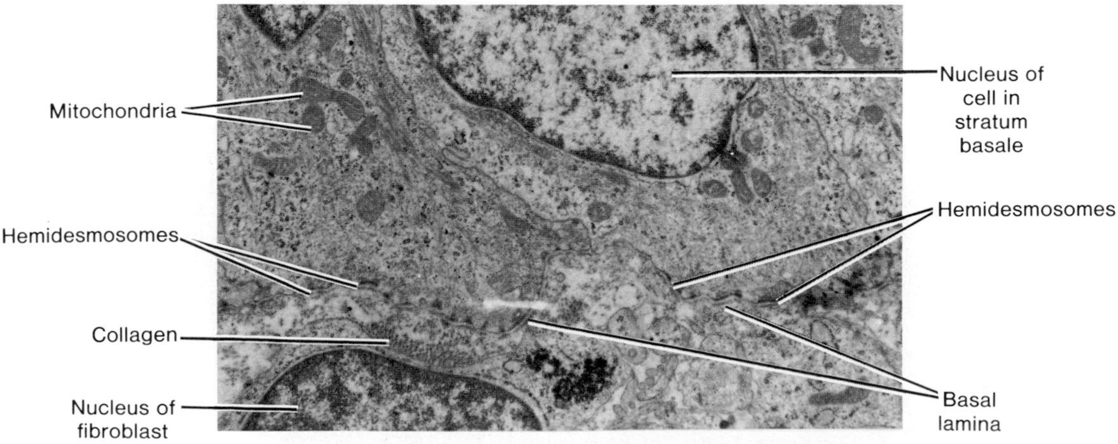

Figure 13-7. Epidermis (thin skin). TEM, ×8000.
Figure 13-8. Interface of epidermis and dermis. TEM, ×7000.

13-9

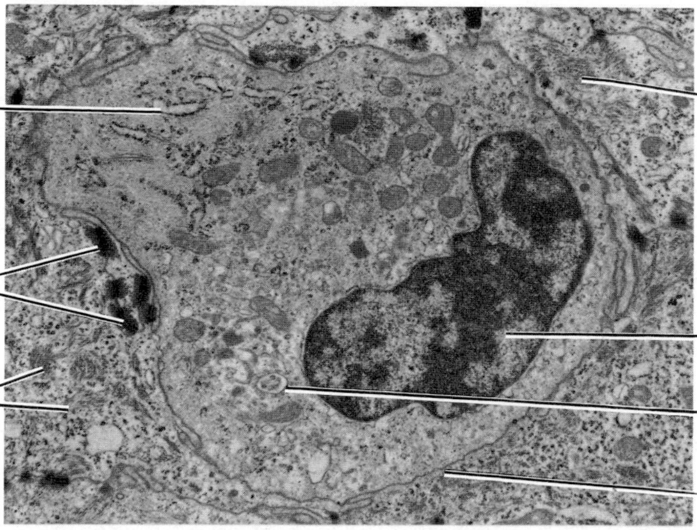

13-10

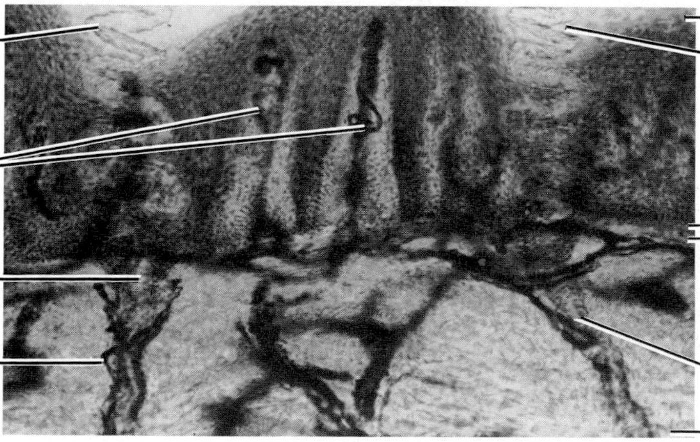

13-11

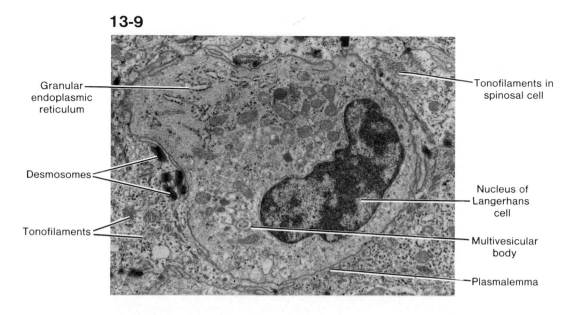

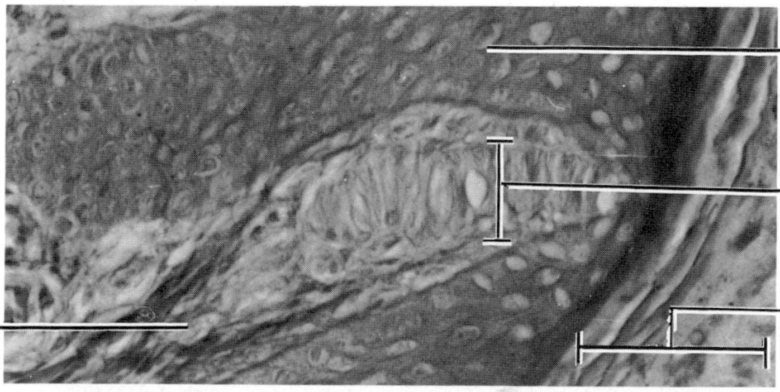

Figure 13-9. Cell of Langerhans (epidermis). TEM, ×10,000.
Figure 13-10. Thick skin (human). LM, ×100.
Figure 13-11. Meissner's corpuscle. LM, ×400.

13-12 Hair

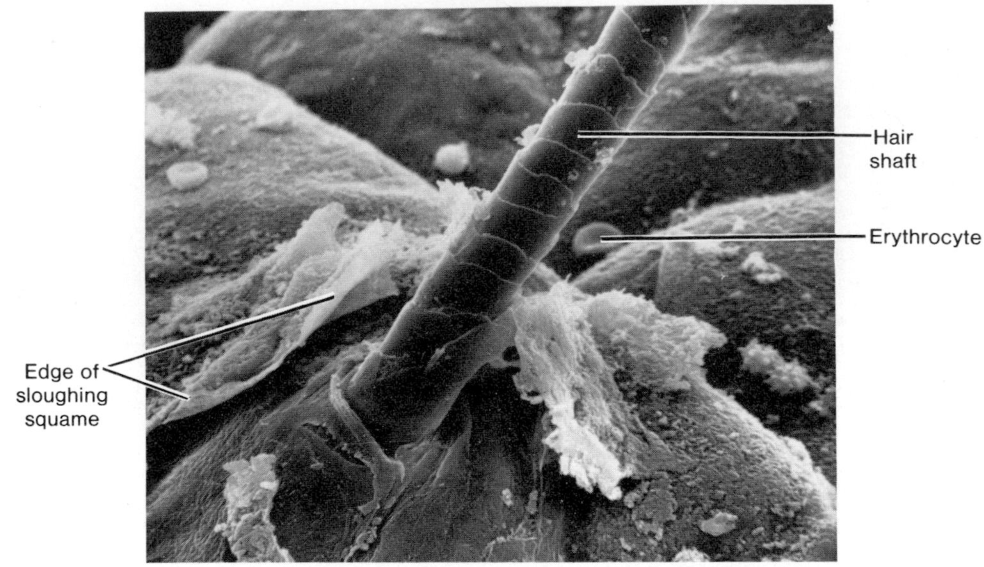

13-13

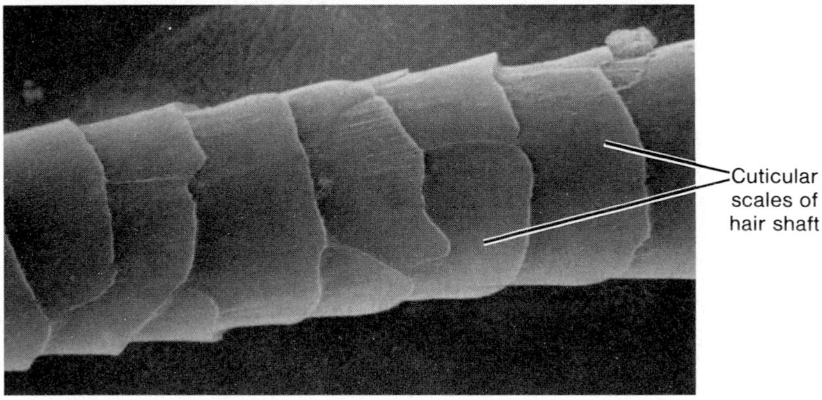

13-14

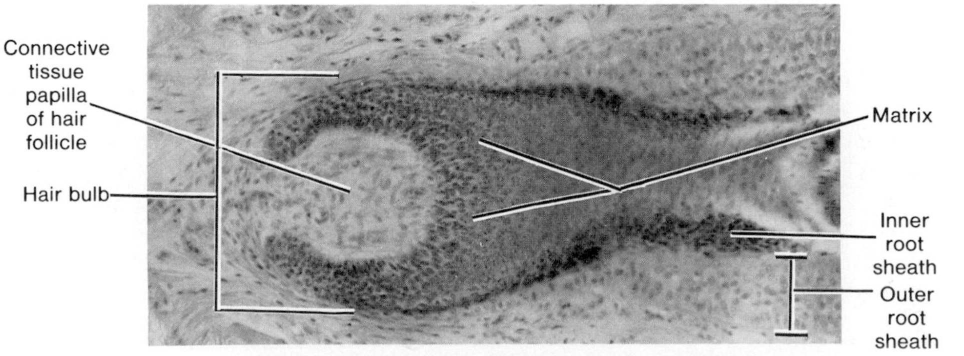

Figure 13-12. Hair shaft (epidermis). SEM, ×1000.
Figure 13-13. Hair shaft. SEM, ×2000.
Figure 13-14. Hair follicle. LM, ×100.

13-15 Glands

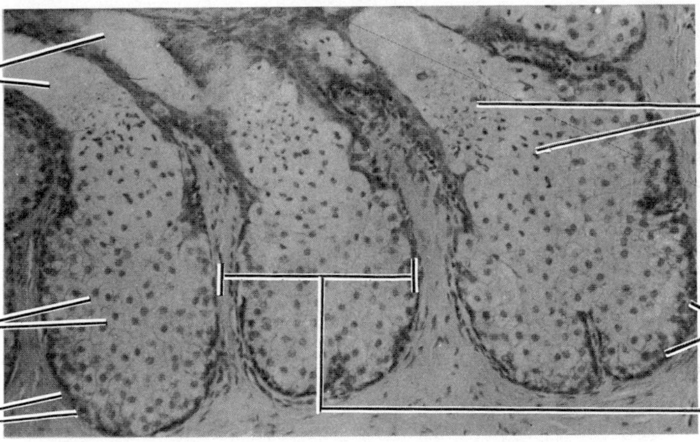

13-16

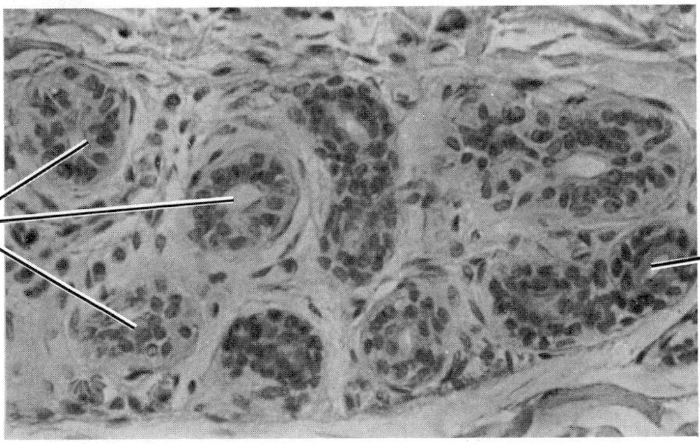

13-17

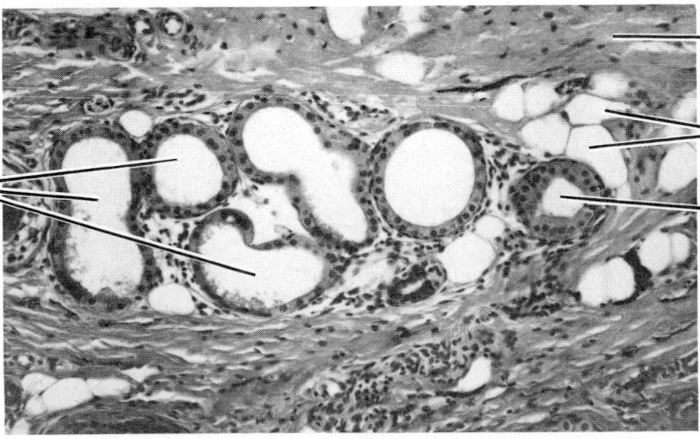

Figure 13-15. Sebaceous gland (human). LM, ×100.
Figure 13-16. Eccrine sweat gland (human). LM, ×250.
Figure 13-17. Apocrine sweat gland (human). LM, ×100.

13–18

Development

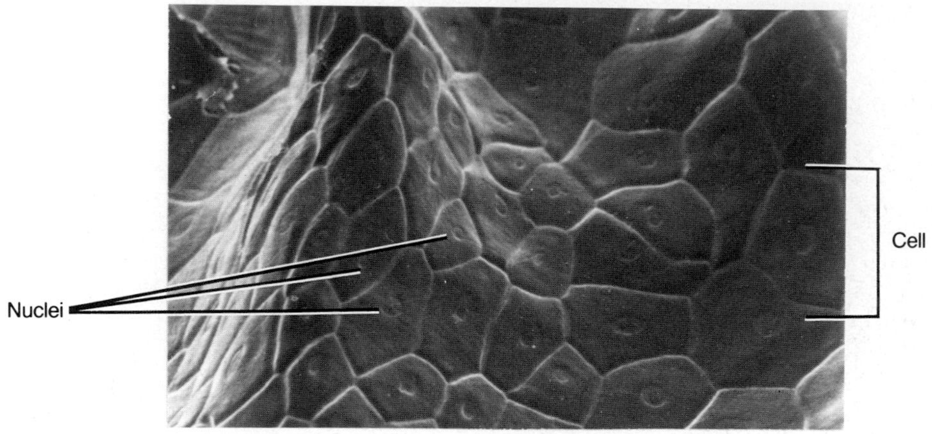

13–19

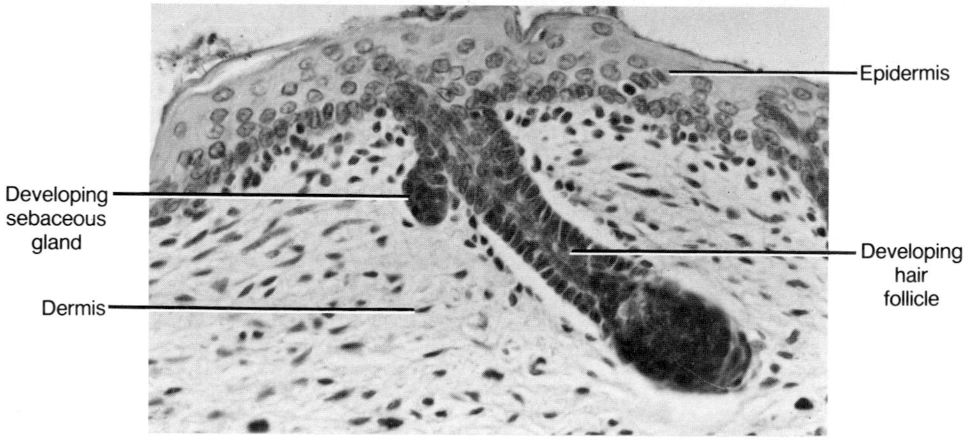

13–20

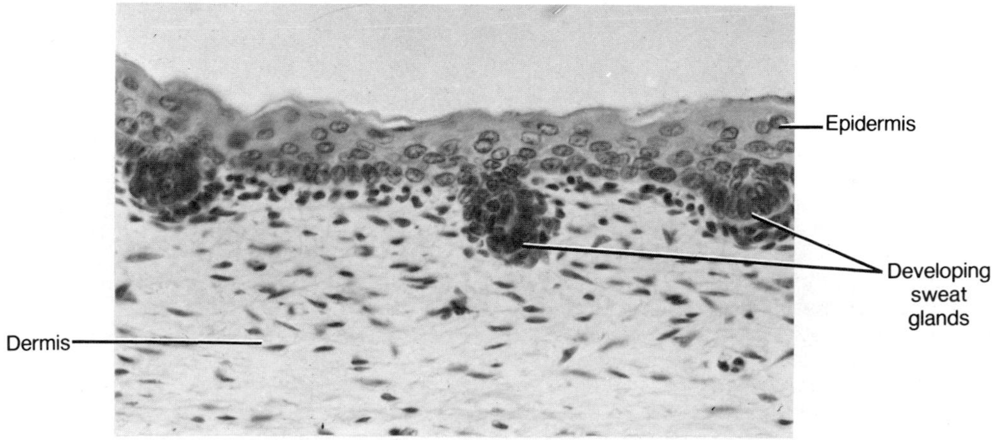

Figure 13-18. Periderm. SEM, ×300.
Figure 13-19. Hair follicle. LM, ×250.
Figure 13-20. Sweat glands. LM, × 250.

14

Respiratory System

The respiratory tract consists of two major parts—a respiratory portion and a conducting portion. Respiratory tissue, located within the lungs, is that part of the tract where the actual exchange of gases occurs between air and blood and is characterized by the close relationship of capillary blood and air chambers. The conducting portion delivers air to the respiratory tissue, and its walls are relatively rigid in order to keep the airways open. This part of the respiratory tract consists of the nose (or nasal cavities), pharynx, larynx, trachea and various subdivisions and branchings of the bronchial tree. Parts of the conducting system are present within the lungs (intrapulmonary), while the remainder are outside the lungs (extrapulmonary).

NOSE

KEY WORDS: pseudostratified ciliated columnar epithelium, goblet cells, olfactory epithelium, lamina propria, venous sinuses, mucoperiosteum, mucoperichondrium

The skin that covers the external surface of the nose extends for a short distance into the vestibule of the nose. Here, stiff hairs with their associated sebaceous glands aid in filtering the inspired air. More posteriorly, the vestibule is lined by nonkeratinized stratified squamous epithelium. Throughout most of the remainder of the nasal cavity, the respiratory passage is lined by a **pseudostratified ciliated columnar epithelium** that contains **goblet cells**, but a specialized **olfactory epithelium** is present in the roof of the nasal cavities.

A layer of connective tissue, the **lamina propria**, underlies the epithelium and is separated from it by a basement membrane. Contained within the lamina propria are mucous glands, serous glands and thin walled **venous sinuses.** The latter are especially prominent in the lamina propria that covers the middle and inferior conchae and serve to warm the inspired air. Lymphatic tissue is present also and becomes prominent near the nasopharynx. The deep layers of the lamina propria fuse with the periosteum or perichondrium of the nasal bones and cartilages and at these sites, the nasal mucosa has been called a **mucoperiosteum** or **mucoperichondrium**, respectively.

The surface of the epithelial lining is

bathed by a film of mucus that is constantly moved toward the pharynx by the action of the ciliated epithelial cells. The mucus is derived from the surface goblet cells but the secretions from the glands within the lamina propria also contribute. The layer of mucus serves to moisten the air and to trap particulate matter. The same type of mucosal covering extends into the paranasal sinuses, but here the epithelium is thinner; there are fewer goblet cells and the lamina propria is thinner and contains fewer glands. Venous sinuses are absent.

Olfactory Epithelium

KEY WORDS: pseudostratified columnar, supporting (sustentacular) cells, olfactory cells, bipolar nerve cells, olfactory vesicle (olfactory knob), olfactory hairs, fila olfactoria, olfactory glands, basal cells

Olfactory epithelium (Fig. 14-1) occurs in the roof of the nasal cavities, where it extends over the superior conchae and for a short distance on either side of the nasal septum. This epithelium also is a **pseudostratified columnar** type, but it lacks goblet cells and is much thicker than the respiratory lining epithelium. Three cell types are present: supporting or sustentacular cells, basal cells and the sensory or olfactory cells.

Supporting (sustentacular) cells are tall with narrow bases and their broad apical surfaces bear long slender microvilli. An oval nucleus is located just above the center of the cell. Beneath the free apical surface, a well developed junctional complex attaches the supporting cells to adjacent olfactory cells.

The **olfactory cells** are the sensory component and are **bipolar nerve cells** evenly distributed among the supporting cells. The cells are spindle-shaped with rounded nuclei located centrally in an expanded area of cytoplasm. Apically, the cell tapers to a single slender process (a modified dendrite) that extends to the surface between the supporting cells, where it expands into a bulb-like **olfactory vesicle**, or **olfactory knob**. Six to eight long **olfactory hairs** extend from the olfactory vesicle and pass parallel to the surface of the epithelium, embedded in a film of fluid. The processes are modified, nonmotile cilia and appear to be the excitable component of the sense organ. For a short distance from their origin, the processes have a typical ciliary structure but then narrow abruptly. At the same time, the microtubules change from doublets to singlets and decrease in number. Basally, the olfactory cell narrows to a thin process, an axon, that passes into the lamina propria where, with similar fibers, it forms small nerve bundles. These collect into the **fila olfactoria,** which ultimately pass to the olfactory bulb of the brain. Also present in the lamina propria are a rich plexus of blood vessels and branched, serous, tubuloalveolar glands. These are the **olfactory glands,** the watery secretion from which serves both to flush the surface of the olfactory epithelium to prevent continuous stimulation by a single odor and as a solvent for odorous materials.

Basal cells are short, pyramidal cells crowded between the bases of sustentacular and olfactory cells. These are undifferentiated cells, capable of giving rise to either of the other two types of cells.

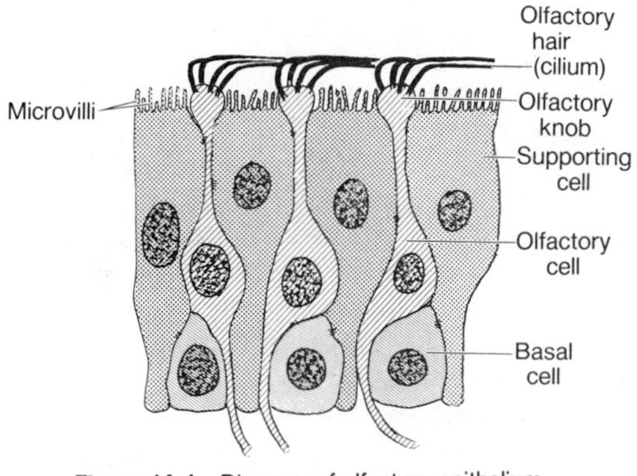

Figure 14-1 Diagram of olfactory epithelium.

PHARYNX AND LARYNX

KEY WORDS: nasopharynx, pseudostratified ciliated columnar epithelium, goblet cells, stratified squamous (nonkeratinized), oropharynx, laryngopharynx, tonsils

The nasal cavities continue posteriorly into the pharynx, which has nasal, oral and laryngeal parts. The most superior part, the **nasopharynx**, is directly continuous with the nasal cavities and is lined by the same respiratory passage epithelium, i.e., **pseudostratified ciliated columnar epithelium** with **goblet cells**. In areas subjected to abrasion, a **nonkeratinizing stratified squamous epithelium** may occur. This type of epithelium is found on the edge of the soft palate and the posterior wall of the nasopharynx, where these surfaces make contact during swallowing and throughout the **oro-** and **laryngopharynx**. The underlying connective tissue contains mucous, serous and mixed mucoserous glands and abundant lymphatic tissue. The latter is irregularly scattered throughout the connective tissue and also forms **tonsillar** structures; these are the pharyngeal tonsils (or adenoids) in the posterior wall of the nasopharynx, the tubal tonsils around the openings of the Eustachian tubes into the nasopharynx and the palatine and lingual tonsils at the junction of the oral cavity and oropharynx.

The larynx connects the pharynx with the trachea. Its framework consists of several cartilages, of which the thyroid, cricoid and arytenoid are hyaline, while the epiglottis, corniculate and tips of the arytenoid cartilages are of the elastic type. This scaffold of cartilages is held together and to the hyoid bone by sheets of dense connective tissue which form the cricothyroid and thyroid membranes. The lining epithelium varies with location. The anterior surface and about one-half of the posterior surface of the epiglottis are covered by stratified squamous, nonkeratinizing epithelium, as are the vocal cords. Elsewhere the larynx is lined by the typical respiratory passage type of epithelium. The epithelium of the epiglottis may contain a few taste buds. The lamina propria of the larynx is thick and contains mucous and some serous or mucoserous glands.

TRACHEA AND EXTRAPULMONARY BRONCHI

KEY WORDS: hyaline cartilage rings, smooth muscle, pseudostratified ciliated columnar cells, goblet cells, brush cells, small granule cells, short cells, adventitia

The trachea and its terminal branches (the primary bronchi) are characterized by the presence of a series of C-shaped **hyaline cartilages** in their walls and these maintain patency of the airway. The spaces between the successive rings are filled with fibroelastic connective tissue and the gaps between the arms of the cartilages are filled with bundles of **smooth muscle**. The gaps are directed posteriorly, and in section the trachea and extrapulmonary bronchi appear flattened at this aspect. The lining consists of a **pseudostratified ciliated columnar epithelium** with **goblet cells**, which rests on a thick basal lamina. Cilia beat toward the pharynx.

In addition to the ciliated and goblet cells, several other cell types have been described in the tracheobronchial epithelium. **Brush cells** contain glycogen granules, show long straight microvilli on their apical surfaces and, basally, make contact with nerve processes. **Small granule cells** are few and scattered. They appear to be part of the diffuse endocrine population of cells, able to take up and store amines and amine precursors. In the depths of the epithelium between the bases of the other cell types are the **short cells.** These are undifferentiated cells that can give rise to goblet and ciliated cells. The lamina propria contains many small seromucous glands and occasional accumulations of lymphatic tissue. External to the cartilage is a fibroconnective tissue coat, the **adventitia**, which contains elastic, collagen and reticular fibers, blood vessels and nerves.

INTRAPULMONARY AIR PASSAGES

KEY WORDS: intrapulmonary bronchi, cartilaginous plates, pseudostratified ciliated columnar, goblet cells, submucosa, simple ciliated columnar, bronchiole, ciliated cuboidal, terminal bronchioles, Clara cells, surfactant

The primary bronchi divide further to give several orders of **intrapulmonary bronchi.** The C-shaped cartilages are replaced by irregular **plates of hyaline cartilage** that completely surround the bronchi. The intrapulmonary bronchi thus are cylindrical and not flattened at one side as are the trachea and extrapulmonary bronchi. Internally the intrapulmonary bronchi are lined by a mucous membrane that is continuous with and identical to that of the trachea and primary bronchi, again, **pseudostratified ciliated columnar** epithelium with **goblet cells**. The underlying lamina propria contains some diffuse lymphatic tissue and is separated from the epithelium by a prominent basal lamina. Beneath the lamina propria, a sheet of irregularly arranged smooth muscle fibers course around the bronchus as open left-handed or righthanded spirals. This muscle layer separates the lamina propria from the fibroconnective tissue of the **submucosa** which lies immediately internal to the cartilages. Mucous and mucoserous glands are present in the submucosa, their ducts penetrating the muscle layer to open onto the epithelial surface. With successive divisions, the intrapulmonary bronchi progressively decrease in size and although they retain the basic structure as outlined above, the layers of their walls become thinner. The smallest bronchi contain isolated cartilage plates and are no longer completely surrounded by cartilage. The epithelium is reduced to **simple ciliated columnar** with **goblet cells**. Mucous and mucoserous glands are present along the bronchial tree as far down as cartilage extends.

When the diameter of the tube reaches about 1 mm, cartilage disappears from the walls and the structure is called a **bronchiole**. Glands and lymphatic tissue also disappear but smooth muscle is relatively prominent. The lining epithelium varies from ciliated columnar with goblet cells in the larger bronchioles to **ciliated cuboidal** with no goblet cells in the **terminal bronchioles**. The latter are the smallest branches of the conducting system. Scattered among the ciliated cells are a few nonciliated cells whose apical surfaces bulge into the lumen and bear a few microvilli. These are the **Clara cells**, also called bronchiolar secretory cells, which are presumed to secrete **surfactant**, a phospholipid that alters the surface tension of the fluid layer over the surface.

RESPIRATORY TISSUE

KEY WORDS: respiratory bronchiole, alveolar duct, alveolar sacs, alveoli, interalveolar septum, alveolar pores, blood-air barrier, pulmonary epithelial cells (pneumonocytes type I), septal cells (pneumonocytes type II), multilamellar bodies, alveolar macrophages

Exchange of gases between air and blood occurs only where these are in close relation. Such a condition is seen first in the **respiratory bronchioles** which form a transition between the conducting and respiratory parts of the respiratory tract. The walls of respiratory bronchioles consist of collagenous connective tissue in which interlacing bundles of smooth muscle and elastic fibers are present. The larger respiratory bronchioles are lined by simple cuboidal epithelium with only a few ciliated cells, and goblet cells are lacking. Many of the cuboidal cells are Clara cells. In the smaller bronchioles, the epithelium becomes low cuboidal without cilia. Budding out from the walls of the respiratory bronchioles are alveoli which represent the respiratory portion of these bronchioles and which become more numerous distally. Respiratory bronchioles end by branching into alveolar ducts.

Alveolar ducts are thin-walled tubes from which numerous alveoli or clusters of alveoli open around the circumference and the wall becomes little more than a succession of openings into alveoli. Appearances of a conduit persist only in the few places where small groups of cuboidal cells intervene between successive alveoli and cover underlying bundles of fibroelastic tissue and smooth muscle. The alveolar ducts terminate in irregular spaces surrounded by alveoli, the clusters of alveoli being termed **alveolar sacs**.

Alveoli are thin walled, polyhedral structures open at one side to permit diffusion of air into their cavities. Adjacent alveoli are separated by a common **interalveolar septum**. The most conspicuous feature of the septum is a rich network of capillaries that bulge the septal wall so that most of the capillary surface is exposed to alveolar air. Reticular and elastic fibers form a tenuous framework for the septa. Small openings in the septal wall, the **alveolar pores**, permit communication and equalization of air pressure between alveoli. On each side, the alveolar wall is covered by an attenuated epithelial lining, beneath which is a basal lamina. In many areas the epithelial basal lamina is separated from that of the capillary endothelium by a space of only 15 to 20 nm. In other regions the two basal laminae are fused. Thus, at its thinnest the **blood-air barrier** consists of the attenuated epithelium of the alveolar lining cell, the fused basal laminae and the endothelial cells of the capillaries within the septal wall.

Several cell types are present in the interalveolar septa. The thin attenuated squamous cells that form a continuous lining for the alveolar wall have been called **pulmonary epithelial cells** or **type I pneumonocytes**. In addition to these are the septal cells, the alveolar phagocytes and the endothelial cells that line the blood capillaries. **Septal cells (type II pneumonocytes)** are rounded or cuboidal and may lie deep to the surface or bulge into the alveolar lumen between the pulmonary epithelial cells. They possess short microvilli on their free surfaces and form junctional complexes with the surface epithelial cells. The most distinctive feature of the septal cells in electron micrographs is the presence of **multilamellar bodies** in their cytoplasm. These consist of thin concentric lamellae and are rich in phospholipid and are thought to be the storage sites of surfactant.

Macrophages are present both within the interalveolar septa and the alveolar lumen. Many contain particles of inhaled dust and have been called "dust cells." Although there still is some disagreement as to the origin of the alveolar phagocytes, the evidence favors an origin from the blood monocytes. The bulk of these cells ultimately are eliminated via the air passages and appear in the sputum; a few may migrate into lymphatics and leave the lungs by this route.

PLEURA

The pleura consists of a thin membrane made up of a layer of collagenous and elastic fibers covered by a single layer of mesothelial cells. The layer lining the wall of the thoracic cavity is the parietal pleura, which reflects from the thoracic walls to cover the surface of the lungs as the visceral pleura. The pleura secretes a small amount of fluid between its two layers to permit friction-free movement.

DEVELOPMENT OF RESPIRATORY SYSTEM

The rudiments of the respiratory passages appear first as endodermal buds (the laryngotracheal groove) in the ventral wall of the pharynx. The groove deepens and its edges fuse to form a tube which gives rise to two distal outgrowths, the lung buds. From these the primary bronchi and lungs eventually develop. The endodermal epithelium of the lung rudiments provides the lining of the respiratory tract while the mesenchyme that covers it develops into the smooth muscle, cartilage, connective tissue and blood vessels of the supporting wall. The lung buds divide and ramify to give the finer divisions of the respiratory tree, ultimately ending in small expansions or infundibula. The minute pouches that develop on the infundibulae become the definitive alveoli.

Throughout their development, the lungs undergo considerable change in appearance and, histologically, three phases can be recognized. The first or glandular phase, is concerned mainly with development of the branching air passages brought about by repeated divisions of the endodermal tube. The tubes are lined by undifferentiated columnar cells that have few organelles but are rich in glycogen. From these develop all of the lining cells of the respiratory tract and the associated glands. The first differentiated cells to appear are globlet and ciliated cells of the trachea and main bronchi. The developing tubes lie in a bed of mesenchyme and at this stage the lung bud has a gland-like appearance. The canalicular phase is marked by rapid growth of the tubular elements to provide the finer twigs of the respiratory tree, and by delineation of the respiratory parts. The terminal buds (infundibula) are less spherical and become intimately related to capillary networks. The cuboidal cells that line the distal airways begin to flatten, denoting the third or alveolar phase. The distal buds become stretched; their epithelium flattens; and thin-walled pockets, the first alveoli, pouch out from the buds. Some distention of alveoli occurs prior to birth, but their full expansion takes place with the onset of respiration.

FUNCTIONAL SUMMARY

The stiff hairs in the vestibule of the nose are believed to help in excluding particulate matter in the inspired air from reaching the remainder of the respiratory passages. Mucus secreted by the goblet cells of the respiratory lining and by the glandular elements in the nose and conducting tubular portion provides a blanket of moisture which aids in trapping particles and preventing drying of the mucosal surface. The secretions also humidify the air as it passes along the conducting passages. The beat of the cilia moves the blanket of fluid toward the mouth, both in the nose and in the lower respiratory passages. The large venous plexuses in the nasal cavity warm the inspired air.

In several species, including man, periodic engorgement of the plexus occurs, alternating on either side of the nasal cavity. This results in a temporary obstruction to air flow on the one side, allowing the mucosa to recover from the drying effects of air. In man the periods of occlusion occur approximately hourly.

The olfactory epithelium serves for the sense of smell, the sensory component being the olfactory cells. The olfactory hairs borne by these cells are nonmotile cilia and are believed to be the excitable element of the sense organ. Glands in this area secrete a watery fluid which serves as a solvent for odorous materials and also flushes the olfactory epithelium to prevent continuous stimulation by a single odor.

Patency of the conducting portions, from the trachea to the smallest intrapulmonary bronchus, is maintained by the cartilage that is present in the walls. In the trachea and main bronchi, the fibroelastic tissue between the cartilages gives pliability and longitudinal extensibility to these structures. This is essential for the accommodations these structures make for the incursions of the lung during breathing. Beginning with the small bronchi, the epithelium progressively simplifies and becomes thinner. Ciliated cells persist farther along the respiratory tree than do goblet cells and may ensure that the sites of gaseous exchange do not become coated with a viscid, mucoid material that would impede the passage of gases. Significantly, cells that produce surfactant begin to appear at about the level at which goblet cells disappear. Surfactant reduces the surface tension of the fluid layer.

During late phases of expiration, bronchioles close so that provision of a nonsticky fluid of decreased surface tension may be important in reopening the bronchioles.

The mucous secretions and cilia of the respiratory tree serve the same defensive functions as in the nasal passages. In addition, the mucosubstances have antiviral and antibacterial properties. The lymphoid tissue associated with the larger respiratory passages gives local immunological protection.

Exchange of gases occurs where air and blood are closely approximated and this occurs in the alveoli. The barrier between the air in the alveoli and the blood in the capillaries of the alveolar septum consists only of a thin film of fluid, an extremely attenuated cytoplasm of the alveolar lining cell, the conjoined basal lamina of these cells and the endothelium of the capillary itself. Surfactant-secreting cells also are present in the alveolar lining. Without surfactant, the alveolus tends to collapse because of the surface tension of the fluid bathing the alveolar epithelium. Particulate matter that reaches the alveoli is removed by the alveolar macrophages.

During the process of respiration, the size of the thoracic cavity is increased in its vertical, anteroposterior and lateral dimensions. Vertically the size of the cavity is increased by a downward movement of the diaphragm and the trachea must accommodate to this increase. The lateral dimensions are increased by a swinging out of the ribs in a "bucket-handle" motion and the bronchi must accommodate to this increase. The anteroposterior dimensions are increased as the sternum moves forward as the result of the "pump handle" action of the ribs.

Each lung is enclosed in a sac formed by the pleural membranes. The outer (parietal) layer is attached to the inner surface of the thoracic wall, the inner (visceral) layer to the surface of the lungs. Between the layers is a thin film of fluid and the space between the two layers of pleura is under a negative pressure. As the thoracic wall moves outward to increase the size of the thoracic cage, the parietal pleura follows passively. The combined effects of surface tension and negative pressure result in the visceral pleura also being drawn outward. Since the visceral pleura is firmly attached to the lungs, these are expanded, the air pressure within the lungs is thus decreased, and air is drawn into the lungs. Expiration of air from the lungs occurs as a result of elastic recoil of the lungs as the thoracic wall relaxes.

Atlas and Table of Key Features for Chapter 14

Table 14.1
Key Histological Features of Respiratory System

Division	Part	Epithelium	Support	Other Features
Extrapulmonary conducting	Nose (a) Main portion	Pseudostratified ciliated columnar with goblet cells (respiratory lining epithelium)	Hyaline cartilage and bone	Lamina propria forms a mucoperiosteum; contains seromucous glands and large venous sinuses
	(b) Olfactory region	Pseudostratified columnar with 3 cell types: basal, supporting, olfactory	Bone of nasal concha	Lamina propria contains serous glands, venous sinuses and nerves; forms a mucoperiosteum
	Pharynx (a) Nasal	Respiratory lining epithelium	Skeletal muscle	Lamina propria contains mucous, serous and mucoserous glands; abundant lymphatic tissue; pharyngeal tonsils
	(b) Oral	Stratified squamous, non keratinized	Striated muscle	As above; palatine tonsils
	(c) Laryngeal	Stratified squamous to middle of posterior surface of epiglottis and vocal cords: respiratory lining epithelium elsewhere	Cartilage; dense regular connective tissue	Epiglottis, corniculate cartilage, tips of arytenoid are elastic cartilage, rest are hyaline; epithelium over epiglottis may contain taste buds
	Trachea and main bronchi	Respiratory lining epithelium	C-shaped hyaline cartilages; fibroelastic connective tissue	Supporting connective tissue divided into lamina propria and submucosa by elastic tissue; seromucous glands in submucosa: scattered lymphatic tissue
Intrapulmonary conducting	Intrapulmonary bronchi	Respiratory lining epithelium in largest; ciliated columnar with goblet cells in smallest	Irregular, discontinuous plates of hyaline catilage decreasing in smaller bronchi	Smooth muscle increasingly prominent as cartilage disappears; mucoserous glands and lymphatic tissue in submucosa
	Bronchioles	Ciliated columnar with goblet cells in largest to ciliated columnar with no goblet cells in smallest; Clara cells appear	Smooth muscle	Connective tissue decreased in amount: no glands or lymphatic tissue present

Table 14.1 (*cont*)

Division	Part	Epithelium	Support	Other Features
Transitional from conducting to respiratory	Respiratory bronchioles	Simple cuboidal, some ciliated, no goblet cells; Clara cells	Thin layer of fibroelastic connective tissue; few smooth muscle cells	Alveoli bud out from wall
	Alveolar ducts	Cuboidal, nonciliated between successive alveoli	Thin, delicate connective tissue	
Respiratory	Alveolar sacs	Thin squamous epithelium: Type II alveolocytes, phagocytes	Elastic and reticular fibers	Formed by clusters of alveoli
	Alveoli	Attenuated squamous cells, Type II alveolocytes, macrophages	Reticular and elastic fibers	Closely approximated to capillaries: blood air barrier consists of cytoplasm of Type I alveolocyte, common basement membrane, cytoplasm of endothelial cells

14-2 Nose

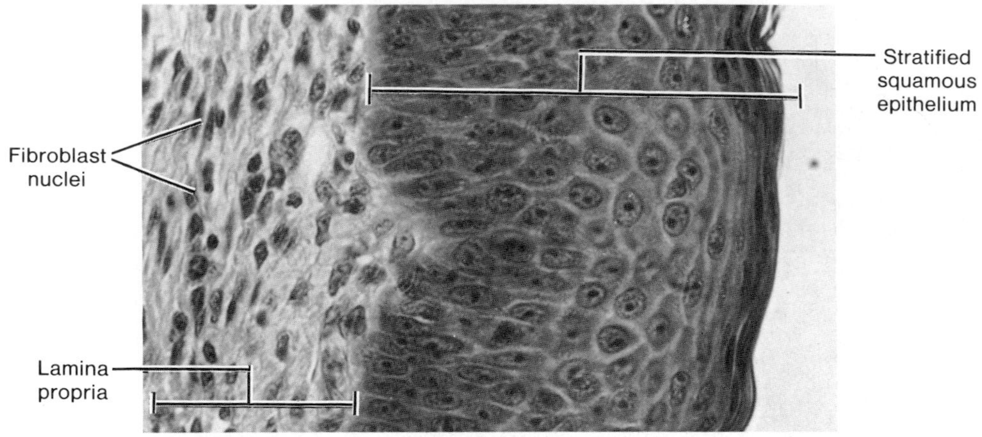

14-3

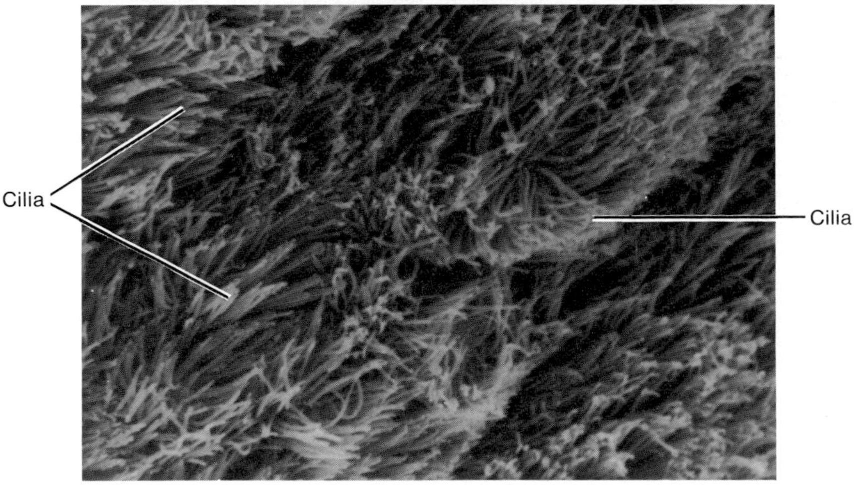

14-4

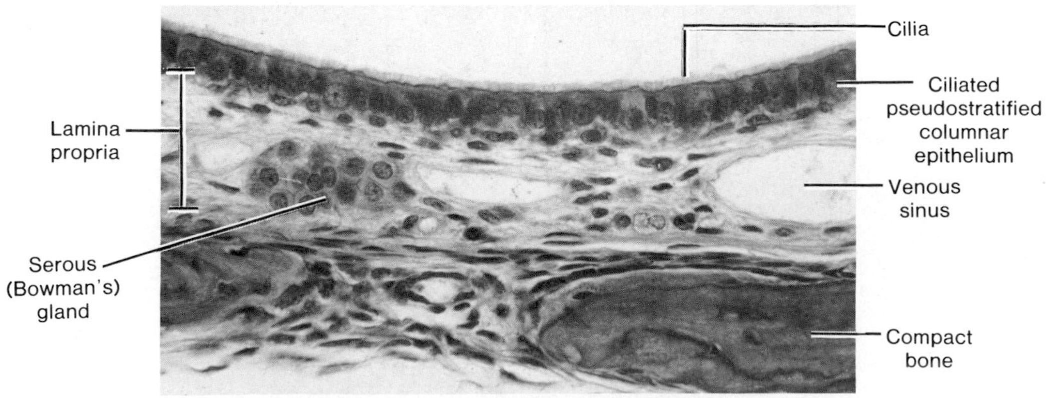

Figure 14-2 Vestibule (human). LM, ×300.
Figure 14-3 Surface of inferior concha. SEM, ×4000.
Figure 14-4 Nasal concha (cross section). LM, ×250.

14-5

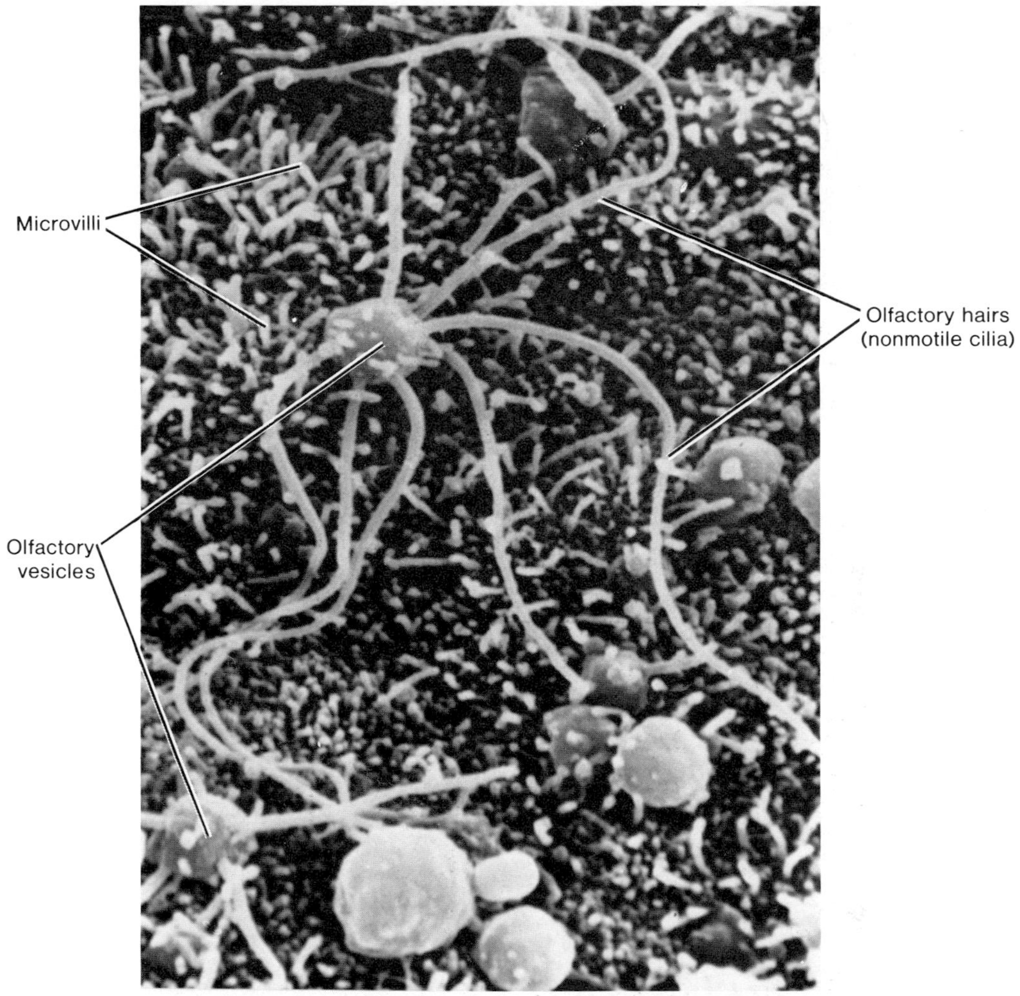

14-6

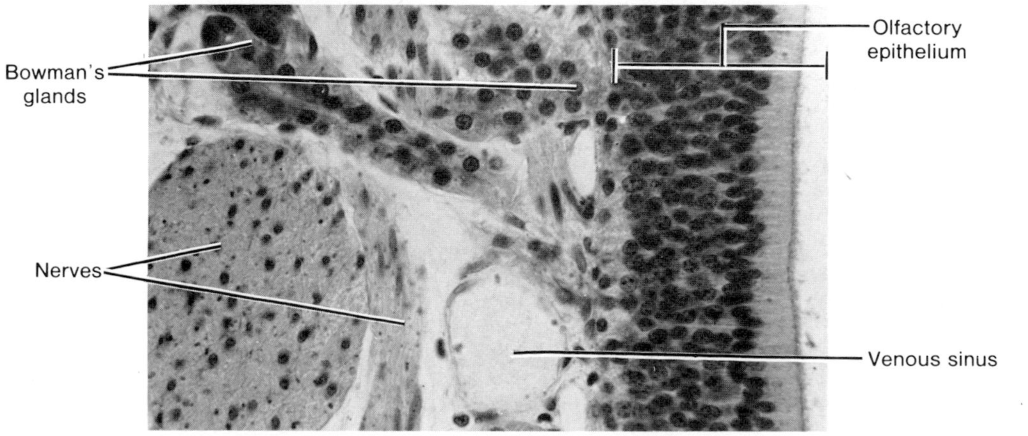

Figure 14-5 Surface of olfactory epithelium (chick). SEM, ×5700.
Figure 14-6 Olfactory epithelium (superior concha). LM, ×250.

14-7 Conducting Airways

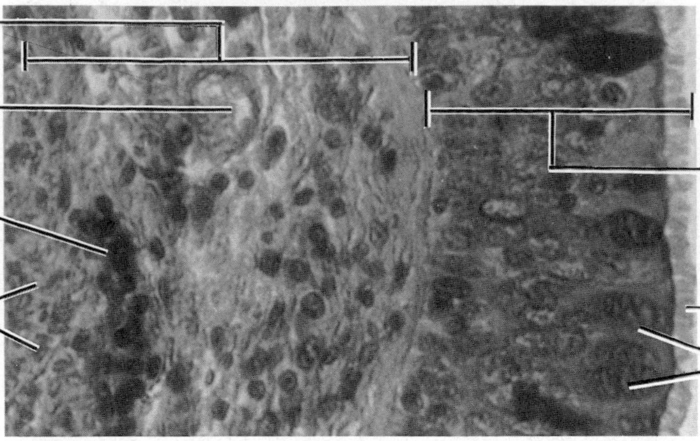
Lamina propria
Venule
Diffuse lymphatic tissue
Cross section of elastic fibers
Ciliated pseudostratified columnar epithelium
Cilia
Goblet cells

14-8

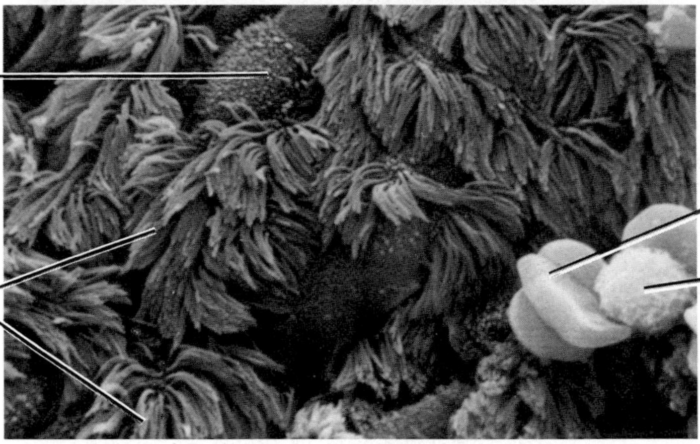
Apex of nonciliated cell
Cilia
Erythrocyte
Lymphocyte

14-9

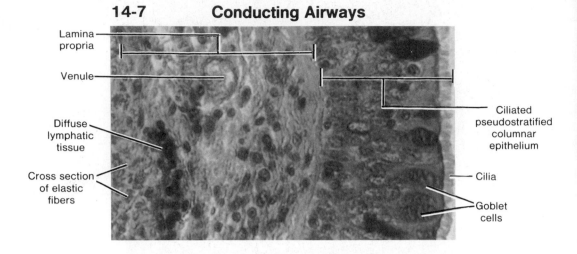

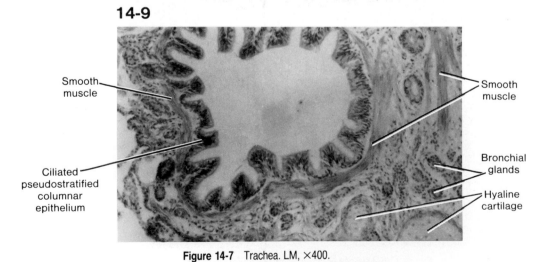

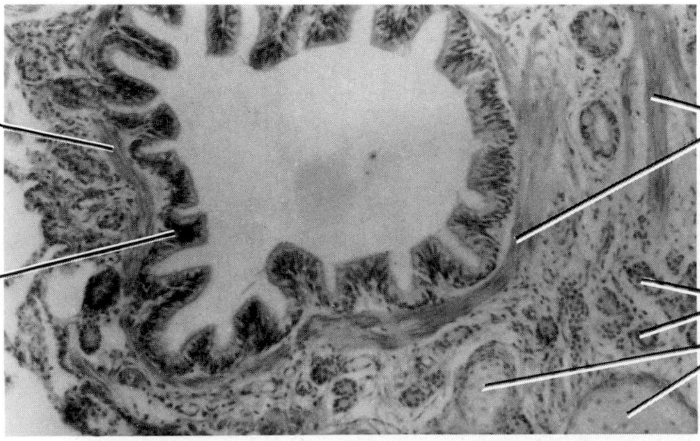
Smooth muscle
Ciliated pseudostratified columnar epithelium
Smooth muscle
Bronchial glands
Hyaline cartilage

Figure 14-7 Trachea. LM, ×400.
Figure 14-8 Surface of trachea. SEM, ×2000.
Figure 14-9 Intrapulmonary bronchus. LM, ×100.

14-10

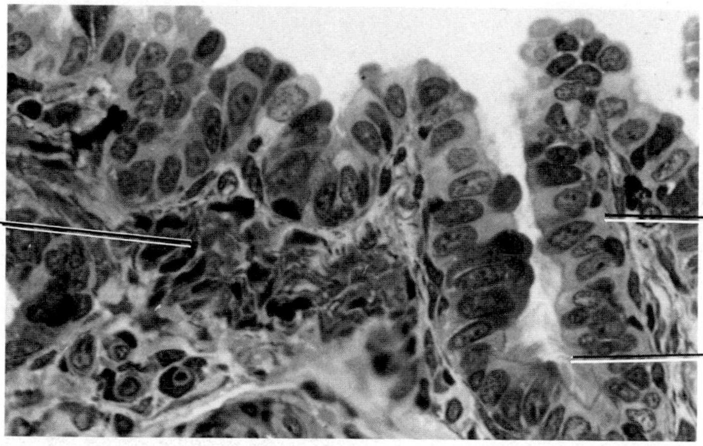
Lamina propria
Ciliated simple columnar epithelium
Cilia

14-11

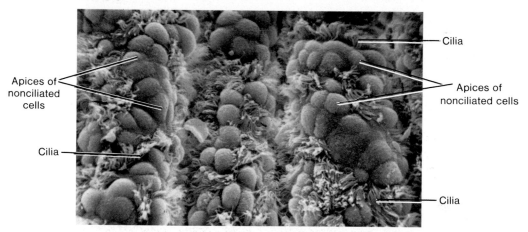

Apices of noncilliated cells
Cilia
Cilia
Apices of noncilliated cells
Cilia

14-12

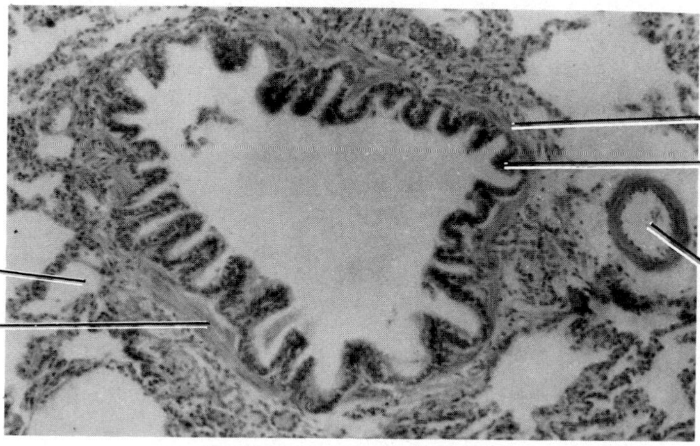
Smooth muscle
Cillated simple columnar epithelium
Pulmonary arteriole
Alveolus
Smooth muscle

Figure 14-10 Bronchiole. LM, ×400.
Figure 14-11 Bronchiole. SEM, ×1000.
Figure 14-12 Bronchiole. LM, ×100.

14-13 Lung (Respiratory Portion)

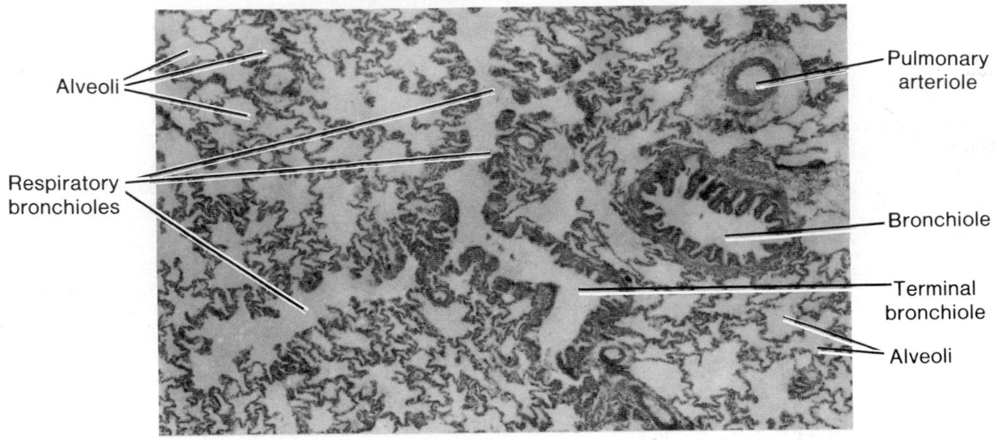

14-14

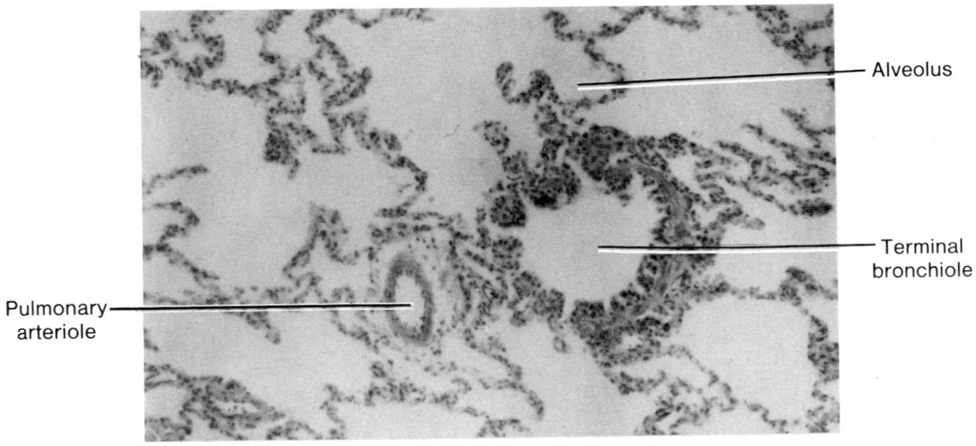

14-15

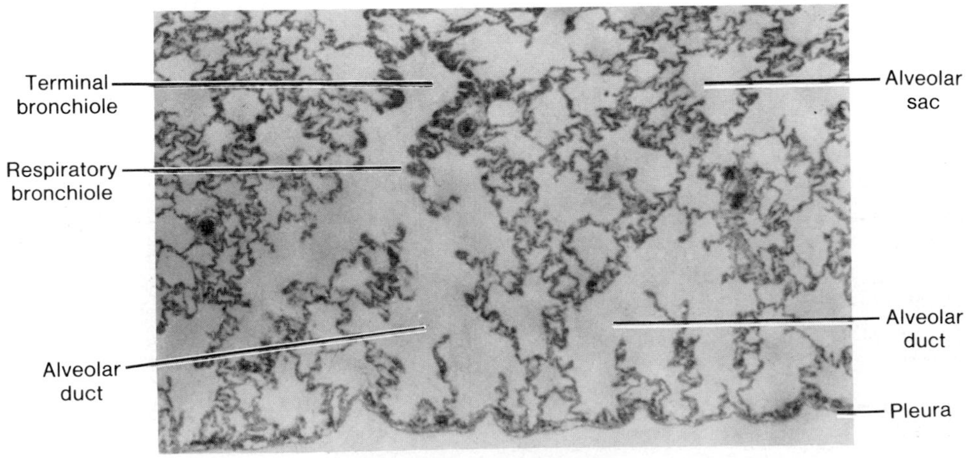

Figure 14-13 Lung. LM, ×40.
Figure 14-14 Lung. LM, ×100.
Figure 14-15 Lung. LM, ×40.

14-16

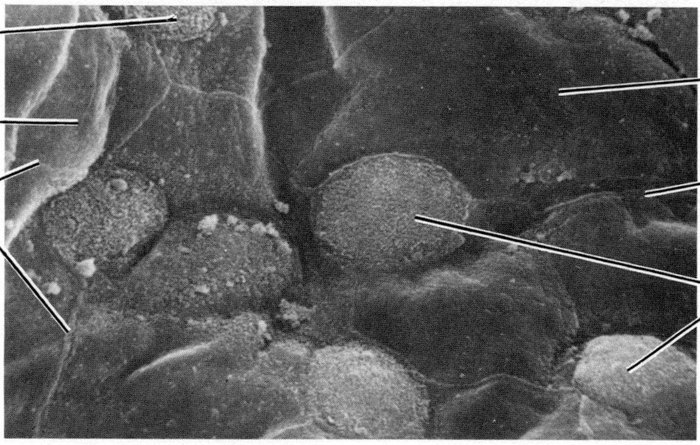

14-17

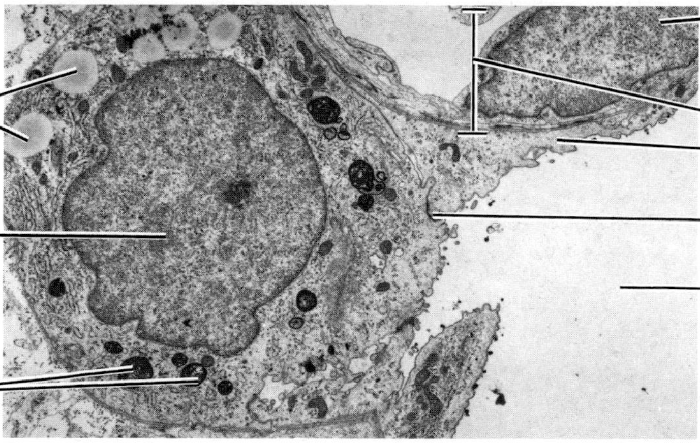

14-18

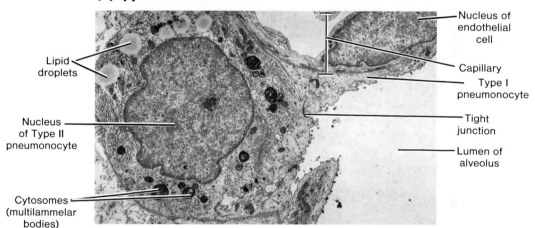

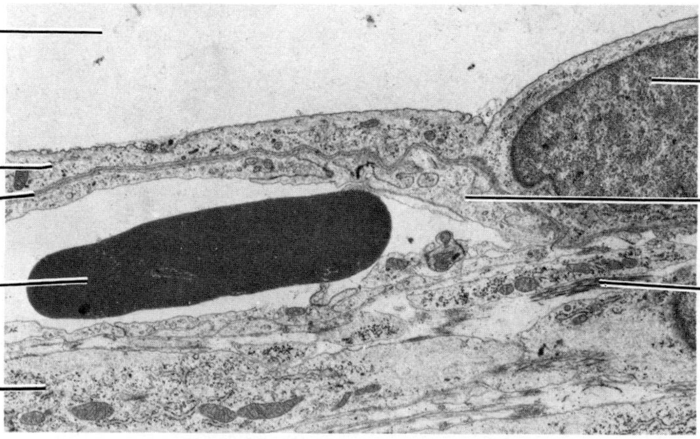

Figure 14-16 Alveolus. SEM, ×2000.
Figure 14-17 Alveolus. TEM, ×4000.
Figure 14-18 Alveolus. TEM, ×4000.

14-19

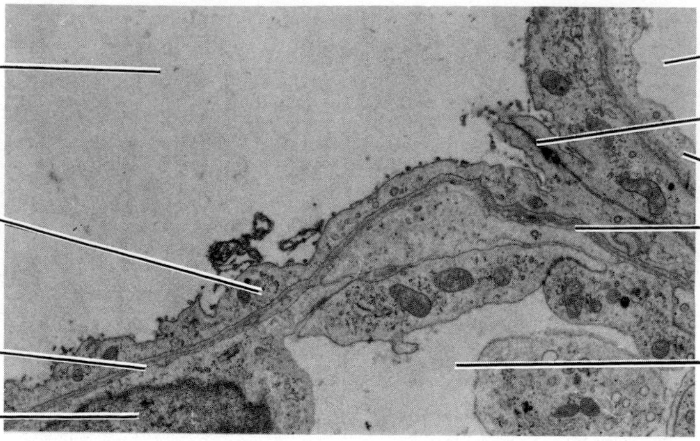

14-20

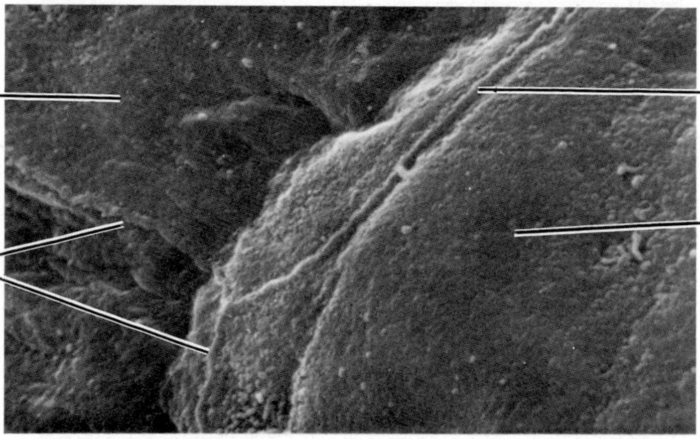

14-21

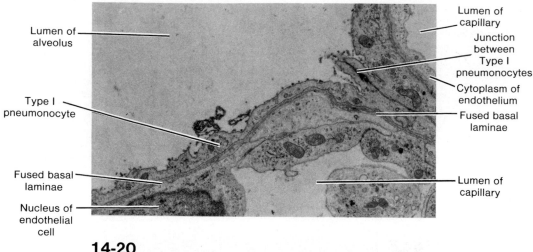

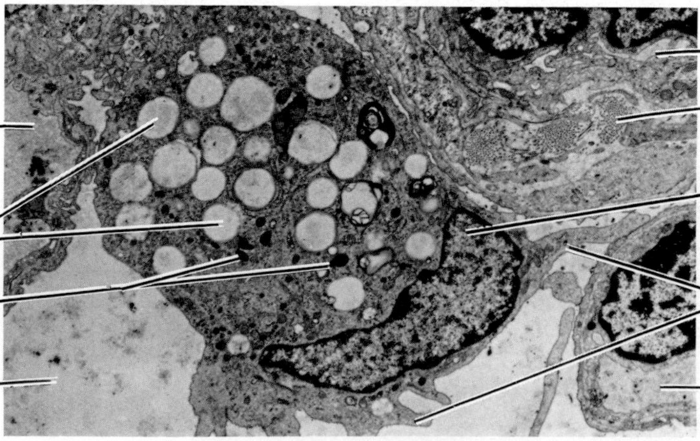

Figure 14-19 Alveolus. TEM, ×5000.
Figure 14-20 Alveolus. SEM, ×10,000.
Figure 14-21 Alveolar macrophage. TEM, ×2500.

14-22 Pleura

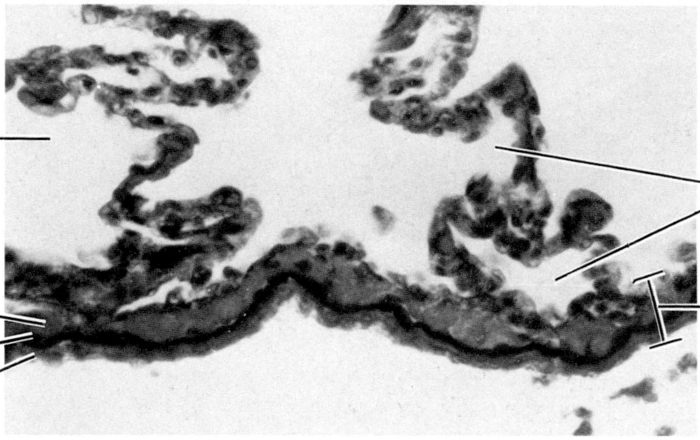

14-23

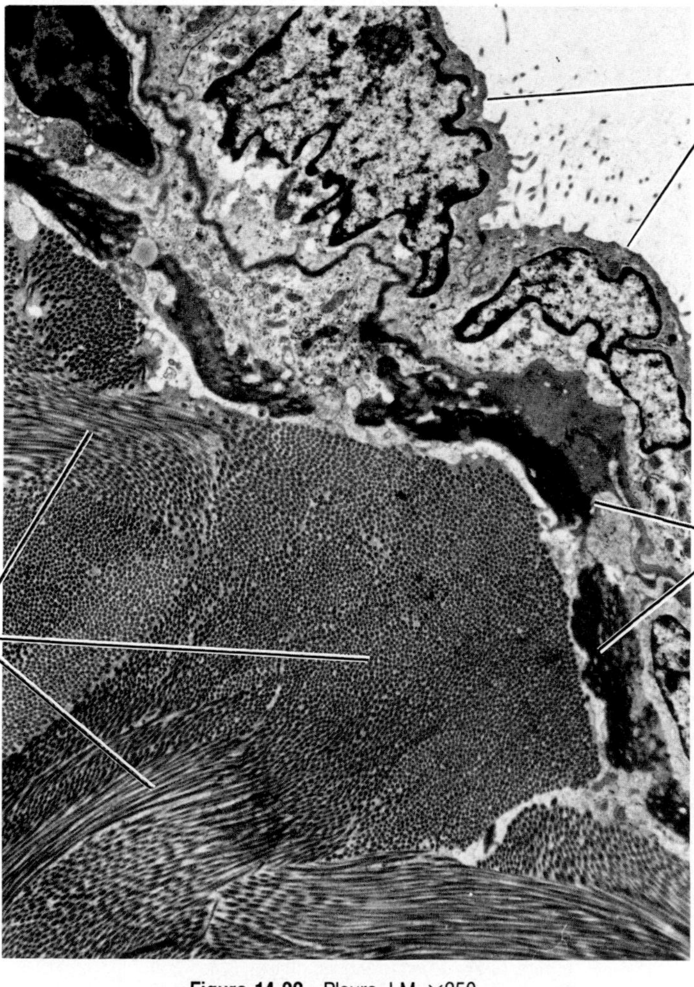

Figure 14-22 Pleura. LM, ×250.
Figure 14-23 Pleura. TEM, ×3000.

14–24 Development

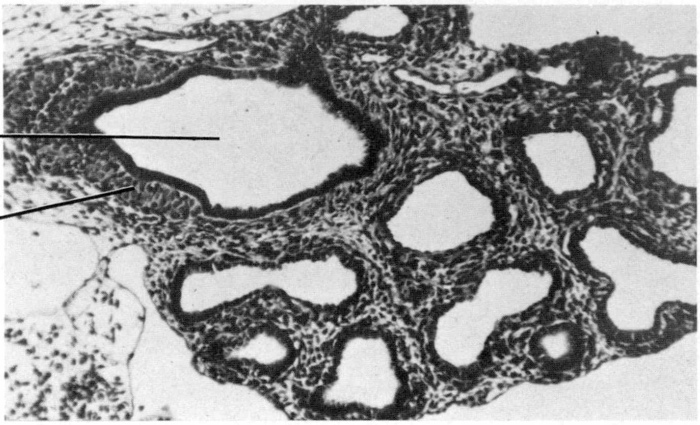

14–25

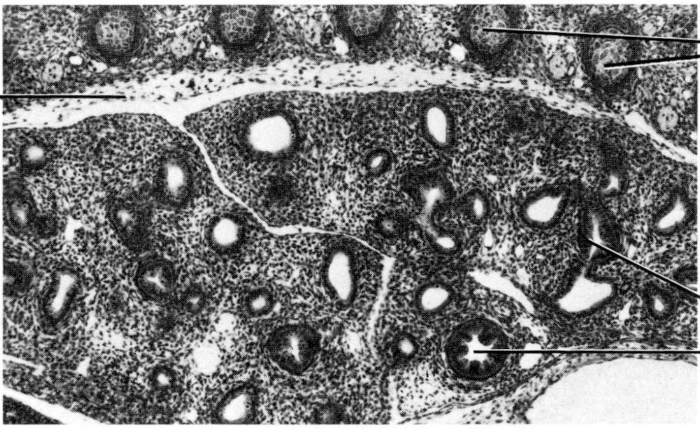

14–26

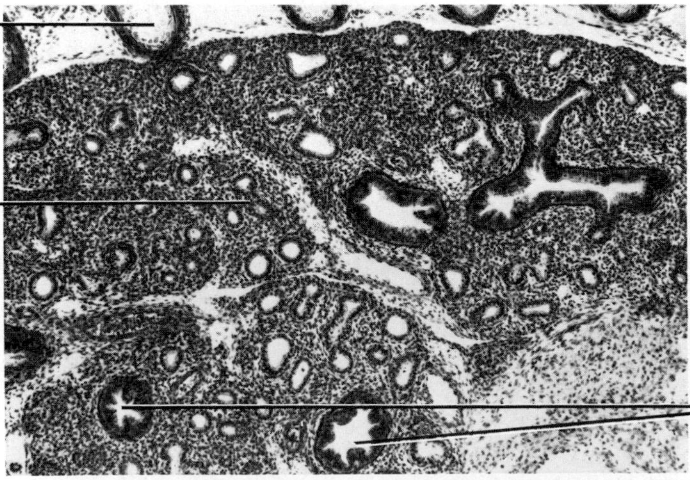

Figure 14-24 Lung (glandular phase). LM, ×250.
Figure 14-25 Lung (glandular phase). LM, ×100.
Figure 14-26 Lung (early canalicular phase). LM, ×100.

15

Digestive System

The digestive tract consists of the oral cavity, pharynx, esophagus, stomach, small intestine, large intestine, rectum and anal canal. In addition to the digestive tract proper, there are associated glands located outside the tract but which are connected to it by ducts.

GENERAL STRUCTURE

KEY WORDS: mucous membrane (mucosa), lining epithelium, lamina propria, muscularis mucosae, submucosa, muscularis externa, adventitia, serosa

Throughout its extent, the alimentary tract shows several features that can be considered to form basic components. The innermost layer of the digestive tract is referred to as a **mucous membrane**, or **mucosa**, and consists of a **lining epithelium** and an underlying layer of fine, interlacing connective tissue fibers, the **lamina propria**. A muscular component of the mucosa, the **muscularis mucosae**, is found only in the tubular portion of the digestive tract. Immediately beneath the mucosa is a layer of coarse, loosely interwoven collagen fibers and scattered elastic fibers. This layer is the **submucosa**, which houses larger vessels and nerves and attaches the mucosa to surrounding structures. It provides the mucosa with considerable mobility, and where it is absent, the mucosa is immobile and firmly attached to underlying structures. In the tubular portion of the tract, a thick layer of smooth muscle, the **muscularis externa**, forms an outer supporting wall which in turn is surrounded either by connective tissue, the **adventitia**, or by a layer of connective tissue covered by mesothelium, the **serosa**.

ORAL CAVITY

The irregularly-shaped oral cavity consists of the lips, cheek, tongue, gingiva, teeth and palate. The mucosa is formed by a stratified squamous epithelium and a rather dense lamina propria. A submucosa may be present in some regions of the oral cavity.

Lip

KEY WORDS: vermillion border, papillae, labial glands

The external surface of the lip is covered by thin skin and contains sweat glands, hair follicles and sebaceous glands. At the **vermillion** (red) **border**, the lip is covered by a nonkeratinized, translucent stratified squamous epithelium that lacks hair follicles and glands. The lamina propria projects into the overlying epithelium to form numerous tall connective tissue **papillae** that contain abundant capillaries. The combination of tall vascular papillae and translucent epithelium accounts for the red hue on this part of the lip. The red portion is continuous with the oral mucous membrane internally and with thin skin externally. Because glands are not associated with the red portion of the lip, it is kept moist by licking.

The inner surface is lined by nonkeratinized (wet) stratified squamous epithelium overlying a compact lamina propria with numerous connective tissue papillae. Between the oral mucosa and the skin are the skeletal muscle fibers of the orbicularis oris muscle. Coarse connective tissue fibers in the submucosa connect it to the underlying muscle. The ducts of numerous mixed mucoserous **labial glands** in the submucosa empty onto the internal surface of the lip and provide lubrication for this region. They can be identified as small bumps when the tongue is pressed firmly against the interior of the lip.

Cheek, Palate, and Gingiva

A similar mucous membrane lines the interior of the cheek, soft palate, floor of the mouth and undersurface of the tongue. The mucosa of the cheek and soft palate, like that of the lip, is attached to underlying skeletal muscle fibers by coarse connective tissue elements of the submucosa, which allows considerable mobility to the oral mucosa in these three regions. Mixed mucoserous glands, adipose tissue, larger blood vessels and nerves are found in the submucosa. The cheek and soft palate contain a core of skeletal muscle, the buccinator and palatine muscles, respectively. Externally, the cheek is covered by typical thin skin. As the noncornified stratified squamous epithelium of the oral cavity reflects over the posterior aspect of the soft palate to enter the nasopharynx, it changes into the typical respiratory-passage epithelium (ciliated pseudostratified columnar).

The hard palate, gingiva and dorsum of the tongue, which are subject to more intense mechanical trauma during chewing, generally lack a submucosa and are covered by cornified stratified squamous epithelium. In these areas the lamina propria of the mucous membrane is immobilized by its attachment to underlying structures. Where the mucosa is attached directly to bone, it is called a mucoperiosteum. The mucosa of the gingiva (gums) is attached directly to the periosteum of the underlying alveolar bone and a similar attachment of mucosa to periosteum is observed in the midline raphe of the hard palate, and where the hard palate joins the gingiva. A submucosa is present under the remainder of the hard palate and contains abundant adipose tissue anteriorly and small mucous glands posteriorly.

Tongue

KEY WORDS: papillae, lingual tonsils, filiform, fungiform, circumvallate, taste buds, serous glands of von Ebner, foliate papillae

The mucous membrane of the tongue is firmly bound to a core of striated muscle and a submucosa is absent. The skeletal muscle forms interwoven fascicles that course in three planes, each perpendicular to the other. The undersurface of the tongue is smooth, whereas the anterior two-thirds of the upper surface shows numerous small protuberances called **papillae**. The dorsal surface of the posterior one-third lacks papillae but shows mucosal ridges and moundlike elevations. The latter are the result of the underlying lymphatic nodules of the **lingual tonsils**.

Four types of papillae are associated with the anterior portion of the tongue: filiform, fungiform, circumvallate and foliate papillae. **Filiform papillae** are 2 to 3 mm in length and contain a conical core of connective tissue that is continuous with the underlying lamina propria. The covering epithelium shows varying degrees of cornification.

Fungiform papillae are scattered singly between the filiform type and in shape resemble a mushroom, hence, their name. They are most numerous near the tip of the tongue and appear as small red dots due to the rich vasculature of their connective tissue cores. **Taste buds** may be associated with this type of papillae.

Circumvallate papillae, the largest of the papillae, are located along the V-shaped sulcus that divides the tongue into anterior and posterior regions. They number 10 to 14 in man. The circumvallate papillae appear to be sunk within the mucous membrane of the tongue and, as their name indicates (vallum, wall), are circumscribed by a wall of lingual tissue but are separated from it by a deep furrow. Each contains a large core of connective tissue that possesses numerous vessels and nerves and, on occasion, may contain a small serous gland. The epithelium over the lateral surfaces of the circumvallate papillae contains numerous taste buds. **Serous glands (of von Ebner)** open into the bottom of the furrow. Their thin serous secretions continuously wash out this furrow and provide an adequate environment for sensory reception by taste buds. **Foliate papillae**, although rudimentary in man, are well developed in some species, such as the rabbit, and contain numerous taste buds. They appear as oval bulges on the posterior, dorsolateral aspect of the tongue and consist of parallel ridges and furrows. Taste buds lie within the epithelium on the lateral surfaces of the ridges, and intrinsic glands of the serous type drain into the bottoms of the adjacent furrows.

Taste Buds

KEY WORDS: taste pore, supporting (sustentacular) cells, neuroepithelial cells, taste hairs

Taste buds are present in the fungiform, circumvallate and foliate papillae, and may be scattered throughout the epithelium of the soft palate, glossopalatine arch, pharynx and epiglottis. They appear as lightly staining oval structures that extend from the basement membrane almost to the surface of the lining epithelium. A small **taste pore** provides for communication with the external environment. Taste buds consist of **supporting (sustentacular) cells**, between which are **neuroepithelial cells**. Both cell types have large microvilli, the **taste hairs**, that project into the taste pore and are embedded in an amorphous, polysaccharide material. Neuroepithelial cells are stimulated by substances entering the taste pore and the sensation is then transmitted to club-shaped nerve endings that pass between both cell types of the taste bud but apparently make synaptic contact only with the neuroepithelial cells. Four taste sensations are perceived: bitter, sweet, salty and sour (acid). Sensations may be detected regionally on the tongue (tip, sweet and salty; sides, sour; area of circumvallate papillae, bitter) but structural variations in taste buds from different regions have not been observed.

SALIVARY GLANDS

KEY WORDS: minor, major salivary glands, saliva

Salivary glands of the oral cavity can be divided into the **minor** and **major salivary glands**; all are compound, tubuloalveolar glands. The major salivary glands are the parotid, submandibular (submaxillary) and sublingual glands. Numerous smaller, intrinsic salivary glands are associated with the oral cavity and constitute the minor salivary glands (Table 15-1) which secrete continuously to moisten the mucosa of the oral cavity, vestibule and lips.

Saliva is a mixture of secretions from both groups of salivary glands and contains water, ions, mucins, immunoglobulins, desquamated epithelial cells and degenerating granulocytes and lymphocytes (salivary corpuscles). The enzymes amylase and maltase also are present and begin the digestion of some carbohydrates. Saliva serves to keep the oral cavity moist, soften ingested material, and cleanse the oral cavity. Some heavy metals are eliminated in salivary secretion and decreased secretion during dehydration helps initiate the sensation of thirst.

Table 15.1.
Minor Salivary Glands

Name	Location	Type of Gland
Labial glands	Upper and lower lips	Mixed
Buccal glands	Cheeks	Mixed
Anterior lingual glands	Tip of tongue	Mixed
Glands of Von Ebner	Near circumvallate papillae	Serous
Posterior lingual glands	Root of tongue	Mucous
Palatine glands	Palate	Mucous

Major Salivary Glands

The major salivary glands consist of the parotid, submandibular and sublingual glands. These lie outside the oral cavity but are connected to it by ducts. The major salivary glands secrete only in response to nervous stimulation. The response is reflexive and can be stimulated by the smell, sight or even the thought of food.

Parotid Gland

KEY WORDS: compound tubuloalveolar, serous, intercellular secretory canaliculi, intercalated duct, striated duct, basal striations, intralobular duct, interlobular ducts

The parotid is the largest of the major salivary glands and is located below and anterior to the external ear. Its primary excretory duct passes through the cheek and opens into the vestibule of the mouth opposite the upper second molar tooth. It is a **compound tubuloalveolar gland** and in man, most domestic mammals and rodents is entirely **serous**. A few mucous cells are present in the parotid glands of carnivores, young puppies and lambs. The adult human parotid shows an abundance of scattered fat cells. A fibrous capsule encloses the gland and connective tissue septa subdivide it into lobes and lobules. A delicate stroma surrounds the secretory units and ducts and contains numerous blood capillaries and scattered nerve fibers. Myoepithelial cells associated with the secretory units lie between the epithelial cells and the limiting basement membrane and may aid in expressing the secretion out of the secretory units and into the duct system.

Alveoli are composed of pyramidal-shaped, serous cells with basally placed oval nuclei, basophilic cytoplasm and discrete, apical secretory granules. Small channels, the **intercellular secretory canaliculi**, are found between serous cells and provide an additional route by which secretory products can reach the lumen.

The initial segment of the duct system is the **intercalated duct**, which is particularly prominent in the parotid gland. It is lined by a simple squamous or low cuboidal epithelium and may be associated with myoepithelial cells. Intercalated ducts are continuous with **striated ducts** which are lined by columnar cells that show numerous **basal striations**. These elaborate infoldings of the basal plasmalemma increase the surface area, while the mitochondria associated with the infoldings provide energy at the base of the cell and play a significant role in fluid and ion transport. The intercalated and striated ducts constitute the duct system *within* the lobule and collectively form the **intralobular duct system**. The remaining ducts are found in the connective tissue *between* lobules and are referred to as **interlobular ducts**. They are continuous with the intralobular ducts and are lined at first by a simple columnar epithelium which becomes pseudostratified and then stratified as the diameter of the ducts increases. The surrounding connective tissue becomes more abundant as these ducts join to form the major excretory duct. The distal portion of the duct is lined by stratified squamous epithelium that becomes continuous with the lining epithelium of the cheek.

Submandibular Gland

KEY WORDS: mixed compound tubuloalveolar gland, serous demilunes (crescents), intercellular canaliculi, striated ducts

The submandibular gland, like the parotid, is **compound tubuloalveolar** and has a fibrous capsule with septa, lobes, lobules, myoepithelial cells and a prominent duct system. It is a **mixed gland,** with the majority of the secretory units being serous in man, horse and ruminants, but in dogs and cats the mucous components are more prominent. In rodents the gland is primarily serous. The mucous tubules usually show **serous crescents** or **demilumes** at their blind ends. Small channels, the **intercellular secretory canaliculi**, pass between the mucous cells and extend between the serous cells of the demilune. Thus, the secretory product of the demilunes has direct access to the lumen of the mucous tubule. Generally, the duct system is similar to that of the parotid, but **striated ducts** are longer and hence are more conspicuous in histological sections of the submandibular gland. The major excretory duct of the submandibular gland empties onto the floor of the oral cavity.

Sublingual Gland

KEY WORDS: composite gland, mixed compound tubuloalveolar gland

The sublingual is a **composite** of **glands** of variable size. Each gland opens independently onto the floor of the mouth or into the excretory ducts of the submandibular gland. The capsule is not well defined, although septa are present. It is a **mixed compound tubuloaveolar gland,** with the majority of the secretory units being mucous in ruminants, swine and rodents. Mixed units are present in small carnivores, man and the horse. Serous cells are, for the most part, arranged as demilunes. Myoepithelial cells are found in relation to the secretory units. Segments of the intralobular duct system are short and not as readily observed as they are in the other two major salivary glands.

TEETH

Two sets of teeth are distinguished in man: primary (deciduous) and permanent teeth. Primary teeth erupt 6 to 8 months after birth and form a complete set of 20 by 2 years of age. They are shed between the 6th and 13th year and gradually are replaced by the permanent set, which numbers 32.

Structure

KEY WORDS: crown, root, neck, socket (alveolus), pulp chamber, apical foramen, enamel, dentin, cementum, pulp, periodontal membrane, gingiva

All teeth show the same histological organization (Fig. 15-1). Each has a **crown** and a **root** and the point where the two meet is called the **neck**. The root fits into a **socket** or **alveolus** of the mandible or maxilla. Each tooth contains a small cavity, or **pulp cavity** that corresponds in shape to the external form of the tooth. The pulp chamber communicates with the alveolar cavity and periodontal membrane through the **apical foramen**, a small opening at the tip of the root. The hard tissues of the tooth consist of **enamel, dentin** and **cementum**. Soft tissues associated with the tooth are the **pulp, periodontal membrane** and **gingiva**.

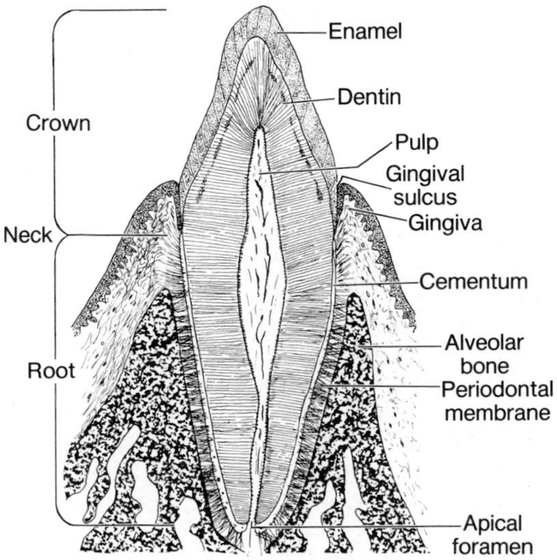

Figure 15.1. Structure of a tooth.

Dentin

KEY WORDS: dentinal tubules, odontoblast, dentinal or Tome's fibers, sheath of Neumann

Dentin forms the bulk of the tooth and surrounds the pulp chamber. It is harder than compact bone and consists of 80% inorganic material and 20% organic substance. Most of the organic material is collagen, while the inorganic component is in the form of hydroxyapatite crystals. Dentin has a radially striated appearance due to numerous minute canals called **dentinal tubules** which pursue an S-shaped course as they extend from the pulp chamber to the dentinoenamel junction. The dentinal tubules contain fine cytoplasmic processes (**dentinal,** or **Tome's, fibers**) of a cell type known as the **odontoblast.** The thin layer of dentin that immediately surrounds each dentinal tubule shows a greater refringence than the remaining dentin and is called the **sheath of Neumann.** The cell body of the odontoblast lies in the pulp cavity immediately adjacent to the dentin. It is this cell which lays down the organic matrix of dentin which is formed throughout life, resulting in a progressive narrowing of the pulp cavity with age. Some areas of dentin remain incompletely calcified and are referred to as interglobular spaces. Dentin is sensitive to cold, pain, touch and hydrogen ion concentration. Sensation is thought to be perceived by the processes of the odontoblasts, which in turn transmit the sensory stimulation to adjacent nerves in the pulp cavity.

Enamel

KEY WORDS: enamel prisms, interprismatic substance, ameloblast

Enamel covers the dentin of the crown and is the hardest substance of the body. It is acellular and consists primarily of calcium salts in the form of apatite crystals. Only 1% of the enamel substance is organic material. Enamel consists of thin rods or **enamel prisms** that are oriented perpendicular to the surface of the dentin and extend from the dentinoenamel junction to the surface of the tooth. Each prism, 6 to 8 μm in diameter, follows a spiralling, irregular course to the surface of the tooth. Between the enamel prisms is the **interprismatic substance**, which also consists of apatite crystals in a small amount of organic matrix. Each enamel prism is the product of a single **ameloblast**, the enamel producing cells which are lost during eruption of the tooth. Thus, new enamel cannot be formed after the tooth has erupted.

Cementum

KEY WORDS: acellular cementum, cementocytes, cellular cementum, Sharpey's fibers

Cementum covers the dentin of the root of the tooth. Nearest the neck of the tooth (the upper one third) the cementum is thin and lacks cells, forming the **acellular cementum**. The remainder, which covers the apex of the tooth, contains the **cementocytes** that lie in lacunae and are surrounded by a calcified matrix similar to that of bone. This type of cementum is referred to as **cellular cementum**. The organic matrix of cementum is elaborated by cementocytes and cementum increases in thickness with age. Coarse bundles of collagen fibers penetrate the cementum as **Sharpey's fibers**, which anchor the root of the tooth to the surrounding alveolar bone of the socket.

Pulp

KEY WORDS: connective tissue, apical foramen

Pulp is the **connective tissue** which fills the pulp chamber. It contains numerous thin, collagenous fibrils embedded in an abundant, gelatinous ground substance. Stellate-shaped fibroblasts are the most prominent cells of the pulp, although mesenchymal cells, macrophages and lymphocytes are found in limited numbers. The cell bodies of the odontoblasts also are found in the pulp, lining the perimeter of the pulp cavity immediately adjacent to the dentin. Blood vessels, lymphatics and nerves enter and exit the pulp cavity through the **apical foramen**.

Periodontal Membrane

KEY WORDS: bundles of collagen fibers, Sharpey's fibers

The periodontal membrane consists of thick **bundles of collagen fibers** that run between the cementum covering the root of the tooth and the surrounding alveolar bone. The fibers extend into the bone and cementum as **Sharpey's fibers**. The orientation of the fibers in the periodontal membrane varies at different levels in the alveolar socket. Although firmly attached to the surrounding alveolar bone, the fibers are not taut and the tooth is able to move slightly in each direction. The periodontal membrane serves as a suspensory ligament for the tooth. In addition to typical connective tissue cells, osteoblasts and osteoclasts may be found where the periodontal membrane enters the alveolar bone. The periodontal membrane has a rich vascular supply and is sensitive to pressure changes.

Gingiva (Gum)

KEY WORDS: gingival ligament, epithelial attachment (epithelial attachment cuff)

The gingiva surrounds each tooth like a collar and is attached to the periosteum of the underlying alveolar bone. Near the tooth, collagenous fibers of the gingival lamina propria blend with the uppermost fibers of the periodontal membrane. Some collagenous fibers extend from the lamina propria into the cervical (upper) cementum and constitute the **gingival ligament**, which provides a firm attachment to the tooth. The keratinized stratified epithelium of the gingiva also is attached to the surface of the tooth and at this point forms the **epithelial attachment** or **attached epithelial cuff**. The attachment of the epithelial cuff to the tooth is maintained by a thickened basal lamina and hemidesmosomes which seal off the dentogingival junction.

PHARYNX

The oral cavity continues posteriorly into the pharynx, which extends from the base of the skull to the level of the cricoid cartilage, where it is continuous with the esophagus. The digestive and respiratory systems merge briefly in the pharynx, which is subdivided into nasal, oral and laryngeal portions. The pharyngeal walls basically consist of three strata: a mucosa, a mucularis and an adventitia.

Oropharynx

KEY WORDS: nonkeratinized stratified squamous epithelium, lamina propria, muscularis, skeletal muscle

The oropharynx is lined by a **nonkeratinized stratified squamous epithelium** and a dense, fibroelastic **lamina propria**. Immediately beneath the lamina propria is a well-developed layer of elastic fibers which is continuous with the muscularis mucosae of the esophagus. Proximally, the elastic layer blends with the connective tissue between the muscular bundles of the pharyngeal wall. A submucosa is present only where the pharynx is continuous with the esophagus and in the lateral walls of the nasopharynx. The **muscularis** of the pharyngeal wall is composed of the **skeletal muscle** of the pharyngeal constrictor muscles which in turn are covered by connective tissue of the adventitia.

TUBULAR DIGESTIVE TRACT

The tubular digestive tract consists of the esophagus, stomach, small intestine, colon and rectum. Each region of the digestive tube consists of the four basic strata or layers, but the components of these layers vary according to the function of the region.

Esophagus

The esophagus is a relatively straight muscular tube about 25 cm long. It is continuous above with the pharynx at the inferior border of the cricoid cartilage and below becomes continuous with the cardia of the stomach.

Mucosa

KEY WORDS: nonkeratinized stratified squamous epithelium, lamina propria, muscularis mucosae, smooth muscle

The mucosa consists of a lining epithelium, a lamina propria and a muscularis mucosae. The epithelial lining is thick and in man consists of a **nonkeratinized stratified squamous epithelium** continuous with the similar epithelium of the oropharynx. At the junction with the stomach, the epithelium shows an abrupt transition to a simple columnar epithelium. In species accustomed to a coarse diet, the epithelium undergoes extensive keratinization, as in ruminants. The **lamina propria** is a loose areolar connective tissue with diffuse and nodular lymphatic tissue scattered along its length. The **muscularis mucosae** consists of longitudinally arranged **smooth muscle** cells in a fine, elastic network. Circularly arranged smooth muscle cells also may be present. The muscularis mucosae is continuous with the elastic layer of the pharynx at the level of the cricoid cartilage.

Submucosa

KEY WORDS: collagenous fibers, elastic fibers, longitudinal folds

This layer consists primarily of coarse **collagenous fibers** and **elastic fibers**. Contained within it are larger blood vessels, lymphatics, nerve fibers, occasional autonomic ganglia and glands. Extensive **longitudinal folds** of the submucosa give the mucosa of the nondistended esophagus a characteristic pleated appearance. During swallowing, the bolus of food smooths out these folds and allows the lumen to increase in size temporarily, to accommodate the material swallowed.

Muscularis Externa

KEY WORDS: skeletal muscle, mixed smooth and skeletal muscle, smooth muscle

The upper quarter of the muscularis externa consists of **skeletal muscle** only. From the lower border of the inferior constrictor muscle of the pharynx, the muscle progressively becomes more regularly arranged into inner circular and outer longitudinal layers. In the second quarter of the human and opossum esophagus a **mixture of skeletal and smooth muscle** is found, while in the distal one half, only **smooth muscle** is present. The muscularis externa of many species, such as the dog, consists only of skeletal muscle. Cells of autonomic ganglia are found between the inner and outer layers of smooth muscle.

Adventitia

A layer of loosely-arranged connective tissue, the adventitia, covers the outer surface of the esophagus and binds it to surrounding structures. Below the diaphragm a short segment of the esophagus is covered by a serosa.

Glands

KEY WORDS: esophageal cardiac, lamina propria, esophageal glands proper, submucosa

Two kinds of glands are present in the esophagus: esophageal cardiac glands and esophageal glands proper. Two groups of **esophageal cardiac glands** usually are described, one group located in the proximal esophagus near the pharynx, the other in the distal esophagus near the cardia of the stomach. Both are compound tubuloalveolar glands of the mucous type and have a restricted location in the **lamina propria**. The **esophageal glands proper** also are mucous, compound tubuloalveolar glands but are confined to the **submucosa** throughout the remainder of the esophagus. Myoepithelial cells are associated with the secretory units in man and a few other species. In some animals, such as the horse and cat, esophageal glands are absent.

Stomach

The stomach forms an expanded portion of the tubular digestive tract between the esophagus and small intestine. In man and many other species, the stomach is divided into the cardia, a short region where the esophagus joins the stomach; the fundus, a dome-shaped elevation of the stomach wall above the esophagogastric junction; the corpus, the large central portion of the stomach, and the pylorus, the narrow region just prior to the gastrointestinal junction. The stomach shows upper concave and lower convex external borders termed the lesser and greater curvatures, respectively. The stomach functions both for the storage and digestion of food, and although storage is not of primary importance in man, it is of considerable importance in ruminants and other herbivorous species. The digestive function of the stomach involves both the mechanical and chemical breakdown of ingested substances.

Mucosa

KEY WORDS: rugae, gastric lining epithelium, simple columnar, gastric pits (foveolae), cardiac glands, gastric glands, pyloric glands

The mucosa of the empty stomach has numerous folds or ridges known as **rugae**. In the distended stomach, rugae for the most part disappear. The **gastric lining epithelium** is **simple columnar** and begins abruptly at the junction with the stratified squamous epithelium of the esophagus, and ends abruptly at the intestinal epithelium of the duodenum. In man, the lining epithelium is similar in structure throughout the stomach. Columnar cells of the gastric lining epithelium are secretory and collectively form the glandular organization called a *secretory sheet*. The neutral mucin produced by the surface epithelium is secreted continuously and forms a mucous film that protects the mucosa from the acid pepsin in the gastric lumen and also lubricates the surface.

The apices of the columnar cells are held in close apposition by tight junctions and the lateral cell membranes show numerous desmosomes. Scattered, stubby microvilli are present on the apical surfaces, and numerous discrete secretory granules fill the apical cytoplasm of the cells. The basal cytoplasm shows profiles of rough endoplasmic reticulum; well-developed Golgi complexes occupy the supranuclear region.

The gastric mucosa contains approximately 3 million minute, tubular infoldings of the surface epithelium, called **gastric pits** or **foveolae**, which are lined by the same simple columnar epithelium that covers the surface. The epithelial cells on the surface are replaced every 4 to 5 days. New cells are derived from a small population of relatively undifferentiated cells located in the bottoms of the gastric pits. Cells from this region gradually migrate upward along the gastric pit to replace cells of the surface epithelium.

A gastric lining of simple columnar epithelium as in man and some other species is not a universal condition. The gastric mucosa of several mammalian forms (monotremes, certain kangaroos, rodents, ruminants, and several herbivorous species) is lined completely, or in part, by stratified squamous epithelium.

Three types of glands are usually found in the gastric mucosa: **cardiac, gastric** and **pyloric glands.**

Cardiac Glands

KEY WORDS: simple branched tubular glands, mucous cells, endocrine cells

The cardiac glands of man begin immediately around the esophageal orifice and extend about 3.4 cm along the proximal stomach, but attain their greatest depth near the esophageal-gastric junction. Here the tubular glands branch freely and appear to be collected into aggregates (lobule-like complexes) by the surrounding connective tissue of the lamina propria. Near the junction with the fundus, the cardiac glands show less branching and the distinct grouping disappears, resulting in a decrease in the thickness of the glandular area. The cardiac glands for the most part are **simple branched tubular glands** that open into the overlying gastric pits. The depth of the gastric pit and length of the cardiac gland are about equal. The secretory units are composed primarily of **mucous cells**, but occasional parietal cells are observed and appear identical to those in the gastric glands. A number of **endocrine cells** of undetermined nature also are present.

Gastric Glands

KEY WORDS: simple branched tubular glands, mucous neck cells, parietal cells, intracellular canaliculi, tubulovesicular system, hydrochloric acid, gastric intrinsic factor, chief (zymogen) cells, pepsinogen, pepsin, endocrine cells

The gastric glands are the most abundant glands of the stomach (approximately 15 million) and are found along the entire corpus of the stomach. They are mainly **simple branched tubular glands** in man, although in some species (rat) most are simple tubular. The glands run perpendicular to the surface of the mucosa and one or several glands may open into the bottom of each gastric pit. The gastric glands are about four times as long as the pits into which they open. Each gastric gland is composed of mucous neck cells, parietal cells, chief or zymogen cells and endocrine cells.

Mucous neck cells occur primarily in the upper portions of the gastric glands, where these open into gastric pits. The cells often appear to be sandwiched between other cell types and are characterized by their irregular shape. Some have a broad apex and a narrow base, others a narrow apex and a wide base. The nucleus is confined to the base of the cell, surrounded by a basophilic cytoplasm. Secretory granules fill the apical cytoplasm. Unlike the mucous cells that line the gastric surface, mucous neck cells produce an acidic mucin.

Although most numerous in the central region of the gastric glands, **parietal cells** also are scattered among mucous neck cells in the upper portion of the gland. They are large, spherical cells whose bases often appear to bulge from the outer margin of the gland into the lamina propria. In routine sections, parietal cells are characterized by the acidophilia of their cytoplasm. Each cell contains a large, centrally placed nucleus, numerous mitochondria, and is characterized by **intracellular canaliculi**. These are invaginations of the plasmalemma that form channels near the nucleus and open at the apex of the cell into the lumen of the gland. Numerous microvilli project into the lumina of the canaliculi, their number and length varying according to the secretory activity of the cell. Immediately adjacent to each canaliculus a series of smooth cytoplasmic membranes form small tubules and vesicles known as the **tubulovesicular system**. Secretion of **hydrochloric acid** occurs along the cell membrane that lines the canaliculi. During acid secretion the tubulovesicular membranes diminish and the canalicular microvilli become more abundant; during acid inhibition the reverse is observed. In addition to hydrochloric acid, parietal cells of the human stomach secrete a glycoprotein, **gastric intrinsic factor**, which forms a complex with dietary vitamin B_{12} in the gastric lumen. This complex is absorbed in the small intestine, and a deficiency of intrinsic factor results in decreased vitamin B_{12} absorption. Vitamin B_{12} is important for the maturation of red blood cells in the bone marrow and lack of this vitamin results in pernicious anemia.

Chief or **zymogen cells** are present mainly in the basal half of the gastric glands and in routine sections stain basophilic. The cells contain abundant granular endoplasmic reticulum in the basal cytoplasm, well-developed Golgi complexes in the supranuclear cytoplasm and apical zymogen granules. Such features characterize a cell involved in protein (enzyme) secretion.

Chief cells secrete **pepsinogen**, a precursor of the enzyme **pepsin**, which reaches its optimal activity at pH 2.0. The acid environment in the gastric lumen is created by the parietal cells. Pepsin hydrolyzes proteins into smaller peptide molecules and is important in the gastric digestion of protein.

Also scattered within the bases of the gastric glands are **endocrine cells**, peptide-producing cells characterized by specific granules enclosed within smooth membranes. The polarization of these cells suggests that they secrete into the blood stream or into the surrounding tissues rather than into the lumen of the gastric gland. The gastrointestinal hormones somatostatin, glucagon, and pancreatic polypeptide, and the amine 5-hydroxytryptamine (5-HT), have been identified in some endocrine cells of the gastric glands.

In some species (koala, wombat, beaver, pangolin, grasshopper mouse) the gastric glands are organized into large, complex glandular structures that are set away from the gastric lumen but communicate with it either by a single or a limited number of large orifices.

Pyloric Glands

KEY WORDS: simple or branched tubular glands, mucous cells, endocrine cells, G cell, gastrin

The pyloric glands are confined to the distal 4 or 5 cm of the stomach. They are **simple or branched tubular glands** composed of a **mucous cell** similar in type to the mucous neck cell of the fundic region. Occasional parietal cells also may be present. The pyloric glands empty into gastric pits, the ratio between the depths of the pit and gland being approximately 1:1 as in the cardiac glands. Numerous **endocrine cells**, primarily **G cells**, are present and these unicellular, endocrine glands produce **gastrin**, a peptide hormone that stimulates acid secretion by the parietal cells in the remainder of the stomach. Endocrine cells that produce somatostatin and 5-HT are present in pyloric glands also. Thus, in addition to the exocrine function of mucus production, the pyloric glands have an important endocrine function as well.

Lamina Propria

The lamina propria of the stomach is obscured by the close approximation of the glands in the gastric mucosa. It consists of a delicate network of collagenous and reticular fibers which surround and extend between the glands and gastric pits. Numerous lymphocytes, some plasma cells, eosinophils and mast cells are found within the lamina propria. Lymphatic nodules also may occur.

Muscularis Mucosae

The muscularis mucosae consists of an inner circular, an outer longitudinal and in some places, an additional outer circular layer of smooth muscle. Slips of smooth muscle also extend into the lamina propria between the glands and extend to the gastric epithelium. The muscularis mucosae gives additional mobility to the gastric mucosa.

Submucosa

The submucosa consists of a coarse connective tissue rich in mast cells, eosinophils and lymphoid cells. This layer contains lymph vessels and the larger blood vessels. Parent blood vessels pierce the stomach wall at the lesser and greater curvatures and supply smaller branches that run around the circumference of the stomach in the submucosa. Smaller branches of the submucosal vessels then enter the mucosa to provide its vascular supply.

Muscularis Externa

KEY WORDS: outer longitudinal, middle circular, inner oblique, pyloric sphincter

The muscularis externa consists of three layers of smooth muscle: **outer longitudinal, middle circular** and **inner oblique** layers. In the pylorus, the middle circular layer increases in thickness and forms the **pyloric sphincter**, which is thought to aid in controlling the emptying of the stomach. Strong contractions of the muscular wall of the stomach result in a churning action that contributes to the mechanical breakdown of ingested material and to gastric emptying.

Serosa

A thin layer of loose connective tissue covers the muscularis externa and is covered on its outer aspect by the mesothelial lining of the peritoneal cavity.

Small Intestine

The small intestine extends between the stomach and colon and is divided into the duodenum, jejunum and ileum. Although there are minor microscopic differences between these subdivisions, all have the same basic organization as the remainder of the digestive tube (i.e., a mucosa, a submucosa, muscularis externa and serosa) and the transition from one segment to another is gradual. The small intestine has several functions, including moving chyme from the stomach to the colon and completing the digestive process by adding enzymes secreted by the intestinal mucosa and accessory glands (liver and pancreas). The primary function, however, is absorption.

Specializations for Absorption

KEY WORDS: plicae circulares, intestinal villi, microvilli, striated border, terminal web

Three structural specializations, plicae circulares, intestinal villi, and microvilli, markedly increase the surface area of the intestinal mucosa to enhance the absorptive process.

Plicae circulares are large, permanent folds which consist of the intestinal mucosa and a central core of submucosa. These large, shelf-like folds sometimes branch and spiral about the lumen of the intestine for one-half to two-thirds of its circumference. Plicae begin in the upper duodenum, reach their maximum development in the proximal jejunum and thereafter diminish in size and disappear in the distal half of the ileum.

The intestinal mucosa also presents numerous finger-like evaginations called **villi** which cover the entire surface of the small intestine. They consist of a central core of connective tissue of the lamina propria, covered by the intestinal epithelium. Villi measure 0.5 to 1.5 mm in length and are best developed in the duodenum and jejunum, where they are broad, spatulate structures. In the ileum they become shorter and appear more finger-like.

The surface area of the small intestine is increased approximately 30-fold by the presence of large numbers of closely packed **microvilli** on the luminal surfaces of the intestinal absorptive cells. The microvilli constitute the **striated border** of light microscopy. Each microvillus represents a cylindrical extension of the plasma membrane enclosing a small core of cytoplasm. Interiorly, each microvillus contains numerous thin actin filaments that extend into the apical cytoplasm of the cell and contribute to the **terminal web**, a network of fine filaments that lies immediately beneath and parallel to, the overlying microvillus border. Near the lateral surface of the cell, the filaments merge with those associated with the junctional complexes. Filaments of the microvilli and terminal web contribute to the cytoskeleton and give mobility to the microvillus border.

Mucosa

KEY WORDS: simple columnar epithelium, villi, intestinal glands

The intestinal mucosa consists of a **simple columnar epithelium**, a lamina propria and a muscularis mucosae. The numerous **villi** of the mucosal lining give a velvet-like appearance to the interior of the small intestine. Emptying between the bases of the villi, are numerous simple, tubular glands called **intestinal glands**. They measure 0.3 to 0.5 mm in depth and extend through the mucosa to the level of the muscularis mucosae, separated from one another by the connective tissue elements of the lamina propria. The intestinal glands contribute secretions to aid in the digestive process, but more importantly, they represent sites for the continual renewal of intestinal epithelial cells to replace those shed at the tips of villi.

Epithelial Lining

KEY WORDS: intestinal absorptive cells, striated border (microvilli), terminal bars, surface coat, goblet cells, endocrine cells, caveolated cells

The epithelium lining the intestinal lumen contains a heterogeneous population of simple columnar cells. The principal type is the **intestinal absorptive cell**. These are tall cylindrical cells that rest on a delicate basement membrane and show prominent

striated borders (**microvilli**) at their free surfaces. Prominent **terminal bars** unite the cells at their apices and desmosomes scattered along the lateral surfaces aid in holding the cells in close apposition. The microvilli that comprise the striated border are covered by a layer of glycoprotein which is elaborated by the intestinal epithelial cells. This glycoprotein layer, which has been termed the **surface coat**, is resistant both to mucolytic and proteolytic agents and is believed to have a protective function as well as being involved in the digestive process.

Although considerable digestion occurs in the intestinal lumen due to the presence of pancreatic enzymes and bile salts, a significant amount of digestive breakdown also occurs on the microvillus surface prior to absorption. Enzymes (disaccharidases, peptidases) that participate in the breakdown of disaccharides and polypeptides are found in or along the plasma membrane of the microvilli. In addition to contributing to the digestive process, the intestinal absorptive cells are actively involved in the absorption of protein, amino acids, carbohydrates and lipid from the intestinal lumen. Absorbed materials passing through the epithelium must enter the cell through the apical plasmalemma. Substances are prevented from entering between intestinal epithelial cells by the zonula occludens which forms a seal around the cell apices. Absorbed sugars and proteins pass through the basal cell membrane and into blood capillaries present in the connective tissue core of the villus.

Lipid absorption is peculiar, both in its pathway through the intestinal absorptive cell and in the fact that it enters lymphatic channels rather than the blood vascular system. Triglyceride is broken down to fatty acid and S-monoglyceride by pancreatic lipase in the intestinal lumen. After passage through the apical cell membrane, resynthesis of triglyceride occurs in the smooth endoplasmic reticulum of the apical cytoplasm. The reformed lipid makes its way to Golgi complexes, where it is complexed with protein to form the lipoprotein droplets known as chylomicrons. Chylomicrons are devoid of limiting membranes and are discharged laterally from the intestinal absorptive cells into the intercellular space at the level of the nucleus, thus bypassing the basal region. They pass down the intercellular spaces, through the basal lamina and enter lymphatic channels (lacteals) by passing between endothelial cells.

Goblet cells are scattered between the intestinal absorptive cells and increase in number distally in the intestinal tract. The mucus secreted by these unicellular apocrine glands serves to lubricate and protect the mucosal surface. The apical regions of goblet cells often are expanded by the accumulation of secretory granules. The base of the cell, on the other hand, is a slender region that contains the nucleus, scattered profiles of granular endoplasmic reticulum and occasional Golgi complexes. Goblet cells lie within the lining epithelium and are united to intestinal absorptive cells by apical tight junctions and by scattered desmosomes along the lateral surfaces.

Also scattered within the intestinal epithelium of both villi and glands are **endocrine cells**. The number of these cells is much less than that of the goblet cells. The endocrine cells secrete peptide hormones (Table 15-2 and Fig. 15-2) that influence gastric secretion, motility, gallbladder contraction and pancreatic function. They are characterized by dense secretory granules, scattered profiles of rough endoplasmic reticulum and an electron lucent cytoplasm.

Occasionally another cell type, the **caveolated cell**, can be seen. This is a pear-shaped cell with a wide base and a narrow apex that protrudes slightly into the lumen. They are held in close apposition to neighboring epithelial cells by tight junctions and desmosomes. Caveolated cells have large microvilli that are characterized by bundles of filaments which extend deep into the supranuclear region. Between the filamentous bundles small elongated channels, the caveolae, extend from the apical cell membrane between microvilli into the deep apical cytoplasm. This cell type is found elsewhere in the gastrointestinal tract and other organs of entodermal origin. They may serve as chemoreceptors in some regions, as in the respiratory system for example, but their function in the intestine is unknown.

Intestinal Glands

KEY WORDS: undifferentiated cells, oligomucous cells, Paneth cells, intraepithelial lymphocytes

Table 15.2.
Hormones and Related Substances of the Alimentary Canal

Hormone	Primary Location of Endocrine Cells	Primary Action
Gastrin	Antrum of stomach (G cell)	Stimulates acid secretion
Secretin	Duodenal and proximal jejunal mucosae (S cell)	Controls pancreatic H_2CO_3 secretion and biliary H_2O/ion secretion
Cholecystokinin (CCK)	Mucosae of duodenum and jejunum (I cell)	Stimulates pancreatic enzyme secretion, gallbladder contraction
Enteroglucagon	Mucosa of ileum (L cell) and fundus (A cell)	Stimulates hepatic glyconeogenesis
Gastric inhibitory peptide (GIP)	Mucosae of duodenum and jejunum (K cell)	Inhibits gastric acid secretion
Motilin	Mucosa of jejunum (one type of enterochromaffin cell, EC_2)	Strong stimulator of motor activity in gut
Vasoactive intestinal polypeptide (VIP)	Gastric, small intestinal and colonic mucosae (D_1 cell)	Stimulates gut motility, H_2O/ion secretion
Somatostatin	Mucosae of stomach, duodenum and jejunum (D cell)	Inhibits the action or release of other hormones (paracrine functions)
Neurotensin	Mucosa of ileum (N cell)	Stimulates contractions of muscularis externa
Serotonin	Mucosae of small intestine and colon (enterochromaffin (EC) cells)	Stimulates gut motility
Histamine	Fundic mucosa of stomach (enterochromaffin-like (ECL) cell)	Stimulates secretion and gut motility, and is a vasodilator
Bombesin-like peptide	Mucosae of stomach and jejunum (P cell)	Stimulates gastric acid secretion and exocrine pancreas secretion
Substance P	Gastric mucosa (EC_1 cell)	Stimulates gut motility

All epithelial cells that line the intestinal surface arise from cells in the intestinal glands. The upper regions of the glands are lined by a simple columnar epithelium similar to and continuous with that which lines the intestinal lumen. It contains absorptive cells, goblet cells, scattered endocrine cells and, on occasion, caveolated cells. **Undifferentiated cells** line the basal half of the intestinal glands and undergo frequent mitoses. Intestinal absorptive cells and **oligomucous cells,** which represent intermediate stages of goblet cell formation, lie in the midgland region. New intestinal epithelial cells are continually formed in the basal region of the intestinal glands, migrate by upward displacement of cells and ultimately come to cover the villi and line the entire intestinal lumen. The oldest intestinal epithelial cells are exfoliated at the tips of the villi. Complete turnover of epithelial cells in the upper half of the intestinal gland and lining of the intestinal lumen occurs every 4 to 5 days. As absorptive intestinal cells migrate up the villus, they increase in height and the striated border becomes a more prominent feature.

In addition to these cell types, small groups of pyramidal-shaped cells with conspicuous granules are found at the bottom of the intestinal glands. These are the **Paneth cells** which, unlike other cells of the intestinal epithelium, form a relatively stable population with only a low rate of turnover. Paneth cells are abundant in man, monkeys, ruminants and several species of rodents, but are absent in cats, dogs and raccoons. Their function is unknown.

Intraepithelial lymphocytes often are seen between and within intestinal epithelial cells that cover villi or line the glands.

Lamina Propria

KEY WORDS: special lymphoid tissue, lymphatic nodules, Peyer's patches, M cell, central lacteals

The connective tissue of the lamina propria forms the cores of the villi and fills the areas between intestinal glands. The intestinal lamina propria is rich in reticular fibers that form a delicate meshwork containing numerous reticular cells, lymphocytes, plasma cells, macrophages and eosinophils, giving the lamina propria a very cellular appearance. The lamina propria of the in-

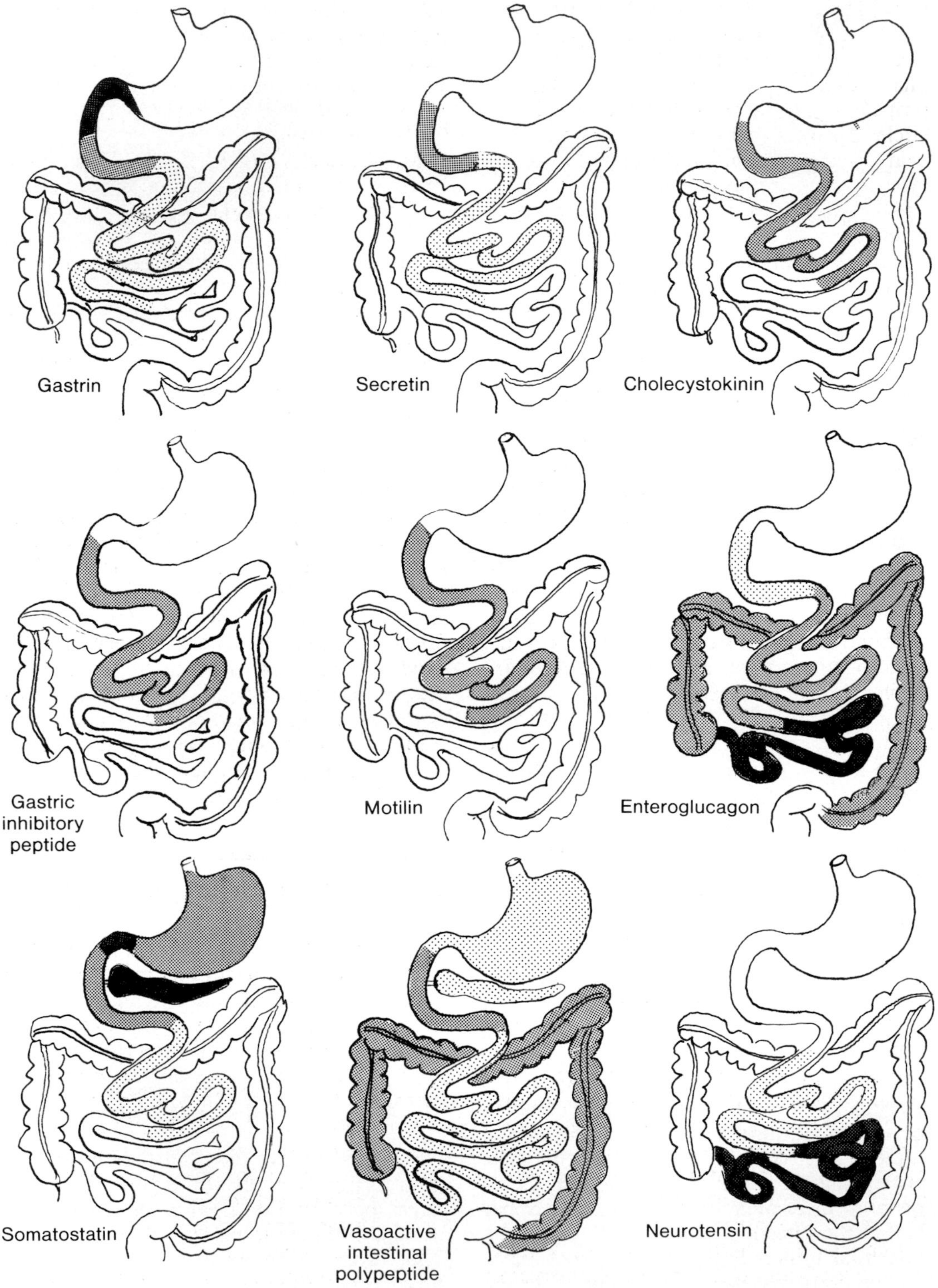

Figure 15.2. Distribution of endocrine cells in man.

testinal tract has been considered to represent a **special type of lymphoid tissue** and forms part of the GALT (gut-associated lymphatic tissue). The free cells of the lamina propria provide a protective sleeve that encircles the intestinal lumen immediately beneath the intestinal epithelium. Lymphocytes are the most numerous of the free cells and provide a vast reserve of immunocompetent cells. In addition, plasma cells elaborate an immunoglobulin which is taken up by intestinal absorptive cells. A protein (secretory piece) synthesized by the epithelial cells is attached to the immunoglobulin intracellularly and the complex is then secreted by the intestinal epithelial cells to provide the surface of the epithelium with a defensive immunological border against bacterial and viral invasion. Lymphocytes often leave the lamina propria and migrate through the overlying intestinal epithelium into the lumen.

Lymphatic nodules of variable size lie in the lamina propria and are scattered along the entire intestinal tract but become larger and more numerous distally. They are particularly numerous and well developed in the ileum and often extend the full thickness of the mucosa. The lymphatic nodules may be solitary or grouped together in aggregates called **Peyer's patches**. These oval structures may be quite large, 20 mm in length, and are visible to the naked eye. Peyer's patches may occupy the full depth of both the mucosa and submucosa.

A peculiar type of epithelial cell, the **M cell**, lies in the intestinal epithelium, where it covers lymphatic nodules. The cell is characterized by the presence of microplicae on its luminal surface, rather than microvilli. M-cells sequester intact macromolecules from the intestinal lumen and transport them in membrane-bound vesicles to intraepithelial lymphocytes. The sensitized lymphocytes then migrate to various aggregates of lymphatic tissue in the lamina propria or mesenteric lymph nodes, transporting information to the sites of antibody formation. The same lymphocyte may return to the lamina propria, where it originated, or may become a plasma cell. The M-cell provides a mechanism by which the immune system can maintain immunological surveillance of the environment of the gut lumen and respond appropriately to any changes. M-cell monitoring of the gut lumen is not unique. Langerhans cells of the epidermis perform a similar function in monitoring the external environment and relaying information to the immune system.

Small arteries which course on the inner surface of the muscularis mucosae break up into capillary networks that supply the intestinal glands. Other small arteries enter the cores of the villi, where they form a dense capillary network immediately beneath the intestinal epithelium. Near the tip of the villus, the capillaries drain into small veins that run downward to anastomose with a venous plexus surrounding the intestinal glands before joining veins in the submucosa.

Lymphatic vessels also are found in the lamina propria and are important in fat absorption. Dilated lymphatic channels begin blindly in the cores of villi near their tips and are referred to as **central lacteals**. Their walls consist of thin endothelial cells surrounded by a basal lamina and reticular fibers. At the bases of the villi, the lymphatic capillaries anastomose with those coursing between intestinal glands and form a plexus prior to passing through the muscularis mucosae. In the submucosa they join larger lymphatic vessels. Vessels that pierce the muscularis mucosae may contain valves.

Muscularis Mucosae

KEY WORDS: inner circular layer, outer longitudinal layer

This well-defined layer of the mucosa consists of **inner circular** and **outer longitudinal layers** of smooth muscle and is intimately associated with thin elastic fibers. Slips of smooth muscle leave the muscularis mucosae and enter the cores of villi to provide the means by which villi contract. Contraction of villi provides the intestinal epithelium covering the villi with a continuous, new environment for maximal absorptive efficiency during digestion. The pump-like action during contraction also aids in moving absorbed materials into the blood and lymphatic capillaries, out of vessels in the lamina propria and into the larger vessels of the submucosa, thereby aiding in the absorptive processes.

Submucosa

KEY WORDS: duodenal glands, branched tubular glands, urogastrone-epidermal growth factor, submucosal plexus

The submucosa consists of coarse collagenous fibers and numerous elastic fibers. It often contains lobules of adipose tissue as well as the cells normally associated with loose connective tissue. In the ileum it may contain large aggregates of lymphoid cells derived from Peyer's patches. The submucosa of the duodenum houses the **duodenal glands**, the ducts of which pierce the muscularis mucosae. In most marsupials, some insectivores and several ungulates (deer, pronghorn, moose, elk, bison, sheep), the ducts empty directly into the intestinal lumen. In all other species, including man, the glands drain into overlying intestinal glands. These **branched tubular glands** are first encountered immediately distal to the muscle mass of the pyloric sphincter and also may be observed in the proximal jejunum in some species. They often are found in the submucosal core of the plicae circulares. The duodenal glands are the only submucosal glands present in the gastrointestinal tract and are found only in mammals.

The glands consist of secretory cells with ultrastructural features of serous and mucous cells. In the rabbit, both serous and mucous cell types are present. The duodenal glands secrete a mucin-containing, alkaline fluid that protects the duodenal mucosa, proximal to entrance of the pancreatic duct, from the erosive effects of acid pepsin secreted by the stomach. Cells of the human duodenal glands show immunoreactivity for **urogastrone-epidermal growth factor**, a peptide which is a potent inhibitor of gastric acid secretion.

Nerve fibers and parasympathetic ganglia form the **submucosal plexus** found in the submucosa of the esophagus, stomach, small intestine and large intestine. This plexus provides motor innervation for the muscularis mucosae and the slips of smooth muscle that enter villi or other regions of the mucosa. Large blood and lymphatic vessels also are found within the submucosa. The large mesenteric vessels pierce the muscularis externa where it is attached to the mesentery, enter the submucosa, branch and run around the circumference of the intestinal tube. The submucosal vessels supply and receive small tributaries from the overlying mucosa.

Muscularis Externa

KEY WORDS: inner circular layer, outer longitudinal layer, myenteric plexus

The muscularis externa consists of **inner circular** and **outer longitudinal layers** of smooth muscle. Both layers take a helical course around the intestinal tract. The fibers in the outer layer form a more gradual helix, giving the impression of a longitudinal arrangement. Between the two layers of smooth muscle are nerve fibers and parasympathetic ganglia that constitute the **myenteric plexus**. This supplies the motor innervation to the muscularis externa of the entire gastrointestinal tract.

Serosa

The muscularis externa is invested by a thin layer of loose connective tissue covered by a layer of mesothelial cells from the peritoneum. At the point of attachment of the mesentery to the intestinal wall, the serosa becomes continuous with both sides of the mesentery and encloses connective tissue elements, blood vessels and nerves.

Ileocecal Junction

The lumen of the ileum becomes continuous with that of the large intestine at the ileocecal junction. Here the lining is thrown into anterior and posterior folds called the ileocecal valves which consist of both mucosa and submucosa and are surrounded by a thickening of the inner circular layer of the muscularis externa.

Large Intestine

The large intestine is approximately 180 cm in length and is subdivided into several regions. The cecum is continuous with the ileum at the ileocecal junction and forms a blind pouch at the proximal end of the colon. It bears the appendix, a small, slender, blind diverticulum of the cecum. The remainder of the colon is divided into ascending, transverse and descending parts, reflecting their anatomical locations. Structurally these show the same features. The large intestine is continuous with the rectum and anal canal, the latter terminating as the anus.

Mucosa

KEY WORDS: lacks villi, absorptive cells, goblet cells, fluid absorption, mucus secretion

The mucosa of the large intestine is **lacks villi** and has a smooth interior surface. The lumen is lined by a simple columnar epithelium which consists of intestinal **absorptive cells** and numerous **goblet cells**. The latter increase in number toward the rectum and in the distal regions of the colon. The epithelium consists primarily of goblet cells.

Intestinal glands of the colon are larger and more closely packed than those in the small intestine and increase in length distally to reach their maximum depth (0.7 mm) in the rectum. The glands contain numerous goblet cells and in the basal half of the glands, proliferating, undifferentiated epithelial cells and endocrine cells are present. Paneth cells usually are absent.

The composition of the lamina propria and muscularis mucosae is the same as that of the small intestine. Scattered lymphatic nodules are present and may protrude through the muscularis mucosae to lie in the submucosa.

Ingested material enters the cecum as a semifluid and becomes a semisolid in the colon. Although no digestive enzymes are secreted by the colon, some digestion does occur as a result of enzymes present in the developing fecal mass as well as through the action of the bacterial flora normally associated with the large intestine. The primary functions of the large intestine are the **absorption of fluid** and the **secretion of mucus** to protect the mucosa from abrasion by the developing fecal mass.

Submucosa

The submucosa of the large intestine is similar to that of the small intestine and contains the larger vessels and components of the nervous system (submucosal plexus). Glands are not present. As in the remainder of the digestive tube, blood vessels pierce the muscularis externa and course around the circumference of the intestinal wall. The large vessels supply tributaries which penetrate the muscularis mucosae to form capillary networks in the lamina propria around the intestinal glands and beneath the surface lining epithelium. The veins follow the same course as the arterial component.

Muscularis Externa

KEY WORDS: taenia coli, haustra, plicae semilunares

The outer longitudinal coat of the muscularis externa of the cecum and colon differs from that of the small intestine in that it forms three longitudinal bands, the **taenia coli**. Between the taenia, the muscle coat is thinner and may be incomplete. The inner circular layer is complete and appears similar to that of the small intestine. Components of the myenteric plexus lie just external to the circular layer as in the small intestine. Due to the tonus of the taenia coli, the wall of the colon is gathered into outward bulges, or **haustra**. Between the haustra are crescentic folds, the **plicae semilunares**, that project into the lumen of the colon.

Serosa

KEY WORDS: adventitia, appendices epiploicae

The serosa is incomplete in the colon and the ascending and descending limbs are retroperitoneal. Here the muscular wall of the colon is attached to adjacent structures by an **adventitia**. Where a serosa is present it may contain large, pendulous lobules of fat called **appendices epiploicae**.

Appendix

The structure of the appendix resembles that of the colon and cecum, but in miniature. The lumen is small and irregular in outline and taenia coli are absent. The lamina propria is extensively infiltrated with lymphocytes and details of the mucosa often are obscured by numerous lymphatic nodules which may occupy both the mucosa and the submucosa.

Rectoanal Junction

KEY WORDS: pectinate line, circumanal glands, rectal columns, anal valves, hemorrhoidal plexus, internal anal sphincter, external anal sphincter

The mucosa of the first portion of the rectum is similar to that of the colon, except that the intestinal glands are slightly longer and the lining epithelium is composed primarily of goblet cells. The distal 2 to 3 cm of the rectum forms the anal canal, which ends at the anus. Immediately proximal to the **pectinate line** the intestinal glands become shorter and finally disappear. At the pectinate line the simple columnar epithelium makes an abrupt transition to noncornified stratified squamous epithelium. Intestinal glands disappear distal to this junction. After a short transtitional zone, the noncornified squamous epithelium becomes continuous with the keratinized stratified squamous epithelium of the skin at the level of the external anal sphincter. Beneath the epithelium of this region are simple tubular, apocrine sweat glands, the **circumanal glands,** which secrete an oily material. Circumanal glands are well developed in some species, particularly during the breeding cycle.

The mucosa of the anal canal proximal to the pectinate line forms large longitudinal folds called **rectal columns** (columns of Morgagni). The distal ends of the rectal columns are united by transverse mucosal folds called **anal valves** and the recess above each valve is termed an anal sinus. It is at the level of the anal valves that the mucularis mucosae becomes discontinuous and disappears.

The submucosa of the anal canal contains numerous veins which form a large **hemorrhoidal plexus**. When distended or varicosed, these vessels protrude into the overlying mucosa and are referred to as internal hemorrhoids or piles. The inner circular layer of the muscularis externa increases in thickness at its termination and forms the **internal anal sphincter**, while the thin outer longitudinal layer breaks up and blends with the surrounding connective tissue of this region. Skeletal muscle fibers circumscribe the distal anal canal and constitute the **external anal sphincter**, which is under voluntary control.

LIVER

The liver is the largest organ in the body and lies in the upper abdominal cavity, immediately beneath the diaphragm on the right side. It is both an endocrine and an exocrine gland, releasing several substances directly into the blood stream and secreting bile into a duct system.

The liver is uniquely situated with respect to the venous blood flow from the gastrointestinal tract. Blood from the portal vein, which drains the gastrointestinal tract, passes through the substance of the liver before entering the systemic circulation. The liver, therefore, receives all of the materials absorbed by the gastrointestinal tract except lipids, which are transported by lymphatics to enter the general circulation. Tributaries of the portal vein empty into hepatic sinusoids that drain into the hepatic veins. The arrangement in the liver of a set of sinusoids between veins is referred to as the hepatic-portal system. The liver also has an arterial supply from the hepatic artery, and both the venous (portal) and arterial (hepatic) bloods percolate through the liver sinusoids and exit by way of the hepatic veins, which join the inferior vena cava for return to the heart.

Organization

KEY WORDS: capsule, hepatocytes, sinusoids, central vein, hepatic lobule, portal area, portal vein, hepatic artery, bile duct, lymphatic channel, liver acinus, portal lobule

The liver is invested by a delicate connective tissue **capsule** that is continuous with the peritoneum. The capsule contains numerous elastic fibers and is covered by a mesothelium, except for a small bare area where the liver abuts the diaphragm.

The liver is composed of epithelial cells, the **hepatocytes,** arranged in branching and anastomosing plates separated by blood **sinusoids**. Both form a radial pattern about a **central vein,** which is the smallest tributary of the hepatic vein. The spoke-like arrangement of hepatic plates about a central vein constitutes the basis of the classical **hepatic lobule**, which appears somewhat hexagonal in cross section with a central vein at the center and portal areas at the corners. The liver consists of about 1 million such units, each approximately 0.7 mm wide and 2.0 mm long.

A **portal area** contains a branch of the **portal vein**, a branch of the **hepatic artery**, a **bile duct** and occasionally a **lymphatic channel**. All are enclosed in a common investment of connective tissue. Blood passes from small branches of the hepatic artery and portal vein into the sinusoids that lie between the plates of hepatocytes. Blood flows slowly through the sinusoids toward the center of the lobule and leaves through the central vein. Hepatocytes nearest the branches of the portal vein and hepatic artery (i.e., at the periphery of the lobule) receive blood with the highest nutritive and oxygen content. Both diminish as blood flows toward the central vein. Due to this arrangement, three distinct zones can be recognized in an hepatic lobule according to their metabolic activity: a zone of permanent function at the periphery, a zone of intermittent activity near the center of the lobule and a zone of permanent repose around the central vein. In the pig, camel and raccoon, the classical lobule is bounded by a delicate connective tissue, but this limiting connective tissue is not observed in man. However, the boundaries of the hepatic lobule can be determined by observing the central vein and then noting the portal areas at the corners of the lobule.

Also related to the blood supply is a smaller unit of liver structure known as the liver acinus or functional unit. The **liver acinus** (Fig. 15-3) is defined as that hepatic tissue supplied by a terminal branch of the hepatic artery and portal vein and drained by a terminal branch of the bile duct. It is represented as a diamond-shaped area with central veins at opposite corners. Branches of the vessels and a branch of the bile duct lie between the two portions of adjacent hepatic lobules that they supply.

The **portal lobule** is centered about a portal canal and consists of the hepatic tissue drained by a bile duct of a portal area. The portal lobule is triangular in shape and contains portions of three adjacent hepatic lobules. A central vein is located at each corner of this unit.

A single layer of small, dark hepatocytes limits the liver parenchyma beneath the capsule and is called the *subcapsular limiting plate.* A similar wall of hepatic cells surrounds the portal areas and forms the periportal limiting plate, which is pierced by tributaries of the hepatic artery, portal vein and bile ductules.

Hepatic Sinusoids

KEY WORDS: discontinuous endothelium, fenestrations, perisinusoidal space, hepatic macrophage, Kupffer cell, lipocytes

Hepatic sinusoids are larger and more irregular in shape than ordinary capillaries. The sinusoidal lining consists of a simple layer of squamous epithelium supported by little if any connective tissue. Three types of cells usually are associated with the sinusoidal lining: endothelial cells, stellate cells

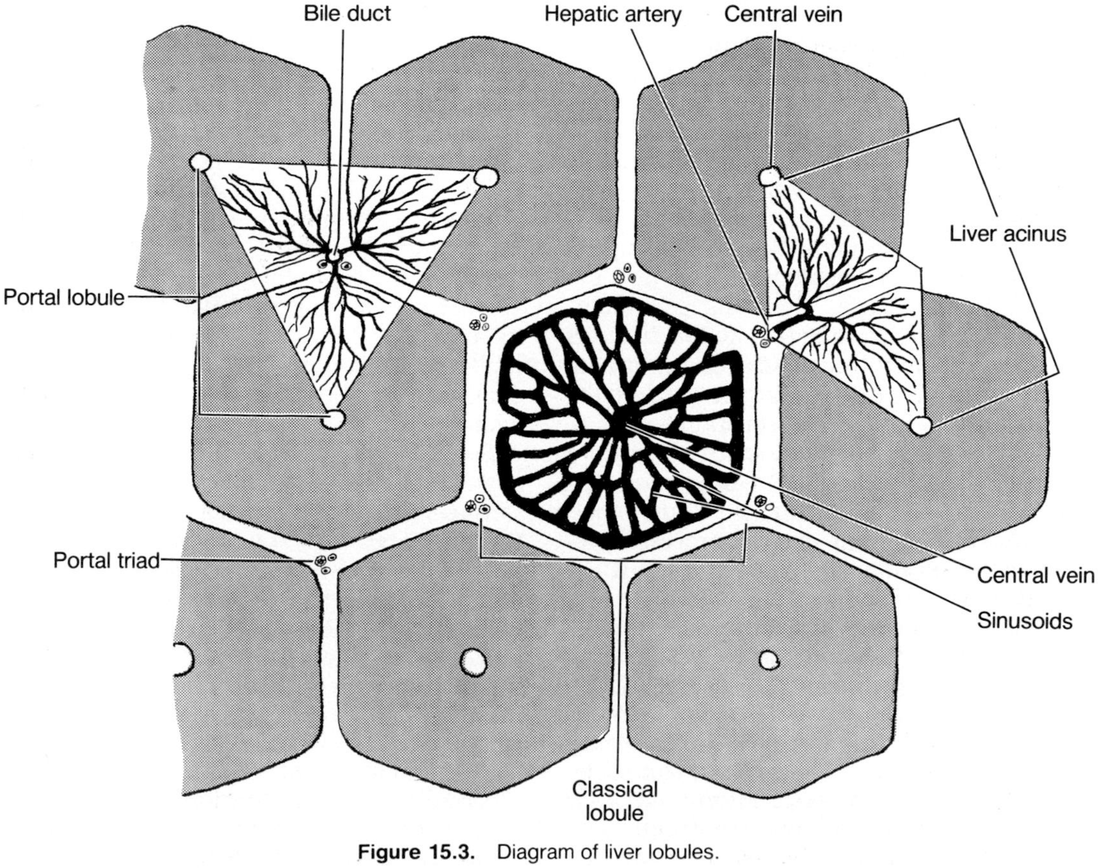

Figure 15.3. Diagram of liver lobules.

(Kupffer cells or hepatic macrophages) and fat-storing cells (lipocytes).

Endothelial cells constitute the major cellular element of the sinusoidal lining and in most species, including man, form a **discontinuous endothelium**. There is no basal lamina and the cells are separated by gaps 0.2 to 0.5 μm wide. The endothelial cells also show numerous intracellular **fenestrations** or pores. There are species differences in the structure of sinusoids and in sheep, goats and cows the endothelium is continuous; the endothelial cells show fewer fenestrations and there is a distinct basement membrane.

Where a discontinuous, fenestrated type of endothelium is present, the sinusoidal lining is separated from the liver cells by a narrow **perisinusoidal space.** Blood plasma flows freely through the endothelium and into the space, but the sinusoidal lining does hold back erythrocytes. Although occasional bundles of reticular fibers and fine collagenous fibers are present in the perisinusoidal space, it contains no ground substance and blood plasma moves freely through it. Because of the direct access of the blood plasma to the surface of hepatocytes, the liver cells are constantly bathed on one surface by plasma that is rich in nutrients absorbed by the gastrointestinal tract. Thus, the perisinusoidal space has considerable significance in the active exchange of nutrients between plasma and liver cells. The degree of activity is reflected in the modifications of the plasmalemma of the hepatocytes that face the perisinusoidal space. Here the cell membrane possesses numerous, well-developed microvilli that project into the perisinusoidal space and increase the surface area of the hepatocyte to facilitate absorption.

Also present in the sinusoidal lining are irregularly shaped cells that expose the greater part of their cytoplasm to the blood in the sinusoid and extend processes between the endothelial cells. This cell is actively phagocytic and is called a stellate cell, **hepatic macrophage** or **Kupffer cell**. Unlike the neighboring endothelial cells, their cytoplasm contains vacuoles, lysosomes, Golgi complexes and short profiles of granular endoplasmic reticulum; phagocytized material also may be present. The cells are part of the mononuclear macrophage system and arise from monocytes of the bone marrow.

The third cell type is located on the side of the sinusoidal lining facing the perisinusoidal space. This cell accumulates lipid and is most numerous in the peripheral and intermediate zones of the hepatic lobule. They have been called **lipocytes** (fat-storing cells, stellate cells or interstitial cells), but their functional significance is unknown.

Hepatocytes

KEY WORDS: polyploid, bile canaliculi

The parenchyma of the liver consists of large polyhedral hepatocytes arranged in plates that radiate from the region of the central vein. The surfaces of an individual hepatocyte either contact an adjacent hepatocyte or border on a perisinusoidal space. The latter surface shows numerous, well-developed microvilli. The plates of hepatocytes are supported by a delicate stroma that consists primarily of reticular fibers.

The nuclei are large, round and usually occupy a central position in the cell. Most cells have a single nucleus, but as many as 25% of the hepatocytes are binucleate. In addition, there is considerable cell-to-cell variation in the size of the nuclei, reflecting the **polyploid** nature of some of the hepatic cells.

The cytoplasm is rich in organelles: arrays of granular endoplasmic reticulum, a moderate amount of smooth endoplasmic reticulum, mitochondria, Golgi complexes, peroxisomes and lysosomes. Inclusions such as glycogen and lipid also are common. Glycogen often appears as dense rosettes called alpha particles, which are made up of smaller beta particles; these alpha particles measure 20 to 30 nm in diameter. The cytoplasm is variable in appearance and changes with the nutritive state of the organism.

Between adjacent hepatocytes are tiny channels, **bile canaliculi,** which course through the parenchyma and terminate in the bile ducts of the portal areas. Bile canaliculi represent an expansion of the intercellular space and their walls are formed by the adjacent cell membranes of two apposing hepatocytes. Short microvilli extend from the cell membranes into the lumen. The plasma membranes along the margins of a canaliculus are joined by occluding junctions similar to the zonula occludens in other epithelia. They form a seal which prevents bile from escaping into the intercellular space between hepatocytes. Golgi complexes of hepatic cells often lie immediately adjacent to the canaliculi. Bile canaliculi are capable of intermittent contraction.

Bile Ducts

KEY WORDS: bile ductules, interlobular bile ducts, extrahepatic ducts, common hepatic duct, common bile duct (ductus choledochus)

Bile canaliculi unite with bile ducts in the portal canals by small, interconnecting channels called terminal **bile ductules.** They are small, have thin walls and their small lumina are surrounded by a low cuboidal epithelium that rests on a distinct basal lamina. The terminal ductules empty into **interlobular bile ducts,** which are surrounded by the connective tissue of the portal area. The lumina of the bile ducts increase in diameter as they course toward the exterior and the lining epithelium increases in height. Interlobular ducts unite to form the **extrahepatic ducts**, the surrounding layers of connective tissue become thicker and the lining epithelium becomes tall columnar. Two large extrahepatic ducts, the left and right hepatic ducts, unite to form the major excretory duct of the liver, the **common hepatic duct**. It is joined by the cystic duct, which drains the gallbladder, to form the **common bile duct (ductus choledochus)**. The latter empties into the duodenum.

The major extrahepatic ducts are lined by a tall columnar, mucous-secreting epithelium. The remainder of the wall consists of a thick layer of connective tissue that is rich in elastic fibers and often contains numerous lymphocytes and occasional migrating granulocytes. Bundles of smooth muscle, running in longitudinal and oblique directions, are present in the common bile duct and form an incomplete layer around the lumen. Near the wall of the duodenum, the smooth muscle forms a complete investment and thickens to form a small sphincter, the sphincter choledochus. Distal to this region, the common bile duct and the major pancreatic duct merge as they pass through the intestinal wall and empty their contents through a common structure called the hepatopancreatic ampulla. As the ducts pass through the duodenal wall, they are surrounded by a common sphincter of smooth muscle.

Bile is produced continuously by the liver and ultimately leaves the organ through the extrahepatic duct system. Resistance at the sphincters forces bile to enter the cystic duct and pass into the gallbladder, where it is stored.

One of the functions of the liver is to store carbohydrate in the form of glycogen. When needed, glycogen is released into the bloodstream as glucose. The liver has functions in protein metabolism, fat metabolism and storage; in the synthesis of fibrinogen, prothrombin and albumin; is an important organ for the storage of several vitamins (primarily A, D, B_2, B_3, B_4 and B_{12}); and plays an important role in detoxifying lipid soluble drugs and alcohol. Detoxified materials are excreted by the hepatocytes into the bile and conducted via the biliary duct system to the intestinal tract for elimination. Bile is a complex exocrine secretion of the liver and contains bile acids, bile pigments, bile salts, cholesterol, lecithin, soaps and neutral fats. Bile salts act as emulsifying agents and are important in the breakdown of fat in the intestinal lumen during digestion. Some bile salts may be reabsorbed in the intestinal tract to be secreted once again into the bile. This reutilization of bile salts is referred to as the enterohepatic circulatory system.

Gallbladder

KEY WORDS: cystic duct, spiral valve, mucous membrane, simple columnar epithelium, muscularis, adventitia, serosa, cholecystokinin

The gallbladder is a blind, sac-like structure on the inferior surface of the liver approximately 4 cm wide and 8 cm long. It is connected to the common hepatic duct by the **cystic duct**, the mucous membrane of which forms prominent, spiraling folds that contain bundles of smooth muscle. These folds make up the **spiral valve,** which prevents the collapse or distention of the cystic duct during sudden changes in pressure. The wall of the gallbladder consists of a mucous membrane, a muscularis and a serosa or adventitia.

The **mucous membrane** consists of a **simple columnar epithelium** and an underlying lamina propria. The oval nuclei are located basally in the cells and the luminal surfaces show numerous short microvilli. The apices of adjacent cells are joined near the lumen by typical zonula occludens junctions. The epithelium rests on a thin basal lamina which separates it from the delicate connective tissue of the lamina propria. The latter contains numerous small blood vessels. Glands are found occasionally in the lamina propria, especially where the gallbladder joins the cystic duct. These small, simple tubuloalveolar glands are thought to secrete mucus. The mucosa of the nondistended gallbladder forms large irregular folds called rugae, which flatten out as the gallbladder fills with bile. The gallbladder has a considerable capacity for distention.

There is no submucosa. The **muscularis** consists of interlacing bundles of smooth muscle which spiral around the lumen of the gallbladder. Gaps between the smooth muscle bundles are filled with collagenous, reticular and elastic fibers.

The surrounding fibroconnective tissue of the **adventitia** is fairly dense and is continuous with the connective tissue of the liver capsule. The free surface of the gallbladder (the surface facing the abdominal cavity) is covered by a **serosa**.

The gallbladder stores and concentrates bile, which is elaborated continuously by the liver. In man the gallbladder may contain 30 to 50 ml of bile. Upon stimulation by **cholecystokinin** the gallbladder wall contracts and the sphincters of the common bile duct and ampulla relax, allowing bile to be released into the duodenum.

In some mammalian species, such as the white tailed deer and the rat, the gallbladder is absent.

PANCREAS

The pancreas is the second largest gland emptying into the gastrointestinal tract. In man it is a retroperitoneal organ about 20 to 25 cm long that extends transversely from the duodenum across the posterior abdominal wall to the spleen. Macroscopically it consists of a head that lies in the C-shaped curve of the duodenum, a slightly constricted neck and a body which forms the major part of the pancreas. It lacks a definite capsule but is covered by a thin layer of areolar connective tissue which extends delicate septae into the substance of the pancreas and subdivides it into numerous small lobules. Blood vessels, nerves, lymphatics and excretory ducts course through the septae. The major excretory duct runs the length of the pancreas in its center, collecting side branches along its course, and generally resembles a herringbone. The duct and its branches provide some structural support for the gland.

The pancreas consists of an exocrine portion, which elaborates numerous digestive enzymes, and an endocrine portion, whose secretions are important in carbohydrate metabolism. Unlike the liver, the exocrine and endocrine functions of the pancreas are performed by different groups of cells.

Exocrine Pancreas

KEY WORDS: compound tubuloacinar (alveolar) gland, pyramidal cells, zymogen granules, digestive enzymes, secretory capillaries

The exocrine pancreas is a large, lobulated, **compound tubuloacinar (alveolar) gland** in which the secretory units are tubular or flask-shaped. A delicate network of reticular fibers surrounds the individual secretory units and provides the supporting stroma. Each acinus consists of a single layer of large **pyramidal-shaped cells** whose narrow apices border on a lumen and broad bases lie on a thin basement membrane. The acinar cells contain a single, spherical nucleus near the base, and one or more nucleoli may be present. The basal and perinuclear cytoplasm is filled with granular endoplasmic reticulum and mitochondria. Extensive Golgi complexes occupy the supranuclear region and are associated with forming zymogen granules. Mature **zymogen granules** are large, spherical, homogenous structures that are limited by a membrane and often fill the apical cytoplasm. The pancreatic acinar cell, as indicated by its morphology, is actively involved in the synthesis and release of proteins (enzymes).

Digestive enzymes of the pancreas are synthesized in the granular endoplasmic reticulum of the acinar cell and pass through the cisternae of this organelle to reach the Golgi complex in small transport vesicles. Precursors of the enzymes are packaged into zymogen granules by membranes of the Golgi complex. The granules then are liberated into the apical cytoplasm, where they accumulate. During release, zymogen granules migrate to the apical cell membrane and discharge their contents into the acinar lumen by exocytosis. The granules also may discharge their contents into fine **secretory capillaries** that lie between adjacent acinar cells and are continuous with the central acinar lumen. Pancreatic acinar cells secrete amylases, lipases, endopeptidases (trypsin, chymotrypsin and elastases) which cleave central peptide bonds and exopeptidases (carboxypeptidases A and B) which cleave terminal peptide bonds. Together these proteolytic enzymes cleave proteins into peptide fragments in the intestinal lumen. The fragments then are reduced to their constituent amino acids prior to absorption.

Deoxyribonuclease and ribonuclease also are produced by pancreatic acinar cells and digest deoxyribonucleoprotein and ribonucleoprotein, respectively. Pancreatic amylase breaks down starch and glycogen to disaccharides, and pancreatic lipase hydrolyzes neutral fat into fatty acid and glycerol.

Duct System

KEY WORDS: centroacinar cells, intercalated duct, intralobular duct, interlobular duct, secretin, cholyecystokinin, enterokinase

An extensive duct system permeates the pancreas. At their beginnings, the ducts extend into acini and are interposed between acinar cells and the lumen. Ductal cells within the pancreatic acini are called **centroacinar cells** and appear as flattened, light-staining cells with few organelles. The wall of the short initial segment of the duct system is lined by centroacinar cells and pancreatic acinar cells and is continuous, outside the secretory unit, with the **intercalated** and **intralobular ducts**. These are tributaries of the **interlobular ducts** found in the loose connective tissue between lobules. The transition from one to the next is gradual. The epithelial lining begins as simple squamous in the intercalated ducts, increases in depth to cuboidal in the intralobular ducts and is columnar in the interlobular ducts. Scattered goblet and endocrine cells also are found in the ductal system. The cells lining the ducts stain lightly and organelles are not a prominent feature of their cytoplasm. Scattered desmosomes are present along the lateral cell surfaces and the apical surfaces bear microvilli. Adjoining cells are united by tight junctions at their apices.

A scanty connective tissue consisting primarily of reticular fibers supports the intercalated and intralobular ducts. The interlobular and major excretory ducts are contained within the interlobular septae and thus are surrounded by a considerable amount of fibroconnective tissue. The interlobular ducts drain into the primary and the accessory pancreatic ducts.

The primary duct courses the entire length of the pancreas and increases in size near the duodenum. Here it runs parallel to the ductus choledochus and often shares a common opening with the latter at the greater duodenal papilla. The openings of both ducts are controlled by the sphincter of the papilla. An accessory duct may lie proximal to the main duct and opens independently into the duodenal lumen. Secretion by the exocrine pancreas is influenced by eating and is under nervous and hormonal control. Two polypeptide hormones, secretin and cholecystokinin, are released from cells of the intestinal mucosa and influence pancreatic secretion.

Secretin elaborated by S-cell in the mucosae of the duodenum and proximal jejunum, stimulates the ductal system of the pancreas to secrete a large volume of fluid that is rich in bicarbonate. In the intestinal lumen, this alkaline secretion neutralizes the acid chyme from the stomach and thus deactivates the gastric enzyme pepsin whose optimal activity occurs at a low pH (2.0). It also establishes the neutral to alkaline environment that is needed for the optimal activity of the pancreatic enzymes.

Cholecystokinin (elaborated by the I-cell of the duodenal and jejunal mucosa) stimulates the secretory units of the pancreas to synthesize and release digestive enzymes. The proteolytic enzymes are secreted as inactive precursors (zymogens) which, in part, are converted to their active forms by an enzyme **enterokinase** from the intestinal mucosa. Pancreatic amylase and lipase are said to be secreted in their active forms. Cholecystokinin also stimulates the gallbladder to contract, thereby adding bile to aid in neutralizing the intestinal contents, and provides bile salts that act as emulsifying agents in the breakdown of neutral fats.

Endocrine Pancreas

KEY WORDS: pancreatic islets, alpha (A) cells, glucagon, beta (B) cells, insulin, delta (D) cells, somatostatin, PP cells, pancreatic polypeptide, exocytosis, fenestrated endothelium

Scattered between the elements of the exocrine pancreas are irregular, elongate masses of pale staining cells known as the **pancreatic islets.** They number approximately 1 million in man and constitute the endocrine portion of the pancreas. As with all endocrine glands, they have a rich vascular supply. The islets are incompletely separated from the surrounding exocrine pancreas by a delicate investment of reticular fibers. In ordinary tissue sections, the pancreatic islets appear to be composed of a homogeneous population of pale staining polygonal cells, but with special stains and in electron micrographs several distinct cell types have been identified (Table 15-3). The majority are alpha (A) and beta (B) cells.

Alpha (A) cells make up about 20% of the islets in man and generally are located at the periphery of the islet. They contain large, dense, spherical granules that are limited by a membrane. Mitochondria are long and slender with a typical internal structure. A few profiles of granular endoplasmic reticulum are scattered within the cytoplasm, and Golgi complexes usually are found near the nucleus.They contain secretory granules that measure about 250 nm in diameter. Alpha cells produce the peptide hormone **glucagon**, which elevates the level of blood sugar. These cells have been implicated in the production of gastric inhibitory peptide, CCK and ACTH-endorphin also.

Beta (B) cells constitute about 78% of the cells of islets and tend to be located near the center of the islet. The secretory granules are smaller than those in alpha cells and show species differences. In man, bat and dog, beta cell granules contain small dense crystals that give them a distinctive appearance. In other species the central cores of B cells vary in shape, through plates, spheres or rosettes. The granular endoplasmic reticulum of beta cells is less extensive and the Golgi complexes are more prominent than in alpha cells. Beta cells produce **insulin**, which acts on the plasmalemma of various cell types (particularly liver, muscle and fat cells) to facilitate the entry of glucose into the cells. The net effect of the movement of blood glucose into cells results in a lowering of the blood glucose level. Insulin also stimulates pancreatic acinar cells.

Several other endocrine cell types are present in small numbers in the islets. The hormone **somatostatin** is secreted by **delta (D) cells** and inhibits hormone secretion by surrounding endocrine cells. **Pancreatic polypeptide** is a hormone secreted by PP cells, and opposes the action of CCK and inhibits pancreatic acinar secretion. Endocrine cells of the types found in the islets (including alpha and beta cells) also are found scattered within the ducts and acini of the exocrine pancreas. The relative numbers of the different endocrine cells may vary according to their locations in the head or body of the pancreas and may relate to the different origins of these two parts. There also is a considerable species variation in the distribution of cells within the islets. In man and most rodents, beta cells tend to be located centrally, while A, D and PP cells are concentrated at the periphery of the islets. A and D cells tend to make up a central location in the islets of the horse and monkey, whereas in teleost fishes and dogs, the various cell types are randomly distributed throughout the islet.

Islet cells are intimately associated with

Table 15.3.
Endocrine Cells of the Pancreas

Lausanne Classification of Cell Types (1977)	Hormonal Substance	Primary Function
A (alpha) cell	Glucagon	Increases blood sugar
B (beta) cell	Insulin	Decreases blood sugar
D cell	Somatostatin	Inhibitor of hormone secretion (paracrine function)[a]
PP cell	Pancreatic polypeptide	Opposes action of CCK
D_4 cell	Vasoactive intestinal peptide (VIP)	Increases blood sugar (vasodilator)
EC cell	Serotonin	Vasoactive agent
	Substance P	Increases motility of gut
	Motilin	Increases motility of gut
G cell[b]	Gastrin	Increases HCl secretion in stomach

[a] Paracrine function. Secretion of somatostatin is directly into the intercellular space from which it diffuses to inhibit the secretion of adjacent endocrine cells.

[b] G cells are present only in some species or restricted to fetal life in others.

surrounding capillaries and their secretory granules often appear to be located near the cell membrane that is adjacent to the vasculature. Secretory granules are released from islet cells by **exocytosis** into the surrounding blood vessels. The capillary endothelium of the islets contains numerous **fenestrations** to facilitate the entry of secretory products into the vasculature. In contrast, the capillary endothelium of the exocrine pancreas generally is not fenestrated.

A significant proportion of the arterial blood enters the pancreas via small inter- and intralobular arteries that first supply the islets. Arterioles derived from these arteries give rise to capillaries at the periphery of the islets, in the region of the alpha, delta and PP cells. The capillaries then run centrally within the islet and then from the islet to supply adjacent acinar cells of the exocrine pancreas. Thus, the islet cells can interact with each other and also influence the functions of the exocrine portion of the pancreas.

DEVELOPMENT OF THE DIGESTIVE SYSTEM

When the three germ layers have formed, the embryo appears as a flattened disk with the yolk sac extending from its ventral surface. This surface of the embryo and the interior of the yolk sac are covered by endoderm which forms the lining for the entire digestive tract. With further development, the embryo and gut endoderm fold to form a cylinder. Folding begins at the ends of the embryo, creating two blind endodermal tubes, both of which are continuous with the lumen of the yolk sac at an area called the intestinal portal. The proximal endodermal tube forms the foregut, which gives rise to the oral cavity, pharynx, stomach and proximal duodenum. The midgut is that part which communicates with the yolk sac and from it the jejunum, ileum, cecum, appendix, and ascending and part of the transverse colon form. The caudal tube becomes the hindgut, which differentiates into the rest of the large intestine.

ORAL CAVITY

Lips. The lips begin as a thickened band, the labial lamina, that grows from the ectoderm over the primitive jaw, into the underlying mesenchyme. The labial lamina thickens then, as the central cells degenerate, splits to form the lips and gums. The cheeks arise by fusion of the upper and lower lips at their lateral angles, thus reducing the original broad mouth opening. Skeletal muscles of the lips and cheek arise from mesenchyme that migrates from the second branchial arch to lie between mucosal and epidermal coverings.

Tongue. The tongue arises from the ventral ends of the branchial arches. An ectoderm-covered oral part from the mandibular arches forms the body of the tongue; an endodermal pharyngeal part from the second branchial arch gives rise to the rest of the tongue. The junction between ectoderm and endoderm is just anterior to sulcus terminalis. Thus, fungiform and filiform papillae are ectodermal; the circumvallate papillae is endodermal in origin. At first the tongue is covered by a cuboidal epithelium which later becomes stratified squamous.

All papillae initially form as elevations of the mucosa. A thickened epithelial ring surrounds each circumvallate papilla, grows into the mesenchyme and splits to form a trench around each papilla. Solid epithelial cords that grow from the bottom of the trench give rise to the glands of von Ebner. Taste buds develop on the dome of each early circumvallate papilla, but are replaced by definitive buds along the sides of the papilla. Taste buds appear as local thickenings of epithelium in which basal cells elongate, grow toward the surface and give rise to supporting and taste cells.

Salivary Glands. The major and minor salivary glands are considered to arise from ectoderm. All begin as epithelial buds that grow and branch, tree-like, to form a system of solid ducts. Terminal twigs, which eventually form intercalated ducts, round out at their ends to form secretory tubules and acini. Canalization of the ducts follows. The sublingual gland differs slightly, in that a series of buds develop from the oral epithelium and each remains a discrete gland. In most species the parotid appears first, followed by the submandibular, sublingual and, still later, by the minor glands. Mesenchyme surrounding the epithelial primordia provides the capsule and septae of the larger glands.

At birth, the submandibular gland of the cat is not fully differentiated and in mice, rats and hamsters acini are lacking and glandular development is not complete until maturity. In the opossum submandibular and pig parotid glands, maturation of ducts precedes that of acinar cells, whereas in the submandibular glands of rats and mice, the converse is true.

Teeth. The teeth have a dual origin: enamel arises from ectoderm, dentin, pulp and cementum from mesoderm. Tooth development begins with the appearance of the dental lamina, a plate of epithelium on which knob-like swellings (enamel organs) appear at intervals. These give rise to enamel and also act as molds for tooth development. The enamel organs grow into the mesenchyme, forming inverted, cup-like structures invaginated at the bases by dental papillae. The latter are condensations of mesenchyme that give rise to the dentin and pulp of the teeth. The enamel organ forms a double-walled sac, of which the outer and inner walls differentiate into outer and inner enamel layers, respectively. Loosely arranged cells, the enamel pulp, lie between the two layers. Cells of the inner layer become ameloblasts and produce enamel prisms, beginning at the interface with the dental papilla. Mesenchymal cells of the papilla adjacent to the inner dental layer enlarge and differentiate into odontoblasts. These form a single layer of columnar cells whose apices face the ameloblasts. Odontoblasts produce predentin that soon calcifies to become definitive dentin. Mesenchyme central to the odontoblasts forms the dental pulp.

Dentin is the first of the hard tissues to appear in the tooth. Thereafter, both enamel and dentin are laid down, beginning at the apex and progressing toward the root. As the enamel and dentinal layers thicken, the odontoblasts and ameloblasts gradually move away from each other. Ameloblasts migrate peripherally, remaining at the outer surface of the enamel, and eventually are lost from the tooth at eruption. Odontoblasts move centrally into the pulp cavity, where they persist. As odontoblasts retreat, they trail fine processes extending through the dentin to the dentinoenamel junction. The entrapped processes are the dentinal fibers contained in fine dentinal tubules.

Mesenchyme around the developing enamel organ differentiates into the loose connective tissue of the dentinal sac. Near the root, the inner cells of the sac become cementoblasts and cover the dentin with cementum. Cells at the exterior of the sac differentiate to produce the alveolar bone that surrounds each tooth. The connective tissue between the external and internal layers of the dental sac gives rise to the periodontal membrane.

Prior to eruption of a tooth, a small crater forms in the gingival epithelium and connective tissue, immediately above the crown. The crater, which expands to accommodate the tooth as it emerges, develops either from focal pressure necrosis as the tooth grows upward, or by means of lytic activity of enzymes produced by the dental epithelium, or both.

DIGESTIVE TUBE

The esophagus, stomach, small intestine and colon initially consist of an endodermal tube surrounded by a layer of splanchnic mesoderm. The endoderm gives rise to the lining epithelium and all associated glands of the digestive tube; mesoderm differentiates into the supporting layers of the gut tube.

Esophagus. The esophagus begins as a short tube connecting the pharynx and stomach. As the neck region and thorax develop, the tube elongates. Initially, the esophagus is lined by simple columnar epithelium which gradually becomes stratified and thickens but unlike birds and reptiles, in mammals the esophagus does not become occluded. Ciliated columnar and occasional goblet cells appear among the squamous cells. In chickens, turkeys, guinea fowl, pigeons, opossum, rats and man, ciliated cells persist only until hatching or birth, whereas in frogs and other amphibians, cilia are retained even in the adult. In man, opossums and carnivores the lining remains a wet, nonkeratinized stratified squamous epithelium, but in rodents and ruminants it becomes cornified.

The first glands to appear are the esophageal cardiac glands, followed by the esophageal glands proper, which continue to develop postnatally. Outgrowths at the base of the epithelium give rise to the ductal system of the glands; the secreting units arise from terminal branches of the ducts.

Stomach. The stomach first appears as a fusiform expansion of the foregut lined by a simple or pseudostratified columnar epithelium of endodermal origin. It may remain simple or, as in rodents, become stratified. Gastric pits arise as simple invaginations of the surface epithelium into underlying mesenchyme. In man, the pits form first along the lesser curvature, then gradually in other regions and, about 3 weeks later, in the pyloric and cardiac areas. Soon after the pits form, oxyntic glands develop, arising from epithelial buds at the bases of the pits. Pyloric and cardiac glands develop similarly but later than oxyntic glands. In species with a forestomach (rodents) or ruminant type of stomach, cornification of the lining epithelium usually occurs before birth.

Intestinal Tract. Development of the intestine and the appearance of villi, glands and the various cell types follows a proximal to distal progression. The intestinal tract begins as a simple, endodermal tube extending from stomach to cloaca. As the intestine elongates, a caudal outgrowth indicates the initial development of the cecum from which the appendix arises as the result of extremely rapid growth at the blind end. In the duodenum, a rapid proliferation of cells in the epithelial lining temporarily occludes the lumen. Later, vacuoles appear in the epithelium, coalesce and restore patency to the lumen. To a lesser degree, similar events occur in the remainder of the small intestine and colon. The lining epithelium is now four to five cells thick, has smooth luminal and basal surfaces and lies on a distinct basement membrane. The underlying mesenchyme has not separated into lamina propria and submucosa.

Proliferation of the epithelium, together with invaginations of the mesenchyme, produces folds or ridges in the mucosa, and as they increase in number, the luminal border becomes irregular. The first villi arise from breakup of these mucosal ridges, and since some folds are covered by stratified cuboidal and others by simple columnar epithelium that covers the forming villi, these villi vary in thickness. Subsequently, new villi form as simple evaginations of epithelium and connective tissue, without formation of mucosal folds. Villi that develop in the colon, cecum and appendix disappear in the second half of fetal life.

Intestinal glands develop as simple tubular downgrowths of the epithelium between villi. Duodenal glands arise from outgrowths of epithelium on the intestinal floor between villi, or from intestinal glands, depending on species.

As villi form, myoblasts differentiate in the mesenchyme to establish the muscularis mucosae. At this time the epithelium is simple columnar and goblet and enteroendocrine cells develop in a proximal-caudal progression; Paneth cells are one of the last cells to appear. The muscularis externa arises before the muscularis mucosae, with the inner coat being established first. Its formation involves differentation and proliferation of smooth muscle from mesenchyme, followed by hypertrophy. Hypertrophy accounts for most of the final increase in thickness of the muscle coat. Plicae circulares form late in man, long after villi have developed.

In most postnatal animals, a well-developed endocytic complex is present in the epithelium cells, covering the villi in the distal ileum. The complex, which usually persists until weaning, consists of numerous vesicles and tubules formed by invaginations of the cell membrane between microvilli. These connect with inclusion-containing vacuoles of various sizes in the supranuclear cytoplasm. The complex is implicated in absorption of macromolecules.

Liver. The liver primordium begins as a thickening of endodermal epithelium in the anterior intestinal portal (future duodenum) of the developing gut wall. A hollow ventral outgrowth appears, lined by a simple columnar epithelium that is continuous with the duodenal lining. This hepatic diverticulum enlarges, grows into the vascular mesenchyme of the septum transversum and then divides. A large cranial portion differentiates into the hepatic parenchyma and associated intrahepatic bile ducts; a small caudal part forms the common bile duct, cystic duct, gallbladder and interhepatic bile ducts. The surrounding mesenchyme forms the capsule and stroma.

At first the hepatic cells are small, irregular in shape and usually contain numerous lipid droplets. They may form an irregular network of cords, separated by islands of hemopoeitic cells, but there is little organization into plates, and sinusoids are not clearly defined. As differentiation proceeds, irregular plates of cells form, extending from the central veins toward the periphery of each forming lobule, and sinusoids become apparent. Early liver growth results mainly from hyperplasia but in some species, hypertrophy also occurs. Lipid is lost from hepatocytes; hemopoeitic activity wanes and finally ceases before or shortly after birth.

Bile canaliculi first appear at 6 weeks in the human embryo, before bile secretion begins. During the next 3 to 4 weeks, the rest of the intrahepatic biliary system forms from hepatocytes near the limiting plates of the lobules. These then connect with interlobular ducts in the portal areas.

The caudal part of the hepatic diverticulum soon becomes a solid cord of cells that gives rise to the cystic duct and gallbladder. Epithelial cords (and blood vessels) grow into the connective tissue between lobules and differentiate into hepatic ducts that unite with the bile ductules; how the two join is unknown.

Pancreas. The pancreas develops from endodermal evaginations of the gut wall in two separate locations on opposite sides of the duodenum. These form the ventral and dorsal pancreatic buds, which fuse after the ventral bud has migrated dorsally. The major excretory duct develops in the ventral bud; the accessory duct arises in the dorsal bud. The parenchyma at first consists of a series of blind tubes of simple columnar epithelium that branch and expand into the surrounding mesenchyme. Acini form at the ends of the smallest ducts, but some also arise as paratubular buds from larger ducts. As ducts and acini form, lobes and lobules gradually take shape, limited by the surrounding connective tissue. Some acinar cells expand proximally along the duct, and some of the terminal ductal cells become incorporated into the acini as centroacinar cells. Further increase in acinar cells occurs mainly by division of differentiated cells and may extend into late postnatal life.

Simultaneously, islet cells differentiate from endodermally-derived progenitor cells within the ductal system. Most islets develop at the ends of the ducts but paratubular outgrowths also occur. As ducts and acini continue to develop near the periphery of the lobules, the previously-formed islets come to be more centrally placed in the lobules: these are the secondary islets. Many islets retain their connections with the ductal epithelium from which they arose but as the exocrine parenchyma increases, continuity of islet and duct is obscured. A few primary islets are found outside the lobule, within the interlobular connective tissue. These represent the first endocrine cells to differentiate from the first tubules, prior to the formation of smaller ducts and acini. Isolated cells or small groups of endocrine cells remain scattered along the ductal system or occur between acinar cells even in the adult.

FUNCTIONAL SUMMARY

The digestive system is morphologically and physiologically adapted to break down ingested materials to their basic constituents, which then are absorbed and used by the organism. The process of mechanical and chemical breakdown of food substances is referred to as digestion.

The oral cavity is specialized to take in food which is then mechanically broken down by the grinding and cutting action of the teeth. The pulverized food is moistened and softened by secretions from the major and minor salivary glands. Digestion of carbohydrates is initiated in the oral cavity by the enzymes amylase and maltase, which are secretory products of the major salivary glands. The chemical breakdown of carbohydrates is short-lived, however, as both enzymes are destroyed by the acid environment of the stomach. Salivary gland secretion also

moistens and cleanses the oral cavity, provides a proper environment for taste and serves as a vehicle to transport heavy metals out of the body. It also initiates the sensation of thirst during dehydration when salivary gland secretion decreases and, therefore, is a factor in maintaining fluid balance. The stratified squamous epithelium that lines the oral cavity protects the underlying structures from abrasion during eating. In regions subjected to excessive abrasion, such as the gingiva and hard palate, the epithelium is cornified.

The tongue is important for chewing and swallowing. In many species (cow, anteater) it functions in the gathering of food. The interior of the tongue, cheek and lips consists of skeletal muscle and is under voluntary control. All three serve to direct food to the teeth during mastication and also provide the needed voluntary control during suckling and speech.

The mixture of saliva and ground food is formed into a semisolid mass called a bolus which, when of the proper consistency, is swallowed. Saliva is important for this activity also and swallowing is difficult, if not impossible, in the absence of moisture in the mouth. During the initial stage of swallowing, the bolus is directed into the oropharynx by several simultaneous, coordinated events. The anterior portion of the tongue is pressed firmly against the hard palate and, simultaneously, the base of the tongue is retracted. Bone in the hard palate provides a rigid platform against which the tongue can press, and prevents collapse of the palate due to pressure exerted against it during swallowing. Formation of a mucoperiosteum prevents sliding and tearing of the mucosa covering the palate. As these events occur, the larynx and pharynx are elevated to receive the bolus. Skeletal muscles associated with the soft palate contract, moving the soft palate upward to seal off the oropharynx and prevent food from entering the nasopharynx and nose. As the pharynx is elevated, its lumen dilates to receive the bolus from the oral cavity. Simultaneously, the musculature of the larynx contracts, closing the entrance to the respiratory tree. Skeletal muscle fibers of the three surrounding constrictor muscles of the pharynx contract about the entering bolus and quickly force it into the upper esophagus.

Skeletal muscle fibers of the upper esophagus are fast-acting and their contraction transports the bolus of food into the central region of the esophagus. Here there is a gradual transition to slow-acting smooth muscle in the muscularis externa. Peristaltic waves are formed by the smooth muscle in the distal one-half of the esophagus and move the bolus into the stomach. Because of the peristaltic movements, materials from the esophagus enter the stomach in spurts. The interior of the esophagus of man is lined by a wet, stratified squamous epithelium which, as in the oral cavity, protects the surrounding structures from the abrasive action of materials as they pass through the lumen. The primary function of the esophagus is to transport food from the oral cavity to the stomach. It secondarily functions to warm or cool ingested materials.

In the stomach the smooth muscle layers of the muscularis externa are so arranged that during contraction, the luminal contents are subjected to a churning action which promotes further mechanical breakdown of food materials. Protein is broken down chemically by pepsin, an endopeptidase which cleaves peptide linkages near the center of the protein molecules. In addition to elaborating hydrochloric acid and pepsin, the gastric mucosa secretes a considerable amount of fluid (approximately 1000 ml of gastric juice after each meal in man). Most of this fluid is reabsorbed in the intestinal tract. In man, the parietal cells also secrete gastric intrinsic factor, which binds to vitamin B_{12}. This complex is then absorbed in the intestine. Vitamin B_{12} is important in erythropoiesis. If gastric intrinsic factor is not produced or present in sufficient quantity, much of the vitamin B_{12} passes through the intestinal tract to be lost in the feces and pernicious anemia results. The gastric mucosa of many suckling mammals also produces rennin, an enzyme that curdles milk, and a gastric lipase which begins the digestion of fat.

The contents of the proximal stomach are semisolid, whereas those in the distal region form a pulp-like, fluid mass called chyme. After reaching the proper consistency, chyme enters the duodenum in small portions. The pyloric sphincter aids in controlling the evacuation of the stomach.

The lining epithelium of the stomach is simple columnar and forms a glandular sheet that secretes a neutral mucin. The epithelium and its secretion protect the stomach from the erosive effects of acid pepsin in the gastric lumen. The mucous secretions of the cardiac and pyloric glands contribute to the protection of the mucosa, where the stomach joins the esophagus and duodenum, respectively. Gastrin-producing endocrine cells are present in large numbers in the pyloric glands and their secretion, gastrin, stimulates acid secretion and gastric motility. Because of the large population of G cells, the pyloric region is not merely a mucus-secreting area, but assumes the status of an endocrine organ. The function and specific identity of endocrine cells in the cardia is unknown.

As the acid chyme enters the duodenum it is again subject to a change in pH. Duodenal glands secrete an alkaline fluid, rich in glycoprotein that protects the proximal duodenal mucosa from insult by acid pepsin from the stomach. The alkaline exocrine secretions of the pancreas and liver elevate the pH to neutral or alkaline and provide an environment optimal for the activities of digestive enzymes secreted by the pancreas. In doing so, the proteolytic enzyme of the stomach, pepsin, is deactivated. Bile salts also are added to the intestinal contents and act as detergents or emulsifying agents to aid in the digestion of fats by pancreatic lipase. Most of the digestive process takes place in the intestinal lumen. The final breakdown of the digested materials to their basic constituents—amino acids, monosugars, monoglycerides and fatty acids—occurs on the luminal surface of the intestinal epithelial cells immediately prior to absorption.

The architecture of the intestinal wall is not specialized for digestion but for absorption of digested materials. Three modifications plicae circulares, villi and microvilli, greatly increase the luminal surface area and facilitate absorption. The efficiency of absorption is further increased by the active movement of villi and by segmental movement of the luminal contents due to the contractions of the muscularis externa. The latter moves intestinal contents back and forth in the intestinal lumen. In addition, peristaltic waves of the muscularis externa move the contents through the lumen of the intestinal tract and along the remainder of the alimentary canal. As materials are absorbed along the intestinal tract, the luminal contents become more concentrated. Correspondingly, there is an increase in the number of goblet cells distally in the small intestine and these provide mucus to lubricate the intestinal mucosa.

Goblet cells are one of the most numerous of the cell types present in the colon and they continue to increase in number towards the rectum. Villi are absent, but intestinal glands remain a prominent feature of the mucosa. The primary function of the colon is the absorption of the fluid remaining in the luminal contents. As the fecal mass develops in the colon, secretion from the large population of goblet cells provides the lubrication necessary to prevent mucosal damage as feces pass through the colon. In the upper rectum the lining epithelium is made up primarily of goblet cells.

The anal canal is lined by a wet stratified squamous epithelium which protects this region from the abrasive effects of the fecal mass during defecation. Smooth muscle of the inner circular layer of the muscularis externa forms the internal anal sphincter and the surrounding skeletal muscle fibers adjacent to the anal orifice form the external anal sphincter, which is under voluntary nervous control.

The organism is protected from a vast, ever present population of microorganisms in the intestinal lumen, by immunoglobulins that form a barrier against bacterial and viral invasion. This barrier is the joint product of the intestinal epithelial cells and the lymphoid cells in the lamina propria. Together with phagocytes, they provide a protective sleeve around the intestinal lumen.

From its exocrine portion, the pancreas provides enzymes that digest carbohydrates, proteins and lipids. The endocrine portion secretes insulin and glucogen, hormones that are instrumental in regulating blood glucose levels, the flow of glucose across cell membranes and glyconeogenesis in the liver. Carbohydrate is stored by the liver as glycogen, which can be released into the blood stream as glucose. This organ also contributes bile salts for the emulsification of fats during digestion, plays an important role in detoxification and supplies proteins that are important in blood coagulation.

The endocrine cells of the gastrointestinal mucosa produce hormones which influence or control gastric secretions, gastrointestinal motility, gastric emptying, gallbladder contraction and pancreatic secretions. How specific gastrointestinal hormones interact with one another or are influenced by other major endocrine organs is unknown at the present time.

Atlas and Table of Key Features for Chapter 15

Table 15.4.
Key Histological Features of the Digestive Tract

	Epithelium	Muscularis Mucosae	Muscularis Externa	Lymphatic Tissue	Glands
Esophagus	Stratified squamous nonkeratinizing	Prominent: longitudinal smooth muscle	Outer longitudinal, inner circular layers. Skeletal in upper one-quarter, mixed in middle one-quarter, smooth in lower one-half	Few nodules, diffuse in lamina propria	1. Esophageal proper, scattered along length of esophagus in submucosa, compound tubuloalveolar, mucus-secreting 2. Esophageal cardiac, proximal and distal ends in lamina propria. Compound tubuloalveolar, mucous-secreting
Stomach					
Cardia	Simple columnar (gastric lining)	Smooth muscle; inner circular, outer longitudinal; a third outer circular layer in some areas	Outer longitudinal, middle circular, inner oblique smooth muscle	Small patches of diffuse lymphatic tissue: rare nodules	Long pits (one-half the depth of mucosa); simple branched tubular; mucous, endocrine, and occasional parietal cells
Fundus	Gastric lining epithelium	Same	Same	Same	Short pits (one-quarter the depth of the mucosa): simple branched tubular; mucous neck, parietal, chief, and endocrine cells
Pylorus	Gastric lining epithelium	Inner circular, outer longitudinal smooth muscle	Same	Occasional small lymphatic nodules in lamina propria	Long pits (one-half the depth of mucosa): simple branched tubular; mucous, occasional parietal and endocrine cells (G cells)
Duodenum	Villi covered by simple columnar absorptive cells with microvillus border: goblet and endocrine cells	Inner circular, outer longitudinal smooth muscle	Inner circular, outer longitudinal smooth muscle. Myenteric plexus between layers	Solitary nodules and diffuse lymphatic tissue	1. Intestinal glands in lamina propria. Simple tubular; absorptive; goblet cells; endocrine and Paneth cells 2. Brunner's glands in submucosa; branched tubular

Small intestine	Villi covered by simple columnar absorptive cells: goblet cells increase in number from upper to lower; endocrine cells present	Same	Same	Nodular lymphatic tissue forms aggregates (Peyers's patches) in ileum	Intestinal glands. Same as for duodenum
Colon	Villi absent. Simple columnar absorptive cells; goblet cells increase in number	Same	Outer longitudinal layer condensed into 3 bands—taenia coli	Solitary nodules and diffuse lymphatic tissue	Intestinal glands: goblet, endocrine and absorptive cells. Paneth cells absent
Rectum	Simple columnar; mainly goblet cells	Same	Inner circular and outer longitudinal	Solitary nodules	Intestinal glands: goblet cells more abundant
Anal canal	At pectinate line becomes stratified squamous, noncornified, then stratified squamous cornified at orifice	Disappears at level of anal columns	Inner circular layer thickens to form internal sphincter. Outer longitudinal layer disappears	Solitary lymphatic nodules	1. Intestinal glands disappear at pectinate line 2. Apocrine sweat glands (circumanal glands)

15-4 Oral Cavity

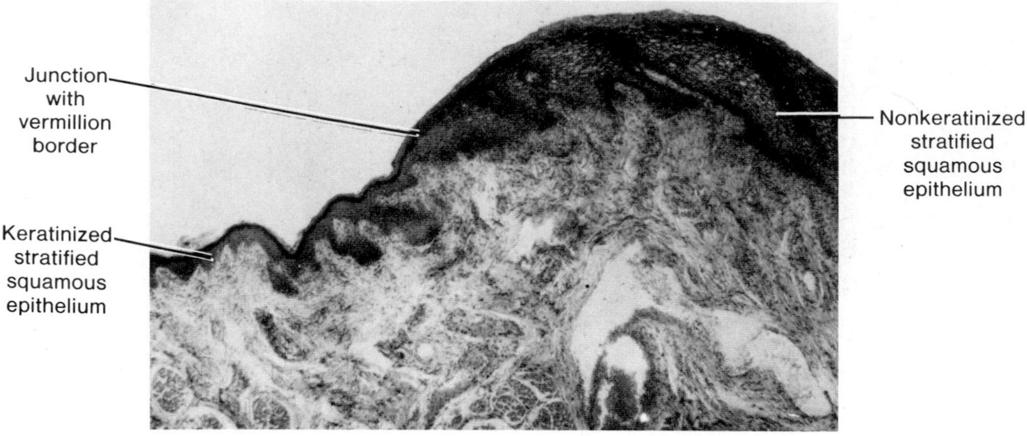

15-5

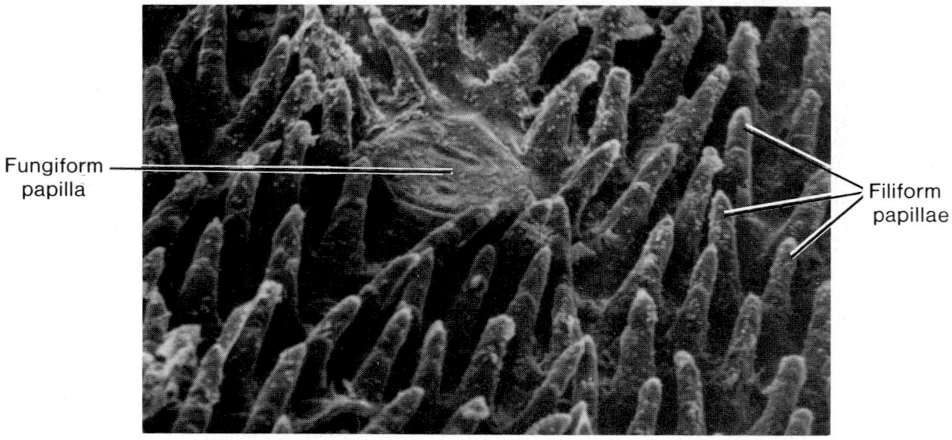

15-6

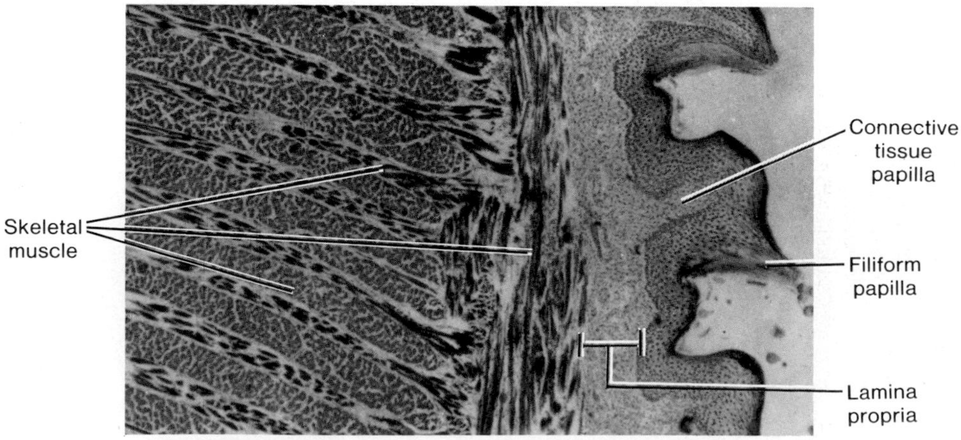

Figure 15.4. Lip. LM, ×100.
Figure 15.5. Dorsal surface of tongue. SEM, ×100.
Figure 15.6. Tongue (filiform papillae). LM, ×100.

15-7

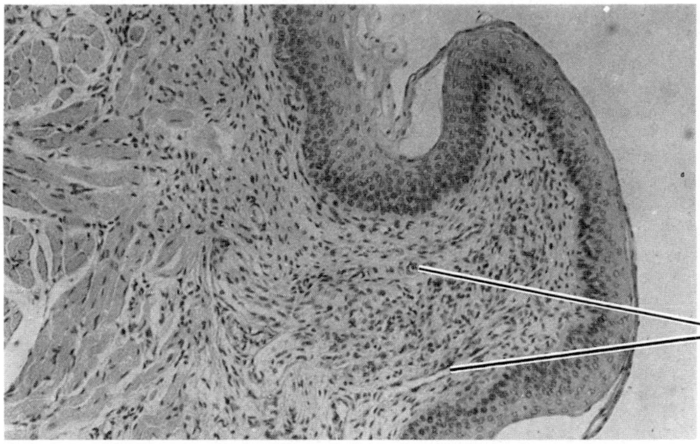

15-8

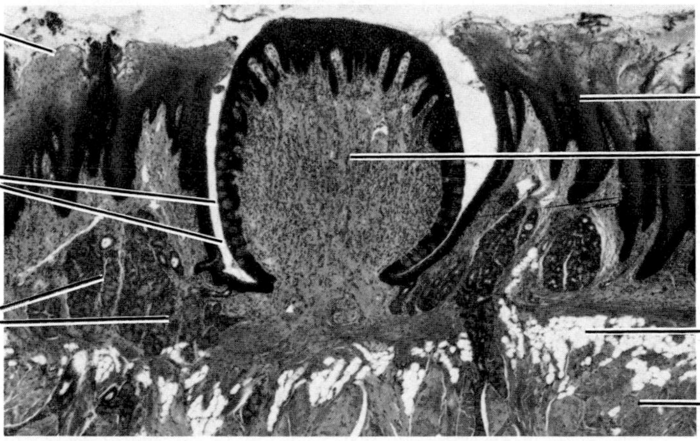

15-9

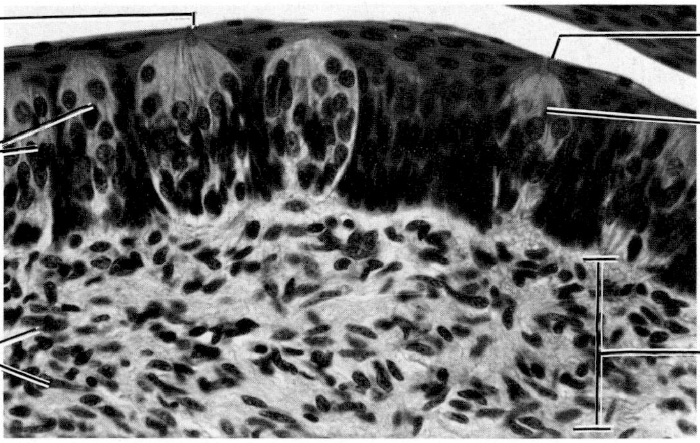

Figure 15.7. Fungiform papilla (tongue). LM, ×250.
Figure 15.8. Circumvallate papilla. LM, ×10.
Figure 15.9. Taste buds (tongue). LM, ×250.

15-10

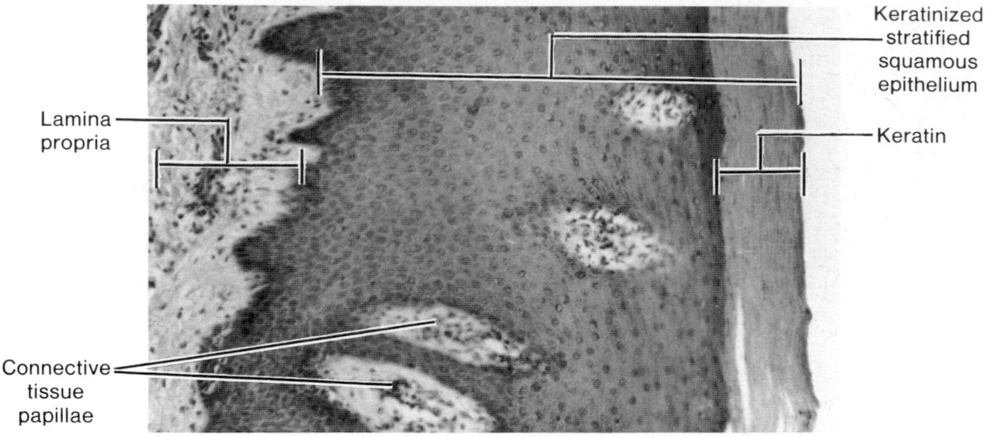

15-11 Salivary Glands

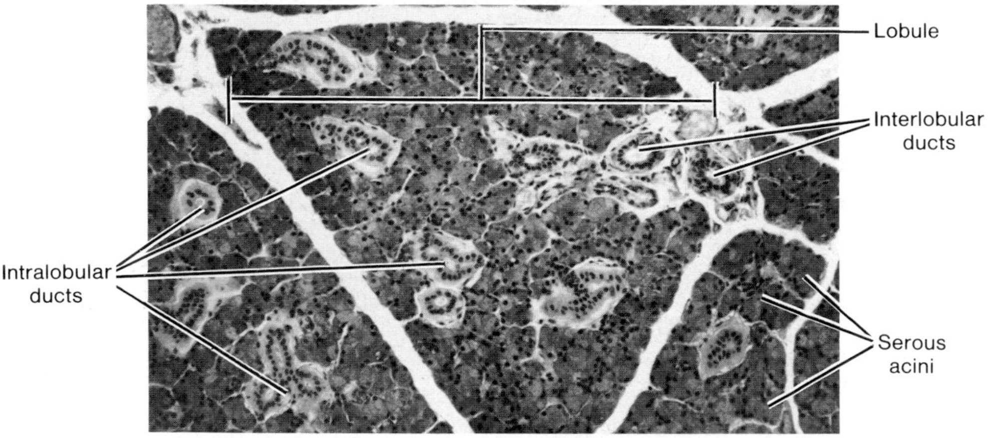

15-12

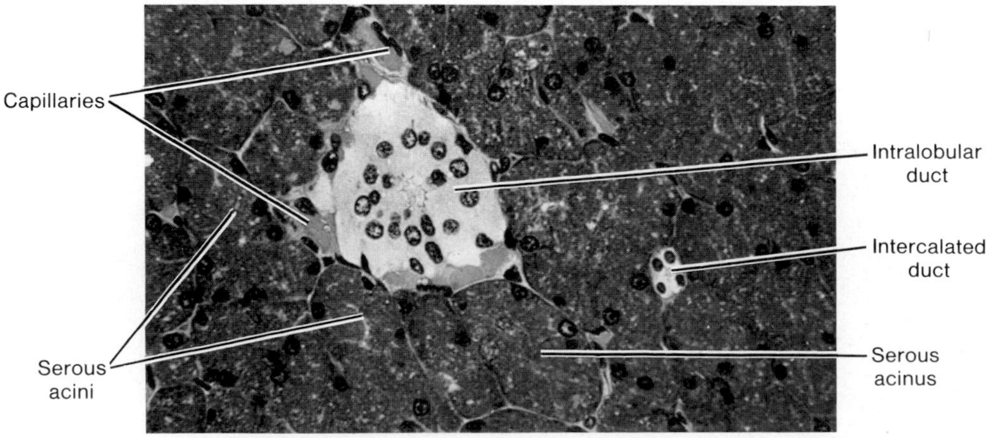

Figure 15.10. Hard palate. LM, ×200.
Figure 15.11. Parotid gland. LM, ×75.
Figure 15.12. Parotid gland. LM, ×250.

15-13

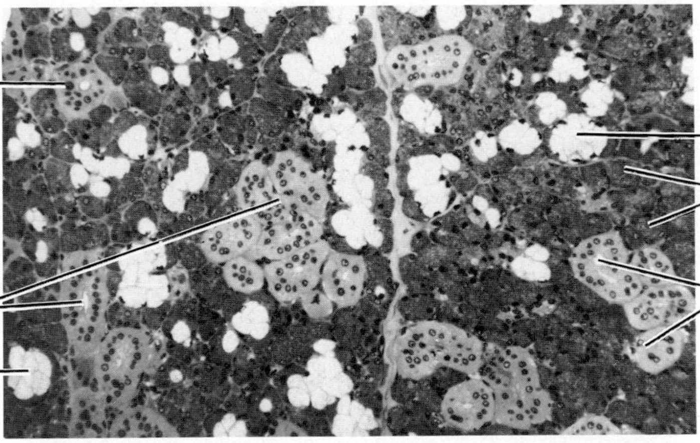

15-14

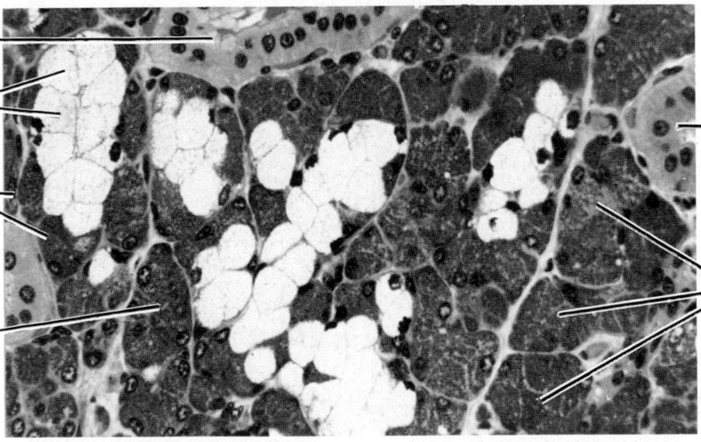

15-15

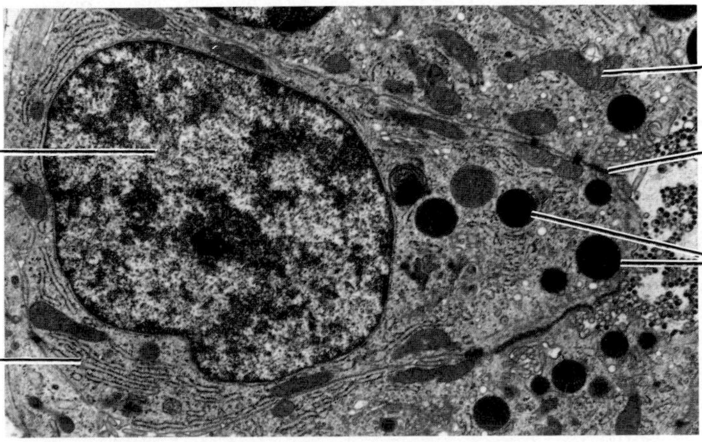

Figure 15.13. Submandibular gland. LM, ×100.
Figure 15.14. Submandibular gland. LM, ×250.
Figure 15.15. Serous acinar cell (submandibular gland). TEM, ×3000.

15-16

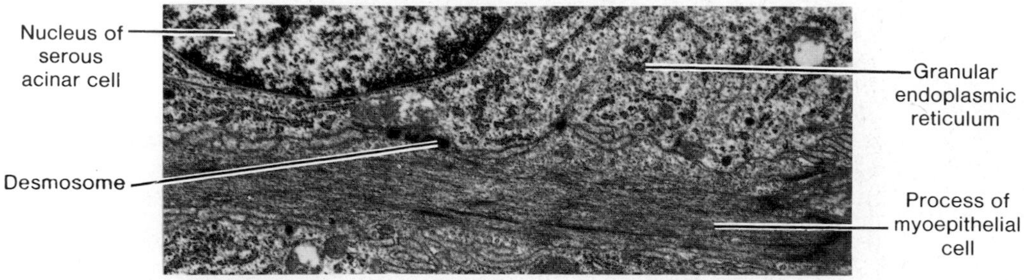

15-17

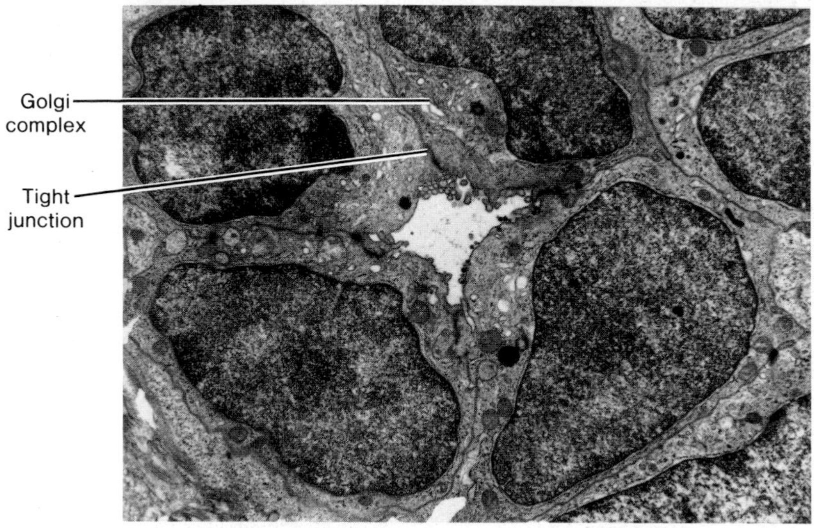

15-18

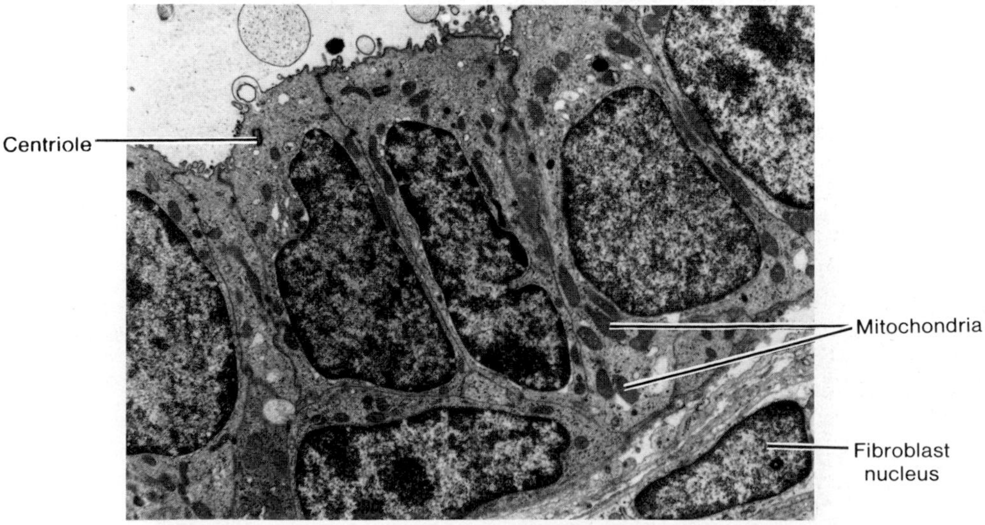

Figure 15.16. Submandibular gland. TEM, ×5000.
Figure 15.17. Intercalated duct (submandibular gland). TEM, ×4000.
Figure 15.18. Intralobular duct (submandibular gland). TEM, ×3000.

15-19

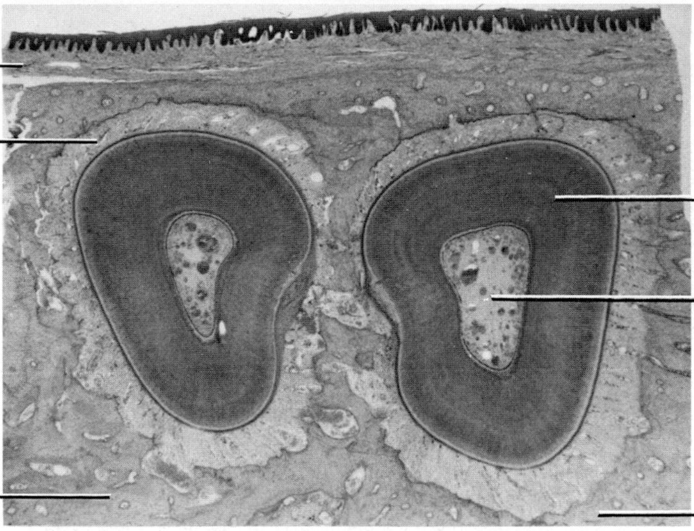

15-20

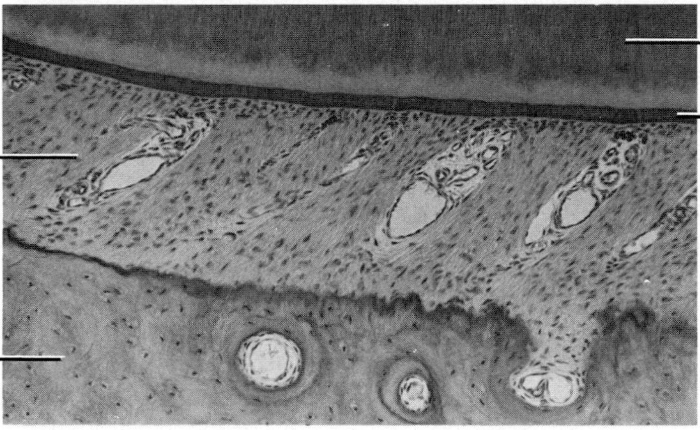

15-21

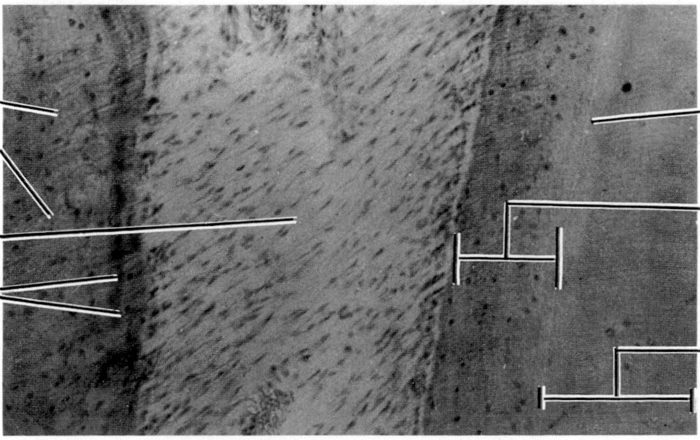

Figure 15.19. Root of tooth. LM, ×30.
Figure 15.20. Tooth. LM, ×250.
Figure 15.21. Tooth. LM, ×250.

15-22

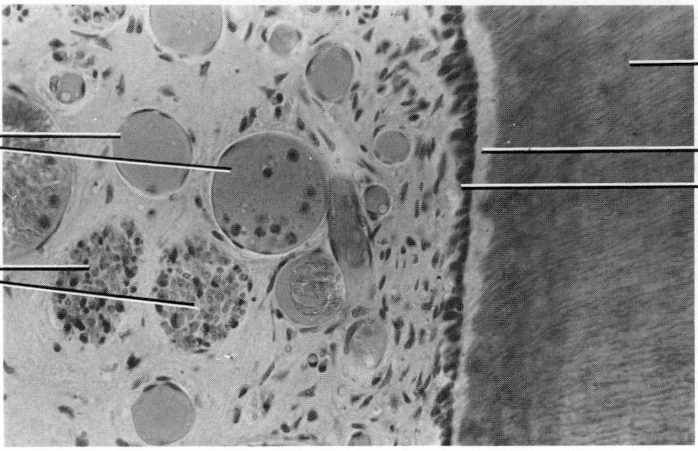

15-23 Esophagus

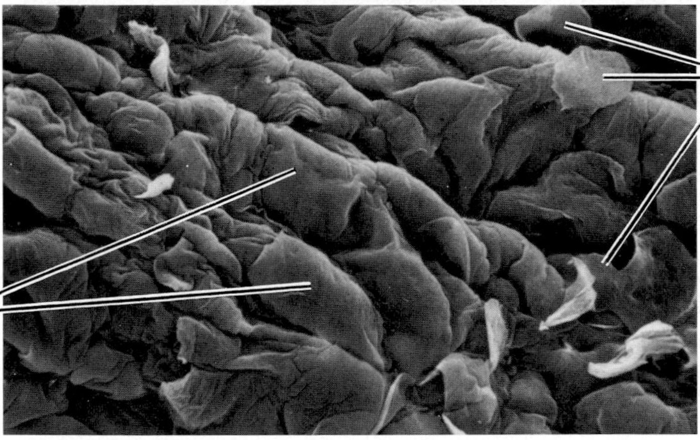

15-24

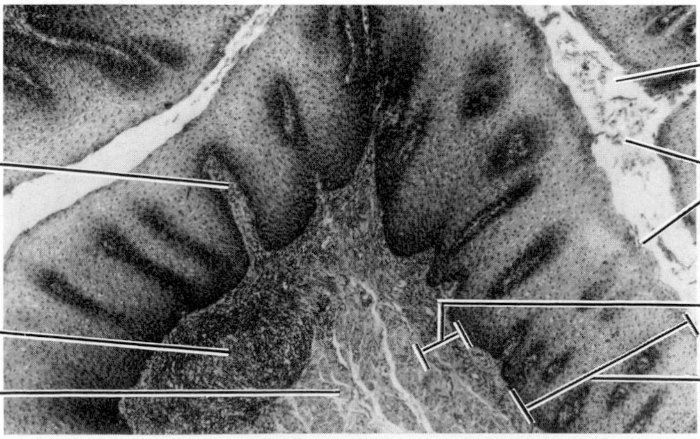

Figure 15.22. Tooth pulp. LM, ×250.
Figure 15.23. Surface of esophagus (human). SEM, ×200.
Figure 15.24. Esophagus (human). LM, ×100.

15-25

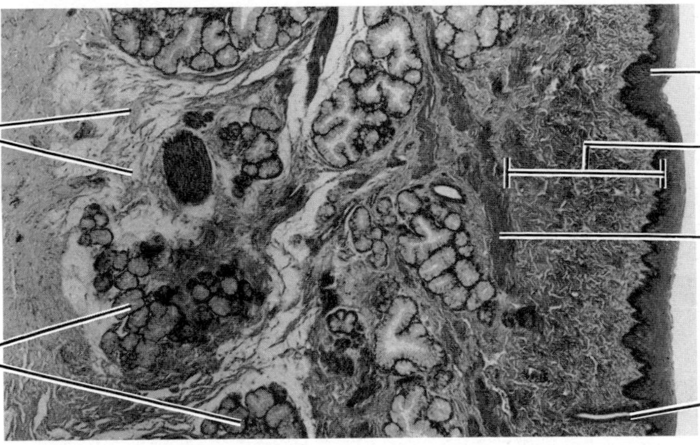

15-26

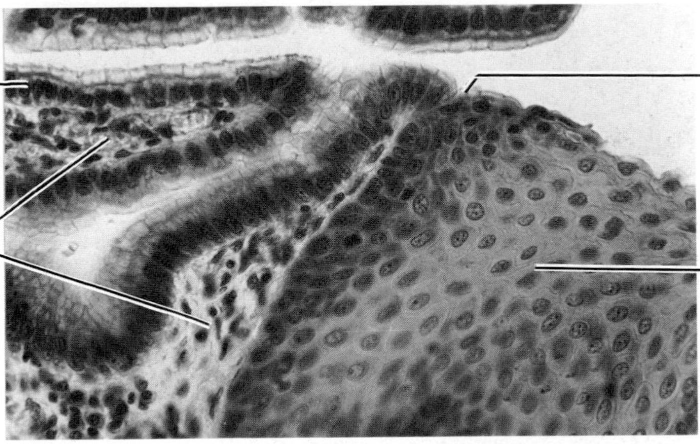

15-27 Stomach

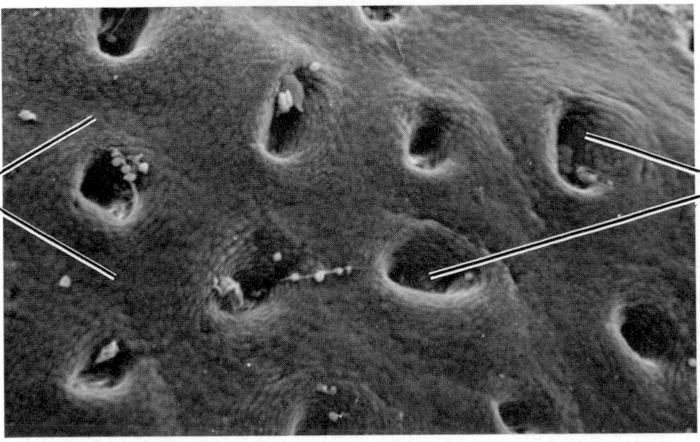

Figure 15.25. Distal esophagus. LM, ×40.
Figure 15.26. Esophageal gastric junction. LM, ×250.
Figure 15.27. Stomach (human). SEM, ×200.

15-28

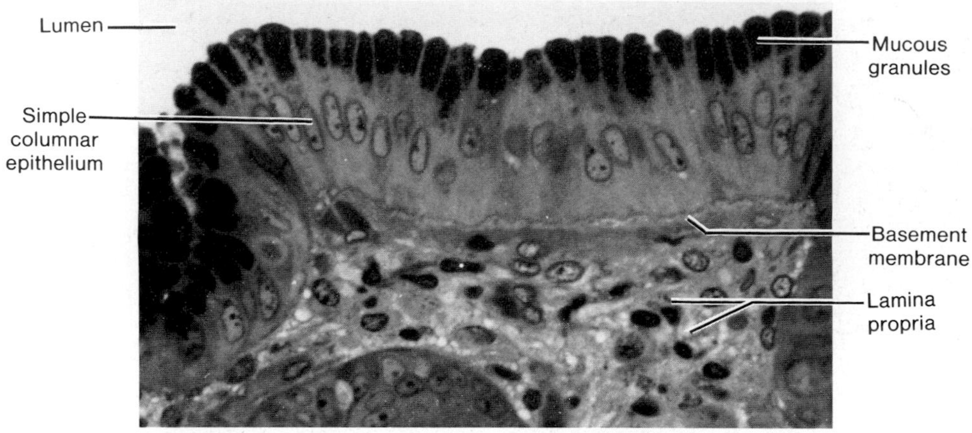

15-29

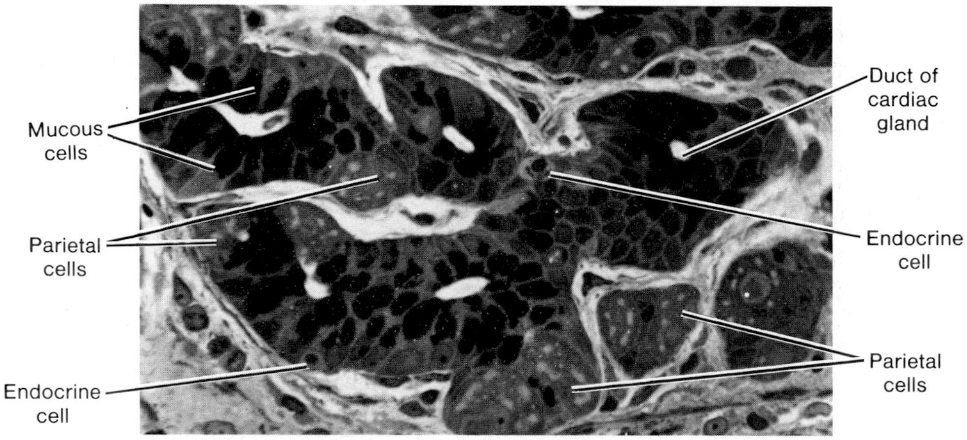

15-30

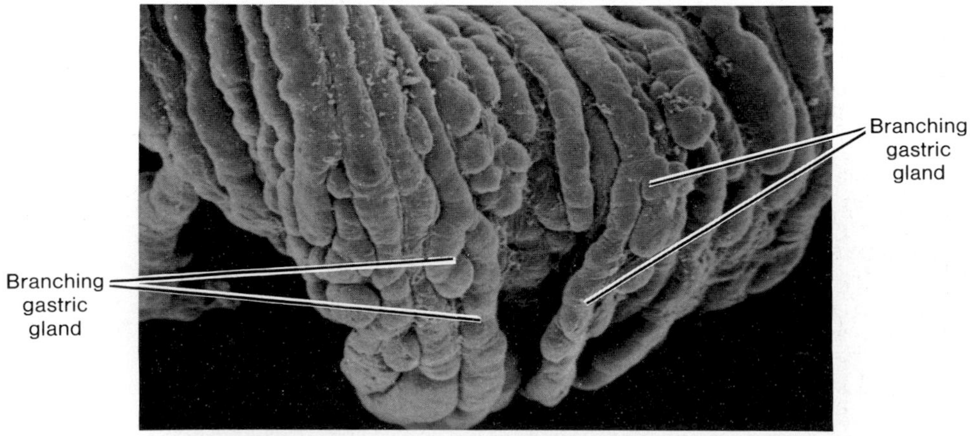

Figure 15.28. Stomach (human). LM, ×500.
Figure 15.29. Cardiac glands (human). LM, ×400.
Figure 15.30. Gastric glands (human). SEM, ×250.

15-31

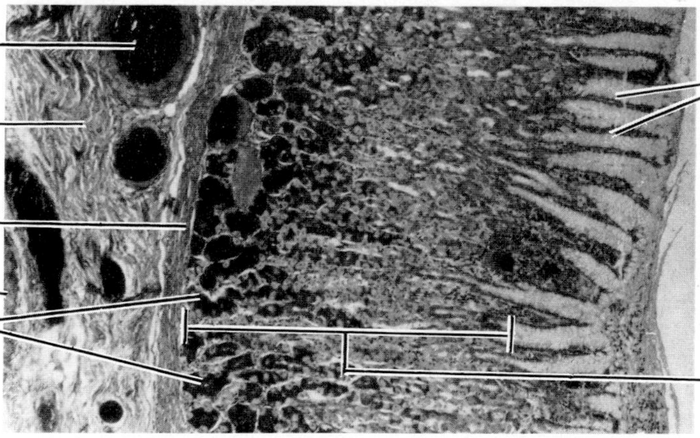

15-32

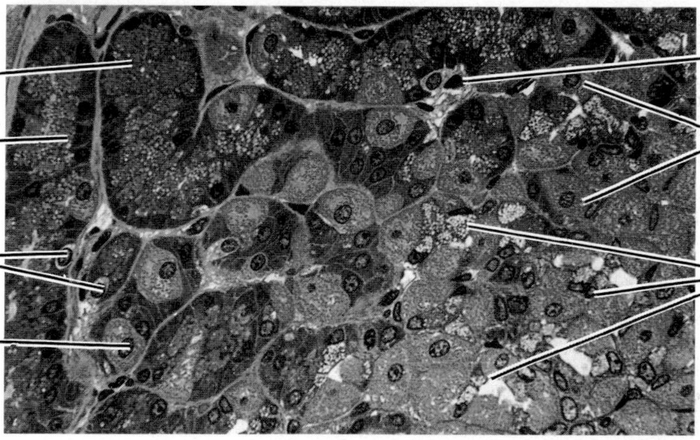

15-33

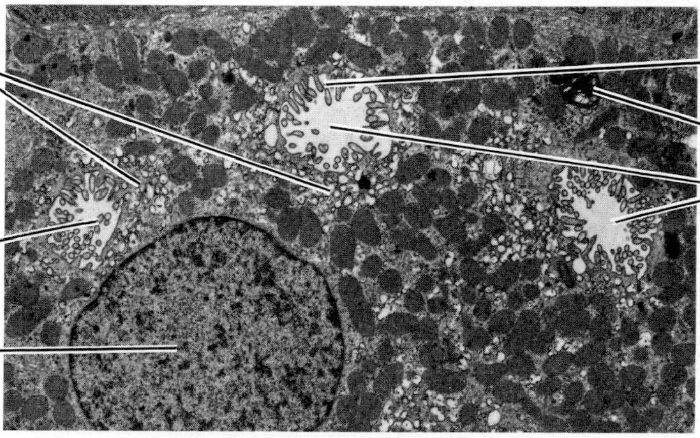

Figure 15.31. Gastric mucosa (human). LM, ×40.
Figure 15.32. Gastric mucosa. LM, ×250.
Figure 15.33. Parietal cells (human). TEM, ×10,000.

15-34

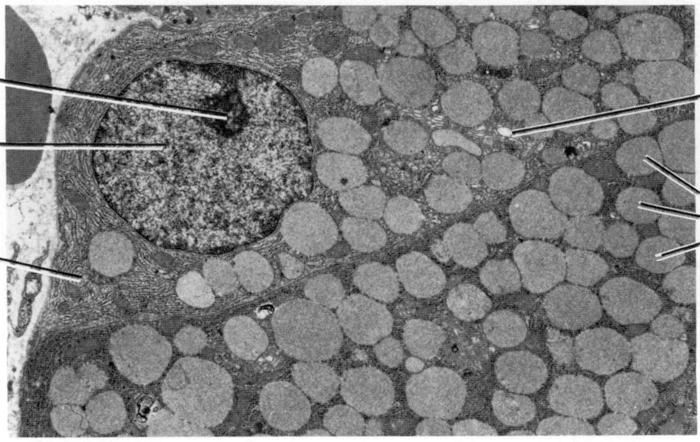

15-35

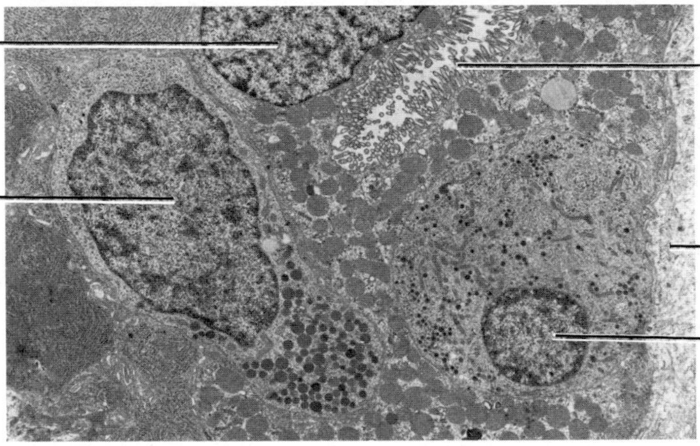

15-36

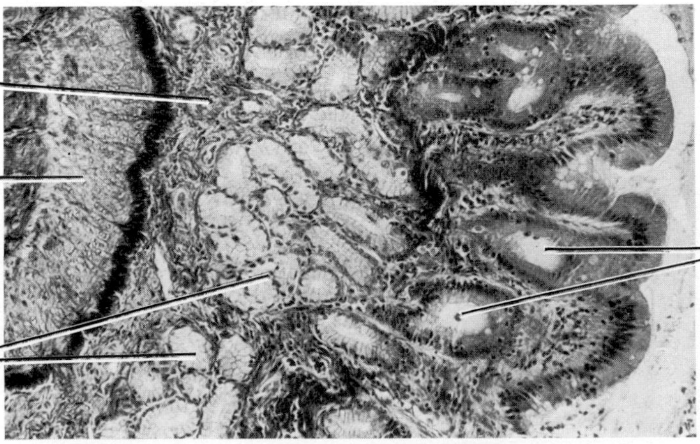

Figure 15.34. Chief cells (human). TEM, ×2000.
Figure 15.35. Endocrine cells (human stomach). TEM, ×2000.
Figure 15.36. Pyloric glands. LM, ×250.

15-37

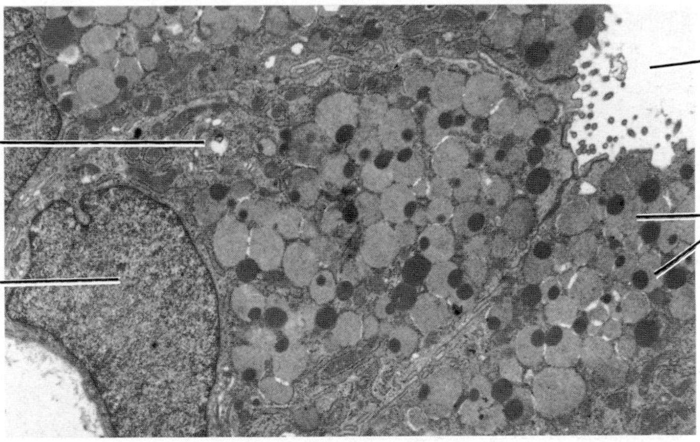
Lumen of pyloric gland
Golgi complex
Secretory granules
Nucleus of mucous cell

15-38 Small Intestine

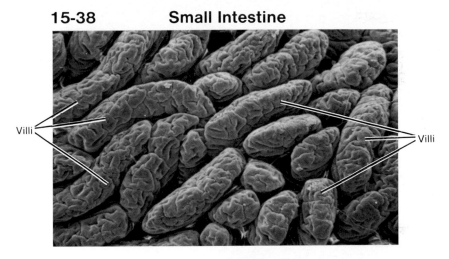

Villi
Villi

15-39

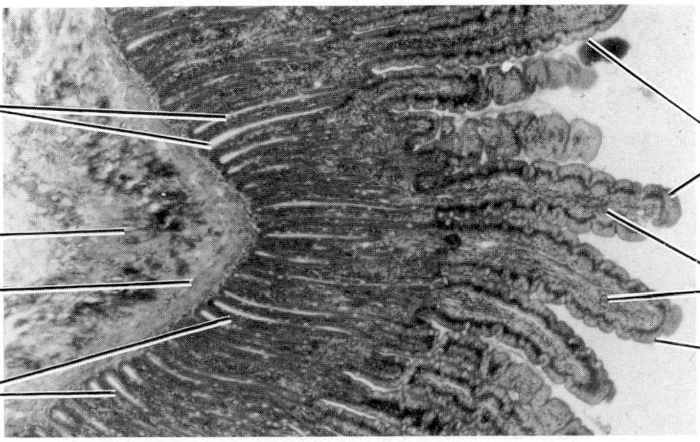
Intestinal glands
Villi
Submucosa
Lamina propria core
Muscularis mucosae
Intestinal epithelium
Intestinal glands

Figure 15.37. Mucous cells of pyloric gland (human). TEM, ×3000.
Figure 15.38. Duodenal villi (human). SEM, ×100.
Figure 15.39. Jejunum. LM, ×40.

15-40

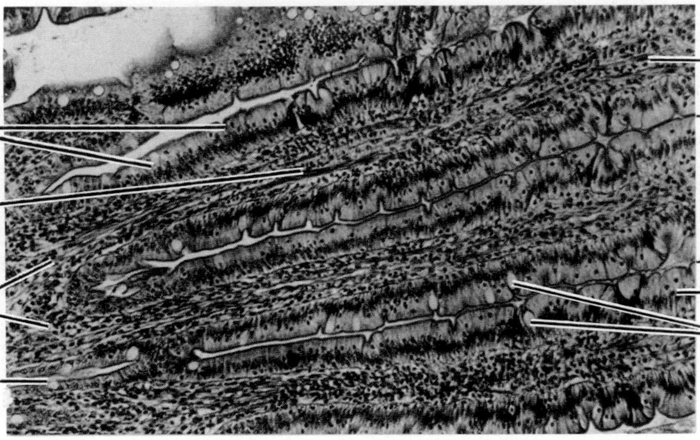

15-41

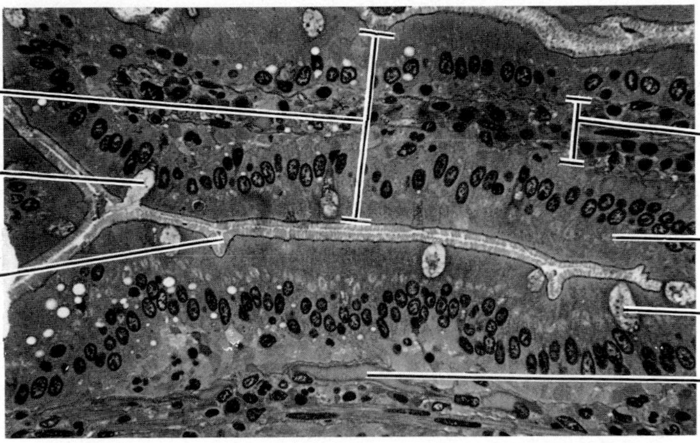

15-42

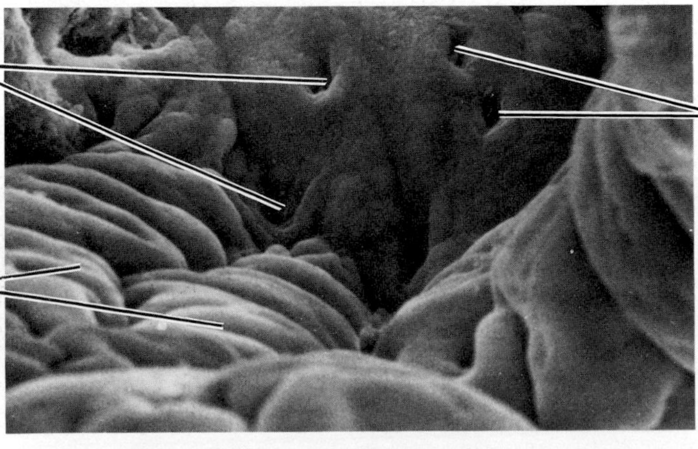

Figure 15.40. Jejunal villi. LM, ×100.
Figure 15.41. Jejunal villi. LM, ×250.
Figure 15.42. Jejunum (human). SEM, ×500.

15-43

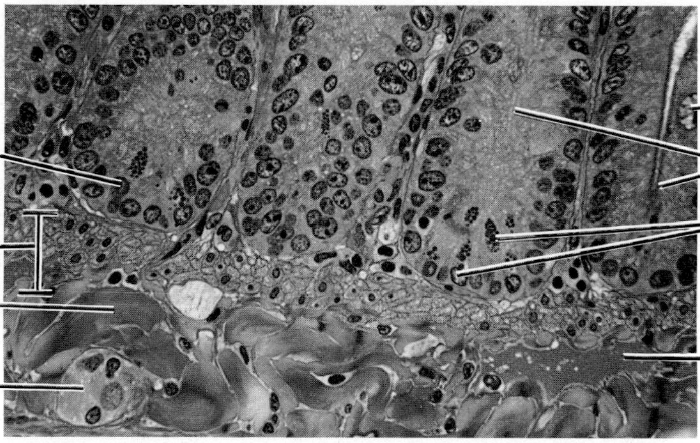

15-44

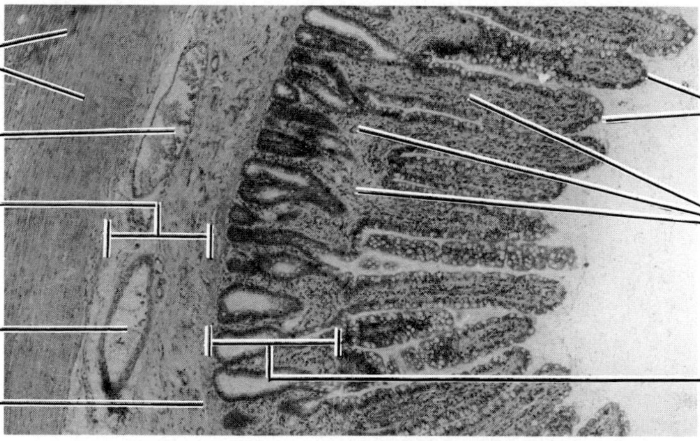

15-45

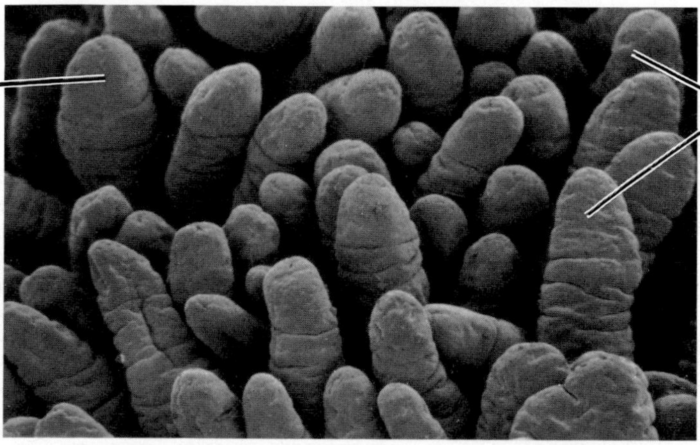

Figure 15.43. Intestinal glands (human). LM, ×250.
Figure 15.44. Ileum (small intestine). LM, ×40.
Figure 15.45. Villi (human ileum). SEM, ×200.

15-46

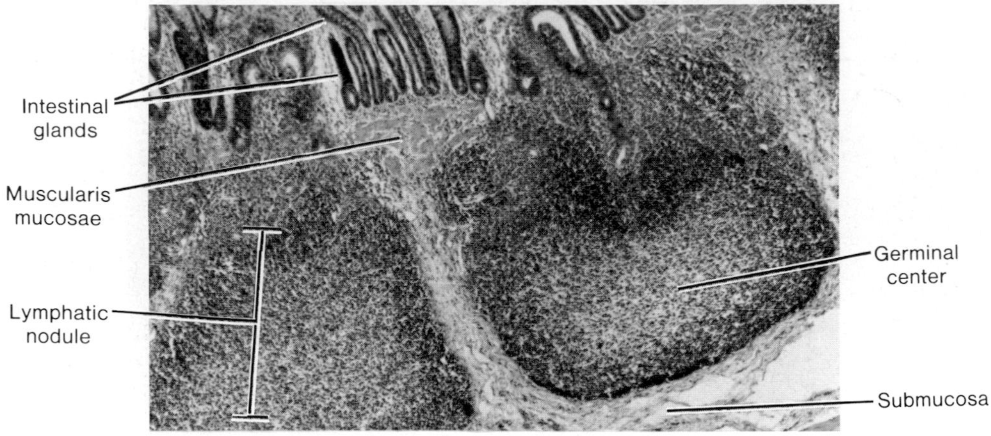

15-47

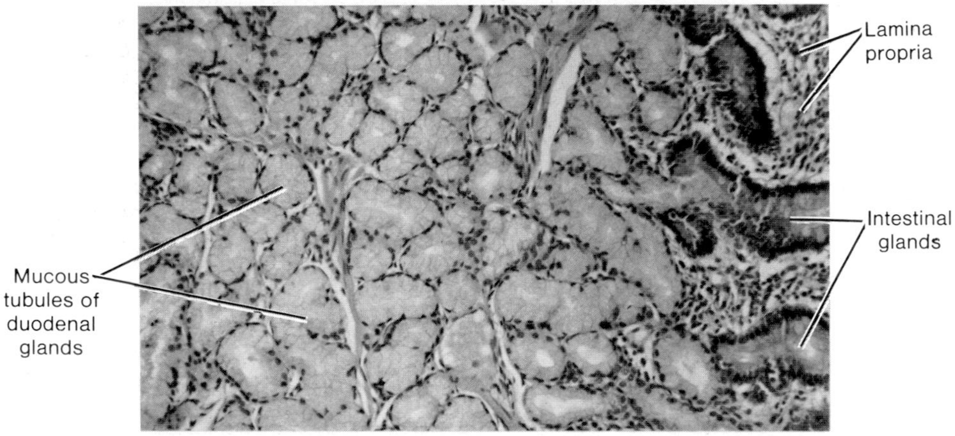

15-48

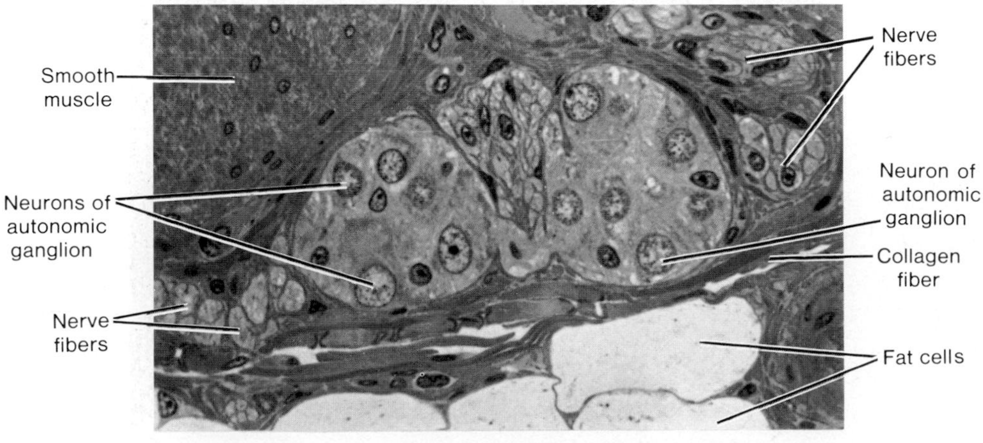

Figure 15.46. Peyer's patch (ileum). LM, ×100.
Figure 15.47. Duodenal glands (human duodenum). LM, ×250.
Figure 15.48. Meissner's plexus (jejunum). LM, ×400.

15-49 Colon

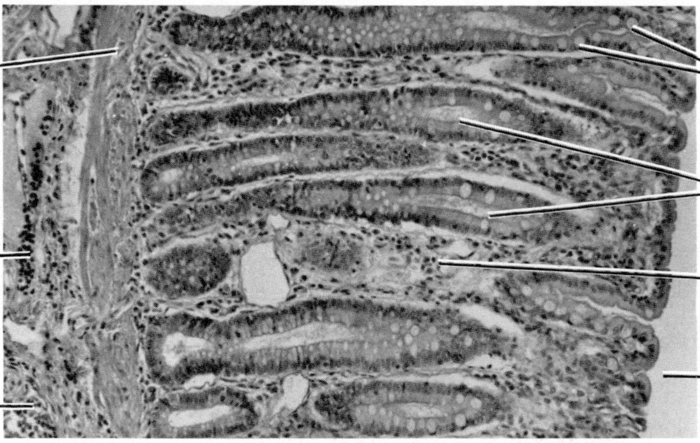

15-50

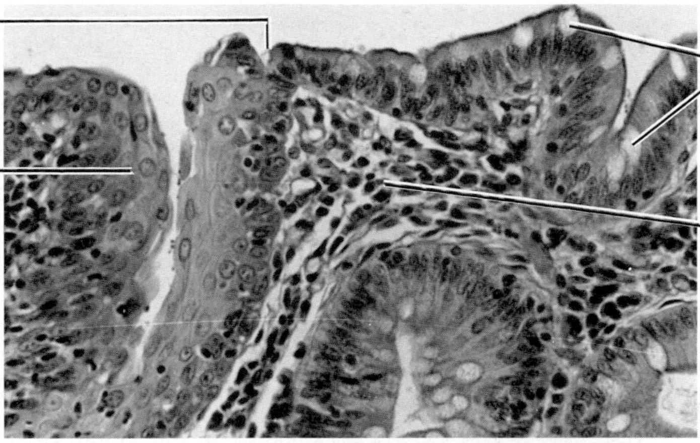

15-51 Anal Canal

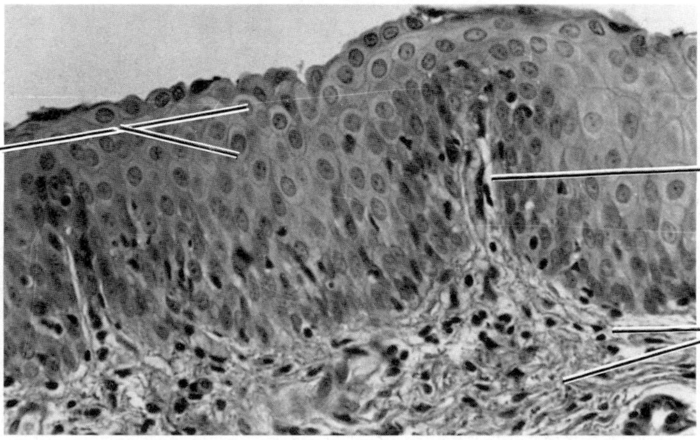

Figure 15.49. Colon (human). LM, ×100.
Figure 15.50. Rectoanal junction. LM, ×250.
Figure 15.51. Anal canal. LM, ×250.

15-52

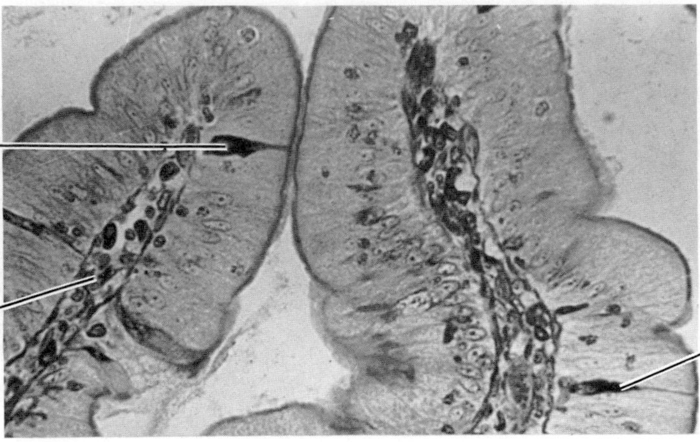

15-53 Liver

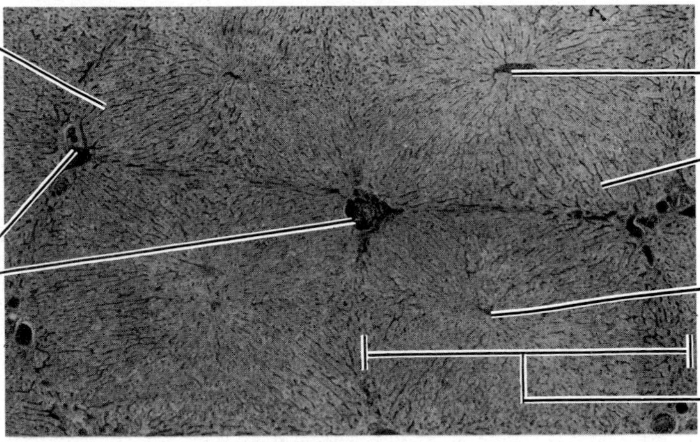

15-54

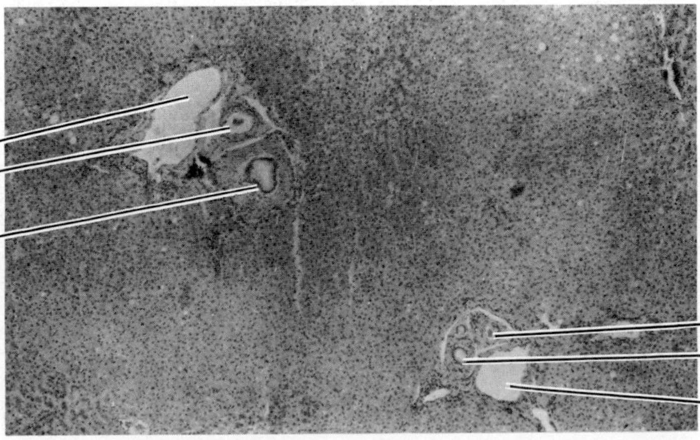

Figure 15.52. Secretin (S) cells, small intestine (PAP technique). LM, ×250.
Figure 15.53. Liver lobules (pig). LM, ×40.
Figure 15.54. Liver (human). LM, ×40.

15-55

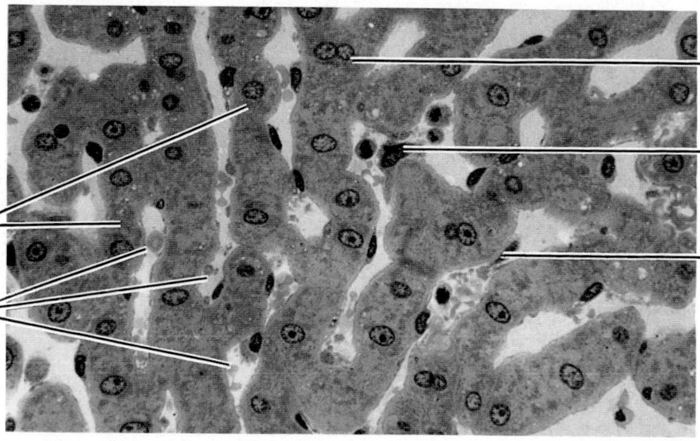

15-56

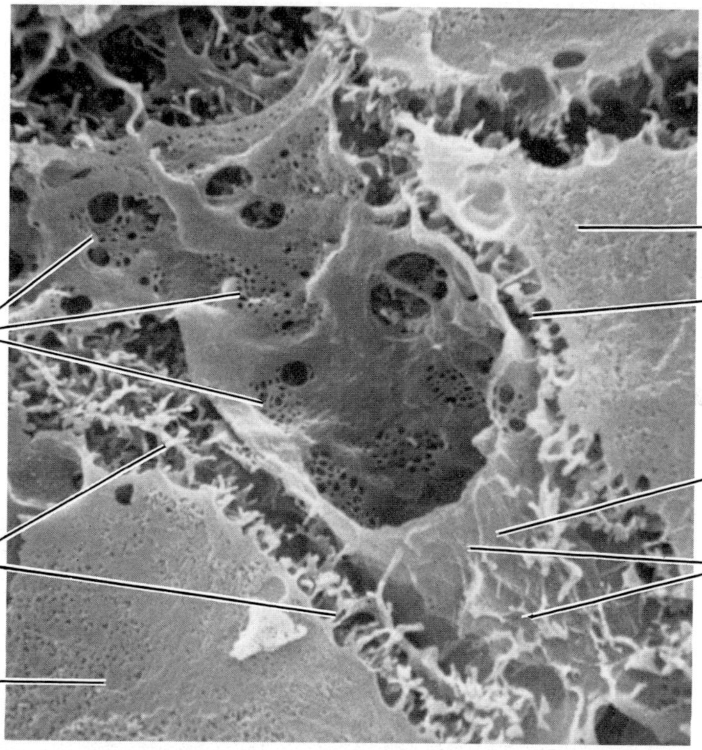

Figure 15.55. Hepatic sinusoids (liver). LM, ×200.
Figure 15.56. Hepatic sinusoid. SEM, ×6000.

15-57

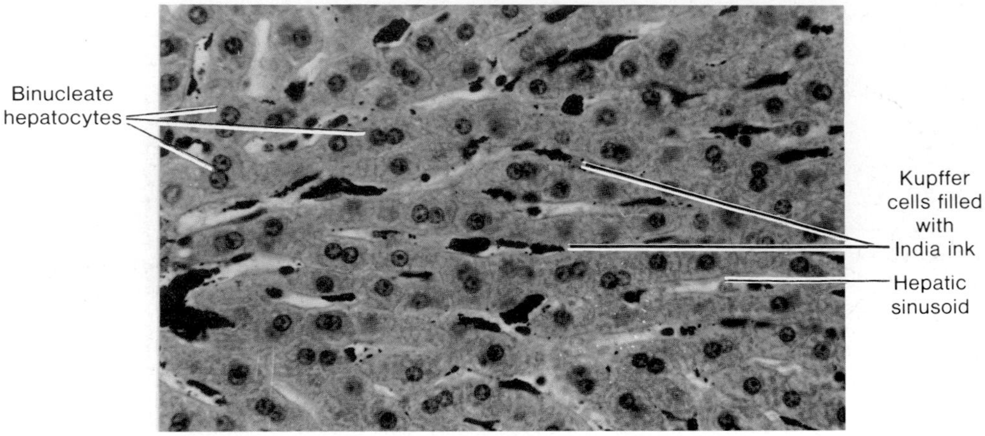

15-58

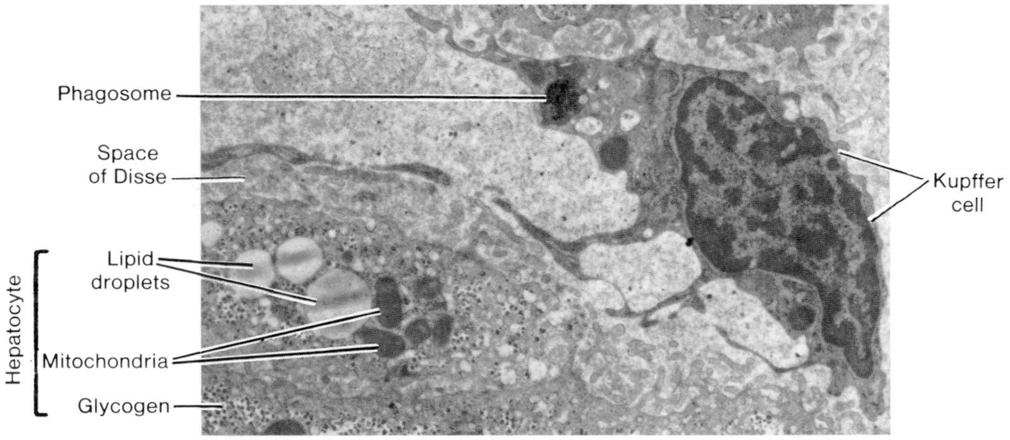

15-59

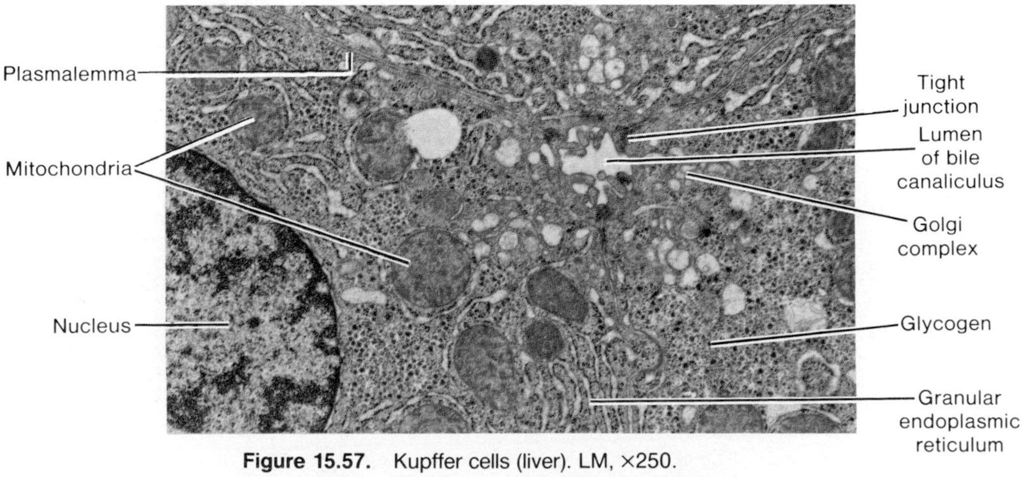

Figure 15.57. Kupffer cells (liver). LM, ×250.
Figure 15.58. Kupffer cell (liver). TEM, ×10,000.
Figure 15.59. Bile canaliculus (liver). TEM, ×6000.

15-60

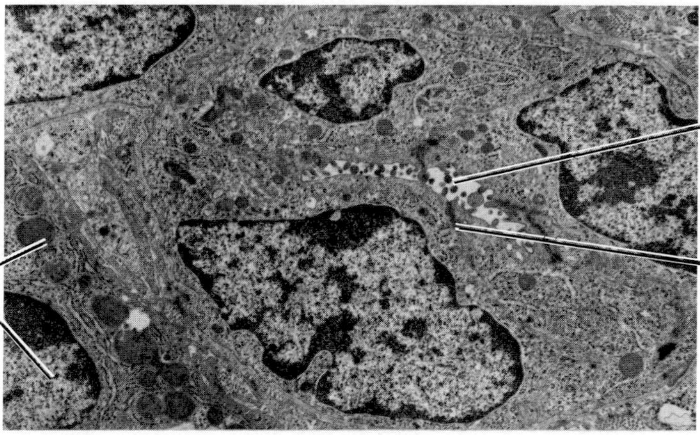

15-61

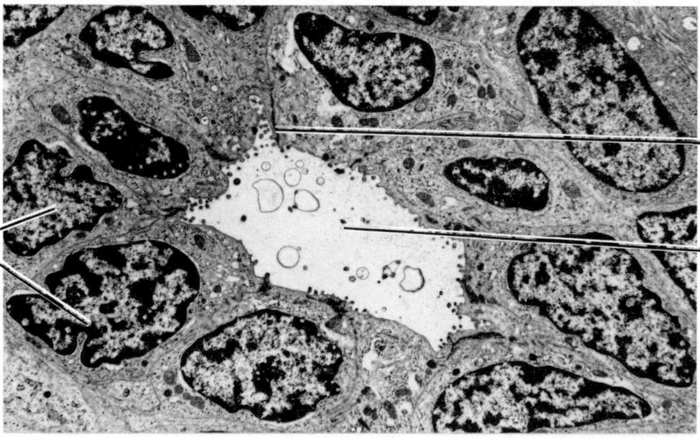

15-62 Gallbladder

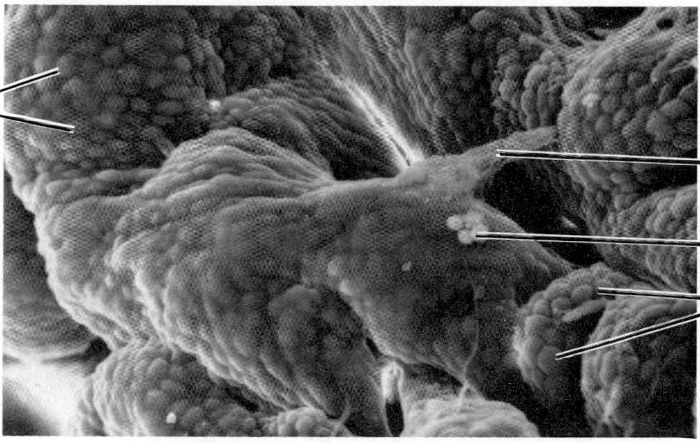

Figure 15.60. Bile ductule (canal of Hering), ×3500.
Figure 15.61. Interlobular bile duct (liver). TEM, ×2000.
Figure 15.62. Surface of gallbladder. SEM, ×500.

15-63

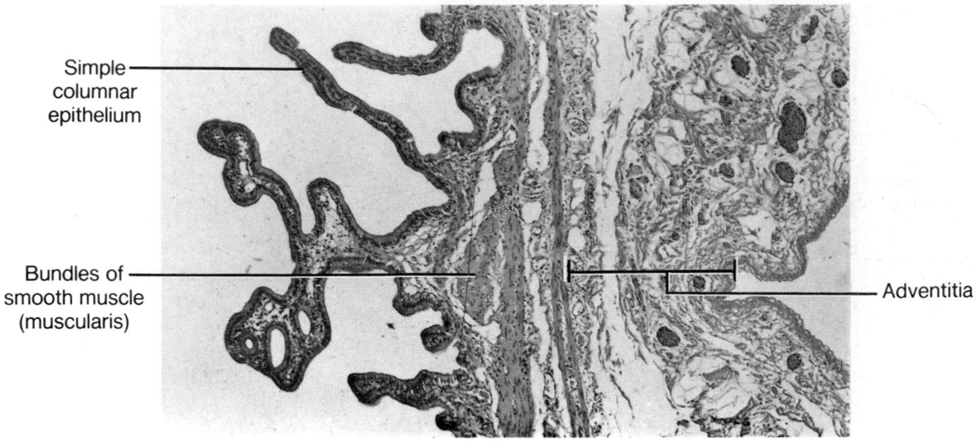

15-64

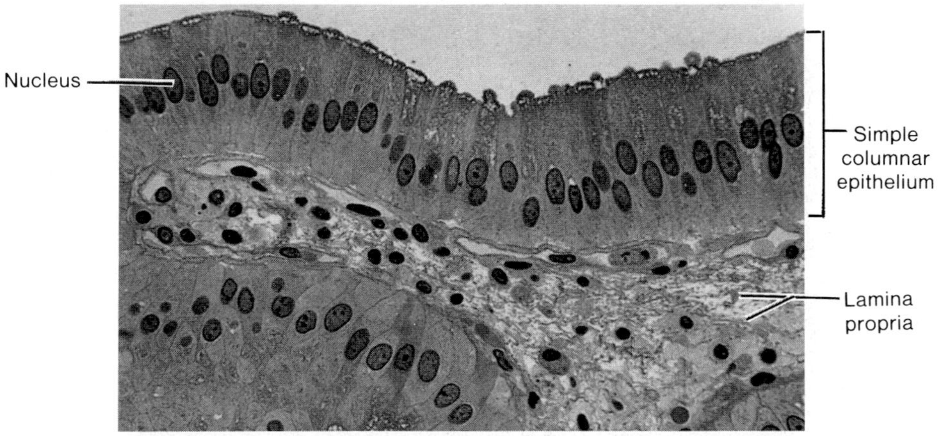

15-65 Pancreas

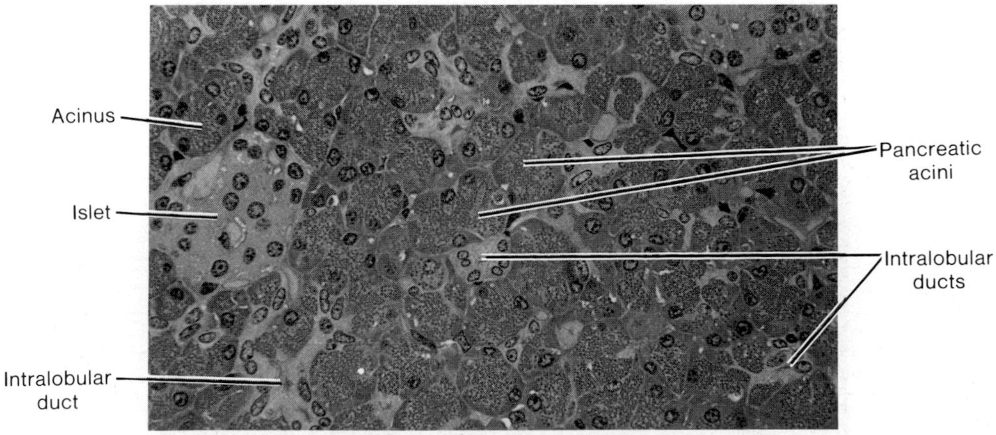

Figure 15.63. Gallbladder. LM, ×40.
Figure 15.64. Gallbladder mucosa. LM, ×250.
Figure 15.65. Pancreas. LM, ×100.

15-66

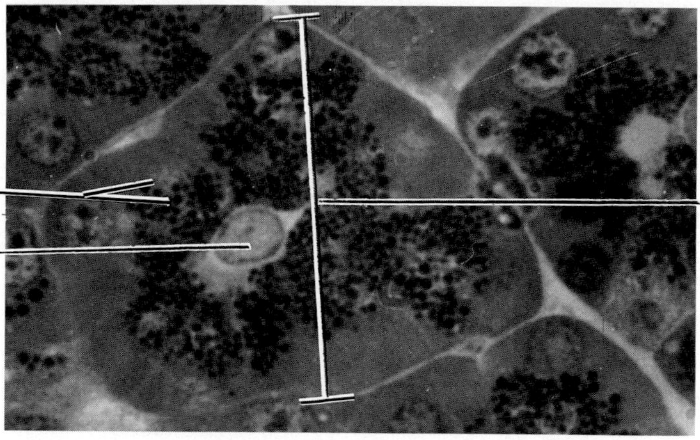

15-67

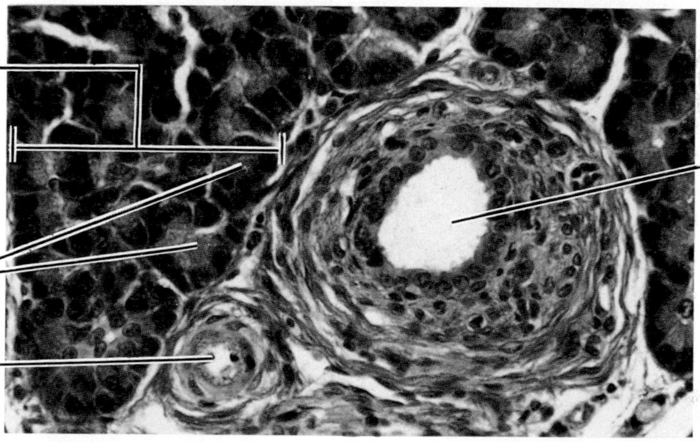

15-68

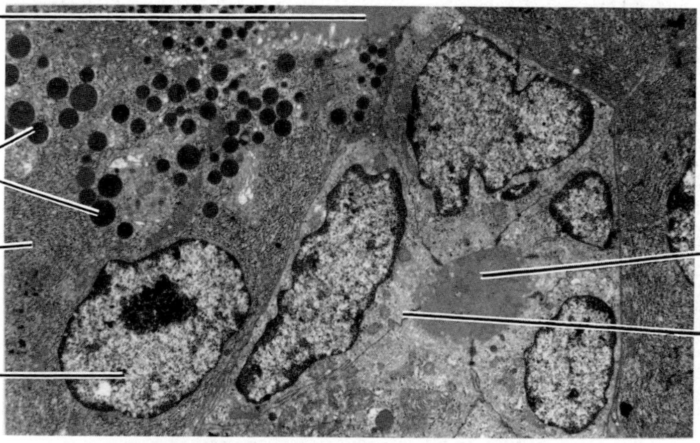

Figure 15.66. Pancreatic acinus. LM, ×1000.
Figure 15.67. Pancreas. LM, ×100.
Figure 15.68. Pancreas. TEM, ×2000.

15-69

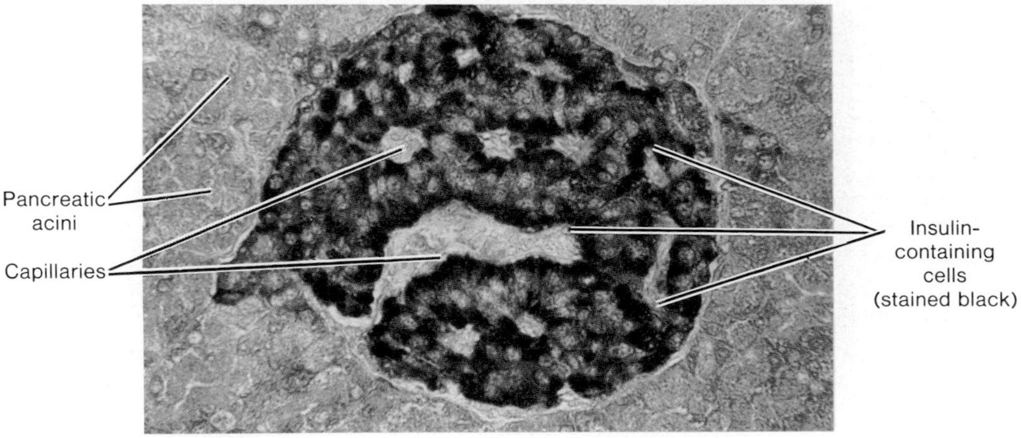

15-70

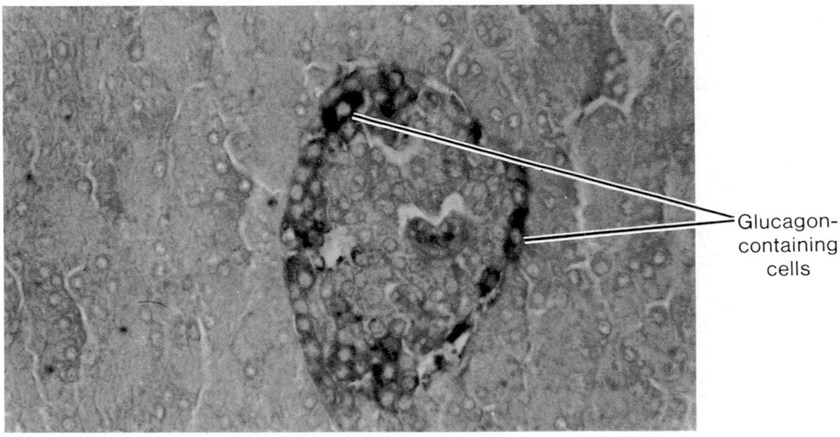

15-71

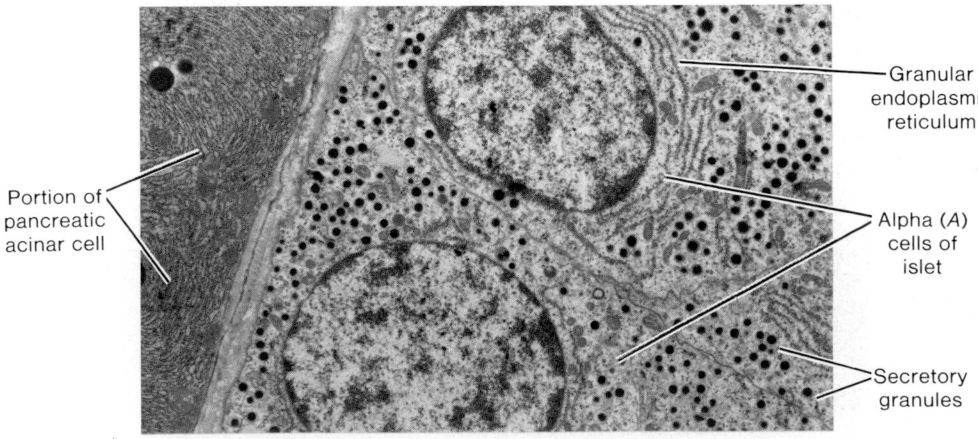

Figure 15.69. Islet stained for insulin (PAP technique). LM, ×250.
Figure 15.70. Pancreas stained for glucagon (PAP technique). LM, ×250.
Figure 15.71. Pancreas. TEM, ×3000.

Development
Tooth

15-72

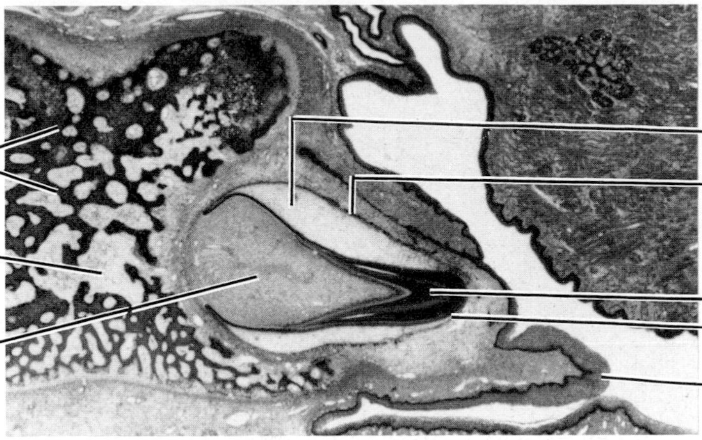

15-73

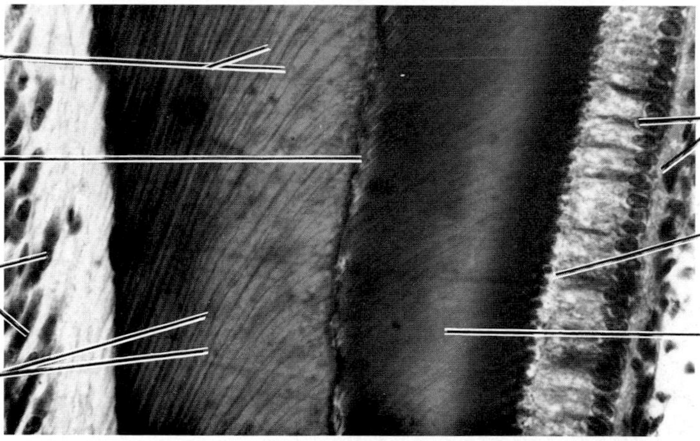

15-74

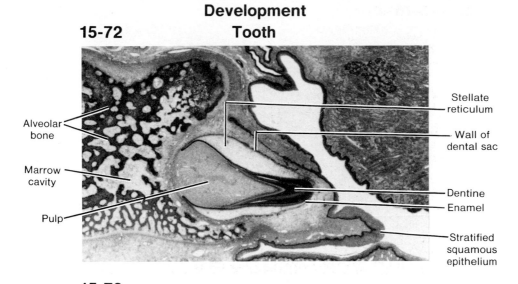

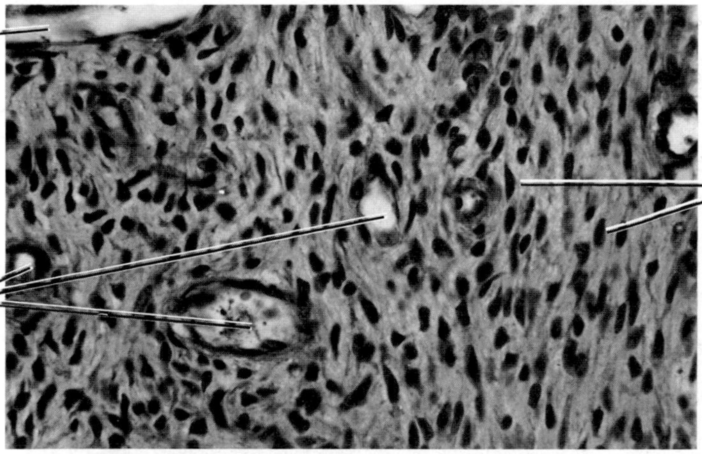

Figure 15.72. Developing tooth. LM, ×10.
Figure 15.73. Developing tooth. LM, ×250.
Figure 15.74. Developing tooth (pulp). LM, ×250

15-75

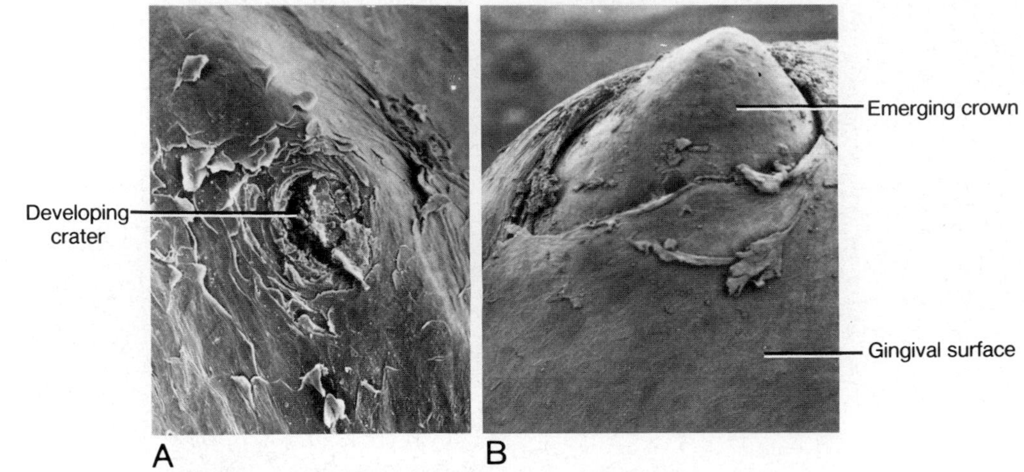

15-76 Submandibular Gland

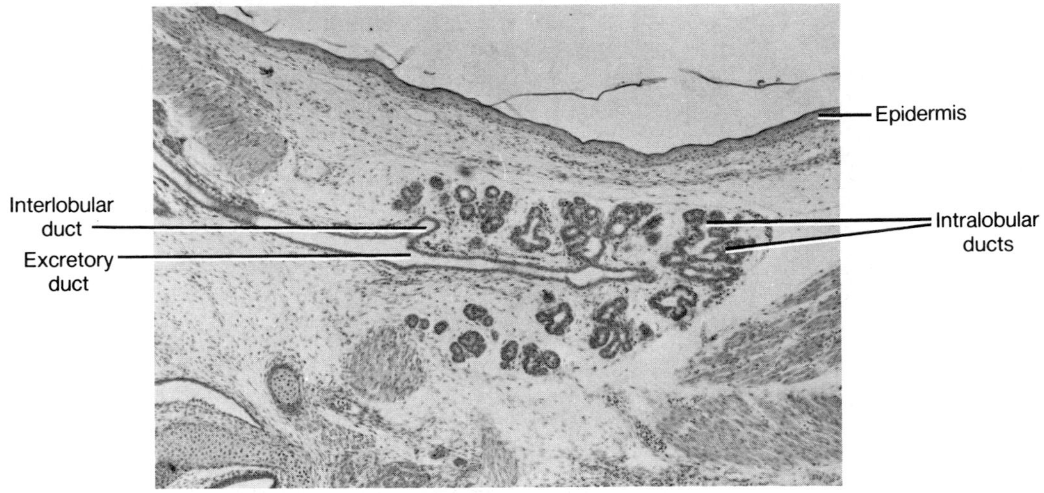

15-77 Esophagus

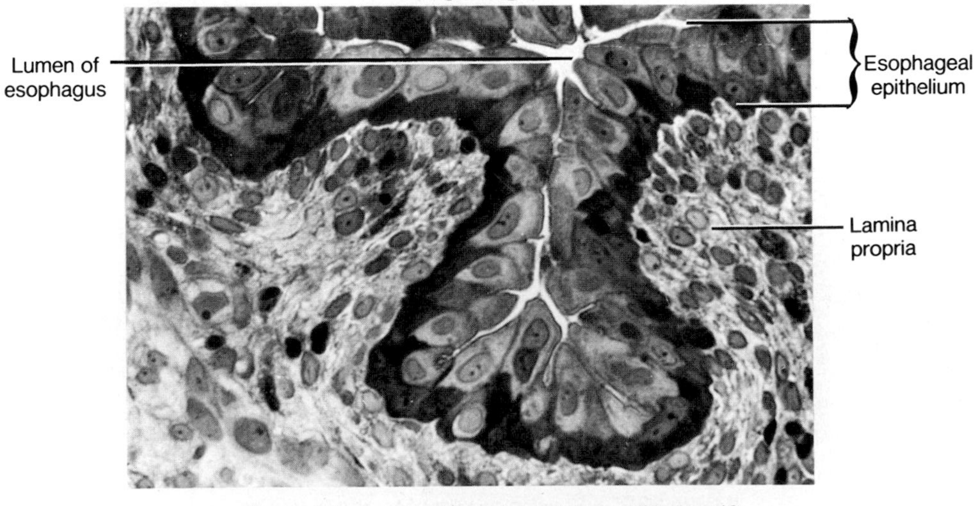

Figure 15.75. Tooth eruption. SEM *A*, ×40; *B*, ×40.
Figure 15.76. Submandibular gland. LM, ×35.
Figure 15.77. Esophagus. LM, ×400.

15-78

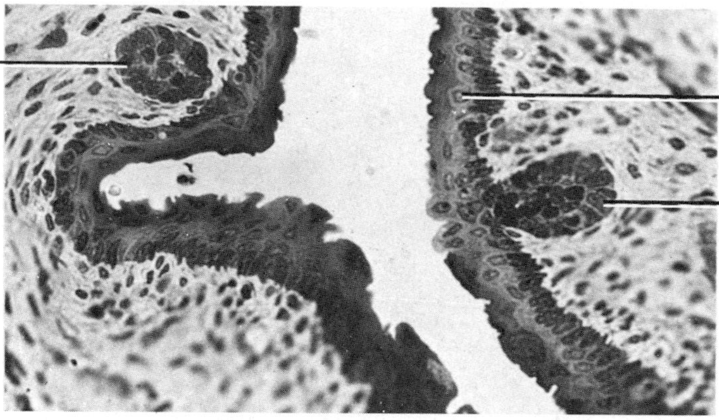

15-79 Stomach

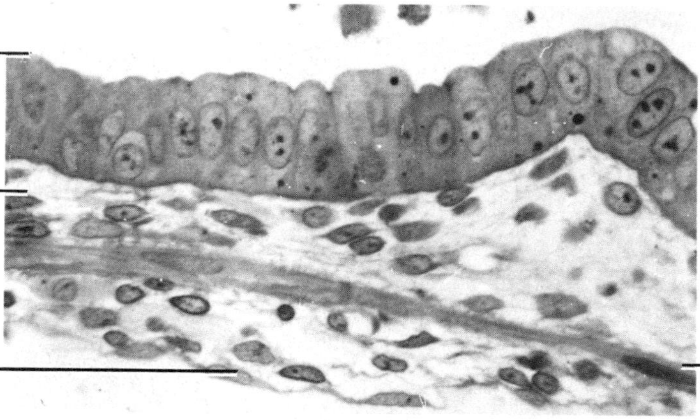

15-80

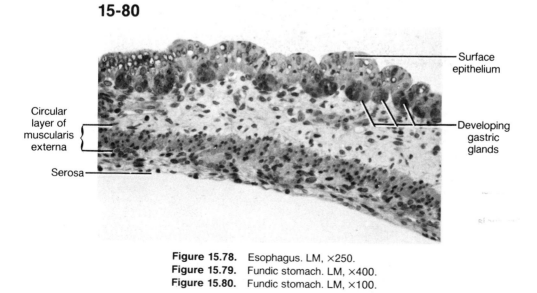

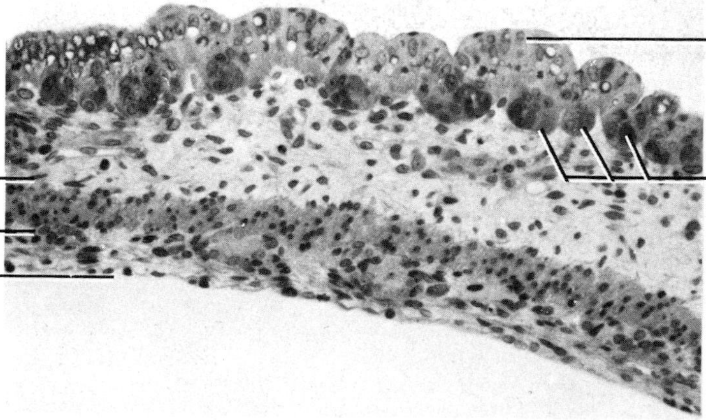

Figure 15.78. Esophagus. LM, ×250.
Figure 15.79. Fundic stomach. LM, ×400.
Figure 15.80. Fundic stomach. LM, ×100.

15-81

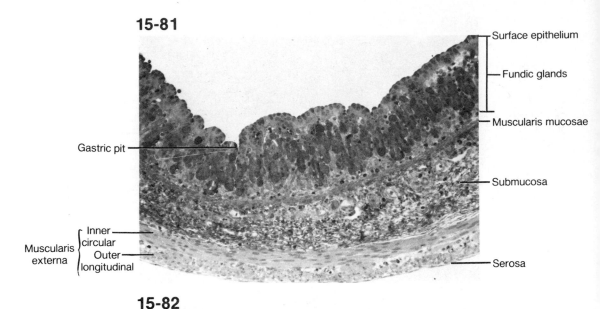

15-82

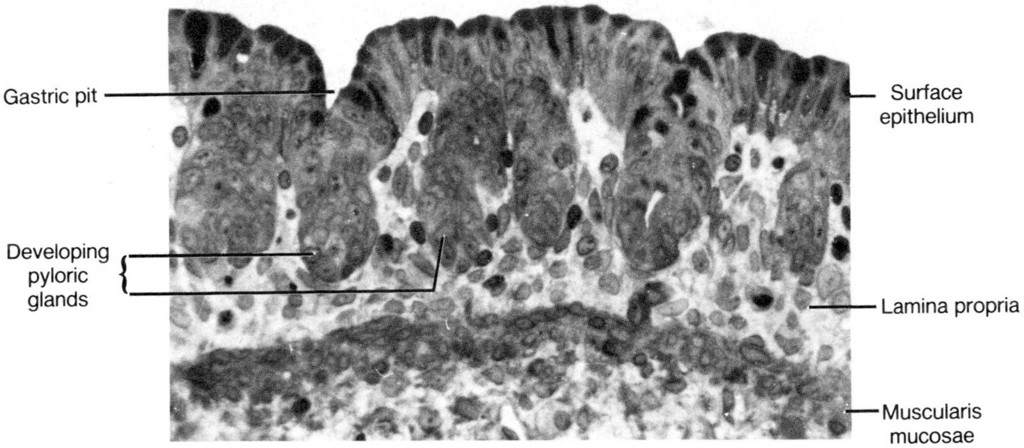

15-83 Small Intestine

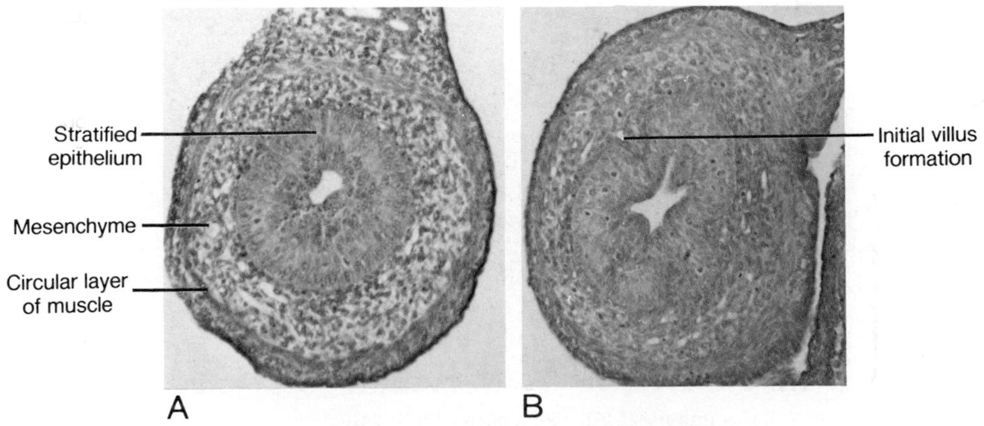

Figure 15.81. Fundic stomach. LM, ×100.
Figure 15.82. Pyloric stomach. LM, ×400.
Figure 15.83. Small intestine. *A* and *B*, ×250.

15-84

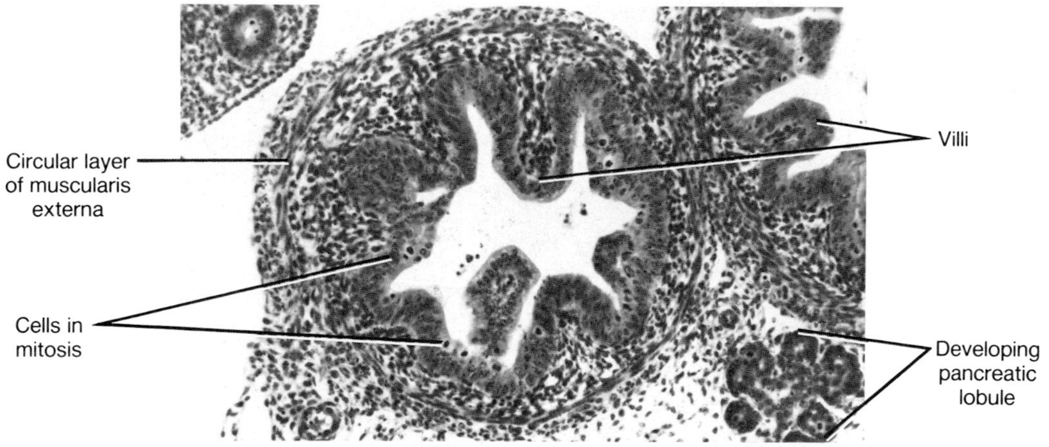

15-85

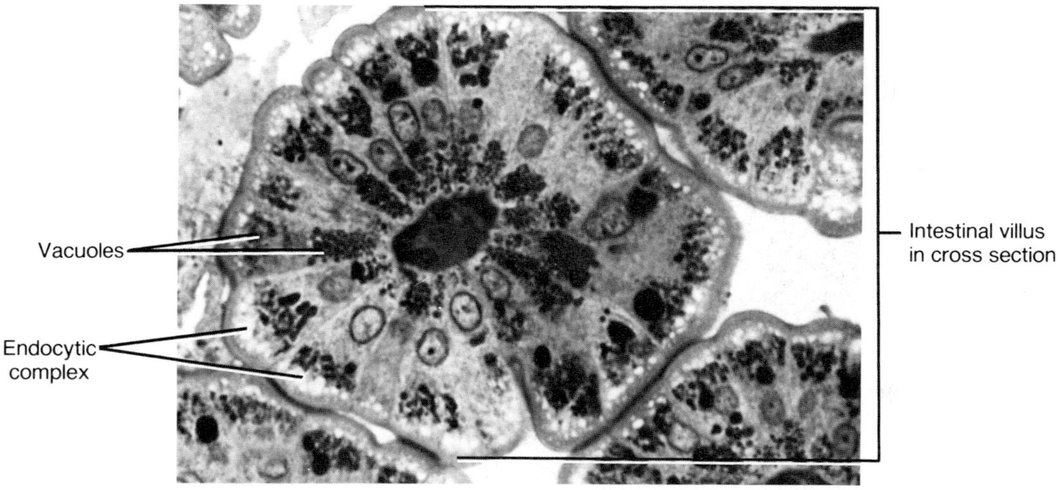

15-86

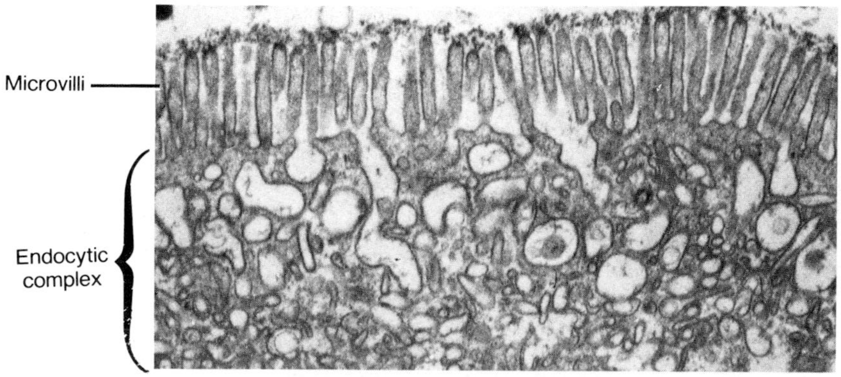

Figure 15.84. Small intestine. LM, ×250.
Figure 15.85. Small intestine. LM, ×500.
Figure 15.86. Small intestine. TEM, ×15000.

15-87

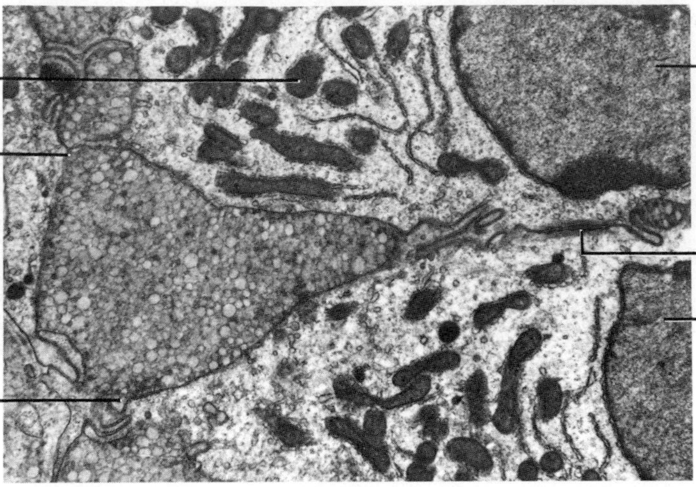

15-88 Colon

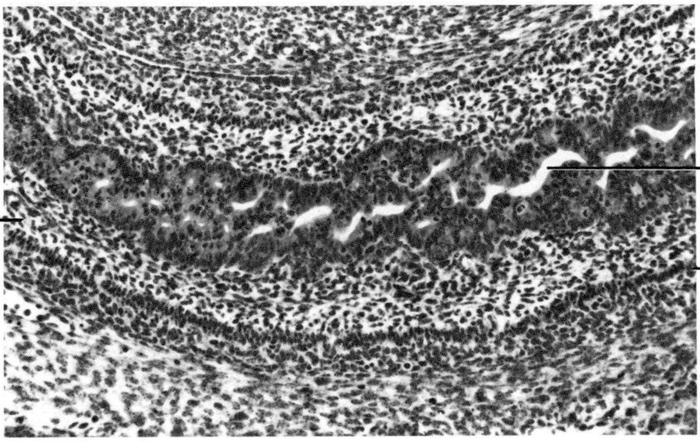

15-89

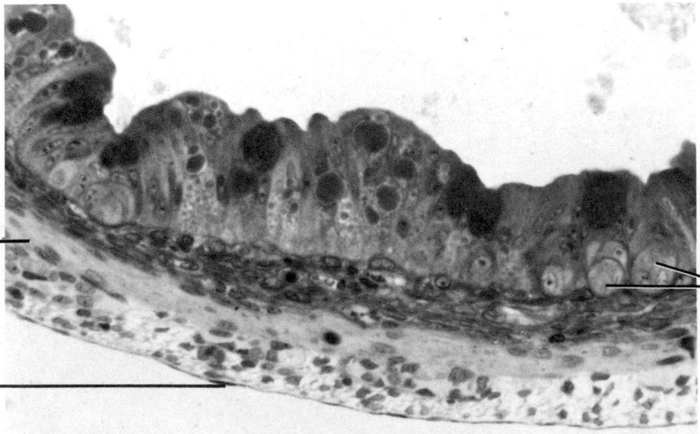

Figure 15.87. Newborn intestinal epithelium. TEM, ×8000.
Figure 15.88. Colon. LM, ×200.
Figure 15.89. Colon. LM, ×350.

15-90

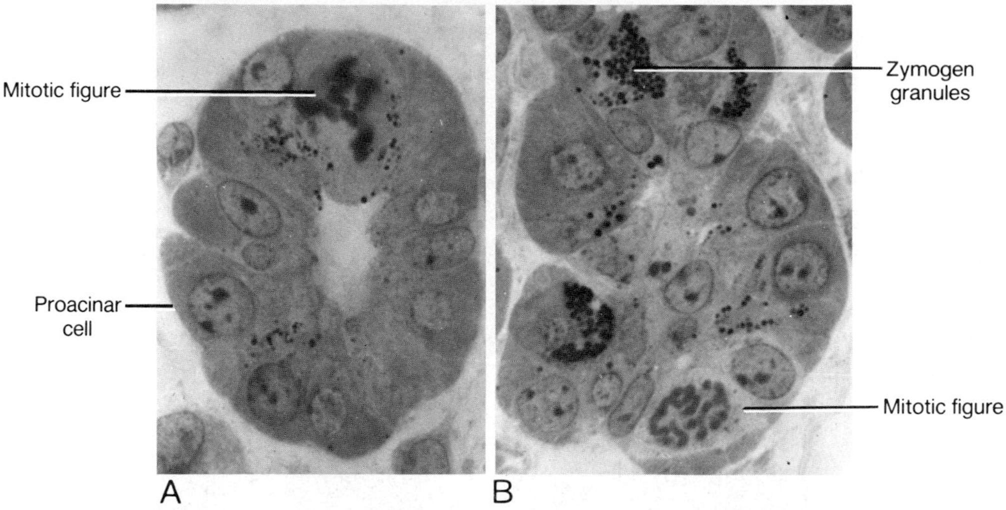

15-91

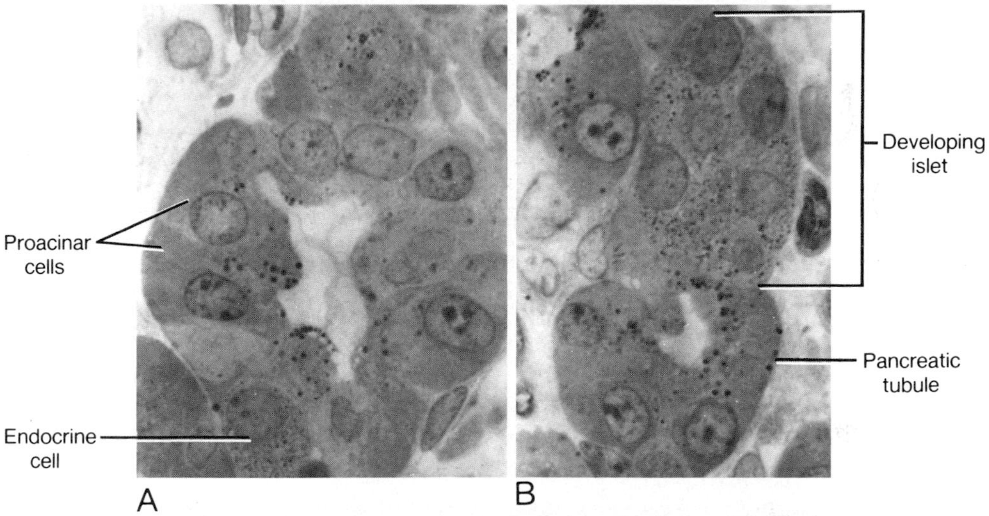

15-92

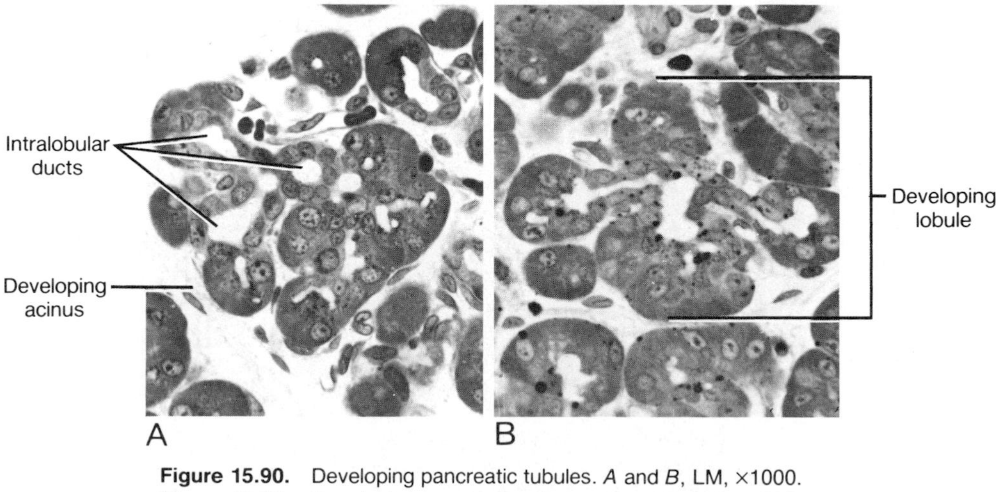

Figure 15.90. Developing pancreatic tubules. *A* and *B*, LM, ×1000.
Figure 15.91. Developing pancreatic tubules. *A* and *B*, LM, ×1000.
Figure 15.92. Developing pancreatic lobules. *A* and *B*, LM, ×250.

15-93

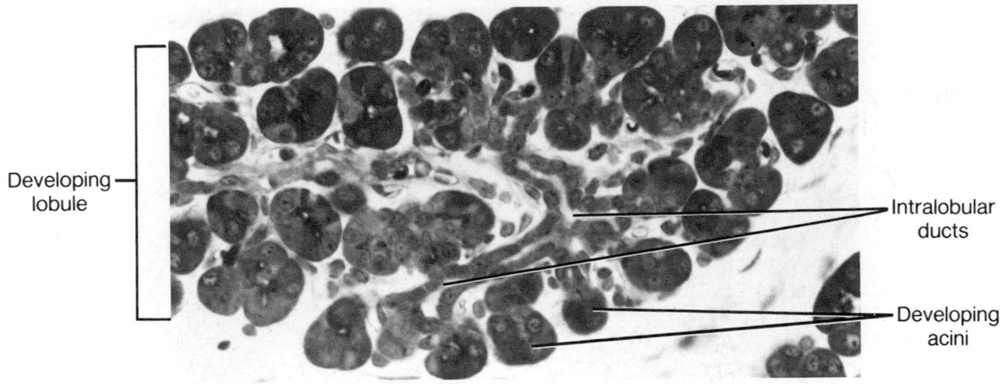

15-94

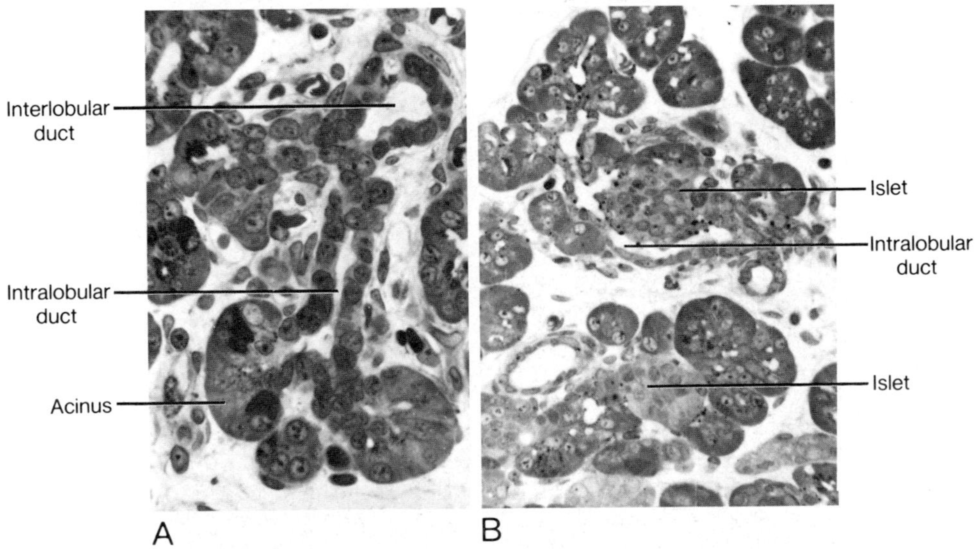

15-95

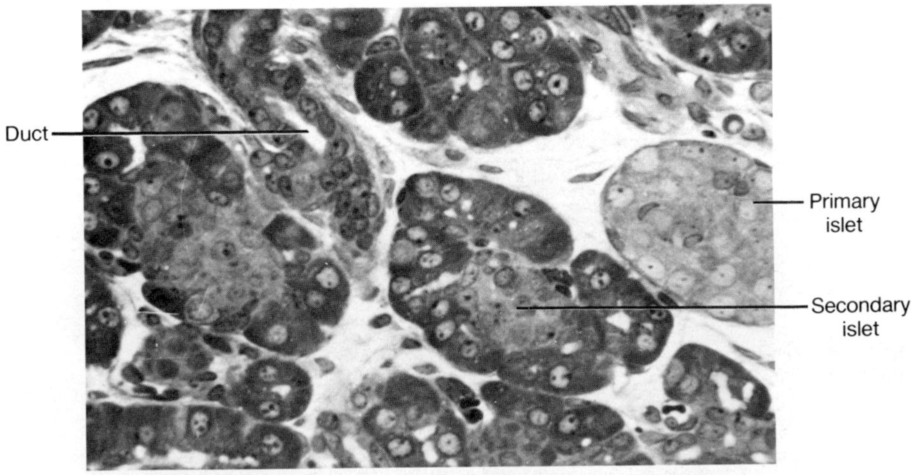

Figure 15.93. Pancreas. LM, ×250.
Figure 15.94. Pancreas. LM, *A*, ×250. *B*, ×100.
Figure 15.95. Pancreas. LM, ×250.

15-96

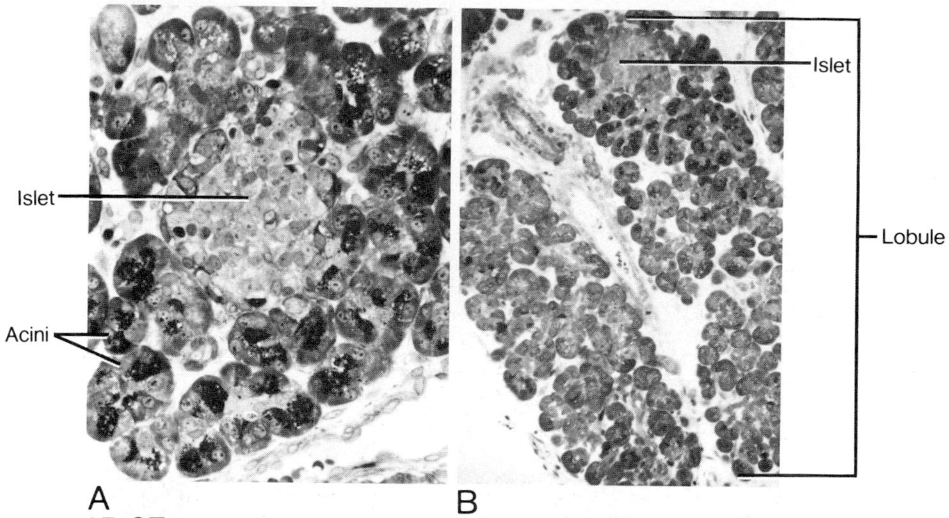

15-97

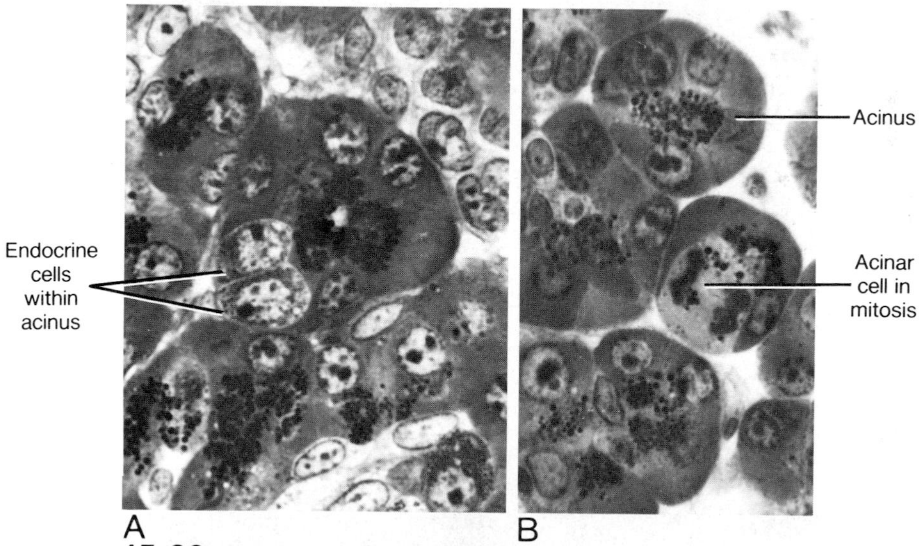

15-98

Liver

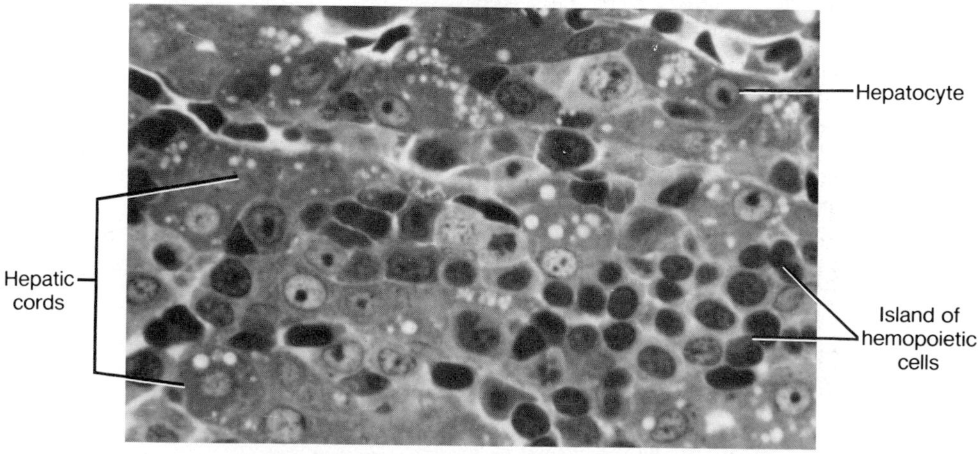

Figure 15.96. Pancreatic lobule. *A* and *B*, LM, ×100.
Figure 15.97. Pancreas. *A* and *B*, LM, ×400.
Figure 15.98. Liver, LM, ×250.

16

Urinary System

The urinary system consists of the kidneys, ureters, bladder and urethra. The kidneys constitute the glandular component while the remainder of the urinary system forms the excretory passages. The ureters conduct urine from the kidney to the bladder, where it is stored temporarily. In turn, the bladder is drained by the urethra, through which the urine ultimately is voided from the body.

KIDNEYS

The kidneys are a pair of compound tubular glands that not only clear the blood plasma of metabolic wastes but also regulate body fluid and salt concentrations, eliminate foreign chemicals and are important in maintaining the acid-base balance of the body. In addition to their excretory function, the kidneys have properties of endocrine organs and release two substances, renin and erythropoietin, directly into the blood stream. Renin is important in regulating blood pressure and sodium ion concentration, whereas erythropoietin influences hemopoietic activity.

Macroscopic Features

KEY WORDS: hilum, renal sinus, renal pelvis, major calyx, minor calyx, renal papilla, cortex, medulla, medullary pyramids, renal columns, medullary ray, renal lobe, renal lobules, multilobular kidney, unilobular kidney

The human kidneys are bean-shaped organs that lie in a retroperitoneal position against the posterior abdominal wall, one on either side of the upper lumbar vertebrae. Each is contained within a thin but strong connective tissue capsule that contains an abundance of fat. The renal artery and the nerves enter the kidney on the medial border at a concavity called the **hilum**, which also serves as the point of exit for the renal vein, lymphatics and ureter. The hilum is continuous with the **renal sinus**, a large, central cavity that is surrounded by the parenchyma of the kidney and filled with a loose areolar connective tissue that normally contains much fat. Branches of the renal artery and vein, nerves, lymphatics and the **renal pelvis**, a funnel-shaped extension of the ureter where it joins the kidney, run through the sinus.

The renal pelvis divides within the renal

sinus to form two or three short tubular structures, the **major calyces**, which in turn subdivide into 8 to 12 smaller units called the **minor calyces.** Each minor calyx forms a cylindrical attachment around a conical projection of renal tissue called a **renal papilla.**

When a hemisection of the kidney is examined macroscopically, the organization of the parenchyma into two distinct regions can be seen readily. The outer region, which forms the **cortex**, is darker, has a granular appearance and forms a continuous layer beneath the capsule. The inner region, or **medulla**, is paler, smoother and consists of from 8 to 20 cone-shaped structures called the **medullary pyramids**, which are separated from each other by inward extensions of cortical tissue. The cortex that passes between and separates adjacent pyramids constitutes a **renal column.** The bases of the pyramids are directed toward the overlying cortex, while their apices are oriented toward the renal sinus and form the renal papillae. From the bases of the pyramids, groups of tubules extend into the cortex, giving it a striated appearance. These striations represent a continuation of medullary tissue into the cortex and constitute the **medullary rays.**

The arrangement of cortex and medulla permits subdivision of the kidney into smaller units, the lobes and lobules. A medullary pyramid, together with its closely associated cortical tissue, makes up a **renal lobe**, while a medullary ray, together with its associated cortical tissue, forms a **renal lobule.** The kidney may consist of several lobes and is then referred to as a **multilobular kidney**; the kidneys of man are of this type. In several species (rat, mouse and rabbit, for example) the **kidneys** are **unilobular** and consist of a single pyramid and its associated cortex.

Microscopic Features

KEY WORDS: uriniferous tubules, nephron, collecting duct

Each renal lobule is made up of numerous epithelial-lined tubules called **uriniferous tubules** (Fig. 16-1). Collectively these constitute the parenchyma of the kidney. Each uriniferous tubule can be divided into a **nephron**, which represents the secretory portion, and a **collecting duct**, the excretory portion that carries urine to the renal pelvis.

Nephron

KEY WORDS: renal corpuscle, proximal tubule, thin segment, distal tubule, loop of Henle

The nephron is the functional unit of the kidney, and during urine formation its various segments participate in filtration, secretion and reabsorption. There are between 1 and 2 million nephrons in each human kidney. A nephron is a blindly ending epithelial tubule that consists of several subdivisions, each of which differs in its structure, function and position within the kidney. A typical nephron consists of a **renal corpuscle**, a **proximal tubule** with convoluted and straight portions, a **thin segment**, and a **distal tubule** which also has a convoluted and a straight portion. Those segments of the nephron between the proximal and distal convoluted tubules, i.e., the straight descending portion of the proximal tubule, the thin segment and the straight ascending portion of the distal tubule, are collectively referred to as the **loop of Henle.**

The renal corpuscle and the proximal and distal convoluted tubules are found only in the cortex, whereas the loop of Henle generally is confined to the medulla or to a medullary ray. The size of the nephrons and the length of their various segments vary according to the position of the parent renal corpuscle in the cortex. Renal corpuscles near the medulla are larger and the thin segment of the loop of Henle, as well as the other segments, are considerably longer than those of nephrons whose renal corpuscles are located in the peripheral regions of the cortex. Nephrons from the subcapsular region have small renal corpuscles and the thin segment of the loop of Henle is short and extends for only a brief distance into the medulla. Those nephrons whose renal corpuscles occupy an intermediate position in the cortex show intermediate features.

Renal Corpuscle

KEY WORDS: glomerulus, glomerular capsule, parietal layer (capsular epithelium), visceral layer (glomerular epithelium), capsular space, vascular pole, urinary pole, podocyte, primary process, secondary process (foot proc-

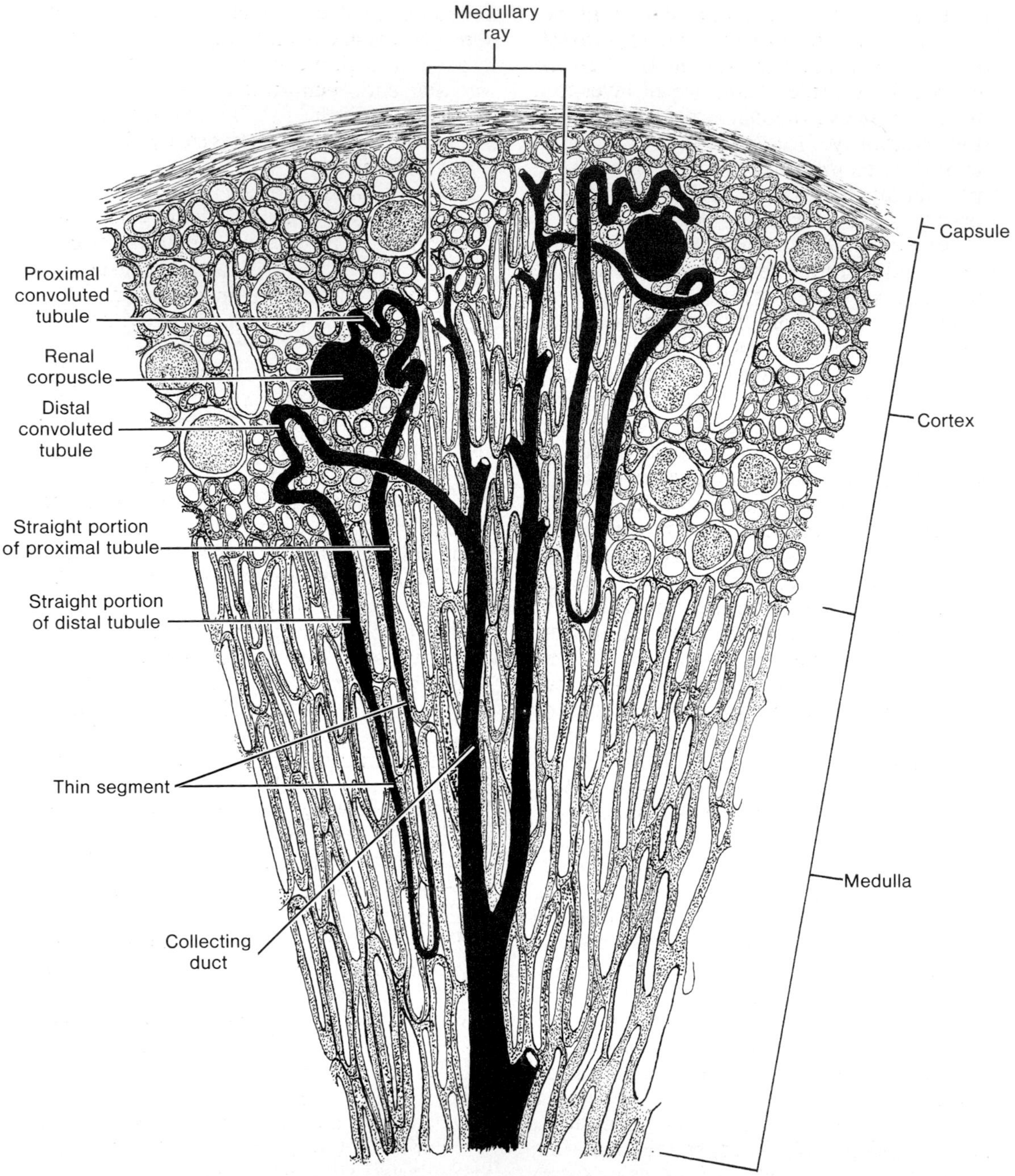

Figure 16.1. Diagram of uriniferous tubules.

esses, pedicles), slit pores (filtration slits), slit membrane, common basal lamina, fenestrated glomerular endothelium, mesangial cells, extraglomerular and intraglomerular mesangium, filtration barrier

A renal corpuscle is roughly spherical in shape and measures 150 to 250 μm in diameter. It consists of a capillary tuft, the **glomerulus**, which projects into a blind expansion of the uriniferous tubule called the **glomerular capsule.** The outer layer of the capsule completely surrounds the glomerulus as the **parietal layer**, which then reflects onto the glomerulus, where it becomes intimately applied to the glomerular capillaries to form a complete investment. This investing layer is called the **visceral layer** of the glomerular capsule. The parietal layer also is known as the **capsular epithelium**, while the visceral layer frequently is referred to as the **glomerular epithelium.** The visceral and parietal layers of the capsule are separated only by a narrow **capsular space.**

Where the afferent and efferent arterioles enter and leave the renal corpuscle is called the **vascular pole**. As the afferent arteriole enters the renal corpuscle, it immediately divides into several primary branches, each of which forms a complex of capillaries (a capillary lobule), which then reunite to form the efferent arteriole. Each glomerulus is made up of several such capillary lobules. On the side opposite the vascular pole, the capsular space becomes continuous with the lumen of the proximal convoluted tubule. This region is known as the **urinary pole.**

The parietal layer of the glomerular capsule consists of a single layer of tightly adherent squamous cells that contain few organelles. Near the urinary pole there is an abrupt transition from this simple squamous form to the large pyramidal cells that line the proximal convoluted tubule. At the vascular pole of the renal corpuscle, the simple squamous epithelium of the capsular epithelium changes to a very specialized cell type known as the podocyte.

Podocytes are large, stellate cells whose cell bodies lie at some distance from the underlying capillaries. The cell bodies are separated from the capillaries by several cytoplasmic extensions, the **primary processes**, that wrap around the underlying glomerular capillaries. The primary processes give rise to numerous **secondary processes (foot processes, pedicles**) that interdigitate with similar processes from adjacent podocytes to invest the capillary loops of the glomerulus. The narrow clefts between the interdigitating foot processes are called **slit pores** or **filtration slits** and measure approximately 25 nm in width. A thin membrane of electron dense material may bridge these gaps and is referred to as a **slit membrane.**

The foot processes of the podocytes and the endothelial cells of the glomerular capillaries share a continuous, **common basal lamina** which measures 0.1 to 0.15 μm in thickness. The basal lamina consists of a mucopolysaccharide matrix that contains type IV collagen. Although initial contact between the glomerular epithelium and the vascular endothelium is necessary to establish the common basal lamina, thereafter it is laid down and maintained by the podocytes themselves.

The **endothelium** of the glomerular capillaries consists of a single layer of attenuated squamous cells. Individual endothelial cells have numerous, large pores or **fenestrae** that measure 50 to 100 nm in diameter. Occasional fenestrae are bridged by a thin diaphragm.

A third cell type, the **mesangial cell**, also is present in the renal corpuscle. These are stellate cells with long cytoplasmic processes that contain numerous filaments. They occupy the region between the afferent and efferent arterioles at the vascular pole and lie in a matrix of amorphous material. The cells constitute the **extraglomerular mesangium** and are continuous with cells of similar appearance, **intraglomerular mesangial cells**, that lie between the glomerular endothelium and the basal lamina. The latter cells are thought to clear away large protein molecules that become lodged on the common basal lamina during the filtration of blood plasma. Mesangial cells also may participate in the removal of older portions of the common basal lamina, on the endothelial side, as it is added to by the podocytes. Mesangial cells are of clinical importance in certain kidney diseases because of their tendency to proliferate.

The renal corpuscle is that portion of the nephron that functions in filtration. The fenestrated glomerular endothelium, the common basal lamina and the foot processes of the glomerular epithelium together form the **filtration barrier** of the renal corpuscle (Fig. 16-2). This barrier permits the passage of water, ions and small molecules from the capillaries into the glomerular space but prevents larger structures such as the formed elements of the blood and large irregular molecules from passing. The capillary endothelial cells prevent the passage of the formed elements, while the common basal lamina restricts the passage of materials with a molecular weight greater than 400,000. Substances of small molecular weight (40,000 or less) traverse the endothelial barrier and the common basal lamina and pass

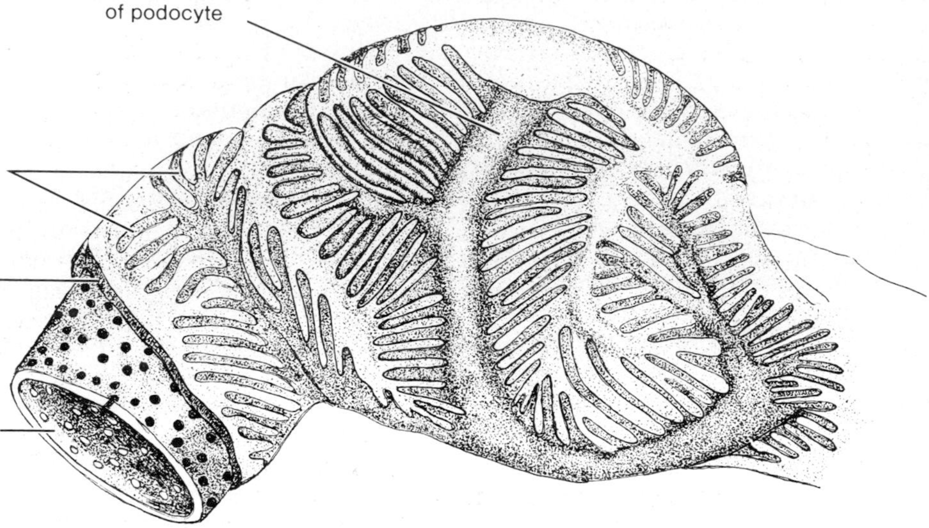

Figure 16.2. Diagram of the filtration barrier.

through the filtration slits of the surrounding glomerular epithelium to enter the capsular space. Although materials with a molecular weight larger than 45,000 or which have a highly irregular shape may pass through the endothelium and common basal lamina, they are unable to traverse the barrier provided by the foot processes of the podocytes. Thus, the glomerular epithelium also is important in limiting the kinds of materials that pass from the blood into the capsular space. Material which collects in the capsular space of the renal capsule is not urine but a filtrate of blood plasma.

The energy for the filtration process is supplied by the hydrostatic pressure of the blood in the glomerular capillaries. This hydrostatic pressure (approximately 70 mm/Hg) provides sufficient force to overcome the colloidal osmotic pressure of substances in the blood (approximately 33 mm/Hg) and the capsular pressure of the filtration membrane (approximately 20 mm/Hg). The resulting filtration pressure (approximately 18 mm/Hg) is great enough to force filterable materials in blood plasma through all three layers of the filtration barrier and into the capsular space.

The hydrostatic pressure exerted within the glomerular capillaries is controlled and made possible by the unusual vascular arrangement associated with the glomerulus. Most vascular areas of the body are supplied by arterioles which form capillaries which then reunite into venules. However, the arrangement of the glomerular capillaries differs in that they are interposed between an afferent arteriole conducting blood to the glomerulus and an efferent arteriole conducting blood away from the glomerulus. The arrangement of capillaries between the two arterioles results in considerable pressure being exerted on the capillary walls. The glomerular pressure can be controlled and regulated by the state of contraction of either arteriole.

As additional filtrate from the blood plasma enters the capsular space, the rise in pressure forces the filtrate into the lumen of the proximal convoluted tubule. Loss of filtrate into the surrounding cortical tissue is prevented by the capsular epithelium which forms a seal around each renal corpuscle.

Proximal Tubule

KEY WORDS: convoluted portion (pars convoluta), straight portion (pars recta), microvillus (brush) border, apical canaliculi, endocytic complex

The proximal tubule begins at the urinary pole of the renal corpuscle and is the longest and largest segment of the mammalian nephron. It is approximately 17 mm in length and makes up the bulk of the cortex. The proximal tubule is divided into a convoluted portion (**pars convoluta**) and a straight portion (**pars recta**). The **convoluted portion** is the longer of the two parts and is the one most frequently observed in sections of the cortex. After following a tortuous course through the cortex in the region of its parent renal corpuscle, the proximal convoluted tubule takes a more direct course through the cortex to become the straight portion of the proximal tubule. It then enters the medulla or a medullary ray, where it turns toward the renal papillae as the first portion of the loop of Henle.

The proximal convoluted tubule is made up of a single layer of large, pyramidal-shaped cells that have a well developed **microvillus (brush)** border. The lateral surfaces of the cells form an intricate system of interdigitating processes and ridges that often extend beneath neighboring cells, and interdigitate with similar processes of the adjacent cells. Thus a complex labyrinth of cell membranes extends into the basal region of the epithelium. Compartmentalization of the lateral and basal regions results in a greater surface area of the cell membrane which facilitates the transport of ions. Each cell of the proximal tubule has a large spherical nucleus, a supranuclear Golgi complex and numerous basal rod-shaped mitochondria which are orientated parallel to the long axis of the cell, closely associated with the lateral ridges and processes.

In typical histological preparations, profiles of the proximal convoluted tubules are the most common tubule in the cortex and usually have a stellate lumen bounded by a distinct brush border. Not all cells of a given tubule show a nuclear profile, due to the large size of the cells, and component cells of the proximal tubule usually have a darkly-staining, granular cytoplasm.

Structurally, the convoluted and straight portions of the proximal tubule are similar, but the cells of the **straight portion** are shorter and the brush border and lateral interdigitations are less well developed than in the convoluted portion. Mitochondria are abundant but are smaller and more randomly scattered throughout the cell.

One of the primary functions of the proximal tubule is absorption of the glomerular filtrate. The brush border, which consists of closely packed, elongated microvilli, markedly increases the surface area available for absorption and the microvilli are embedded in a coat of extracellular proteoglycan that may contain enzymes that facilitate the absorptive process. The apical surfaces of the cells absorb sugars and amino acids from the luminal contents in a manner similar to that of intestinal epithelial cells. Normally, all of the glucose in the glomerular filtrate is absorbed in the proximal convoluted tubule. If blood-glucose levels exceed the absorptive capacity of the enzymes controlling the absorption of glucose, the remainder spills over into the urine resulting in glycosuria.

Protein is absorbed in the proximal tubule by a system of invaginations, called **apical canaliculi**, that give rise to a series of small vesicles which contain protein that has been sequestered from the lumen. The vesicles coalesce to form larger vacuoles. These three elements, namely, the tubular invaginations, the vesicles and the vacuoles, form the **endocytic complex** and it is this complex that is actively involved in protein absorption. The larger protein-containing vacuoles condense and ultimately fuse with lysosomes, the acid hydrolases of which reduce the absorbed protein to its constituent amino acids, which then are released back into the blood stream.

Over 80% of the sodium chloride and water in the glomerular filtrate is absorbed in the proximal tubule. Sodium ion is actively transported from the lumen and chloride ion and water follow passively, with no expenditure of energy by the cell, to maintain osmotic balance. The driving force that moves sodium ion is an active ATPase sodium pump located along the lateral cell membranes which form the complex intercellular space. Other inorganic ions and vitamin C also are absorbed by the proximal convoluted tubule.

In addition to absorption, the proximal convoluted tubule secretes organic acids and bases destined to be eliminated in the urine. Hence, this region of the nephron functions as an exocrine gland. Hydrogen ion also is secreted into the lumen in exchange for bicarbonate ions.

Thin Segment

KEY WORDS: simple squamous epithelium, central cilium

The simple cuboidal epithelium of the straight descending portion of the proximal tubule (the initial segment of the loop of Henle) changes abruptly in the thin segment to become an attenuated, **simple squamous epithelium.** The luminal diameter of the nephron also decreases markedly, from 65 μm in the descending portion to about 20 μm in the thin segment. The thin segment is confined largely to the medulla of the kidney and constitutes the thin limb of the loop of Henle.

The nuclei of the epithelial cells lining the thin segment occupy a central position and cause this region of the cell to bulge into the lumen of the tubule. Ultrastructurally, the cytoplasm shows fewer organelles and the lateral cell membranes have elaborate infoldings which interdigitate with those of adjacent cells. Near the hairpin loops, such interdigitations are less well developed. Typical junctional complexes unite adjacent cells at their apices and the cells rest upon a basal lamina of moderate thickness. The basal cell membrane is relatively smooth. On the luminal surface, the brush border of the proximal tubule is replaced by short, scattered microvilli and each cell bears a single **central cilium.**

The length of the thin segment varies considerably with each nephron and is dependent upon the position of the parent renal corpuscle in the cortex. In nephrons whose renal corpuscles are located in the outer cortex adjacent to the capsule, the thin segments are very short or, in some cases, absent. The longest thin segments are associated with those nephrons whose renal corpuscles are located in the juxtamedullary region of the cortex, and the thin segments of these nephrons may extend almost to the tip of the renal papillae.

Distal Tubule

KEY WORDS: straight portion, macula densa, pars maculata, juxtaglomerular cells, convoluted portion, basal striations, acidification, aldosterone

The distal tubule is divided into three regions: a straight portion (pars recta), a portion that contains the macula densa (pars maculata), and a convoluted portion (pars convoluta).

The **straight portion** of the distal tubule begins as a transition from the thin segment of the nephron. In several species, this transition is abrupt but in man it occurs more gradually. The epithelium increases in height to become cuboidal, but lacks the brush border and apical canaliculi of the proximal tubule. A few microvilli are present, however. Interdigitating processes are present on the lateral surfaces of the cells, and these contain numerous mitochondria. The straight portion of the distal tubule also forms the thick ascending limb of the loop of Henle and completes the looping course of this structure as it ascends through the medulla. It then reenters the cortex to return to the parent renal corpuscle.

As it reaches the renal corpuscle, the distal tubule becomes closely related to the afferent arteriole. The portion of the tubule that contacts the arteriole contains a group of specialized cells which form the **macula densa** (dense spot) and that segment is called the **pars maculata.** The cells are taller and narrower than adjacent tubular cells, so that their nuclei are closer together and more prominent. Cells of the macula densa are polarized toward the basal surface, i.e., the Golgi membranes and occasional granules are found basal to the nucleus, facing the basal cell membrane. The macula densa is related to a modified region of the afferent arteriole, the **juxtaglomerular cells,** which are considered to represent an endocrine portion of the kidney. This feature, together with the polarization of the cells of the macula densa, suggests that the macula densa monitors the luminal fluid in the distal tubule.

The macula densa marks the division between the ascending or straight portion and the **convoluted portion** of the distal tubule, which runs a somewhat tortuous course in the cortex near the renal corpuscle of its origin. The distal convoluted tubule is shorter (5 to 7 mm) than the proximal convoluted tubule and because of this, fewer profiles of the distal tubules are found in histological preparations. The lumen of the distal tubule is generally wider than that of proximal tubules; the cells are shorter and lighter staining; nuclear profiles usually are seen in each cell, in part because many are binucleate and a brush border is lacking.

Electron micrographs show elaborate infoldings of the basal cell membrane that often extend deeply into the cells of the distal tubule. Numerous elongate mitochondria lie parallel to the long axis of the cell in association with basal infoldings, resulting in the prominent **basal striations**, which can be seen with the light microscope. The cells of the distal tubule show a few luminal microvilli and often possess a single central cilium that projects into the lumen. Although their precise function is unknown, these cilia may serve as receptors to sense changes in the luminal contents.

The distal tubule is the principal site for **acidification** of urine and it is here that further absorption of bicarbonate occurs in exchange for hydrogen ions. Approximately one-half of the bicarbonate in the glomerular filtrate is absorbed previously in the proximal tubule. The distal tubule also is the site where ammonia is converted to ammonium ion and thus, this segment of the nephron plays an important role in the acid base balance of the body.

The steroid hormone, **aldosterone**, promotes sodium ion transport from the lumen of the distal tubule in exchange for potassium ion. Inadequate concentrations of aldosterone result in a serious loss of sodium in the urine.

Loop of Henle

KEY WORDS: straight portion of proximal tubule, thin segment, straight portion of distal tubule, countercurrent multiplier system

The loop of Henle is interposed between the proximal and distal convoluted tubules and consists of the **straight portion of the proximal tubule**, the **thin segment**, and the **straight portion of the distal tubule.** Only the kidneys of mammals and birds contain nephrons that have well established loops of Henle. In dessert animals the loops and the renal papillae are long whereas in aquatic species, the loops are less developed and the renal papillae are short. The loops descend in the medulla for variable distances, form a hairpin loop, and then ascend parallel to the descending limb, back through the medulla to the cortex.

The loop of Henle is essential for the production of hypertonic urine and therefore is important in the conservation of body water. The loop acts as a **countercurrent multiplier system** and aids in concentrating urine. The descending thin segment is permeable both to sodium ions and to water, whereas the cells of the ascending limb are the site of a "sodium pump" that actively moves sodium from the tubular lumen into the surrounding interstitium. There is some evidence however, that the ion actively being pumped is chloride, and that sodium ion follows passively. The ascending limb is relatively impermeable to water. Thus, sodium ions are "trapped" in the interstitial substance of the medulla, resulting in an increase in the osmotic concentration around the tubules that course through the medulla. Sodium ions may passively diffuse into the descending thin segment from the surrounding interstitium, only to be pumped out again by the ascending limb as the cycle repeats itself over and over. In this manner, a sodium trap is formed and maintained to establish an osmotic gradient that increases in strength toward the renal papillae. This gradient is important for conservation of water and formation of hypertonic urine by the distal tubules and collecting ducts.

Collecting Ducts

KEY WORDS: initial segment, arched portion, medullary ducts, papillary ducts, area cribrosa, principal cells (light cells), dark cells (intercalated cells), antidiuretic hormone (ADH), renal interstitium

The preceding segments of the nephron, together with the collecting ducts, make up the uriniferous tubule. The collecting ducts can be subdivided depending on their location in the kidney. The **initial segment** is found in the cortex and includes short connecting portions that unite the distal tubules of cortical nephrons to the collecting ducts, and **arched portions** that are formed by the confluence of several connecting portions from juxtamedullary nephrons. The arched portions originate deep within the cortex, ascend in the cortex, and then form an arch to descend within a medullary ray.

Medullary collecting **ducts** are found primarily in the medulla. As the ducts pass through the medulla they converge to form larger, straight collecting ducts known as **papillary ducts**. These terminate at the tip of a renal papilla. The numerous orifices emptying at this point give a sieve-like appearance to the external surface of the renal papillae and this area often is called the **area cribrosa.** The external surface of the renal papillae is covered by transitional epithelium.

Two cell types are present in the lining epithelium of the collecting duct system: **principal cells** (**light cells**) and intercalated cells (dark cells). The light cells generally are cuboidal, have centrally-placed round nuclei and a lightly staining cytoplasm. Perhaps their most characteristic feature is the very distinct cell boundaries. Ultrastructurally, the light cells show scattered, short microvilli on their apical cell membranes, scattered mitochondria and some infolding of the basal plasmalemma. They also contain a single, centrally-placed cilium. Scattered between the light cells are the **dark cells (intercalated cells)**, which contain a greater number of mitochondria and have a more intensely staining cytoplasm. The apical cytoplasm of the dark cell also contains a large number of small vesicles. The apical cell membrane shows microplicae and lacks a central cilium. The function of each of these cell types in the collecting tubule is unknown. As the collecting tubules pass through the medulla, the component cells gradually increase in height and in the papillary ducts become tall columnar.

The collecting ducts conserve water and produce hypertonic urine. As the ducts pass through the medulla to the tips of the papillae, they pass through the increasingly hypertonic environment established and maintained by the loops of Henle. The permeability of the collecting ducts to water is controlled by **antidiuretic hormone** (**ADH**). In the presence of ADH, the collecting ducts become permeable to water, which is drawn from the tubules by osmosis as the result of the hypertonic environment maintained in the medullary interstitium. The loss of water from the tubular contents results in a concentrated, hypertonic urine. In the absence of antidiuretic hormone, due to injury or disease, the kidney cannot concentrate or form hypertonic urine. This condition, diabetes insipidus, results in the production of copious amounts of dilute urine, which results in severe dehydration of the individual.

The **renal interstitium** fills the space between the tubular elements of the kidney. The cortical interstitium is relatively scant except around blood vessels and consists of fine collagen bundles, fibroblasts and scattered phagocytic cells. The medullary interstitium is more abundant and its cells are orientated parallel to the long axis of the tubules. These interstitial cells are characterized by long, branching processes that loop around and encircle adjacent tubules and blood vessels. The medullary interstitium also contains an intercellular matrix and small bundles of collagen.

Juxtaglomerular Apparatus

KEY WORDS: juxtaglomerular cells, renin, angiotensinogen, angiotensin I, converting enzyme, angiotensin II, aldosterone, erythropoietin, macula densa, extraglomerular mesangium

The juxtaglomerular apparatus consists of the juxtaglomerular cells in the wall of the afferent arteriole, the macula densa of the distal tubule and the extraglomerular mesangium. The **juxtaglomerular cells** (J-G cells) are found within the muscular wall of the afferent arteriole as it enters the renal corpuscle at the vascular pole and appear to be highly modified smooth muscle cells. They contain a number of secretory granules, well-developed Golgi complexes and abundant granular endoplasmic reticulum. The J-G cells produce the enzyme **renin** which, when released into the blood, acts on a plasma protein known as **angiotensinogen** and converts it to **angiotensin I.** An enzyme from the lung called **converting enzyme** then converts angiotensin I to the polypeptide **angiotensin II**, which acts upon the zona glomerulosa of the adrenal cortex and stimulates it to release aldosterone. **Aldosterone** influences the distal tubule to transport sodium ion from the lumen in exchange for potassium ion. Angiotensin II also acts as a potent vasoconstrictor and elevates blood pressure. The juxtaglomerular apparatus of some species also produces another humoral agent, **erythropoietin**, that is released into the blood stream and stimulates red blood cell formation in the bone marrow.

The location of the **macula densa**, its basal

polarization and its orientation toward the adjacent J-G cells suggest that there may be an interaction between these two cell groups. The macula densa may function to "sense" the sodium ion concentration in the distal tubule and thereby influence the activity of the J-G cells.

The **extraglomerular mesangium** forms a loose mass of cells between the afferent and efferent arterioles. Component cells may contain granules, but their exact role in the function of the juxtaglomerular apparatus is unknown.

Vascular Supply

KEY WORDS: renal arteries, segmental arteries, interlobar arteries, arcuate arteries, interlobular arteries, intralobular arteries, afferent arteriole, efferent arteriole, peritubular capillary network, vasa recta, vascular countercurrent exchange system

The vascular patterns of the kidney are complex and show regional specializations related to the organization and function of the various parts of the nephron. The **renal arteries** arise from the abdominal aorta and usually divide into anterior and posterior divisions before reaching the renal sinus. These divisions pass anterior and posterior to the renal pelvis to enter the renal sinus and give rise to **segmental** branches which divide further to form **interlobar arteries** that course between renal lobes. At the corticomedullary junction, these arteries divide into several **arcuate arteries** that arch across the base of each medullary pyramid and give off the **interlobular arteries** which pass into the cortex between the lobules. The interlobular arteries run peripherally in the cortex, giving rise to a system of **intralobular arteries** that enter renal lobules and provide the **afferent arterioles** supplying the glomeruli of the renal corpuscles. As the **efferent arteriole** leaves the renal corpuscle of a cortical nephron, it immediately breaks up to form a **peritubular capillary network** that supplies the convoluted tubules. The main circulation of the renal cortex is unique in that the same arterioles give rise to two distinct, sequential capillary beds—the glomerular and peritubular capillaries. Efferent arterioles from juxtamedullary nephrons, on the other hand, form long straight capillaries called **vasa recta** that descend into the medullary pyramid and form hairpin loops. Like the loops of Henle, the loops of the vasa recta are staggered throughout the medulla. The walls of the vasa recta are thin and the endothelium of the ascending (venous) limb is fenestrated. The vasa recta run in close proximity to the loops of Henle, thus permitting an interchange between these two elements. The vasa recta function as a **vascular countercurrent exchange system** that removes excess water and ions. The osmotic gradient is not disrupted due to the slower flow rate and smaller volume in the vasa recta. Blood flow through the vasa recta is in the opposite direction to the flow of fluid through the loops of Henle and this also aids in preventing the disruption of the osmotic gradient.

The venous drainage of the kidney is similar to and follows the same course as the arterial supply. However, there is no venous equivalent to the glomerulus or to the afferent or efferent arterioles. The venous system of the medulla begins in the ascending or venous limb of the vasa recta, which drains into interlobular or arcuate veins. In the peripheral cortex capillaries unite to form the small veins which assume a star-like pattern as they drain into interlobular veins. The renal veins drain into the inferior vena cava. The left renal vein differs in that it is much longer and receives the venous drainage from the left gonad.

EXTRARENAL PASSAGES

The extrarenal passages consist of the minor and major calyces, the renal pelvis, ureter, urinary bladder and urethra. They serve to convey urine (or temporarily store it in the case of the bladder) to the outside, where it is voided from the body. With the exception of the urethra, all have a similar basic structure consisting of a mucosa, a muscularis and an adventitia. All three layers are thinnest in the minor calyces and increase in depth distally to reach their maximum thickness in the bladder.

Calyces, Renal Pelvis, Ureter, and Urinary Bladder

KEY WORDS: mucosa, transitional epithelium, lamina propria, muscularis, inner longitudinal muscle, middle circular muscle, outer longitudinal muscle, adventitia

The thickness of the wall of the excretory passage gradually increases from the upper to lower parts, but except for this, the calyces, renal pelvis, ureters and bladder all show a similar structure. The lumen is lined by a **mucosa** consisting of **transitional epithelium** which rests on a **lamina propria**. There is no submucosa and the lamina propria blends with the connective tissue of the well-developed muscular coat.

Transitional epithelium covers the external surfaces of the renal papillae and reflects onto the internal surfaces of the surrounding minor calyces. It also is continuous with the epithelium of the papillary ducts and thus provides a complete epithelial lining that prevents escape of urine into the neighboring tissues. In the major and minor calyces, the transitional epithelium is two to three layers thick, increasing in the ureter to four or five cell layers and in the bladder to six, eight or more layers of cells. The surface cells are large and rounded in shape and in the relaxed condition have convex or dome-shaped borders that protrude into the lumen. The superficial cells sometimes contain large, polyploid nuclei.

Transitional epithelium shows considerable change in its morphology when distended. During the propulsion of urine down the ureter or in the filled bladder, the epithelium is stretched and flattened by the pressure of the luminal contents. The distended transitional epithelium temporarily assumes the appearance of a thin, stratified squamous epithelium. When the intraluminal pressure is relieved, the epithelium again assumes its nondistended appearance. The transitional epithelium acts as an impermeable barrier to the diffusion of salts and water to and from the urine.

In the relaxed bladder the apical cytoplasm of the superficial cells contains fine filaments and fusiform vesicles that are limited by a membrane of the same thickness as the apical cell membrane. These vesicles are thought to represent reserve surface membrane that is used during distension. Transitional epithelium lies on a very thin basement membrane that usually is not observed with the light microscope.

Beneath the surface epithelium is the lamina propria, which consists of a compact layer of fibroelastic connective tissue. Some diffuse lymphatic tissue also may be present.

The **muscularis** begins in the minor calyces as two thin layers of smooth muscle. The inner layer of longitudinal muscle begins at the attachment of the minor calyx to the renal papilla. The outer layer of muscle spirals around the renal papilla to form a thin muscular coat. The walls of the minor calyces contract periodically around the renal papillae and aid in moving urine from the papillary ducts to the calyces and then into the renal pelvis. The muscularis of the renal pelvis and upper two-thirds of the ureter consist of the same two layers and differ only in thickness. An additional outer, longitudinal layer of smooth muscle usually is present in the lower one-third of the ureter. The muscularis of the urinary passageways consists of bundles of smooth muscle separated by abundant fibroconnective tissue.

The distal ends of the ureters, the intramural portion, pass obliquely through the wall of the bladder to empty into its lumen. The circular layer of smooth muscle disappears and the contractions of the longitudinal layers help dilate the lumen of the distal ureter so that urine can enter the bladder. Peristaltic waves periodically pass along the ureter to convey the urine to the bladder, into which urine enters in small spurts. As the bladder fills, the pressure of its contents keeps the intramural portions of the ureter closed due to their oblique course in the bladder wall and the ureters open only when urine is forced through them. Reflux of urine into the ureters is prevented by a valve-like flap of the bladder mucosa that lies over the ureteral orifices.

The muscularis of the urinary bladder is moderately thick and consists of an **inner longitudinal layer**, a **middle circular layer**, and **an outer longitudinal layer.** The middle circular layer is the most prominent. It spirals around each ureteral orifice, increasing in thickness around the internal urethral orifice, to form the internal sphincter of the bladder.

The muscularis is surrounded by a coat of fibroelastic connective tissue, the **adventitia**, which attaches the extrarenal passage to the surrounding structures. In the renal pelvis it blends with the capsule of the kidney. On the superior surface of the bladder this fibroelastic coat is covered by peritoneum. The adventitia contains numerous blood vessels, lymphatics and nerves. The blood vessels pierce the muscularis, provide it with capillaries and then form a plexus of small vessels in the lamina propria. A rich capillary layer lies immediately beneath the epithelium. Nerve fibers as well as small ganglia also are found in the adventitia. These fibers and neurons represent both the sympathetic and parasympathetic divisions of the autonomic nervous system. The parasympathetic fibers are important for micturition.

Male Urethra

KEY WORDS: prostatic urethra (pars prostatica), membranous urethra (pars membranacea), sphincter urethrae, penile urethra (pars cavernosa), fossa navicularis, glands of Littre, intraepithelial glands

In the male, the urethra conveys urine from the urinary bladder to the outside and serves for the passage of seminal fluid during ejaculation. The male urethra is approximately 18 to 20 cm in length and is described in three segments. The first segment is 3 to 4 cm in length and lies within the prostate (an accessory sex gland) and therefore is referred to as the **prostatic urethra (pars prostatica).** This part of the urethra is lined by transitional epithelium similar to that which lines the bladder. The **membranous urethra (pars membranacea)** is very short (1.5 cm) and extends from the apex of the prostate to the root of the penis. The membranous urethra passes through the pelvic diaphragm to pierce the skeletal muscle of the urogenital diaphragm immediately prior to entering the penis. Skeletal muscle surrounding this portion of the urethra forms the external sphincter of the bladder (also known as the **sphincter urethrae**) and is under voluntary control during micturition.

The third and longest segment (approximately 15 cm) is the **penile urethrae (pars cavernosa),** which runs longitudinally through the corpus cavernosa urethrae and terminates at the tip of the glans penis. The membranous and penile portions of the urethra are lined by stratified or pseudostratified columnar epithelium, although patches of stratified squamous epithelium are often found in the penile portion. The penile urethra has a distal enlargement, the **fossa navicularis**, lined by stratified squamous epithelium. The mucous membrane of the urethra has small depressions or invaginations called lacunae of Morgagni that are continuous with the branched tubular **glands of Littre.** These glands are lined by the same epithelium as the luminal surface but contain **intraepithelial nests** (glands) of clear, mucus-secreting cells. The lamina propria underlying the epithelium of the urethra is a highly vascular, loose fibroconnective tissue rich in elastic networks. The mucosa is bounded by two coats of smooth muscle, an inner longitudinal layer and an outer circular layer.

Female Urethra

The female urethra is shorter than the male (3 to 5 cm in length) and is lined by stratified squamous epithelium, although patches of stratified or pseudostratified columnar may be found. Glands of Littre also are present throughout its length. As in the male, the surrounding lamina propria is a vascular fibroelastic connective tissue that contains numerous venous sinuses. The surrounding muscularis, like the ureter, consists of an inner longitudinal layer of smooth muscle bundles and an outer circular layer. The female urethra is surrounded by skeletal muscle fibers of the urogenital diaphragm (sphincter urethrae) at its orifice.

DEVELOPMENT OF THE URINARY SYSTEM

The urinary and reproductive systems arise in common from mesoderm of the urogenital ridge. In reptiles, birds and mammals, a nonfunctional pronephros, a mesonephros functional in the fetus and a metanephros, the definitive kidney, arise successively, each caudal to the last with some overlapping. A functional adult pronephros occurs only in chordates such as *Amphioxus* and myxinoid fishes. Except for lacking loops of Henle, pronephric and mesonephric nephrons resemble those of the metanephros. Although the nephron and collecting tubules form continuous structures in the definitive kidney, each has a separate origin, unlike other exocrine glands where secretory units and ducts form from the same primordium.

Mesonephroi are drained by mesonephric ducts which regress in the female but in the male are incorporated into the reproductive tract. By a series of subdivisions, an outgrowth of the duct, the ureteric bud, gives rise to the ureters, renal pelvis, major and minor calyces, papillary ducts and collecting tubules. The ureteric bud extends into the metanephric blastema, a mass of mesoderm that gives rise to the nephrons. The looser, more external layer of mesoderm forms the interstitial tissue and capsule of the kidney.

Proliferation of mesoderm in the subcapsular nephrogenic zone results in solid, ovoid masses in which the mesenchymal cells adjacent to collecting tubules form double-layered caps. The rest of the cell mass forms a primitive renal vesicle located between a main collecting tubule and one of its branches. Cells of the renal vesicle and collecting tubule do not make contact. Each renal vesicle gives rise to a nephron unit. The single-layered vesicle lengthens and two indentations appear, transforming it into an S-shaped tubule. The space between the middle and lower limbs of the S fills with mesodermal cells and a capillary. Together, the vessel and lower limb of the tubule evolve into a renal corpuscle. The capillaries lie immediately adjacent to the concave, external surface of the lower limb and as they expand into the tubule, they acquire an epithelial covering and form the glomerular capillaries. The parietal layer of the glomerular capsule, which originates from the opposite side of the tubule, constricts around the point of entry of the capillary loops and establishes the vascular pole. Where the tubule surrounds developing capillaries, the columnar cells share a basal lamina with the endothelial cells.

The provisional glomerular epithelial cells show numerous desmosomes and zonular adherens-like structures that maintain contact between the epithelial cells, while the capillary loops expand. The attachments occur mainly along the central, lateral regions of the cells, rather than at their apices, thus maintaining cell-to-cell union as the glomerular epithelium changes from simple cuboidal to a layer of podocytes. The attachments are transitory and generally are lost as the podocytes evolve. With development, podocytes become cuboidal with finger-like processes extending from their basal surfaces towards adjacent cells. The cells begin to separate from each other and their foot processes increase in size, mingling with others to cover the expanding capillaries.

The opposite ends of the S-shaped tubules unite with nearby collecting tubules and the lumina become continuous. The tubules elongate, become U-shaped and give rise to proximal and distal tubules and loops of Henle. The latter are the last segments to form and are not numerous until late in development.

Initially, development of the kidney is concerned with the formation of nephrons and this is followed by a period of growth and differentiation of established nephrons. In man, nephrogenesis is complete by the 35th week, but there is much species variation: in the guinea pig it is not complete until birth and in marsupials, not until late in postnatal life.

Early in development, the digestive and urogenital systems open into a common space, the cloaca. Later, a wedge of mesenchyme, the urorectal septum, divides the cloaca into a dorsal rectum and a ventral bladder and urogenital sinus. The endodermal lining of the newly-formed bladder becomes stratified and the surrounding mesenchyme differentiates into the muscular wall of the bladder.

FUNCTIONAL SUMMARY

The kidney serves as an organ of excretion, is both an endocrine and exocrine gland, is a target organ of other endocrine glands and plays an important role in the acid-base balance of the organism.

The uriniferous tubules perform three separate functions in the formation of urine: filtration, secretion and selective absorption. The tubules do not synthesize and release new materials in

significant amounts but eliminate excess water and waste products of metabolism that are being transported in the blood plasma. After filtration of the plasma, metabolic waste products such as urea, uric acid and creatinine are not absorbed but remain in the tubular lumen and form constituents of the urine that will be eliminated from the body.

The renal corpuscles filter the blood plasma, and in man, the kidneys produce about 125 ml of glomerular filtrate each minute. Approximately 124 ml of this amount are absorbed by the remainder of the uriniferous tubule, resulting in the formation of about 1 ml of urine. The total glomerular filtrate in man, during a 24-hour period, is between 170 to 200 liters, of which about 99% is absorbed. The filtration process is driven by the hydrostatic pressure of blood, which is sufficient to overcome the colloidal osmotic pressure of the plasma and the capsular pressure at the filtration membrane. The resulting filtrate contains ions, glucose, amino acids, small proteins and the nitrogenous waste products of metabolism. Blood cells and proteins of large molecular weight are prevented from entering the capsular space by the filtration barrier.

The glomerular filtrate is reduced to approximately 15% of its original volume in the proximal convoluted tubule. In addition to the obligatory absorption of sodium chloride and water, glucose, amino acids, proteins and ascorbic acid are actively absorbed in the proximal convoluted tubules. Bicarbonate also is absorbed here in exchange for the secretion of hydrogen ions. Exogenous organic bases and acids are actively secreted into the lumen by the epithelium of the proximal convoluted tubule, thus fullfilling the requirements of an exocrine gland. Most of the materials that have passed through the filtration barrier are immediately reabsorbed by the epithelium of the uriniferous tubules and placed back into the circulation. Those materials in excess of the body's needs plus the metabolic wastes pass along the tubular lumen and are excreted in the urine.

The loop of Henle is an essential element of the uriniferous tubule for the conservation of water and the production of hypertonic urine. An active sodium pump mechanism resides in the cells of the ascending limb of the loop and provides and maintains a gradient of osmotic pressure that increases from the base of the medulla to the papillary tip. The loops of Henle with their hairpin loops act as a counter current multiplier system to maintain this osmotic gradient.

The distal tubule is the principal site for the acidification of urine and is the site for further absorption of bicarbonate in exchange for the secretion of hydrogen ions. It therefore plays an important role in acid base balance. The conversion of ammonia to ammonium ions also occurs in the distal convoluted tubule. The active absorption of sodium ion in the distal convoluted tubule is referred to as facultative absorption and is under the control of the steroid hormone, aldosterone, which acts to increase the rate of sodium ion absorption and potassium ion secretion. If aldosterone is absent, large amounts of sodium are lost in the urine. Parathyroid hormone also acts on the tubular components of the nephrons to promote the absorption of calcium ion and to inhibit the absorption of phosphate ion from the forming urine.

The collecting ducts pass back through the hypertonic environment of the medulla. The permeability of the collecting ducts to water is controlled by antidiuretic hormone (ADH). In the presence of ADH the collecting ducts become permeable to water which, by osmosis, leaves the lumen to enter the surrounding interstitium. The flow of water out of the tubular fluid thus produces a hypertonic urine. If the concentration of ADH in the blood is low, a larger volume of dilute urine will result because the permeability of the collecting ducts to water is decreased.

The endocrine portion of the kidney is the juxtaglomerular apparatus which elaborates an enzyme, renin, which is released into the blood stream. Renin acts on the plasma globulin angiotensinogen to form an inactive protein called angiotensin I. A converting enzyme from the lung converts angiotensin I into angiotensin II and the latter stimulates the zona glomerulosa of the adrenal cortex to release aldosterone. Aldosterone stimulates the distal tubule of the nephron to absorb sodium ions in exchange for potassium ions. Angiotensin II also is a potent vasoconstrictor and raises blood pressure. The renin-angiotensin system is influenced by blood flow through the kidney and is an important factor in hypertension. The juxtaglomerular apparatus in some species also produces a blood-borne factor called erythropoietin which stimulates erythropoiesis in the bone marrow.

A minor calyx is attached around each renal papillae and represents the beginning of the extrarenal passageways. The minor calyces undergo periodic, rhythmic contractions that aid in moving urine from the papillary ducts into the extrarenal system. The walls gently contract around each renal papillae and transport the urine to the renal pelvis. Periodic contractions of the muscular walls propel small volumes of urine from the renal pelvis through the ureter to the urinary bladder. Here it is temporarily stored until a sufficient volume is obtained for urine to be evacuated through the urethra. Contraction of the muscularis of the bladder wall, together with the voluntary relaxation of skeletal muscle forming the sphincter urethrae, accomplish this process during micturition.

Atlas and Table of Key Features for Chapter 16

Table 16.1.
Key Histological Features of the Kidney

	Primary Location	Features of Epithelium	Other Features
Proximal convoluted tubule	Cortex	Large granular, dark-staining cells; brush border, not all cells show a nuclear profile	Stellate or irregular lumen
Distal convoluted tubule	Cortex	Light-staining columnar cells; each cell shows nuclear profile	Smooth luminal surface
Renal corpuscle (Bowman's capsule, glomerulus)	Cortex	Light-staining simple squamous, glomerular endothelium; thick basal lamina	Vascular and urinary poles
Thin segment (loop of Henle)	Medulla	Light-staining tubule lined by simple squamous epithelium	Narrow lumen
Thick segment (loop of Henle)	Medulla	Light-staining cuboidal cells	Lumen patent
Collecting tubule	Medulla	Light-staining columnar cells, distinct cell boundaries	

Table 16.2.
Key Histological Features of Extrarenal Passages

	Epithelium	Supporting Wall
Ureter (proximal 2/3)	Transitional (4–5 cell layers)	Inner longitudinal and outer circular smooth muscle
Ureter (distal 1/3)	Transitional (4–5 cell layers)	Inner longitudinal, middle circular and outer longitudinal smooth muscle
Male Urethra		
(a) Pars prostatica	Transitional	Prostate
(b) Pars membranacea	Transitional	Skeletal muscle (sphincter urethrae)
(c) Pars cavernosa	Stratified and/or pseudostratified columnar; patches of wet stratified squamous in fossa navicularis	Erectile tissue of corpus cavernosum urethrae
Female urethra	Stratified columnar; stratified squamous	Inner longitudinal, outer circular smooth muscle

16-3 Kidney

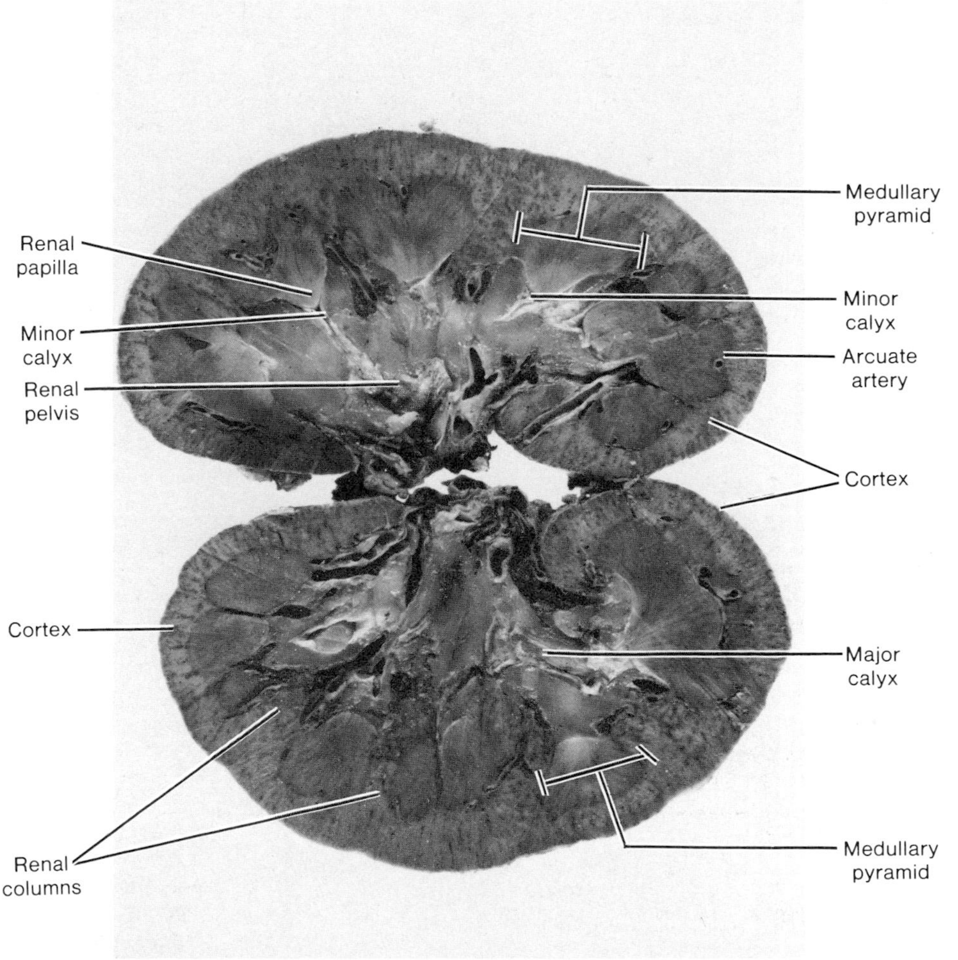

16-4

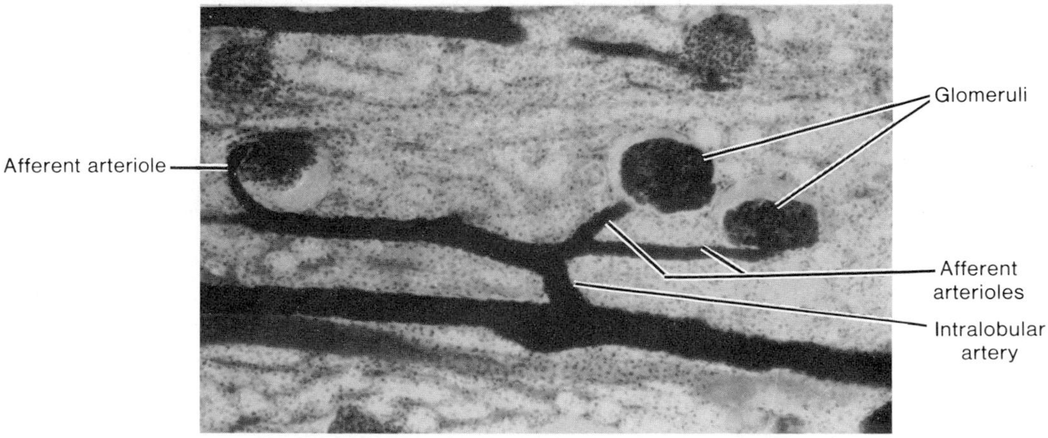

Figure 16.3. Multilobular kidney (human). Actual size.
Figure 16.4. Renal cortex. LM, ×100.

16-5

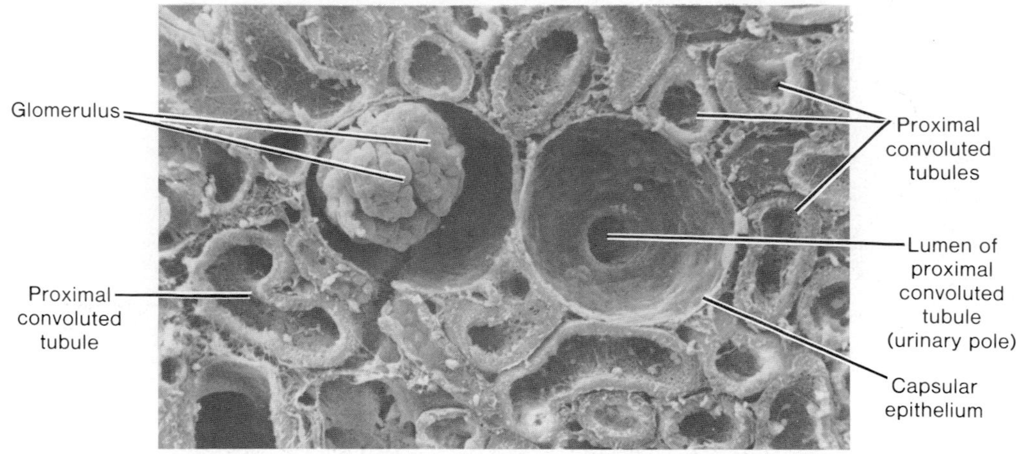

16-6

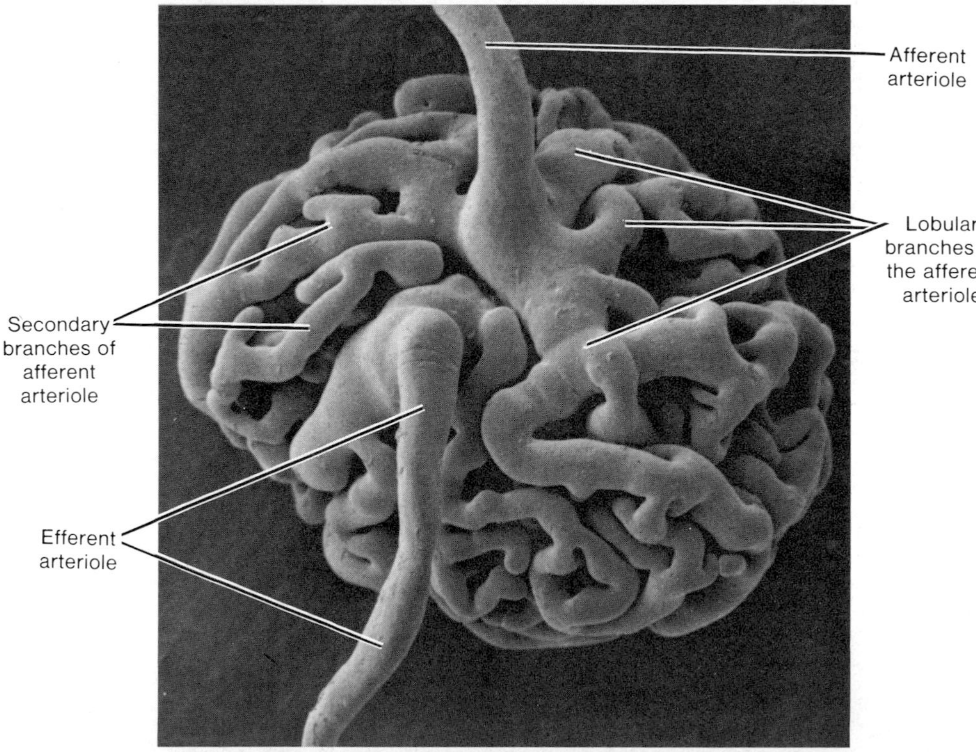

Figure 16.5. Renal cortex. SEM, ×250.
Figure 16.6. Cast of glomerulus. SEM, ×800.

16-7

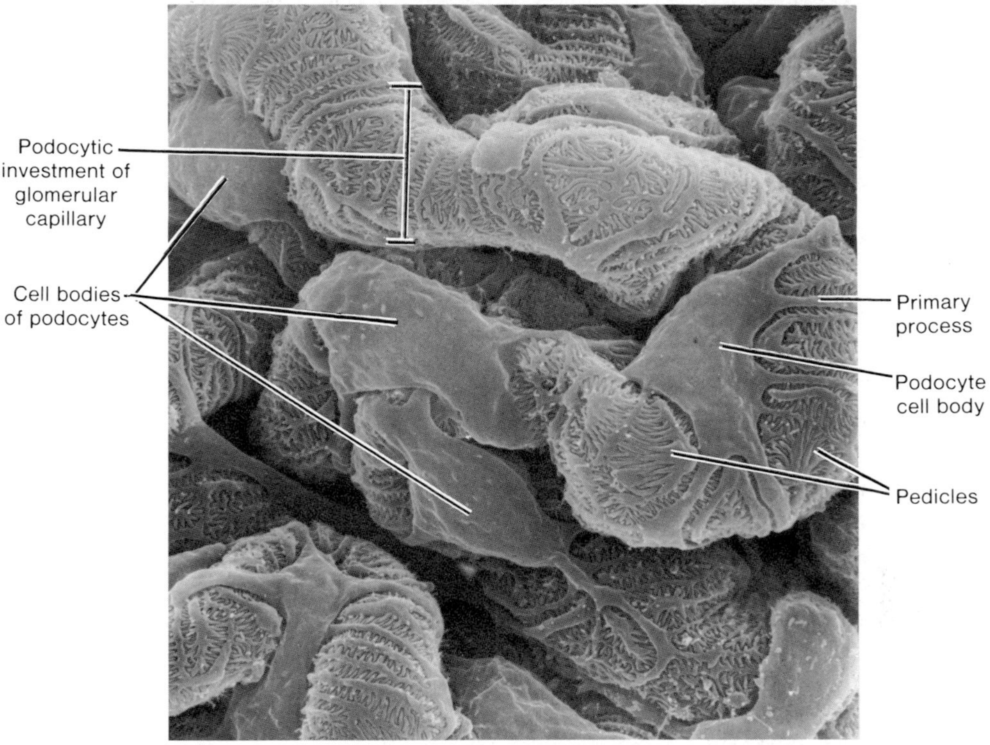

16-8

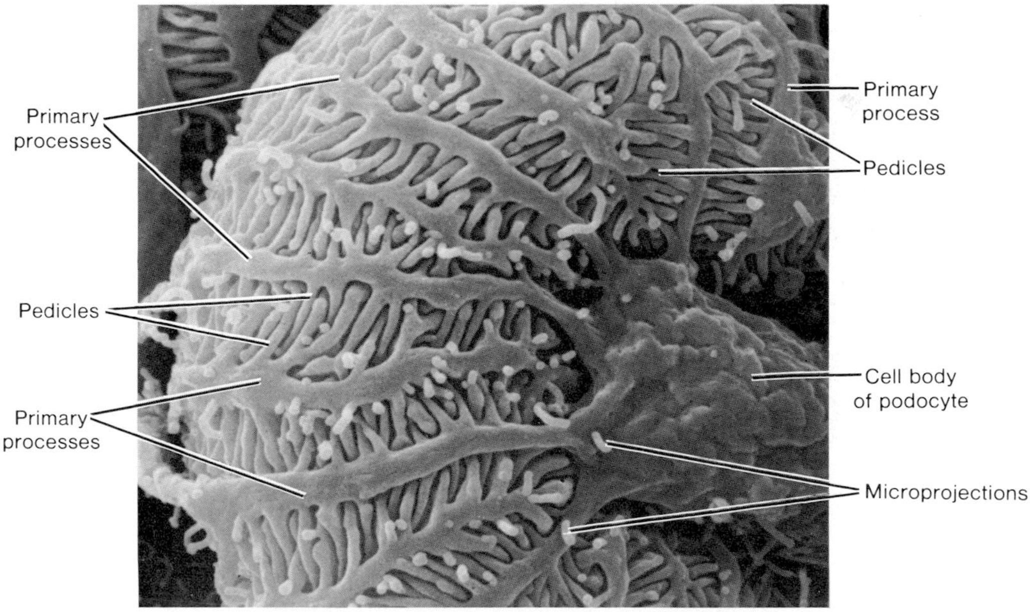

Figure 16.7. Glomerular epithelium. SEM, ×2300.
Figure 16.8. Glomerular epithelium. SEM, ×7600.

16-9

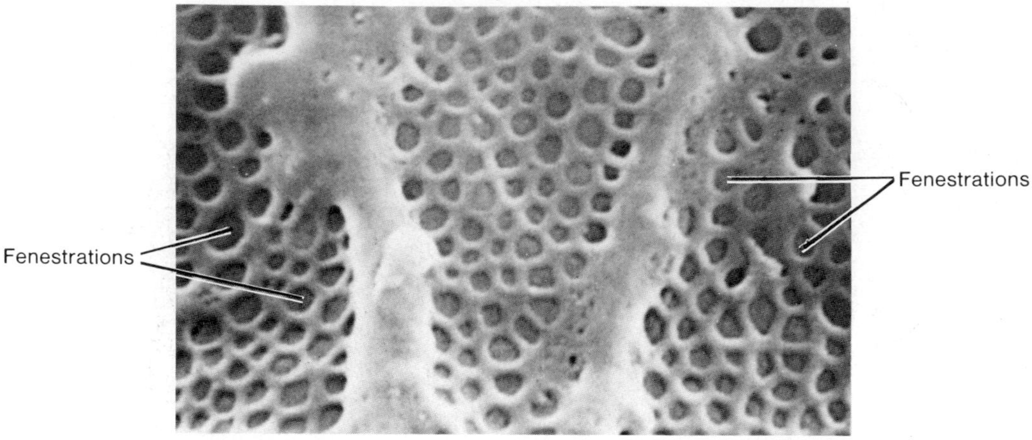

16-10

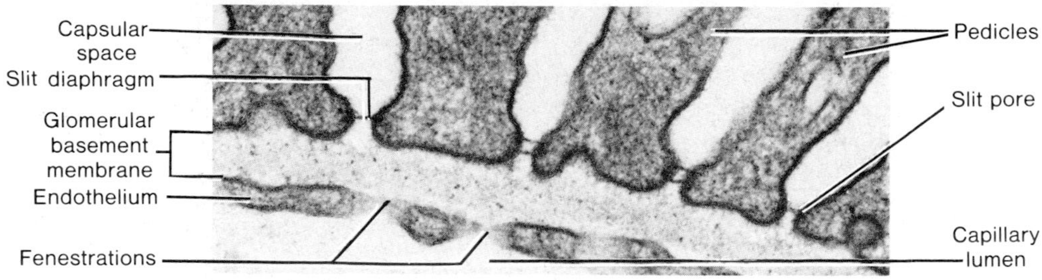

16-11

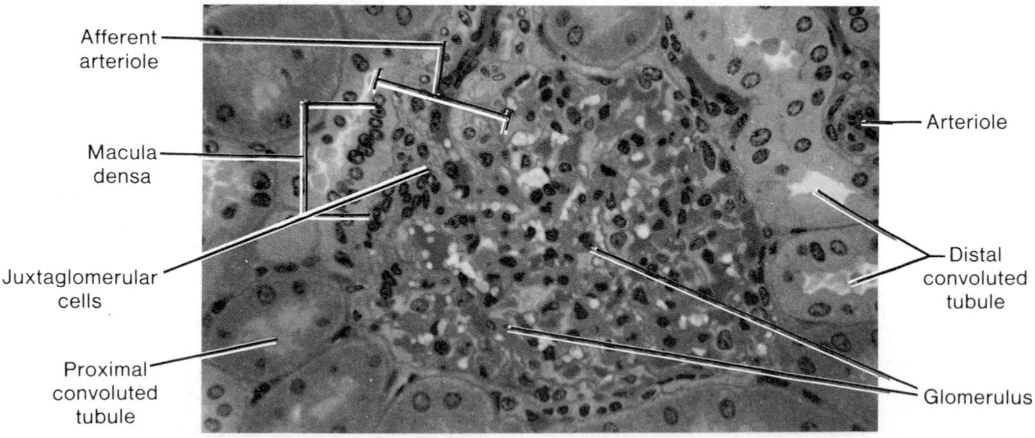

Figure 16.9. Fenestrated glomerular endothelium. SEM, ×35,000.
Figure 16.10. Filtration barrier. TEM, ×80,000.
Figure 16.11. Renal corpuscle. LM, ×250.

16-12

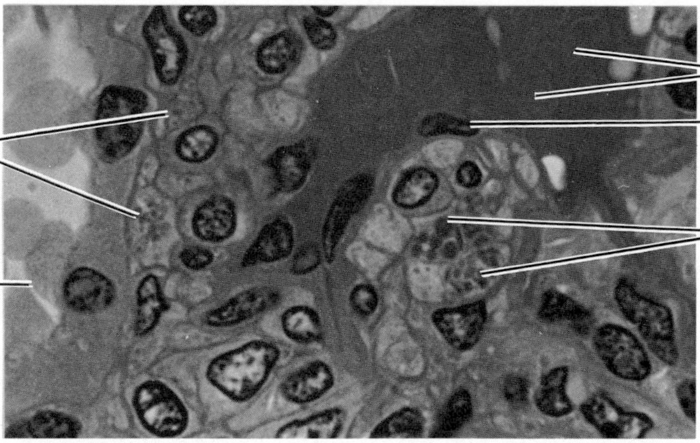

16-13

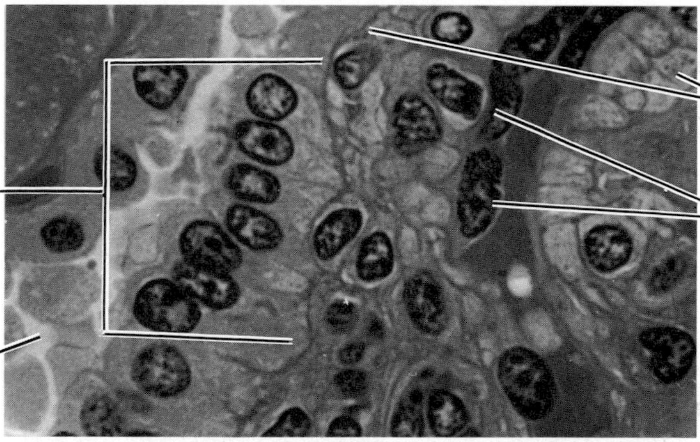

16-14

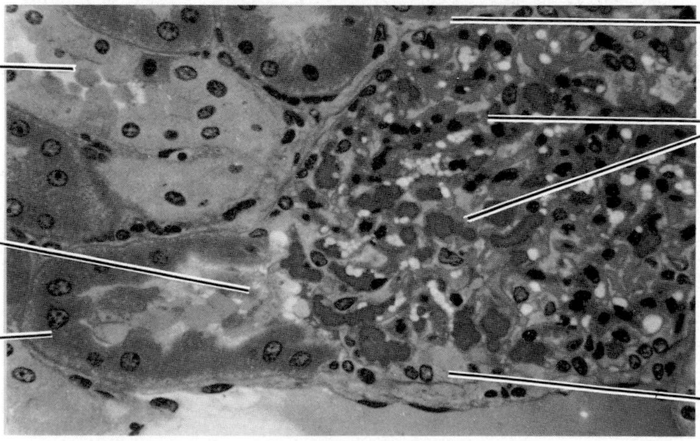

Figure 16.12. Juxtaglomerular cells. LM, ×1000.
Figure 16.13. Juxtaglomerular apparatus. LM, ×1000.
Figure 16.14. Renal corpuscle. LM, ×250.

16-15

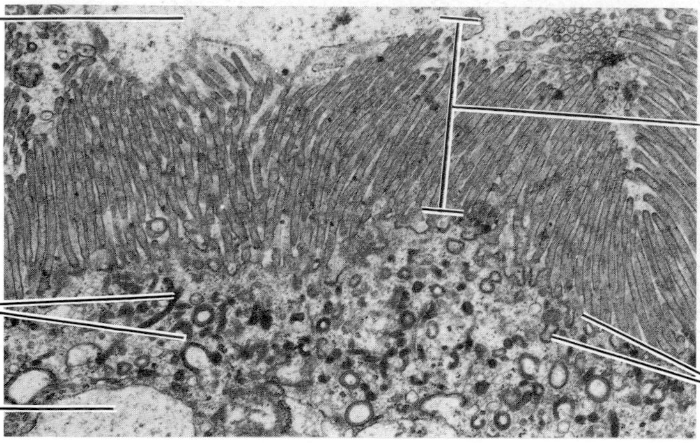

16-16

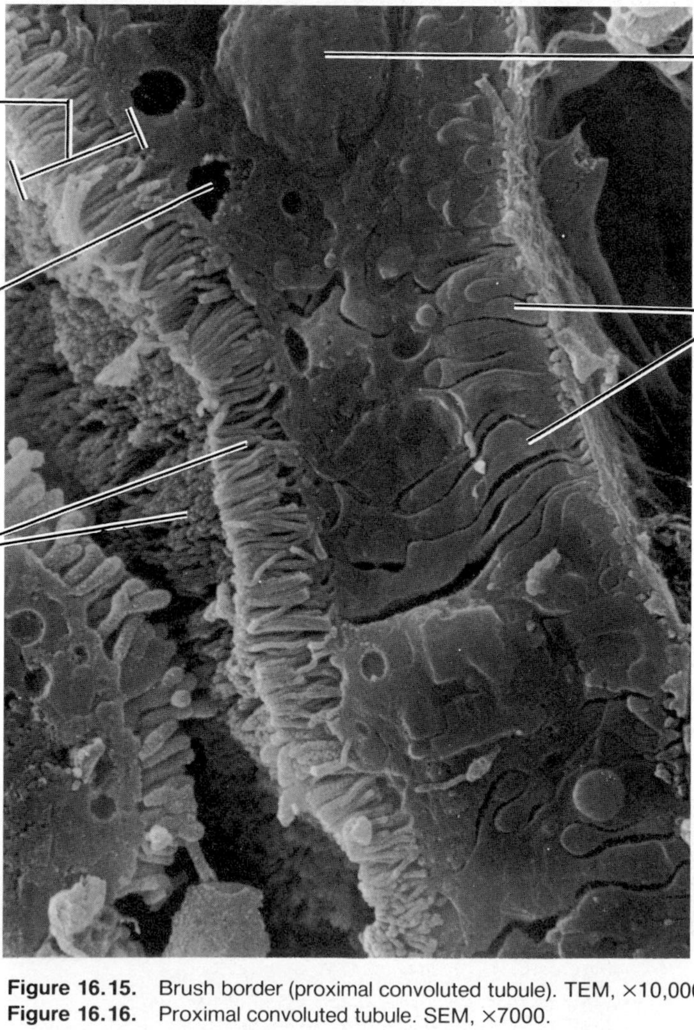

Figure 16.15. Brush border (proximal convoluted tubule). TEM, ×10,000.
Figure 16.16. Proximal convoluted tubule. SEM, ×7000.

16-17

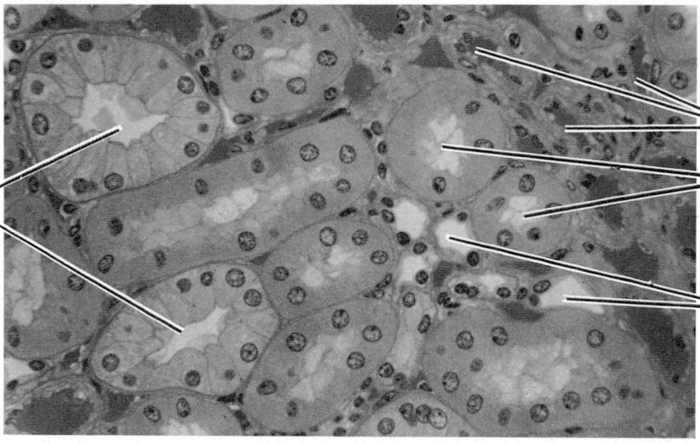

16-18

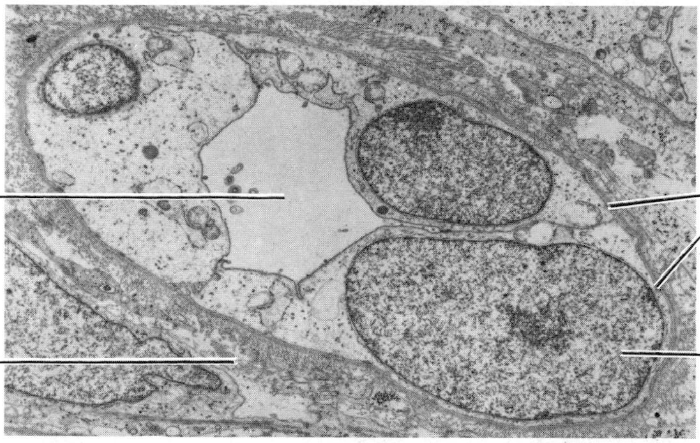

16-19

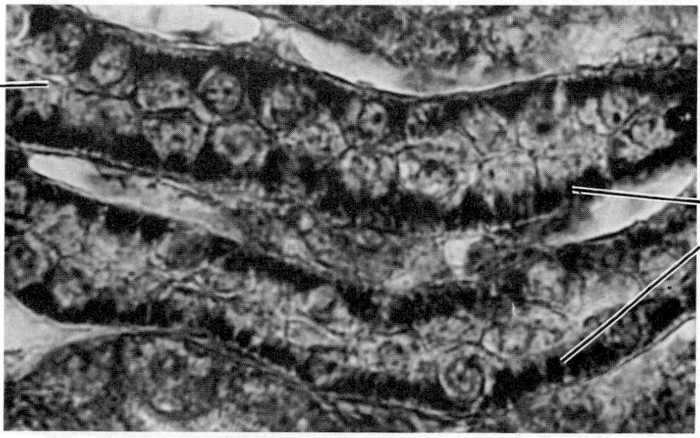

Figure 16.17. Kidney medulla. LM, ×250.
Figure 16.18. Loop of Henle. TEM, ×3000.
Figure 16.19. Distal convoluted tubule. LM, ×400.

16-20

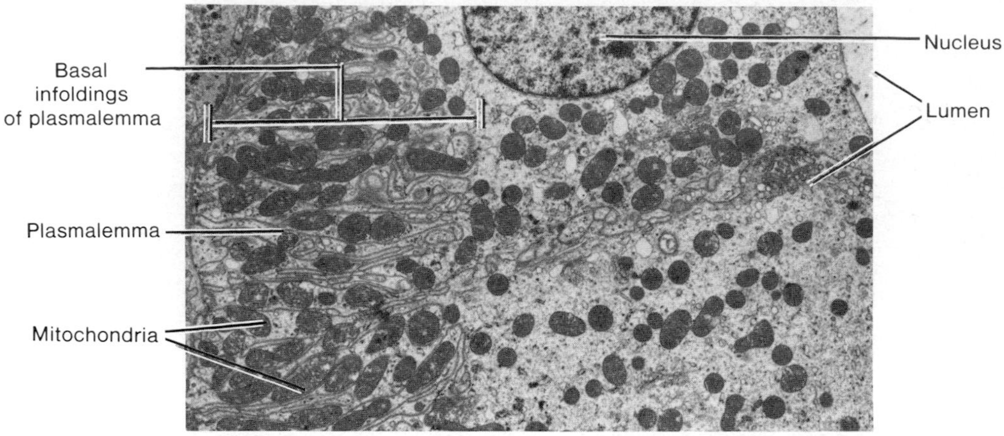

16-21

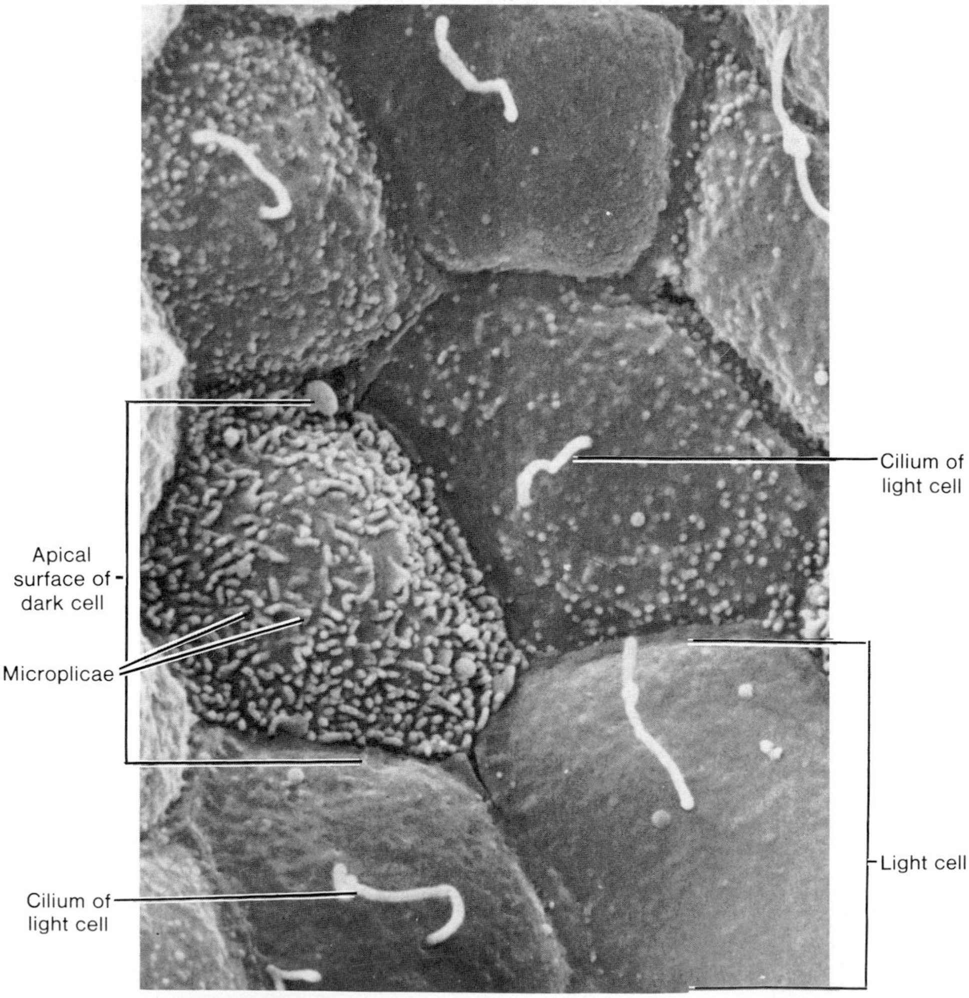

Figure 16.20. Distal convoluted tubule. TEM, ×3000.
Figure 16.21. Collecting tubule (human). SEM, ×8000.

16-22

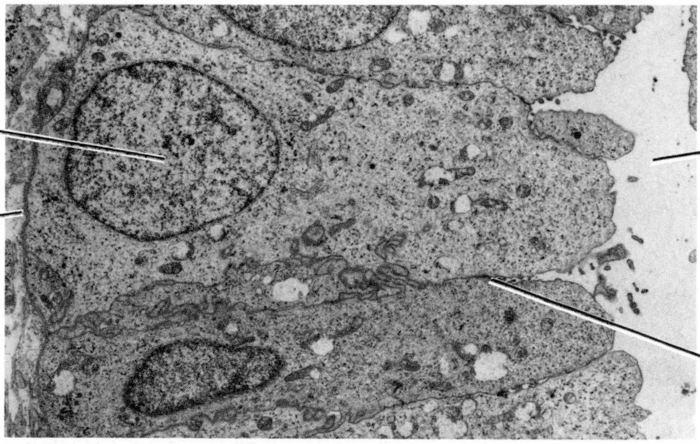

16-23

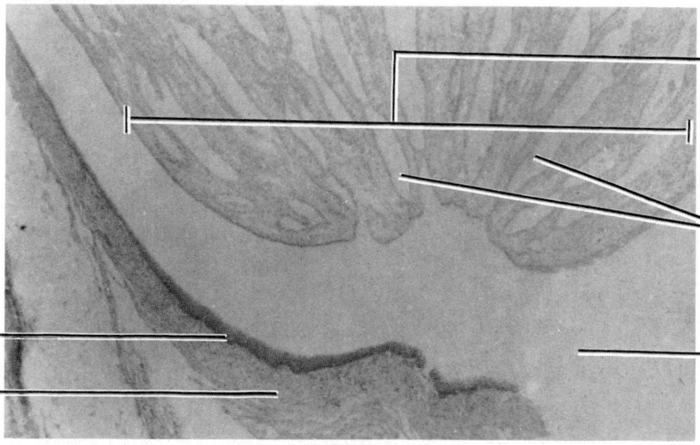

16-24 Ureter

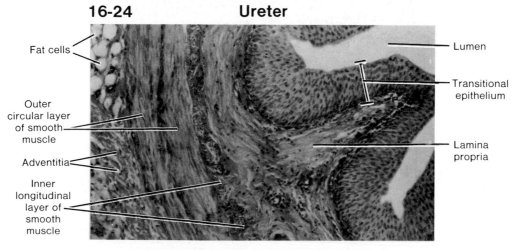

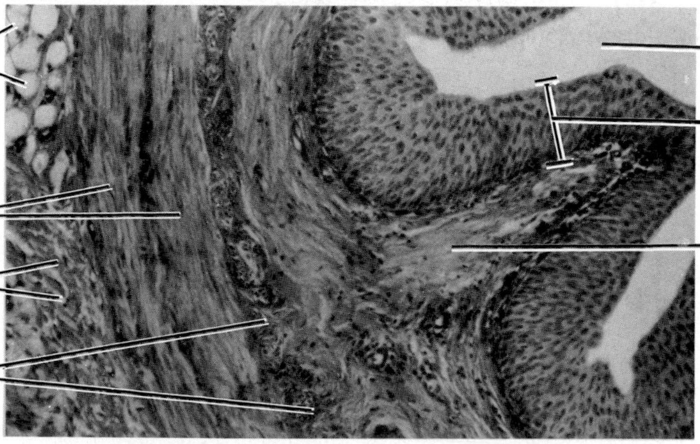

Figure 16.22. Collecting tubule. TEM, ×2000.
Figure 16.23. Minor calyx. LM, ×40.
Figure 16.24. Ureter. LM, ×100.

16-25 Urinary Bladder

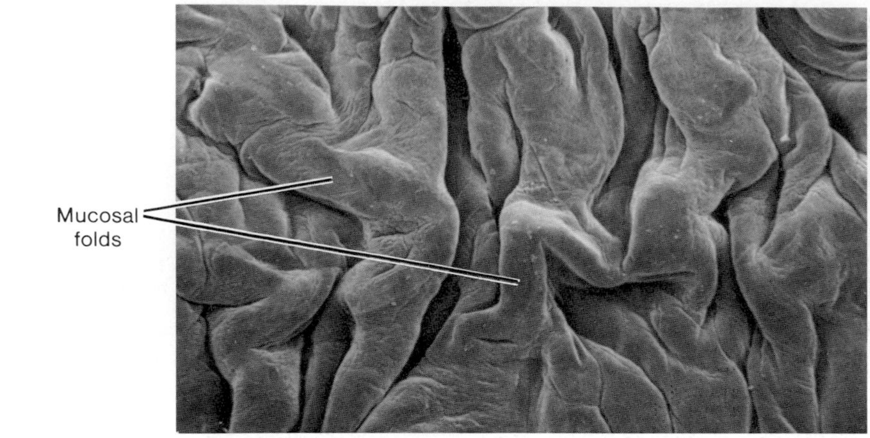

16-26

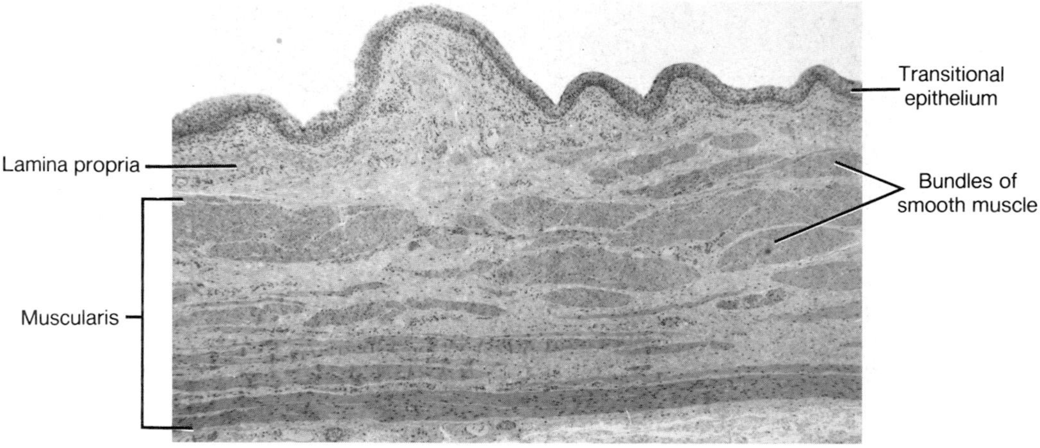

16-27

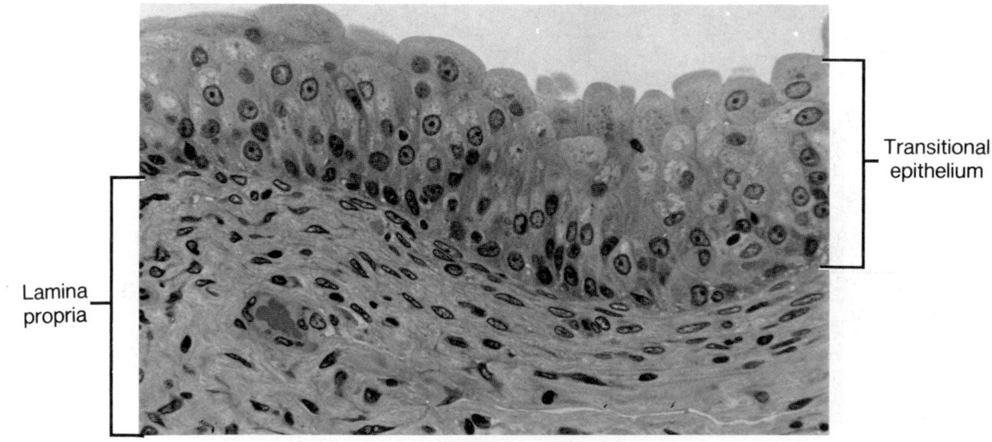

Figure 16.25. Mucosal surface. SEM, ×20.
Figure 16.26. Bladder wall. LM, ×100.
Figure 16.27. Bladder epithelium. LM, ×250.

16-28 Urethra

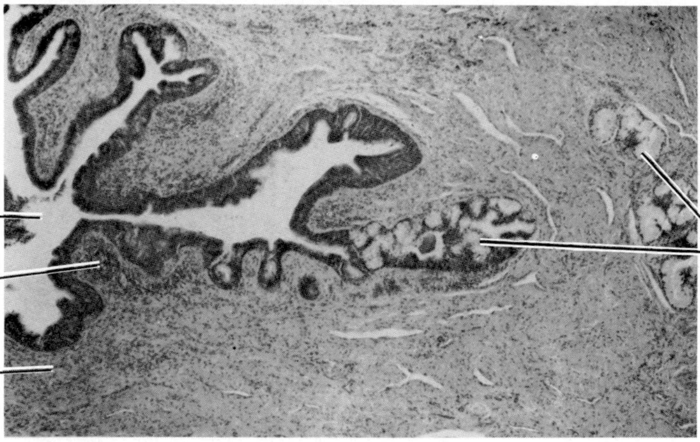

16-29 Development

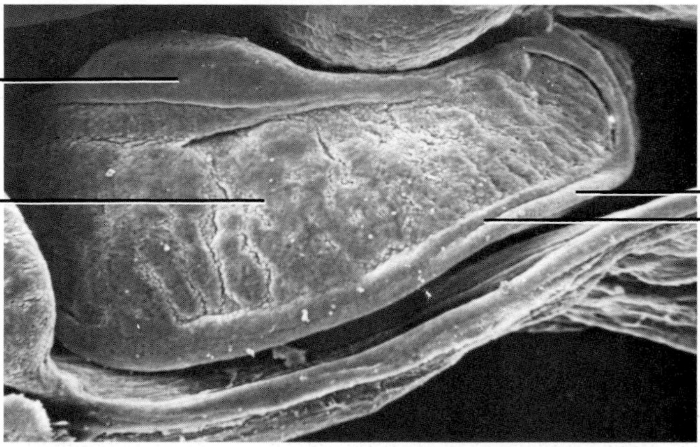

16-30

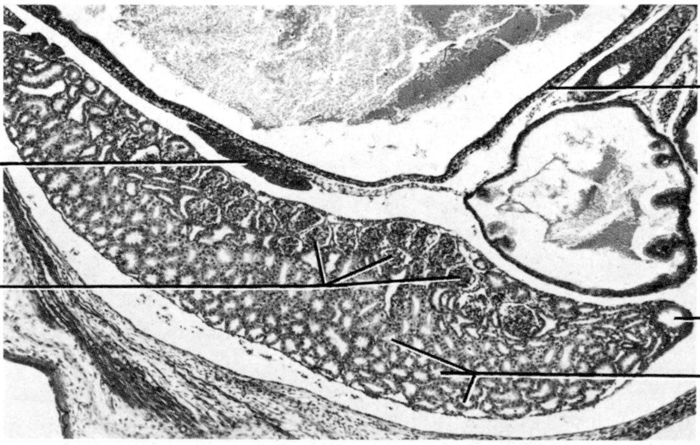

Figure 16.28. Penile urethra. LM, ×100.
Figure 16.29. Mesonephros. SEM, ×50.
Figure 16.30. Mesonephros. LM, ×20.

16-31

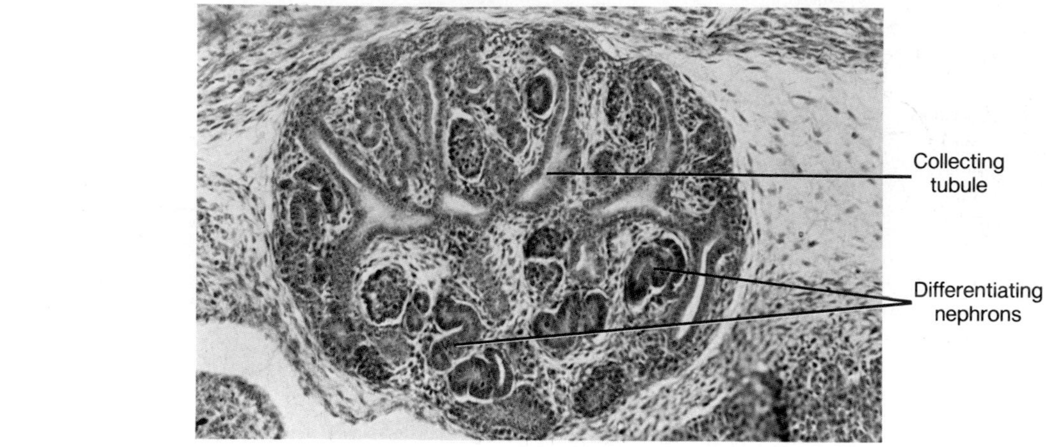

16-32

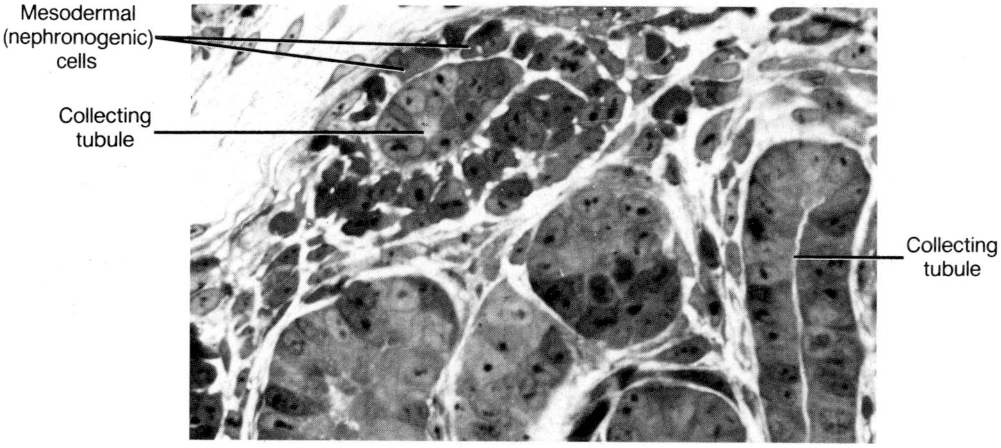

16-33

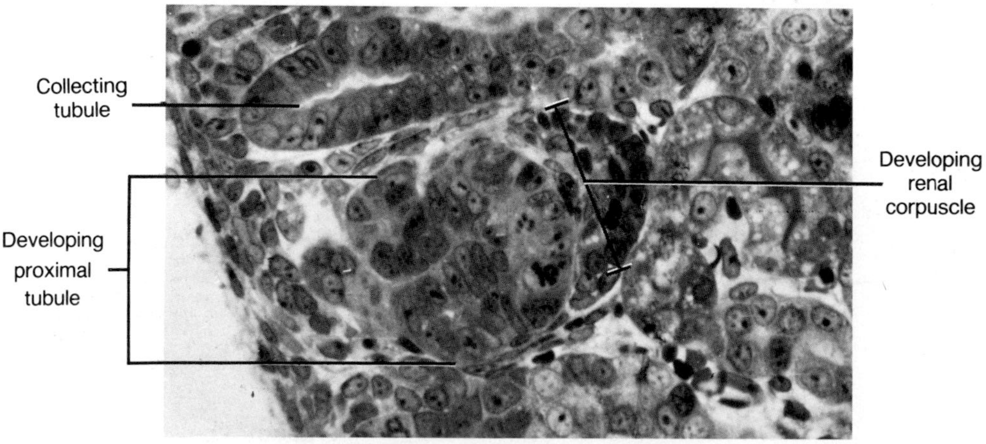

Figure 16.31. Metanephros. LM, ×100.
Figure 16.32. Metanephros. LM, ×400
Figure 16.33. Metanephros. LM, ×400.

16-34

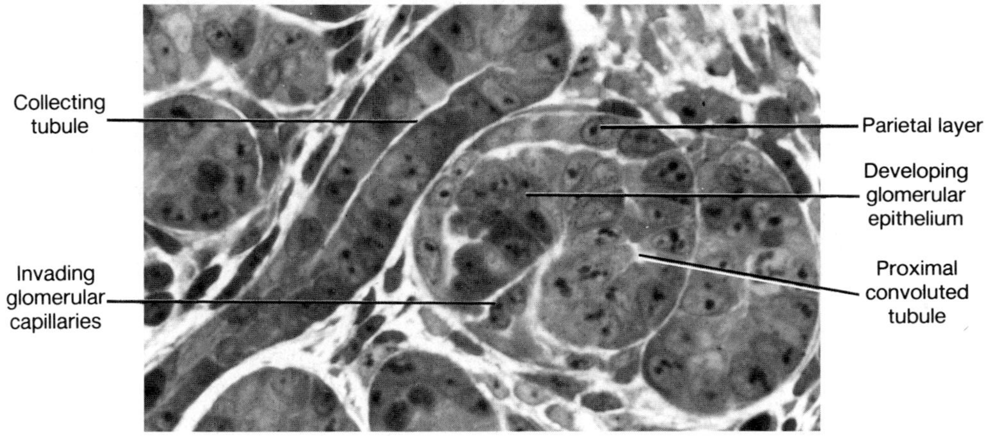

16-35

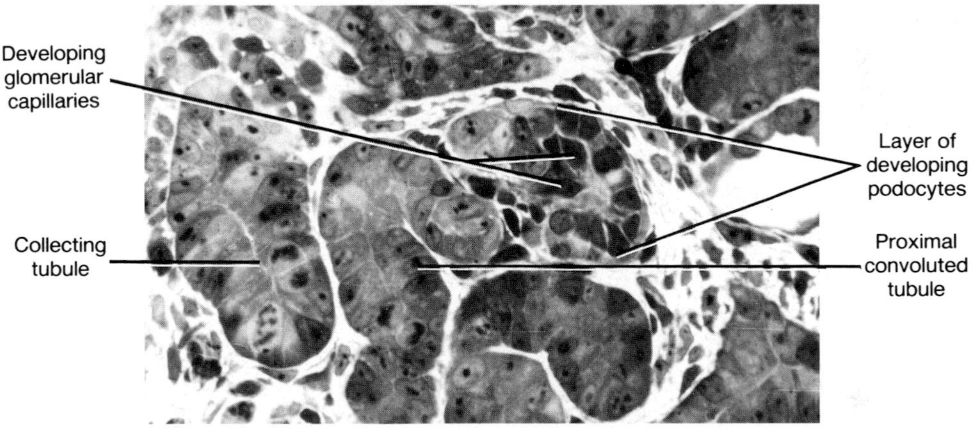

16-36

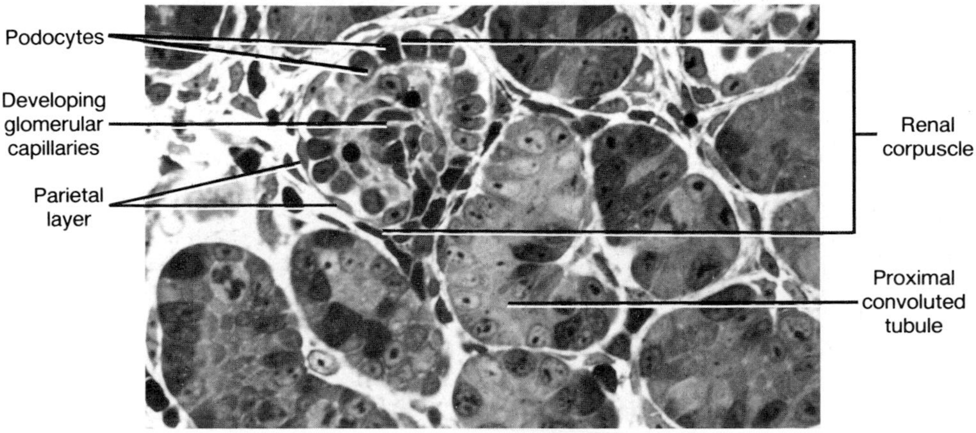

Figure 16.34. Metanephros. LM, ×400.
Figure 16.35. Metanephros. LM, ×400.
Figure 16.36. Metanephros. LM, ×400.

16-37

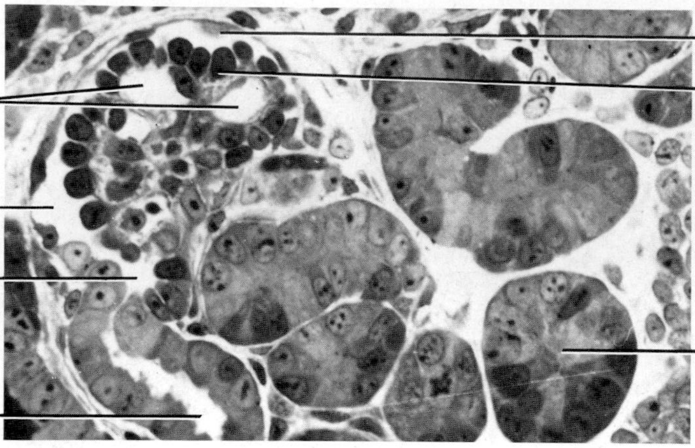

16-38

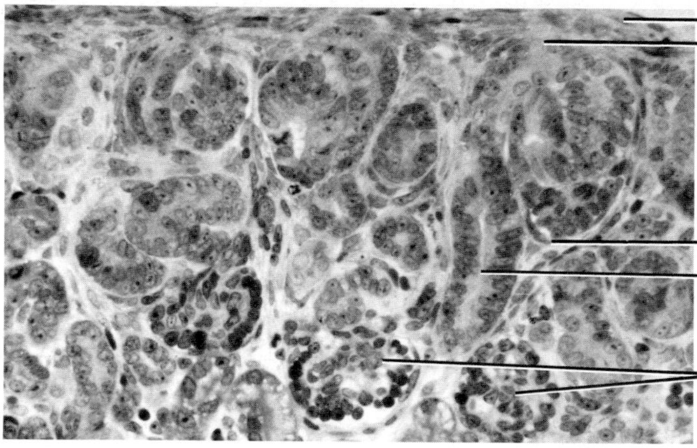

16-39

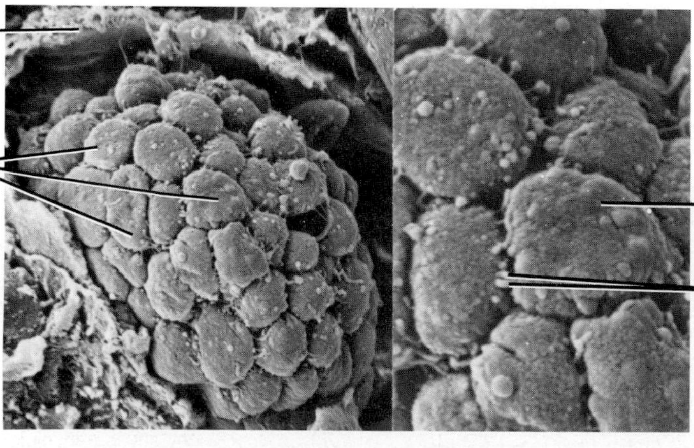

Figure 16.37. Metanephros. LM, ×400.
Figure 16.38. Metanephros. LM, ×250.
Figure 16.39. Renal corpuscles. SEM, *A*, ×1200; *B*, ×4000.

17

The Reproductive Organs

In mammals the male and female reproductive organs produce the gametes, provide a mechanism by which the gametes can be brought together to yield a new individual and in the female, house and nourish the zygote until birth of the new individual.

The generative organs for the production of the male gametes (the sperm) are the testes, while in the female the ovary is the site of production of the equivalent female gametes, the ova. The gametes cannot contain the diploid or somatic number of chromosomes since their fusion would then result in a doubling of the chromosomes with each new generation. Thus, the gametes contain only half the somatic number of chromosomes and this reduction to the haploid number is brought about by a special form of cell division called meiosis.

MEIOSIS

KEY WORDS: two cell divisions, one DNA replication, first meiotic division, separation of homologous chromosomes, second meiotic division, separation of chromatids

Meiosis is characterized by **two cell divisions** but only **one replication of DNA**. Chromosomal DNA is duplicated during interphase, prior to the first division, and results in a double or tetraploid amount of DNA contained within the diploid number of chromosomes. This is no different from that which occurs during the replication of DNA prior to ordinary mitosis. The **first meiotic division** brings about the **separation of** the **homologous chromosomes**, and while this results in halving of the number of chromosomes, each chromosome contains a double amount of DNA so that the content of DNA within the resulting cell remains diploid. A **second meiotic division** then occurs without a period of DNA replication; sister **chromatids are separated** at this time to yield cells with the haploid number of chromosomes and the haploid amount of DNA.

The stages of meiotic division are the same as those of ordinary mitosis, namely: prophase, metaphase, anaphase and telophase.

Prophase I

KEY WORDS: leptotene, zygotene, synapsis (conjugation), bivalent, pachytene, tetrad, diplotene, crossing over, chiasmata, recombination, diakinesis

The first meiotic prophase is long, complex and varies markedly from that of mitotic division. It customarily is divided into five stages: leptotene, zygotene, pachytene, diplotene and diakinesis.

In **leptotene** the chromosomes begin to condense and become visible as individual, slender threads which resemble those of the early prophase of somatic mitosis. In many animals the ends of the chromosomes become oriented to the side of the nucleus nearest the centrosome, with the bodies of the chromosomes extending in loops into the interior of the nucleus.

At **zygotene**, the homologous chromosomes come together to form pairs in which the chromosomes lie side by side, aligned point-for-point along their lengths. Because of their close apposition at this stage, the homologous chromosomes appear to be present in the haploid number. This pairing phenomenon is called **synapsis** (or **conjugation**) and each pair of homologous chromosomes forms a **bivalent**.

The chromosomes continue to contract and at **pachytene** are much shorter and thicker. Each chromosome of the bivalent begins to split lengthwise and can be seen to consist of two chromatids; the bivalent therefore contains four chromatids and is frequently referred to as a **tetrad**.

In the **diplotene** stage each chromosome becomes completely split into its constituent chromatids, which remain held together only by their centromeres (kinetochores). The homologous chromosomes move apart slightly and thus the tetrad formation is more obvious. At points along their lengths, the homologous chromatids make contact with one another and exchange segments, this exchange being called **crossing over**. The physical regions where the contacts are made are called **chiasmata**. The exchange of segments between the homologous chromatids results in a reassortment or **recombination** of the genetic material. The chromosomes continue to shorten and thicken and the nucleolus begins to fragment and disappear.

Diakinesis is marked by an even greater contraction of the chromosomes which are scattered throughout the cell. The homologous chromosomes are still paired but are joined only at the chiasmata. At the end of prophase I, the nuclear membrane and nucleoli have disappeared and the tetrads have begun their migration to the equator of the cell.

Metaphase I

This stage is similar to that of the metaphase of mitotic division, except that pairs of chromosomes (bivalents) and not single chromosomes are arranged about the spindle. The homologous pairs are aligned so that the members of each pair lie on either side of the equatorial plate with the centromeres of the homologous chromosomes facing opposite poles.

Anaphase I and Telophase I

These stages are similar to those of mitotic cell division. However, in the meiotic anaphase I the centromeres are not split, so that rather than chromatids separating and moving to opposite poles, whole chromosomes (each containing two chromatids) are separated. Reconstitution of the nuclei and cytoplasmic divisions occur at telophase I to yield two new cells. However, since the positioning of the bivalents on the equatorial plate at metaphase is random, there is a random assortment of maternal and paternal chromosomes in each of the telophase nuclei.

Meiotic Division II

KEY WORDS: no DNA synthesis, splitting of centromeres, separation of chromatids

The second meiotic division is more like that of mitosis and occurs after a brief interphase during which there is **no synthesis of DNA**. In some species, the cells produced at the end of the first division enter directly into metaphase II and bypass the second prophase. The **centromeres split** at metaphase and the **chromatids separate** during anaphase. Unlike mitosis, however, the sister chromatids are not identical, due to the crossing over which occurred during the first meiotic prophase. Following telophase and cytokinesis, four haploid cells result.

Differences in the Meiotic Divisions of Male and Female Germ Cells

The mechanical events of meiosis are the same regardless of whether sperm or ova are produced, but there are marked differences in the net production of these two gametes and in the time at which meiosis is initiated. In the male, four viable, functioning, sperm are produced from each germ cell that enters meiosis, whereas the same events in the female yield only a single functioning ovum. Following the first and second meiotic divisions, the cytoplasm is distributed equally among developing sperm, but in the formation of ova, the bulk of the cytoplasm is passed to only one cell. The remaining ova, called polar bodies, receive so little cytoplasm that they are unable to survive.

The time at which meiotic division is initiated in the male and female germ cells is remarkably different. In the human female the germ cells begin their meiotic divisions in the embryo, and by the 5th month of intrauterine life, the developing ova are in the diplotene stage of the first meiotic division. However, the division is not completed until just prior to ovulation, hence, many of the ova remain in the diplotene stage for several decades. The second meiotic division and formation of the second polar body occurs only after fertilization. In contrast, meiotic division in the male germ cells is not initiated until puberty, and once the cell enters meiosis it is carried to completion with no prolonged period of interruption.

A diagrammatic representation of meiotic division is shown in Figure 17-1.

FUNCTIONAL SUMMARY

One of the major consequences of meiotic division is a reduction in the number of chromosomes in the sperm and ova to half that present in somatic cells. This ensures that upon union of the gametes, the normal diploid number of chromosomes will be maintained. A second consequence of great importance is the provision of genetic variation as the result of the exchange of genetic material between homologous chromosomes and from the random distribution of homologous chromosomes between the daughter cells during meiosis. The unequal division of the cytoplasm during the formation of ova provides one cell with sufficient cytoplasmic material to nourish the zygote formed at fertilization.

MALE REPRODUCTIVE SYSTEM

The male reproductive system consists of the gonads (testes), their excretory ducts, the accessory sex glands and the penis. The gonads supply the male germ cells, or gametes (the sperm), which are conducted to the exterior by the excretory system, including the penis. The accessory glands contribute secretions that together with the sperm form the semen.

Testes

The testes are compound tubular glands which in most mammals, including man, lie within a scrotal sac suspended from the body by a spermatic cord. The testes are dual organs that serve as exocrine glands, producing a holocrine secretion, spermatozoa, and as endocrine organs for production of the male sex hormone testosterone.

Structure

KEY WORDS: tunica vaginalis, tunica albuginea, mediastinum testis, septula testis, lobuli testis, seminiferous tubules, tunica vasculosa, interstitial tissue, interstitial cells (of Leydig), crystals of Reinke

Each testis is invested anteriorly and laterally by a simple squamous epithelium (mesothelium) known as the visceral layer of the **tunica vaginalis**. On the posterior aspect of the testis, this mesothelium reflects onto and lines the scrotal sac to form the parietal layer of the tunica vaginalis. The serous cavity between visceral and parietal layers allows the testes to move freely and reduces the

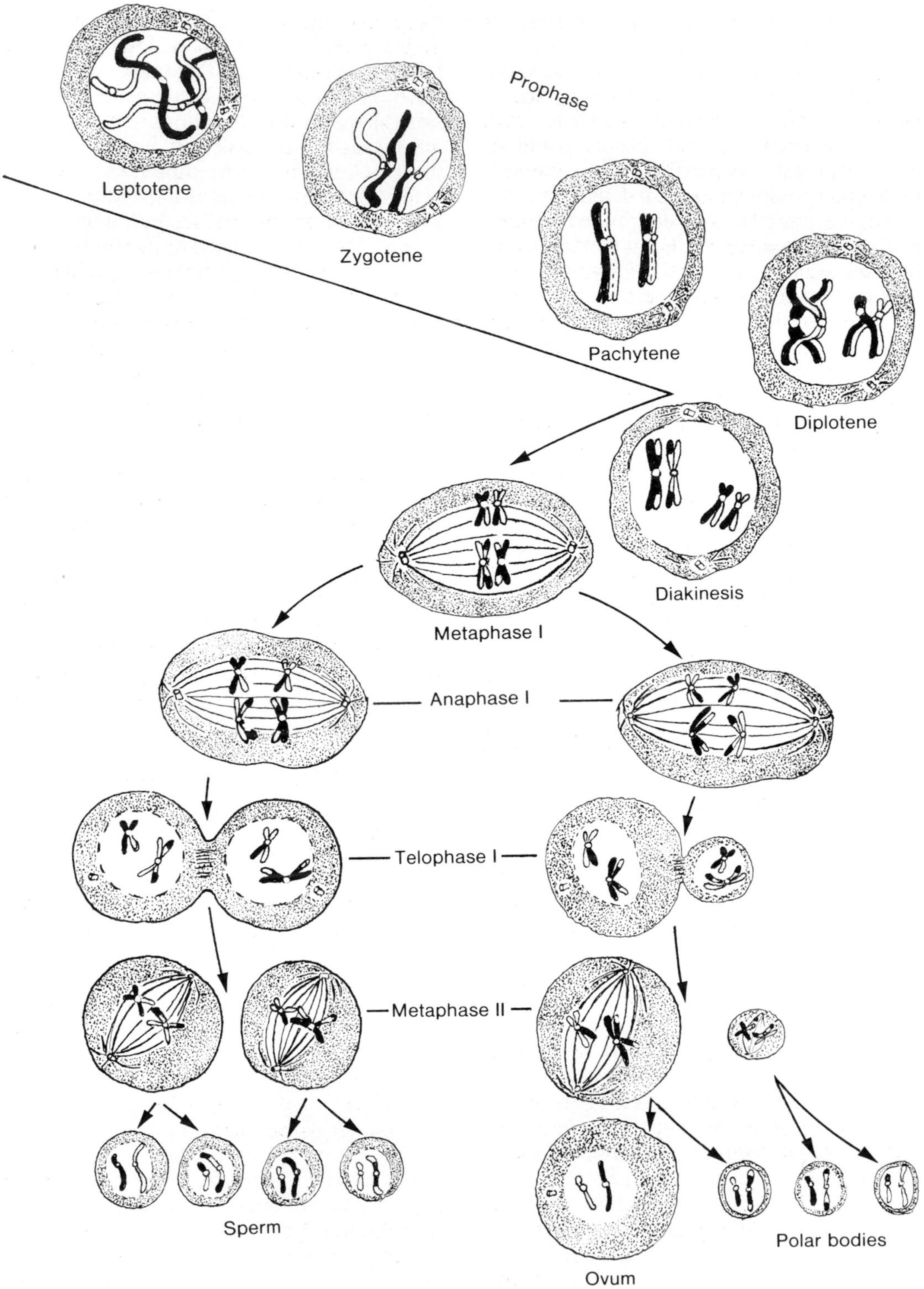

Figure 17-1. Diagrammatic representation of meiotic division.

chance of injury from increased pressure on the external surface of the scrotum.

A thick, fibrous capsule, the **tunica albuginea**, lies immediately beneath the visceral layer of the tunica vaginalis, separated from it only by a basal lamina. The tunica albuginea consists of dense fibroelastic connective tissue and contains scattered smooth muscle cells which in man are concentrated in the posterior region. Here the tunica albuginea thickens and projects into the testis to form the **mediastinum testis**. Connective tissue partitions, the **septula testis**, extend from the mediastinum into the interior of the testis and subdivide it into approximately 250 pyramidal-shaped compartments called the **lobuli testis**. The apices of these compartments are directed toward the mediastinum and each lobule contains one to four convoluted **seminiferous tubules**. These represent the exocrine portion of the testis, the secretory product being entire cells (spermatozoa).

The inner region of the tunica albuginea, the **tunica vasculosa**, consists of a loose connective tissue containing numerous small blood vessels which supply the testis. The connective tissue extends into each lobule and fills the spaces between the seminiferous tubules, where it forms the **interstitial tissue** of the testis. The interstitial tissue is rich in extracellular fluid and contains numerous small blood vessels and lymphatics that form a plexus around the seminiferous tubules.

In addition to fibroblasts and small bundles of collagen fibers, the interstitial tissue contains macrophages, mast cells, mesenchymal cells and large, polyhedral cells that measure 15 to 20 μm in diameter. These are the **interstitial cells (of Leydig).** They commonly occur in groups and constitute the endocrine portion of the testis, producing the male steroid hormone testosterone. The interstitial cells usually contain a single large, spherical nucleus, although binucleate cells are not uncommon. In electron micrographs the cytoplasm is seen to contain abundant smooth endoplasmic reticulum, well developed Golgi complexes and numerous mitochondria. In many species the mitochondrial cristae are tubular rather than lamellar.

Testosterone is essential for the proliferation and differentiation of germ cells, for the structural development of the excretory ducts and accessory sex glands of the male and for maintaining these structures in a functional state. Testosterone influences other tissues and is responsible for the development and maintenance of the secondary sex characteristics—growth of the beard, low pitch of the voice, muscular build, and male distribution of hair. Production of testosterone by the interstitial cells is controlled by a gonadotrophic hormone called interstitial cell stimulating hormone (ICSH), secreted by cells in the anterior pituitary.

Most of the enzymes involved in the synthesis of testosterone are located in the smooth endoplasmic reticulum, although the enzymes for one step (the conversion of cholesterol to pregnenolone) are found in the mitochondria of the interstitial cells. In man the interstitial cells are characterized by the presence of large cytoplasmic crystals known as the **crystals of Reinke**. These proteinaceous crystals are highly variable in shape and size but are seen readily with the light microscope and in electron micrographs present a highly ordered structure. The crystals occur in the testes of most postpuberty individuals and vary considerably in abundance. Their functional significance is unknown.

Seminiferous Tubules

KEY WORDS: peritubular tissue, myoid or peritubular contractile cells, germinal epithelium, Sertoli cells (supporting cells), spermatogenic cells

Each testicular lobule contains one to four highly convoluted seminiferous tubules that measure 150 to 250 μm in diameter and 30 to 70 cm in length. A seminiferous tubule consists of a complex stratified epithelium, the germinal or seminiferous epithelium, surrounded by a layer of peritubular or boundary tissue.

The **peritubular tissue** immediately surrounds the basal lamina of the germinal epithelium and consists of collagenous fibers and flattened cells that, depending on the species, may contain numerous actin-like cytoplasmic filaments; these are the **myoid** or **peritubular contractile cells**. In some primates and several other species (bull, ram, boar), the peritubular tissue contains three to five strata of myoid cells which are said to be contractile and may be responsible for the rhythmic contractions observed in the seminiferous tubules. This propulsive action aids in moving sperm and testicular fluid from the seminiferous tubules into the excretory duct system.

The **germinal epithelium** of the adult is unique among epithelia in that it consists of a fixed, stable population of **supporting cells**, the **Sertoli cells**, and a proliferating population of differentiating **spermatogenic cells**. The forming germ cells slowly migrate upward along the lateral surfaces of the supporting cells to be released at the free surface into the lumen of the seminiferous tubule.

Sertoli Cells

KEY WORDS: crystalloids, basal compartment, adluminal compartment, blood-testis barrier, androgen-binding protein

The Sertoli cell is a tall columnar cell that spans the germinal epithelium from the basal lamina to the luminal surface. This cell has an elaborate shape with numerous lateral processes that form recesses or concavities surrounding differentiating spermatogenic cells. The apical portion of sustentacular cells also envelops developing germ cells and releases them into the lumen of the seminiferous tubule. The expanded basal portion of the cell contains an irregularly-shaped nucleus characterized by a large, prominent nucleolus that is readily visible with the light microscope. The basal cytoplasm contains abundant smooth endoplasmic reticulum while a large, well developed Golgi complex occupies the supranuclear region. The cytoplasm contains numerous lipid droplets, lysosomes, thin elongate mitochondria, scattered profiles of rough endoplasmic reticulum, glycogen and a sheath of fine cytoplasmic filaments that envelops the nucleus and separates it from adjacent organelles. Microtubules and cytoplasmic filaments also are present, their number depending on the state of activity of the Sertoli cells. Human Sertoli cells are characterized by membrane-bound inclusions called the **crystalloids** of Charcot-Bottcher; their function is unknown.

Tight junctions occur between adjacent Sertoli cells near their bases and subdivide the germinal epithelium into basal and adluminal compartments. The **basal compartment** extends from the basal lamina of the germinal epithelium to the tight junctions. The **adluminal compartment** lies between the tight junctions and the lumen of the seminiferous tubule. Each compartment contains a separate, distinct population of spermatogenic cells. The tight junctions between interstitial cells appear to form, in part at least, a **blood-testis barrier** (Fig. 17-2). Germ cells in the basal compartment are contained

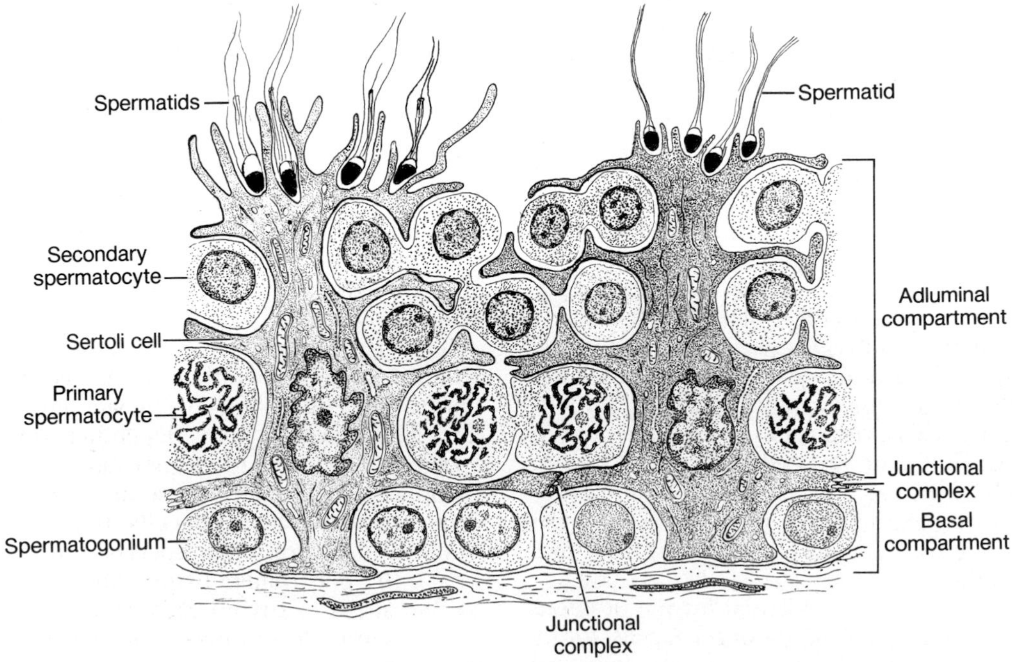

Figure 17-2. Germinal epithelium.

within an environment that has access to substances within the blood, while the germ cells in the adluminal compartment reside in a specialized environment that is maintained and controlled by the Sertoli cells. A number of plasma proteins are present in the basal compartment that are not found in the luminal contents of the seminiferous tubule which, however, are rich in other amino acids and ions. Sertoli cells are thought to provide all the nutrients for the avascular germinal epithelium.

In addition to secreting testicular fluid, Sertoli cells release **androgen-binding protein**, synthesis of which is thought to be stimulated by a pituitary gonadotropin, the male equivalent of follicle-stimulating hormone (FSH). By binding with testosterone, this particular protein serves to concentrate the hormone in the adluminal compartment and provide this region with the high concentration of male hormone necessary for the normal differentiation and development of germ cells. The blood-testis barrier helps to confine the high concentration of testosterone within the adluminal compartment. Many of the developing germ cells in the adluminal compartment are haploid and might be interpreted as foreign material by the body if released into surrounding tissues. The tight junctions between Sertoli cells may prevent the haploid germ cells from entering the general body tissues and thus prevent the development of an antibody response to the organism's own germ cells. Although tight junctions are thought to contribute to this barrier, other factors may be involved, although these are poorly understood.

Sertoli cells phagocytose degenerating germ cells in the seminiferous epithelium and take up the residual cytoplasm that normally is shed during the release of germ cells into the seminiferous tubule. In addition to providing mechanical support and nutrition for the developing germ cells, Sertoli cells also control the movement of germ cells from the basal lamina through the epithelium and play an important role in their release into the tubular lumen. The microtubules and actin-like filaments in the cytoplasmic processes of the Sertoli cell may provide these processes with the needed mobility.

Numerous gap junctions occur between adjacent Sertoli cells and are thought to facilitate communication between cells along a specific segment of a seminiferous tubule during the migration and release of germ cells.

Endocrine control of testicular functions is shown in Figure 17-3.

Spermatogenic Cells

KEY WORDS: spermatogenesis, spermatogonia type A and type B, primary spermatocyte, secondary spermatocyte, spermatids.

The spermatogenic cells of the germinal epithelum consist of spermatogonia, primary spermatocytes, secondary spermatocytes and spermatids. These are not separate cell types but represent stages in a continuous process of differentiation called **spermatogenesis.** The term encompasses the entire sequence of events in the transformation of the diploid spermatogonia at the base of the germinal epithelium into the haploid spermatozoa that are released into the lumen of the seminiferous tubules.

Spermatogonia lie in the basal compartment of the germinal epithelium, immediately adjacent to the basal lamina. The cells

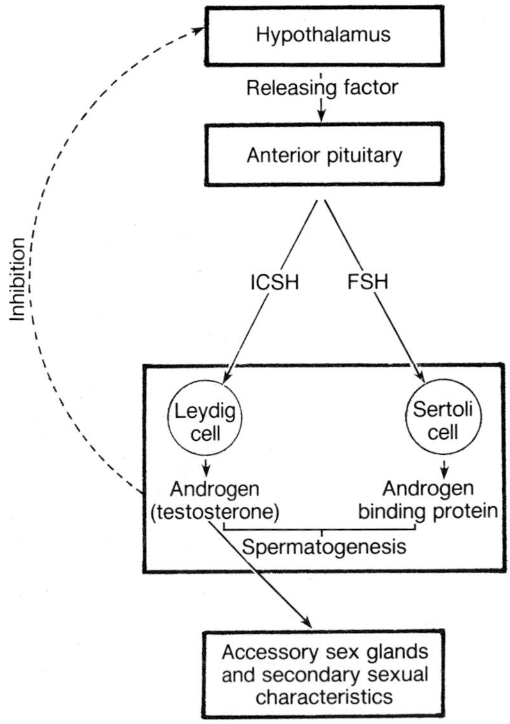

Figure 17-3. Endocrine control of testicular functions.

measure 10 to 12 μm in diameter, are round or ellipsoidal, and the nucleus of each spermatogonium contains the diploid number of chromosomes. Two forms of spermatogonia are generally described—type A and type B spermatogonia. **Type A spermatogonia** replicate by mitosis and provide a reservoir of stem cells for the formation of future germ cells. During mitotic division some type A spermatogonia give rise to intermediate forms that eventually produce **type B spermatogonia**, which are committed to the production of primary spermatocytes.

The **primary spermatocytes** at first resemble type B spermatogonia, but as they migrate from the basal lamina of the germinal epithelium, they become larger and more spherical in outline, and the nucleus enters the initial stages of division. Primary spermatocytes usually are found in the central zone of the germinal epithelium; how these large cells pass from the basal to the adluminal compartment is unknown.

The type of cell division occurring in primary spermatocytes is the reduction division of meiosis. The product of the first meiotic division is the **secondary spermatocyte**, in which the number of chromosomes has been reduced by one-half. The secondary spermatocytes lie nearer the lumen than the primary forms and are about one-half their size. Unlike the long extended division of the primary spermatocytes, the secondary spermatocytes divide quickly (by mitosis) to produce **spermatids**, the nuclei of which contain the haploid number of chromosomes and the haploid amount of DNA. Because they divide quickly after being formed, secondary spermatocytes are observed only rarely in the germinal epithelium. The spermatids are about one-half the size of the secondary spermatocyte. Numerous spermatids in different stages of maturation border the lumen of the seminiferous tubule.

The meiotic divisions during the formation of male germ cells are unique in that not only is the genetic material reduced by one-half, but division of the cytoplasm, although equal, is incomplete. Thus, the cells resulting from a single spermatogonium remain in cytoplasmic continuity throughout the different stages of differentiation. The continuity between individual spermatozoa is finally broken when they are released by the Sertoli cells into the lumen of the seminiferous tubule.

Spermiogenesis

KEY WORDS: acrosome, acrosomal vesicle, head cap, axoneme, implantation fossa, connecting piece, annulus, middle piece, head

The elaborate sequence of events by which spermatids differentiate into the slender, motile spermatozoa is referred to as spermiogenesis. Newly formed spermatids are round cells with central, spherical nuclei, well developed Golgi complexes, numerous mitochondria and a pair of centrioles. Each of these components of the spermatid undergo marked changes during spermiogenesis.

At the onset of spermiogenesis, numerous small granules appear in the Golgi membranes and eventually coalesce into a single structure called the **acrosome**. The forming acrosome is limited by a membrane, the **acrosomal vesicle**, which also is derived from the Golgi complex and is closely associated with the outer layer of the nuclear envelope. The acrosomal vesicle expands, then collapses to form a **head cap** over the anterior one-half of the nucleus. The acrosome, which contains hydrolytic enzymes, remains contained within the acrosomal membrane.

As these events occur, the two centrioles migrate to a position near the nucleus on the side opposite the forming acrosome. From the distal centriole, nine peripheral doublets plus a central pair of microtubules begin to form the **axoneme** of the tail; the proximal centriole becomes closely associated with a caudal region of the nucleus known as the **implantation fossa**.

As the axoneme continues to develop, nine longitudinally oriented coarse fibers extend around it. They blend with nine short, segmented columns that form the **connecting piece** which unites the nucleus (head) with the tail of the spermatozoon. The **annulus**, a ring-like structure, forms near the centrioles and migrates down the forming flagellum. Randomly distributed mitochondria now migrate to the flagellum and become aligned in a tight helix between the centrioles and the annulus. This spirally arranged, mitochondrial sheath characterizes the **middle piece** of the tail of a mature spermatozoon.

Simultaneously, marked changes also occur in the nucleus, which becomes condensed, elongated and slightly flattened. Together with the acrosome it forms the sperm **head**. The bulk of the cytoplasm is now associated with the middle piece of the evolving spermatid, and as differentiation nears completion, the excess cytoplasm is shed as the residual body, leaving only a thin layer of cytoplasm to cover the spermatozoon. The residual cytoplasm is phagocytosed by Sertoli cells as the spermatozoa are released into the lumen of a seminiferous tubule. Although the spermatozoa appear morphologically mature, they are nonmotile and are incapable of fertilization at this time.

In most species, spermatids at specific stages of differentiation are always associated with spermatocytes and spermatogonia, which also are at specific stages of development. A series of such associations occurs along the length of the same seminiferous tubule and the distance between two identical germ cell associations is referred to as a wave of seminiferous epithelium. Although this wave of activity is not observed in man, the fundamental pattern of cycling in the germinal epithelium is the same as in other mammals. The time taken for spermatogonia to become spermatozoa is relatively constant and species specific; in man it is about 64 days. If germ cells fail to develop at their normal rate, they degenerate and are phagocytosed by adjacent Sertoli cells.

Spermatozoa

KEY WORDS: head, tail, acrosomal cap, neck, capitulum, middle piece, principal piece, end piece, capacitation

Spermatozoa that lie free within the lumina of the seminiferous tubules consist of a **head**, which contains the nucleus, and a **tail** which eventually will give motility to the free cell. The chromatin of the nucleus is very condensed and reduced in volume, providing the functionally mature sperm with greater mobility. The condensed form of chromatin also protects the genome while the spermatozoon is enroute to fertilize the female germ cell. The **acrosomal cap** covers the anterior two-thirds of the nucleus and contains lysozomes that are important for penetration of the ovum during fertilization. The size and shape of the nucleus varies tremendously in different species.

The sperm tail measures about 55 μm in length and consists of a neck, middle piece, principal piece and end piece. The structural details of the different segments are best observed with the electron microscope.

The **neck** is that region where the head and tail of the sperm unite. It contains the connecting piece which joins the nine outer dense fibers of the sperm tail to the implantation fossa of the nucleus. The region of the connecting piece that joins the implantation fossa is expanded slightly and is called the **capitulum**. The **middle piece** extends from the neck to the annulus and consists of the axoneme, the nine coarse fibers and the helical sheath of mitochondria. The **principal piece** is the longest portion of the tail and consists of the axoneme and the nine coarse fibers (2 + 9 + 9) enclosed by a sheath of circumferential fibers. The circumferential fibers join two longitudinal thickenings of this sheath, located on opposite sides. The **end piece** represents the shortest segment of the tail and consists only of the axoneme surrounded by the cell membrane. The structure of a spermatozoan is shown in Figure 17-4.

The final step in the physiological maturation of spermatozoa takes place in the female reproductive tract and is called **capacitation**. The final activation of spermatozoa requires from 1 to 6 hours to complete, depending on the species, and is characterized by changes in the acrosomal cap and respiratory metabolism of the spermatozoa. Capacitation substantially increases the percentage of spermatozoa capable of fertilization, but the mechanism of this activation is unknown.

Excretory Ducts

The excretory ducts comprise a complex system of tubules that link each testis to the urethra, through which the exocrine secretion, the semen, ultimately is conducted to the exterior. The duct system consists of the straight tubules (tubuli recti), rete testis, ductuli efferentes, ductus epididymidis, ductus deferens, ejaculatory ducts and prostatic, membranous and penile urethrae.

Tubuli Recti

KEY WORD: simple columnar epithelium

Near the apex of each testicular lobule, the seminiferous tubules join to form a short, straight tubule called the tubuli recti

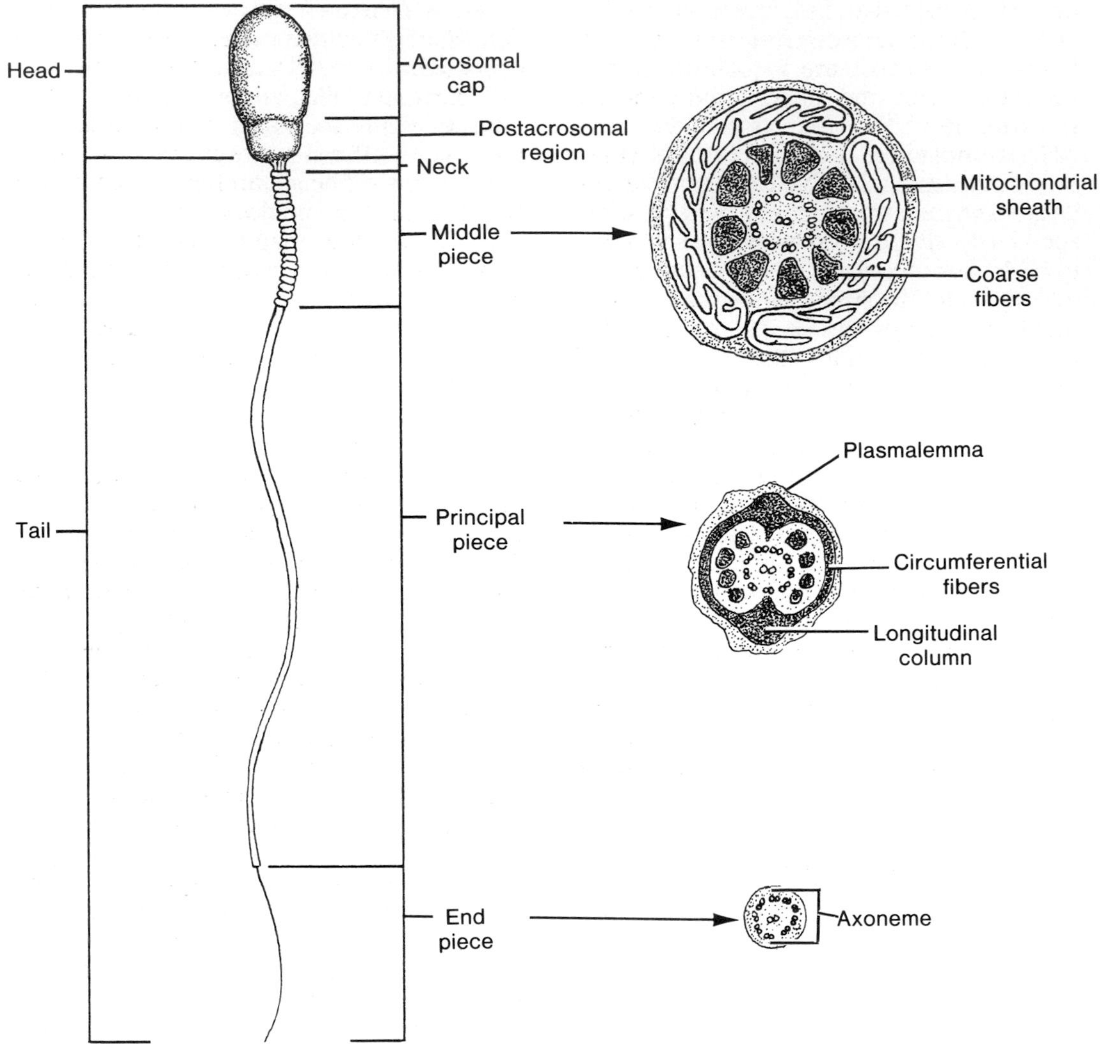

Figure 17-4. Structure of a spermatozoan.

(straight tubule). The lining epithelium is devoid of germ cells and consists only of Sertoli cells. This **simple columnar epithelium** lies on a thin basal lamina and is surrounded by a loose connective tissue. The tubuli recti are short and their lumina are continuous with a network of anastomosing channels in the mediastinum, the rete testis.

Rete Testis

KEY WORD: simple cuboidal epithelium

The rete testis is lined by **simple cuboidal epithelium.** The luminal surfaces of the component cells show short microvilli and each cell bears a single cilium. The epithelium lies on a delicate basal lamina and the channels of the rete testis are surrounded by a dense bed of vascular connective tissue. The rete testis of some species may lie axially in the testis and drain surrounding seminiferous tubules along its entire length.

Ductuli Efferentes

KEY WORDS: initial segment, head of epididymis, tall and short columnar, ciliated and nonciliated cells

In man, 10 to 15 ductuli efferentes emerge from the mediastinum on the posterior-superior surface of the testis and unite the channels of the rete testis with the ductus epididymidis. The ductules follow a spiraled, convoluted course and together with their supporting connective tissue constitute the **initial segment** of the **head of the epididymis**. The luminal surface of the efferent ductules shows a characteristic, irregular contour due to the presence of alternating groups of **tall and short columnar** cells. Both **ciliated and nonciliated cells** are present. Each contains the organelles normally associated with epithelia as well as supranuclear granules that are lysosomal in nature. The nonciliated cells, which show numerous microvilli on their apical free surfaces, are thought to absorb much of the testicular fluid that is present in this segment of the ductal system. Cilia on the other cell type beat toward the epididymis and help to move the nonmotile sperm and testicular fluid in that direction.

The epithelium lies on a basal lamina and is bounded by a layer of circularly arranged smooth muscle which thickens toward the duct of the epididymis. Cilia are not found beyond the ductuli efferentes and the movement of sperm through the remainder of the duct system depends on the contractions of the muscular wall.

Ductus Epididymidis

KEY WORDS: pseudostratified columnar, principal cells, stereocilia basal cells, smooth muscle, three-layered coat

The efferent ductules gradually unite to form a single ductus epididymidis which measures 5 to 7 m in length. This highly coiled duct, together with its associated vascular connective tissue, forms the remainder of the head, the body and the tail of the epididymis. The epithelial lining is **pseudostratified columnar** and consists of principal cells and basal cells.

The **principal cells** are the most numerous and are very tall (80 μm) in the proximal segment of the ductus epididymidis but gradually decrease in height distally and measure only 40 μm near the junction with the ductus deferens. Long, nonmotile microvilli inappropriately called **stereocilia** extend from the apical surface of the principal cells. A remarkably large Golgi complex occupies a supranuclear position in the cell and an abundance of granular endoplasmic reticulum fills the basal region. Lysosomes, multivesicular bodies and numerous coated vesicles also are present. One of the functions of the principal cell is absorption and the proximal portion of the ductus epididymidis and the ductuli efferentes together absorb over 90% of the testicular fluid produced by the seminiferous epithelium.

Basal cells are small, round cells that lie on the basal lamina interposed between the bases of the principal cells. They have a light-staining cytoplasm with few organelles. Scattered intraepithelial lymphocytes often are seen in the epithelium of the ductus epididymidis.

The epididymal epithelium lies on a basal lamina and is surrounded by a thin lamina propria and a thin layer of circularly arranged **smooth muscle** cells. Near the ductus deferens, the muscle layer thickens and becomes **three-layered** (inner longitudinal, middle circular, outer longitudinal), continuous with that of the ductus deferens. The regional differences reflect differences in the mobility of the ductus epididymidis. Proximally, the duct shows spontaneous peristaltic contractions that slowly transport spermatozoa through the epididymis while distally, the peristaltic contractions are reduced and this region serves to store sperm. Spermatozoa become physiologically mature during their course through the epididymis. Those entering the proximal portion of the ductus epididymidis are largely incapable of fertilization and swim in a weak, random fashion. In contrast, spermatozoa from the distal portion are capable of fertilizing ova and show strong, unidirectional motility. How the ductus epididymidis contributes to the maturation of spermatozoa is unknown. In some marsupial species, such as the North American opossum, the sperm pair in the epididymis.

Ductus Deferens

KEY WORDS: mucosa, pseudostratified columnar, stereocilia, lamina propria, muscularis, adventitia, ampulla

The ductus deferens unites the ductus epididymis with the prostatic urethra. It is characterized by a thick wall consisting of a mucosa, a muscularis and an adventitia. The **mucosa** is thrown into longitudinal folds that project into the lumen and consists of a **pseudostratified columnar** epithelium resting on a thin basal lamina. The epithelium exhibits **stereocilia** on its luminal surface. The surrounding **lamina propria** is dense and contains numerous elastic fibers. The **muscularis** is the dominant feature of the ductus deferens and consists of three layers of smooth muscle arranged longitudinally in the inner and outer layers and circularly in the middle layer. The muscularis is surrounded by the loose connective tissue of the **adventitia**, which blends with neighboring structures and serves to anchor the ductus deferens in place. Powerful contractions of the muscular wall expel sperm from the distal ductus epididymidis and rapidly transport them through the ductus deferens during ejaculation.

Near its termination, the ductus deferens dilates to form the **ampulla.** Here the lumen expands and the mucosa is folded, creating a labyrinth of pocket-like recesses. The lining epithelium is similar to that elsewhere in the ductus deferens. The muscular coat of the ampulla is thinner, with less distinct layers than are seen in other parts of the ductus.

Smooth muscle cells in the muscularis of the ductus deferens are unique in that each cell (fiber) receives direct sympathetic innervation. This accounts for the rapid, forceful contractions of the ductus at the time of ejaculation.

Ejaculatory Duct

KEY WORDS: pseudostratified or simple columnar epithelium

A short, narrow region of the ductus deferens extends beyond the ampulla and joins the duct of the seminal vesicle. This combined duct forms the ejaculatory duct, which empties into the prostatic urethra. It measures about 1 cm in length and is lined by a **pseudostratified or simple columnar epithelium.** The mucosa forms outpocketings similar to but less well developed than those in the ampulla. The remainder of the wall of the ejaculatory duct consists only of fibrous connective tissue.

Prostatic Urethra

KEY WORDS: transitional epithelium, colliculus seminalis, prostatic utricle

The ejaculatory duct penetrates the substance of the prostate gland and opens into the prostatic portion of the urethra. The prostatic urethra is lined by a thin, **transitional epithelium** and bears a dome-shaped elevation called the **colliculus seminalis** on its posterior wall. A small blind invagination, the **prostatic utricle**, lies on the summit of the colliculus and represents a remnant of the Müllerian duct in the male. The two ejaculatory ducts, one draining each testis, empty into the prostatic urethra on either side of the utricle. Numerous ducts from the surrounding prostatic glands also empty into this portion of the urethra.

Accessory Sex Glands

Male accessory sex glands include the seminal vesicles, prostate and bulbourethral glands. The secretion from each of these glands is added to the testicular fluids and forms a substantial part of the semen.

Seminal Vesicles

KEY WORDS: folds, honeycombed appearance, pseudostratified columnar epithelium

The seminal vesicles are elongated, saclike structures that lie posterior to the prostate gland. Each joins with the distal end of the ductus deferens to form the ejaculatory duct. The mucosa of the seminal vesicles is thrown into numerous complex primary **folds** which give rise to secondary and tertiary folds. These project into the lumen to subdivide it into many small, irregular compartments that give the lumen a **honeycombed appearance.** All of the compartments communicate with the central lumen, although in sections the impression is one of individual chambers.

The mucosal folds are lined primarily by a **pseudostratified columnar epithelium** consisting of rounded basal cells interposed between cuboidal or columnar cells; regions of simple columnar epithelium also may be present. The mucosal cells contain numerous granules, some lipid droplets and lipochrome pigment which first appears at sexual maturity and increases with age. The ultrastructural features indicate a cell that is active in protein synthesis and the cytoplasm contains abundant granular endoplasmic reticulum, a prominent supranuclear Golgi complex and conspicuous, dense, secretory granules in the apical cytoplasm.

The epithelium rests on a thin lamina propria of loose connective tissue with many elastic fibers. A muscular coat is present and consists of an inner layer of circularly arranged smooth muscle and an outer layer in which the muscle fibers have a longitudinal orientation. Both layers of muscle are thinner than in the ductus deferens. External to the muscle coat is a layer of loose connective tissue rich in elastic fibers.

The secretion from the seminal vesicles provides a substantial portion of the total ejaculate. It is a yellowish, viscid secretion that contains much fructose and prostaglandins and provides an energy source for sperm. In sections the secretions appear as deeply staining, coagulated masses, often with a net-like structure. The seminal vesicles are testosterone-dependent and removal of the hormone, as by castration, results in an involution and loss of secretory function of the seminal vesicle.

Prostate

KEY WORDS: composite gland, compound tubuloalveolar, capsule, septa, prostatic concretions

The prostate is the largest of the accessory sex glands of the male and surrounds the urethra at its origin from the bladder. It is a **composite** gland, consisting of 30 to 50 small, **compound tubuloalveolar** glands from which 20 or more ducts drain independently into the prostatic urethra. These small glands appear to form three strata around the urethra and consist of the periurethral mucosal glands, the submucosal glands and the main or principal prostatic glands which lie peripherally and make up the bulk of the prostate. The entire gland is contained within a vascular, fibroelastic **capsule** that contains many smooth muscle fibers in its inner layers. Broad **septa** extend into the gland from the capsule and become continuous with the dense fibroelastic tissue which separates the individual glandular elements.

The secretory units of the glands are very irregular and vary greatly in size and shape. The glandular epithelium differs from gland to gland and even within a single alveolus. It usually is simple columnar or pseudostratified columnar but may be low cuboidal or squamous in some of the larger saccular cavities. The epithelium is limited by an indistinct basal lamina and rests on a layer of connective tissue that contains dense networks of elastic fibers and numerous capillaries. The cells contain abundant granular endoplasmic reticulum and many apical secretory granules. The lumina of the secretory units may contain spherical bodies, the **prostatic concretions**, which are believed to result from a condensation of secretory material. The concretions may become calcified and appear to increase with age.

The prostatic secretion is a thin, milky fluid with a pH of 6.5 and is rich in zinc, citric acid, acid phosphatase and proteolytic enzymes. One of these enzymes, fibrinolysin, is important in the liquefaction of semen. In several species of rodents, some of the prostatic glands are specialized to provide a secretion that coagulates the seminal fluid to form a vaginal plug which prevents loss of sperm from the female reproductive tract. These modified glandular units have been called coagulating glands. Like the seminal vesicles, the development and functional maintenance of the prostate is dependent upon testosterone.

The connective tissue surrounding the individual glandular units contains much smooth muscle which aids in the discharge of the prostatic fluid during ejaculation.

Bulbourethral Glands

KEY WORDS: compound tubuloalveolar, simple cuboidal to simple columnar

The bulbourethral glands are a pair of pea-sized glandular structures located in the urogenital diaphragm close to the bulb of the urethra. They are **compound tubuloalveolar** glands whose long ducts drain into the proximal part of the penile urethra. Each gland is limited by a connective tissue capsule from which septa, containing elastic fibers and smooth and skeletal muscle cells, extend into the glands to divide them into lobules.

The ducts and secretory portions are irregular in size and shape, and at their terminations, the secretory parts may form cyst-like enlargements. The glandular epithelium varies from **simple cuboidal to simple columnar**, depending on the functional state, but in distended alveoli the epithelium may be flattened. The active cells show a lightly stained cytoplasm filled with mucinogen granules that confine the nucleus to the base of the cell. Excretory ducts are lined by a simple columnar epithelium which becomes pseudostratified columnar near the urethra. In the smaller ducts the epithelium appears to be secretory. The surrounding connective tissue contains an incomplete layer of circularly arranged smooth muscle cells.

The product of the bulbourethral glands is a clear, viscid fluid that is rich in amino sugars and contains sialoprotein. It is secreted in response to erotic stimulation and serves as a lubricant for the penile urethra.

Semen

The final product formed by the exocrine secretions of the testes, and accessory glands is a whitish fluid called the seminal fluid or semen. The average ejaculate in man consists of about 3 ml of semen which, in addition to approximately 300 million sperm, contains degenerating cells exfoliated by the ductal system, occasional wandering cells from connective tissues, pigment granules and prostatic concretions. Hyaline bodies of unknown origin, lipid granules, fat and protein also are present in the semen.

External Genitalia

In the male, the two structures that comprise the external genitalia are the scrotum and the penis.

Scrotum

KEY WORDS: skin, dartos tunic, spermatic cord, pampiniform plexus

The scrotum is a pendulous, cutaneous pouch situated at the base of the penis and below the pubic symphysis. It is divided into two compartments, each of which houses a testis, an epididymis and the lower part of a spermatic cord. The scrotum consists only of skin and a closely associated dartos tunic.

The scrotal **skin** is thin, pigmented and commonly thrown into folds. It contains numerous sweat glands, sebaceous glands which produce an odorous secretion, and some coarse hairs, the follicles of which are visible through the skin. The **dartos tunic** underlies the skin and forms the septum which divides the scrotum into its two compartments. It is firmly attached to the skin and consists largely of smooth muscle and collagenous connective tissue. The appearance of the scrotum varies with the state of contraction or relaxation of the smooth muscle. Under the influence of cold, exercise or sexual stimulation the muscle contracts and the scrotum appears short and wrinkled.

The **spermatic cord** consists of several thin layers of connective tissue that are acquired from the anterior abdominal wall as the testes descend from the abdominal cavity into the scrotal sac during development. It contains the ductus deferens, nerve fibers, lymphatic channels, the testicular artery and the **pampiniform plexus** of testicular veins. As the testicular artery nears the testis, it becomes hightly convoluted and is surrounded by the venous plexus. The close proximity of the surrounding, cooler, venous blood causes the arterial blood to lose heat and provides a thermoregulatory mechanism for precooling the incoming arterial blood. In this way the temperature of the testes in the scrotal sac is maintained a few degrees below body temperature, a condition necessary for the production of germ cells. The temperature can be elevated by drawing the testes closer to the abdominal wall, an action brought about by contraction of the layer of striated muscle (cremaster muscle) which invests the spermatic cord.

The testes of some animals, such as the elephant, descend into the scrotum only during each breeding season and thereafter return to the abdominal cavity and are inactive. In man, failure of the testes to descend (cryptorchidism) results in sterility.

Penis

KEY WORDS: erectile tissue, corpora cavernosa penis, pectiniform septum, tunica albuginea, cavernous spaces, corpus cavernosum urethrae (corpus spongiosum), glans penis, prepuce

The penile urethra serves as a common channel for conducting both urine and seminal fluid to the exterior. It is contained within a cylinder of **erectile tissue**, the corpus cavernosum urethrae (corpus spongiosum), that lies ventral to a pair of similar erectile bodies called the corpora cavernosa penis. Together, these three structures make up the bulk of the penis, the copulatory organ of the male.

The **corpora cavernosa penis** begin as separate entities along the rami of the pubis on either side and join at the pubic angle to form the shaft of the penis. They are united by a common, connective tissue septum called the **pectiniform septum**, and each corpus is surrounded by a thick, fibrous sheath, the **tunica albuginea.** Trabeculae of collagenous and elastic fibers with numerous smooth muscle cells extend into the corpora from the tunica albuginea and divide the central regions of the corpora cavernosa into numerous **cavernous spaces**; those near the center are larger than those at the periphery. These spaces are endothelial-lined vascular spaces and are continuous with arteries that supply them, and with draining veins. The cavernous tissue of each corpus cavernosum penis communicates with the other through numerous slitlike openings in the pectiniform septum.

The ventrally placed **corpus cavernosum urethrae** (**corpus spongiosum**) ends in an enlargement, the **glans penis**, which forms a cap over the ends of the corpora cavernosa penis. Structurally the corpus spongiosum is similar to the corpora cavernosa penis, but the tunica albuginea is thinner and contains more elastic fibers and smooth muscle cells. Similarly, the trabeculae are thinner and these also contain more abundant elastic tissue.

The three corpora are bound together by a subcutaneous connective tissue which contains numerous smooth muscle cells but is devoid of fat. The shaft of the penis is covered by a thin, mobile skin that shows a slight increase in pigmentation. The skin covering the distal shaft, unlike the root, is devoid of hair but does contain scattered sweat glands. In contrast, the hairless skin of the glans penis fuses with the underlying connective tissue and is nonmobile. Unusual sebaceous glands not associated with hair follicles also are found in this region. The glans penis is covered by a fold of skin called the **prepuce** or foreskin, the inner surface of which is moist and resembles a mucous membrane. Numerous free nerve endings are found in the epithelium of the glans penis and prepuce and in the subepithelial connective tissue of the urethra and skin. Encapsulated endings associated with the skin (Meissner's corpuscles) and deeper layers of the dermis (genital corpuscles and corpuscles of Vater-Pacini) also are found.

A section through the penis is shown in Figure 17-5.

Arterial Supply

KEY WORDS: helicine arteries, intimal ridges

The principal arterial supply to the penis is from two arteries that lie dorsal to the corpora cavernosa penis and deep arteries which course within the erectile tissue of these structures. Branches from the dorsal arteries penetrate the tunica albuginea and enter the cavernous tissue, where the arteries branch and either form capillary plexuses or course distally in the cavernous tissue. These arteries, called **helicine arteries**, are highly convoluted in the flaccid condition and follow a spiral course through the trabeculae of the cavernous tissue. The intima of most of these arteries, even before they enter the cavernous tissue, have long, ridge-like thickenings that project into and partially occlude, the lumen. These **intimal ridges** are most frequent where vessels branch and consist of a loose connective tissue that contains numerous smooth muscle cells. Blood from the large central lacunae drains peripherally toward the smaller vascular spaces and finally into a plexus of veins at the periphery.

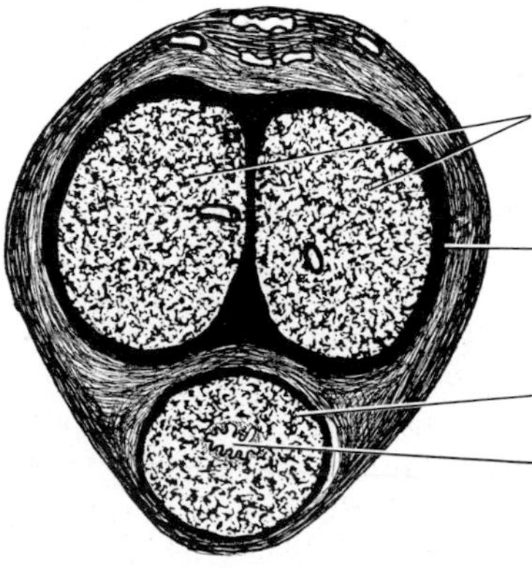

Figure 17-5. Section through the penis.

The veins course along the interior of the tunica albuginea, pierce the limiting tunic and ultimately drain into the deep dorsal vein of the penis.

The arterial blood supply to the corpus spongiosum is similar to that of the two corpora cavernosa penis, except that the venous drainage differs. In this body the veins beginning at the lacunae have large openings and immediately pierce the tunica albuginea to drain to the exterior.

The structure and arrangement of the blood vessels in the cavernous tissue provides the mechanism for erection. During erotic stimulation there is a relaxation of tonus in the smooth musculature of the arterial and trabecular walls. Blood pressure overcomes the elastic resistance of the arteries; the helicine arteries dilate and straighten out as they become filled and the vascular spaces of the cavernous tissue quickly fill with blood. The lacunae of the cavernous tissue, especially those located near the center, become engorged with blood, thus compressing the small peripheral spaces and veins against the interior of the tunica albuginea, retarding egress of blood. As blood accumulates in the erectile tissue of the corpora cavernosa penis, the tissues become rigid and enlarged. The erectile tissue of the corpus spongiosum does not attain the degree of rigidity of the corpora cavernosa penis because there is less compression of the venous drainage and the tunica albuginea is thinner and more yielding. The lesser rigidity of the corpus spongiosum allows the urethra to remain patent, an essential for the passage of seminal fluid during ejaculation.

After cessation of sexual activity, the smooth muscle in the arteries and cavernous tissue regains its tonus. The intimal ridges once again partially occlude the lumina of the arteries, thus reducing the volume of incoming blood. Excess blood remaining in the vascular spaces of the erectile tissue is forced out by the contraction of smooth muscle cells in the trabeculae and by the recoil of surrounding elastic tissue. Gradually, the normal route of blood flow through the penis is restored and the penis returns to its flaccid condition.

DEVELOPMENT OF THE MALE REPRODUCTIVE SYSTEM

The indifferent gonad arises within the urogenital ridge, a thickened area of mesoderm that contains primordia for the kidneys and gonads. Proliferation of peritoneal epithelium (mesothelium) on the ventromedial aspect of the ridge gives rise to a longitudinal thickening, several cells deep, called the genital ridge. The latter runs parallel to the mesonephric ridge. The indifferent gonad consists of a superficial epithelium and an internal gonadal blastema made up of ill-defined cords of cells derived from the superficial epithelium.

Testes. In the male, the gonad rounds up, increases in size and acquires features—a network of branched (testis) cords and a tunica albuginea—that identify it as a testis. With appearance of the tunica albuginea, the germinal epithelium reverts to a typical peritoneal mesothelium and no longer plays a part in testicular development. Primordial germ cells migrate from the yolk sac during the 5th week of gestation in the human and give rise to gonocytes. Together with cells from the gonadal blastema, they form the testis cords: by the 3rd month in man, fetal spermatogonia also are present. The testis cords extend radially toward the mesorchium (gonadal mesentery) and a dense region of the blastema that will become the rete testis. The two become continuous and the testis cords elongate and differentiate into seminiferous tubules. Where they join the rete testis, the tubules remain straight and form the tubuli recti. The seminiferous tubules contain only spermatogonia and sustentacular (Sertoli) cells. The number of sustentacular cells remains constant from birth but from about 10 years of age to puberty, spermatogonia increase markedly in number. The full sequence of spermatogenic cells, from spermatogonia to spermatid, does not appear until puberty.

The mesenchymal tissue in which the testis cords develop, forms the septuli tests, connective tissue of the mediastinum testis and tunica albuginea. Cells in the mesenchymal stroma differentiate into interstitial cells (of Leydig). These are large and abundant from the 4th to 6th months in man, but then regress, only to increase again in size and number, at puberty.

Ducts. Specific development of exocrine ducts does not occur in the male. Rather, as the mesonephric kidney degenerates and is resorbed, its ducts are incorporated into the reproductive system and transformed into genital ducts. In some amphibians the mesonephric system persists, the upper region being associated with the testis and the lower part with the kidney. Thus, in these species, the mesonephric duct conducts sperm and urine to the cloaca. In higher animals this arrangement begins but, as the mesonephros is resorbed, the cranial mesonephric tubules are modified and unite with tubules of the rete testis. These efferent ductules are continuous with mesonephric ducts whose proximal region becomes highly convoluted to form the ductus epididymis. In the opossum, efferent ductules evaginate from the proximal part of the mesonephric duct and unite with the rete testis in a manner reminiscent of the ureteric bud and its subdivisions during differentiation of the metanephros.

Distally, the mesonephric duct remains straight, forming the ejaculatory duct and ductus deferens which, near its distal end, dilates to form the ampulla. Just beyond the ampulla, the epithelium of the ductus evaginates to provide the primordia for the seminal vesicles: the muscle coats are derived from surrounding mesenchyme. In man the vesicles attain the general adult form by the 7th fetal month and slowly grow until puberty, after which the adult proportions are reached.

Prostate. The prostate develops from multiple outgrowths of the urethral epithelium, above and below the entrance of the ejaculatory ducts. Some 60 glands develop in man, organized into five groups that will become the lobes of the prostate. The mesenchyme into which the prostatic glands grow provides the fibromuscular stroma. The gland remains small until puberty when, under the influence of testosterone, development of the prostate is completed.

Glands. The bulbourethral glands also arise as buds of endodermal epithelium, but in the region of the urogenital sinus that forms the membranous urethra. The outgrowths evaginate through the investing mesenchyme to lie within the urogenital diaphragm. Mucous cells appear at about 4 months in man. The bulbourethral glands, also influenced by testosterone, grow throughout puberty. The **urethral glands** (of Littre) are simple outgrowths of the epithelium that lines the urethra.

External Genitalia. Early in development, the cloacal membrane becomes surrounded by mesenchyme and forms two folds that unite anteriorly to form the cloacal swelling. From the anterior part of the swelling, the genital (urethral) folds develop, while the posterior part forms the anal folds. The cloacal swelling increases in size and gives rise to a genital tubercle, at which time the genital swellings become visible just lateral to the genital folds. In the male, the swellings are called scrotal swellings which move caudally, fuse, and form the scrotum.

The genital tubercle elongates to form the phallus, pulling the genital folds forward as its does. The folds form the lateral walls of the urogenital groove, which extends along the caudal surface of the phallus. The genital folds close over, fuse, and form the penile urethra, the tip of which lacks an orifice. Ectodermal cells at the tip grow inward as a solid cord that later canalizes to establish continuity with the remainder of the urethra. Corpora cavernosa penis and urethrae develop from paired and single mesenchymal columns, respectively. The latter forms around the penile urethra within the shaft of the penis and also gives rise to the glans. The external genitalia develop slowly after birth, then grow rapidly during puberty.

FUNCTIONAL SUMMARY

The primary function of the male reproductive system is to provide the necessary haploid germ cells for the procreation of the species. The production of spermatozoa occurs in the germinal

epithelium of the seminiferous tubules and represents the exocrine (holocrine) secretion of the testis. Both spermatogenesis and spermiogenesis are dependent upon high concentrations of testosterone, the endocrine secretion of the testis produced by interstitial cells.

The germinal epithelium essentially consists of two major classes of cells: a mobile population of germ or spermatogenic cells and a stable population of supporting Sertoli cells. The seminiferous epithelium is unique in that it is divided into basal and adluminal compartments which differ markedly, not only in their cellular content but also in their environments. The basal compartment contains the stem cells (spermatogonia) and newly formed primary spermatocytes exposed to an environment which is similar to that of blood plasma. The primary spermatocytes soon migrate into the adluminal compartment where, along with secondary spermatocytes, spermatids and spermatozoa, they are in contact with an environment that is rich in ions, contains certain amino acids not found in the basal compartment and has a high concentration of testosterone.

Sertoli cells are responsible for establishing and maintaining these two different environments. The tight junctions between the Sertoli cells constitute, in part at least, a blood-testis barrier. Any substances that enter or leave the adluminal compartment must pass through the cytoplasm of the Sertoli cells. Under the influence of a gonadotrophic hormone, Sertoli cells release androgen-binding protein that complexes with testosterone to maintain a high concentration of hormone in the adluminal compartment. The blood-testis barrier also serves to prevent the escape of the developing sperm out of the adluminal compartment into the general body tissues. If this were to occur, the haploid germ cells might be interpreted as foreign elements, resulting in an immunologic response directed against the forming germ cells in the germinal epithelium and, thus, causing sterility.

Development of the germ cells occurs in the adluminal compartment, in the embrace of the complex cytoplasmic processes of the Sertoli cells. As spermatogenic cells develop and differentiate, the Sertoli cell is thought to actively move them along their lateral surfaces toward the lumen, into which they are released from the apical surface of the Sertoli cell. Gap junctions provide a means of communication between Sertoli cells and allow for the coordinated release of spermatozoa from a given segment of a seminiferous tubule.

A considerable amount of testicular fluid is produced by the germinal epithelium and serves as a vehicle for the transport of spermatozoa out of the seminiferous tubules and into the excretory duct system.

Testosterone is present, not only in the adluminal compartment of the seminiferous tubules but also in the proximal duct system of the reproductive tract as far as the upper regions of the ductus epididymis. Thus, there exists the unusual circumstance of an endocrine secretion of the testis (testosterone), not only entering the blood stream but also passing through the lumen of the proximal duct system to have an effect on the proximal ductus epididymis. Systemic concentrations of testosterone are necessary for the development and functional maintenance of the remainder of the excretory duct system, the accessory sex glands and the male secondary sex characteristics.

Spermatozoa released into the seminiferous tubules are nonmotile and are moved into the tubuli recti and rete testis by the flow of testicular fluid and by the shallow peristaltic movements of the seminiferous tubules. The presence of a ciliated epithelium, coupled with a progressive increase in smooth muscle in the walls of the ductuli efferentes, contributes to the movement of spermatozoa into the proximal epididymis.

Most of the testicular fluid is absorbed in the ductuli efferentes and in the proximal ductus epididymidis. Sperm entering the ductus epididymidis exhibit weak, random motions and for the most part are incapable of fertilization. In contrast, spermatozoa from the distal epididymis show strong unidirectional motility and are capable of fertilization. Sperm are slowly propelled through the long ductus epididymidis by peristaltic contractions of its muscular wall. During their passage through the epididymis, spermatozoa of some species show continued differentiation of the acrosome and sperm head as well as a progressive increase in their fertilizing capacity. Thus, sperm require the environment provided by the ductus epididymidis to become physiologically mature and viable. Although the maturation process is androgen-dependent, the mechanism by which the various segments of the epididymis control and regulate the physiological maturation of spermatozoa is unknown. The distal ductus epididymidis functions to store sperm. Because of its thick muscular wall, it can contract forcibly and, in coordination with the wall of the ductus deferens, empty the stored sperm into the prostatic urethra.

During ejaculation the three primary accessory sex glands contribute successively to the seminal fluid. The bulbourethral glands and intraepithelial urethral glands secrete fluids which lubricate the urethra during sexual excitement and erection of the penis. At the onset of ejaculation, muscular tissue of the prostatic stroma contracts, discharging the secretory product into the prostatic urethra. Its abundant thin secretion is slightly acidic and contains acid phosphatase. Sperm, together with their suspending fluid, are expelled from the distal ductus epididymidis and ductus deferens. The last component added to the ejaculate is the viscous secretion of the seminal vesicles. This secretion is rich in the sugar fructose, an important energy source for the active, motile spermatozoa. Seminal vesicles also secrete high concentrations of prostaglandins, but their exact role in the female tract is unknown. The final phase of physiological maturation of spermatozoa, capacitation, occurs in the female reproductive tract and substantially increases the percentage of spermatozoa that are capable of fertilization.

Atlas and Table of Key Features for Chapter 17

Table 17-1
Key Histological Features of Male Reproductive Tract

	Epithelial Lining	Support	Muscle
Seminiferous tubule	Germinal epithelium containing spermatogenic cells (spermatogonia, 1° and 2° spermatocytes, spermatids) and Sertoli cells	Peritubular connective tissue: collagen fibers and myoid cells	
Tubuli recti	Simple columnar	Loose connective tissue	
Rete testis	Simple cuboidal. Short microvilli, single cilium on each cell	Dense, vascular connective tissue.	
Ductuli efferentes	Tall, ciliated columnar and short ciliated or nonciliated cuboidal. Lining has irregular contour.	Loose connective tissue between tubules	Thin, circular smooth muscle
Ductus epididymis	Pseudostratified columnar: tall principal cells with stereocilia; short basal cells	Thin lamina propria	Circular smooth muscle
Ductus deferens	Pseudostratified columnar, thrown into longitudinal folds: stereocilia	Dense lamina propria: collagen and elastic fibers. Adventitia of loose connective tissue.	Three layers: inner longitudinal, middle circular, outer longitudinal smooth muscle
Ampulla of ductus deferens	Pseudostratified columnar with stereocilia. Complex folds form extensive pocket-like recesses.	Lamina propria and adventitia less well defined.	Thinner, less distinct layers of smooth muscles
Ejaculatory duct	Pseudostratified or simple columnar. Forms pockets but less prominent than in ampulla	Dense collagenous connective tissue with many elastic fibers	
Seminal vesicles	Honeycombed appearance: pseudostratified columnar with regions of simple columnar	Thin lamina propria with many elastic fibers. External layer of loose connective tissue rich in elastic fibers	Inner circular outer longitudinal smooth muscle
Prostate	Variable. Usually simple columnar or psuedostratified columnar. Low cuboidal or squamous may occur	Vascular connective tissue with dense network of elastic fibers	Smooth muscle fibers in connective tissue surround individual gland units
Bulbourethral glands	Varies. Simple cuboidal to simple columnar. Flattened in distended alveoli. Ducts lined by simple columnar, pseudostratified near urethra	Fibroelastic connective tissue around each glandular structure	Smooth and skeletal muscle fibers in interstitial tissue between glandular elements
Corpora cavernosa penis	Endothelium of vascular spaces	Fibroelastic connective tissue	Smooth muscle cells in trabeculae between cavernous spaces
Corpora cavernosa urethrae	Cavernous spaces lined by endothelium, penile urethrae lined by pseudostratified columnar, nonkeratinized stratified squamous	Fibroelastic connective tissue rich in elastic fibers	Smooth muscle cells more abundant

Testis

17-6

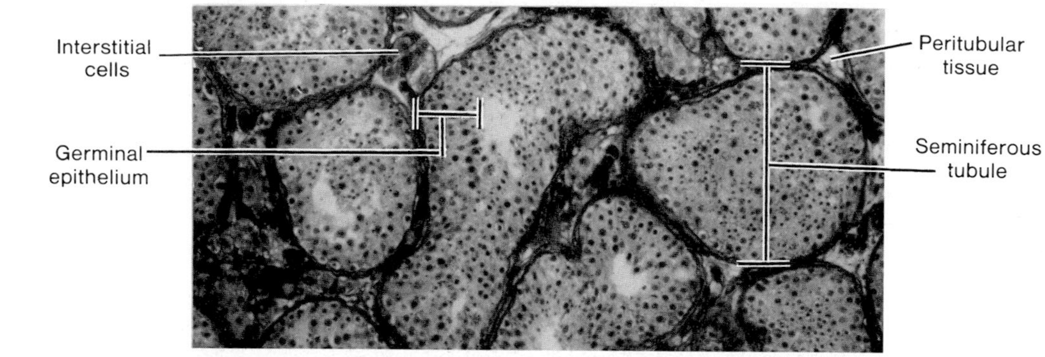

17-7

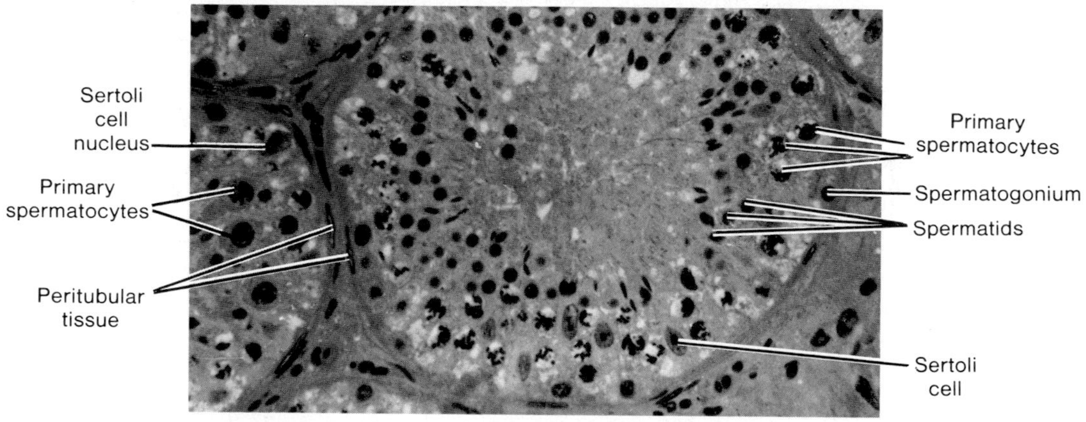

17-8

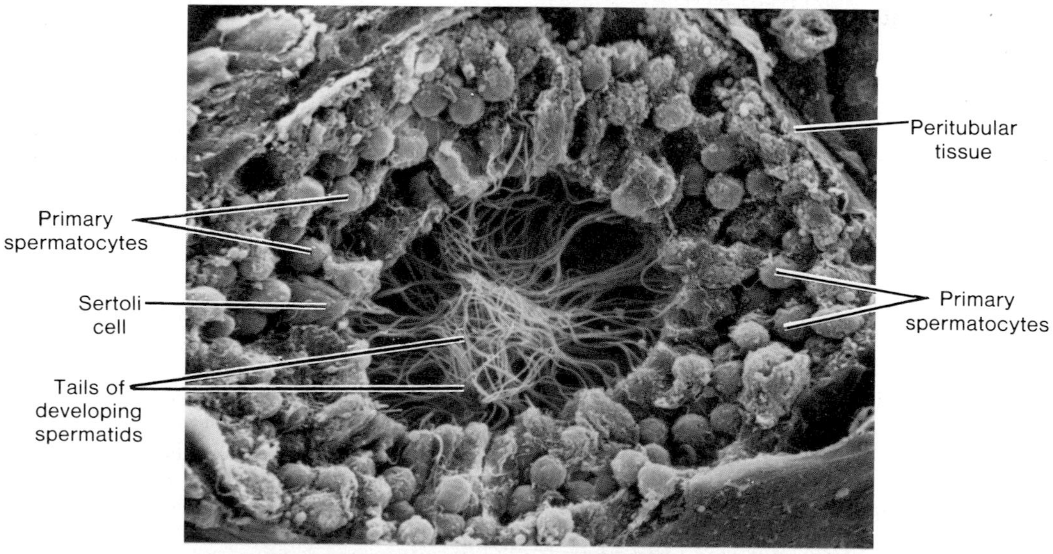

Figure 17-6. Seminiferous tubules (human). LM, ×100.
Figure 17-7. Seminiferous tubule. LM, ×250.
Figure 17-8. Seminiferous tubule. SEM, ×500.

17-9

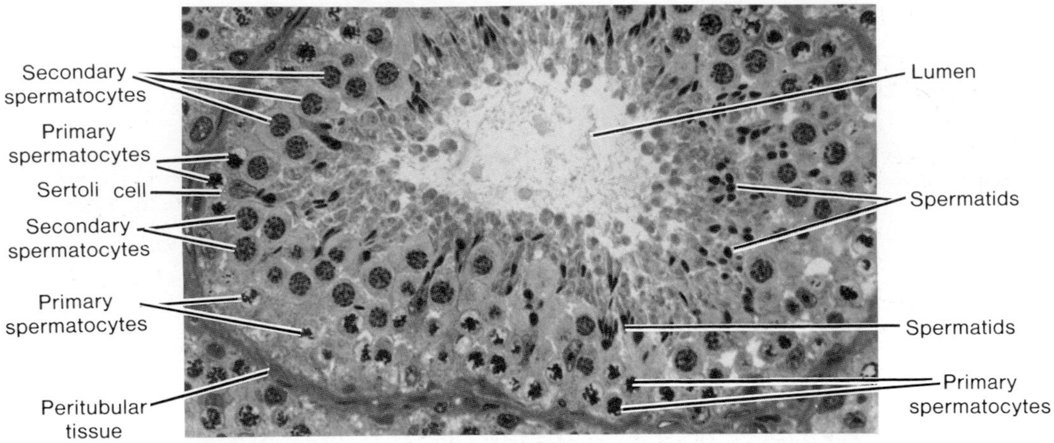

17-10

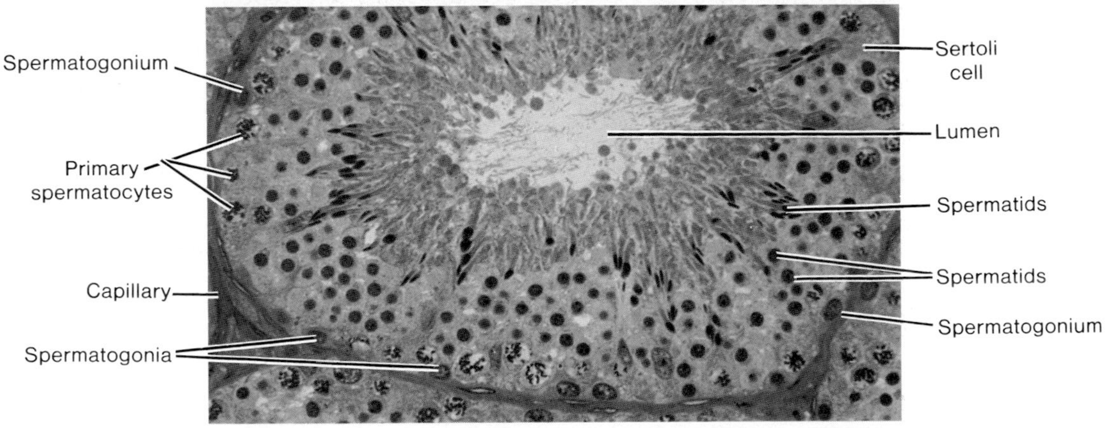

17-11

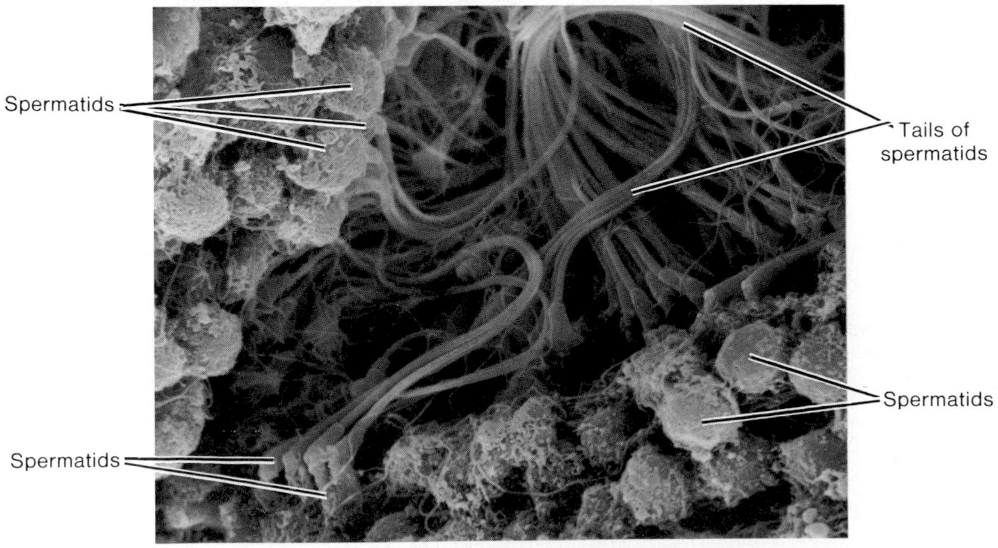

Figure 17-9. Germinal epithelium. LM, ×250.
Figure 17-10. Germinal epithelium. LM, ×250.
Figure 17-11. Germinal epithelium. SEM, ×2000.

17-12

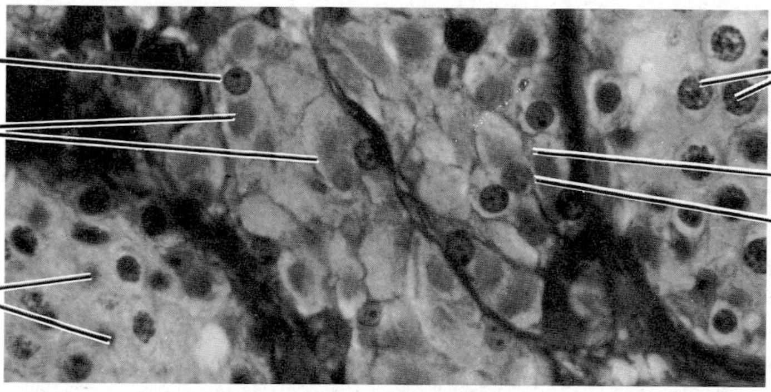

17-13 **Excretory Ducts**

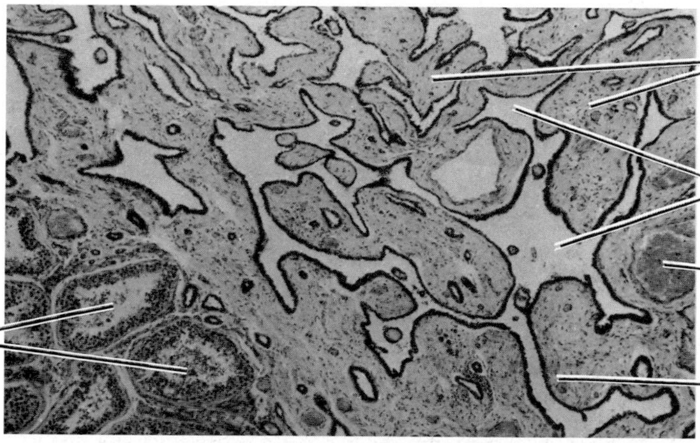

17-14

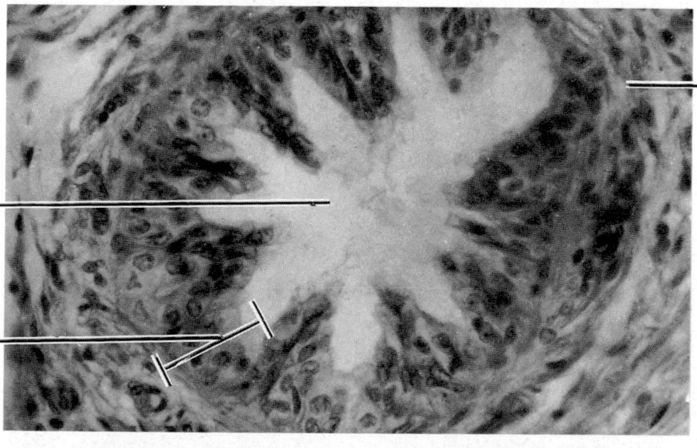

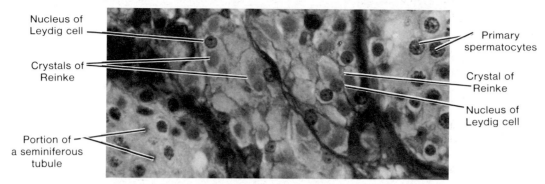

Figure 17-12. Interstitial tissue (human). LM, ×400.
Figure 17-13. Rete testis (human). LM, ×40.
Figure 17-14. Ductuli efferentes (human). LM, ×250.

17-15

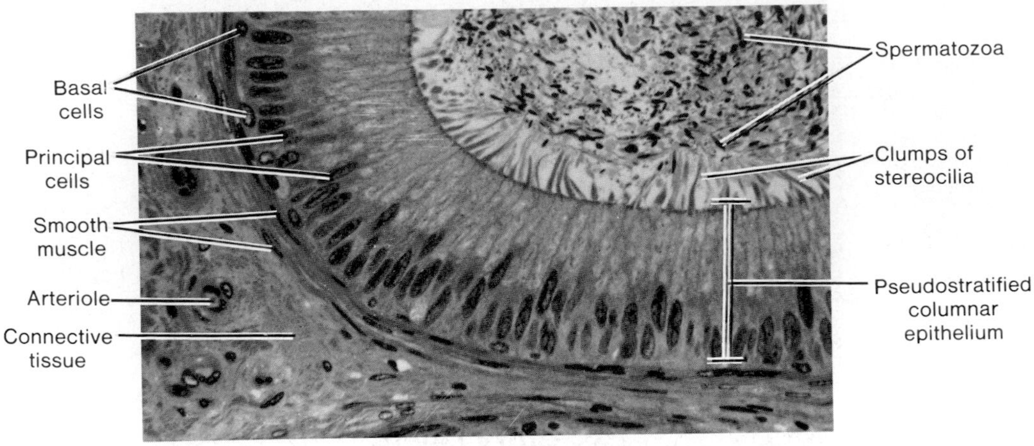

17-16

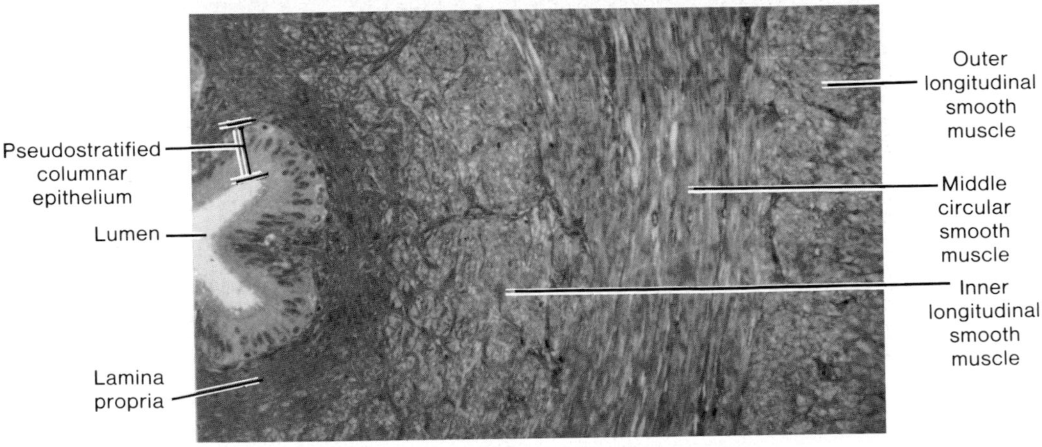

17-17

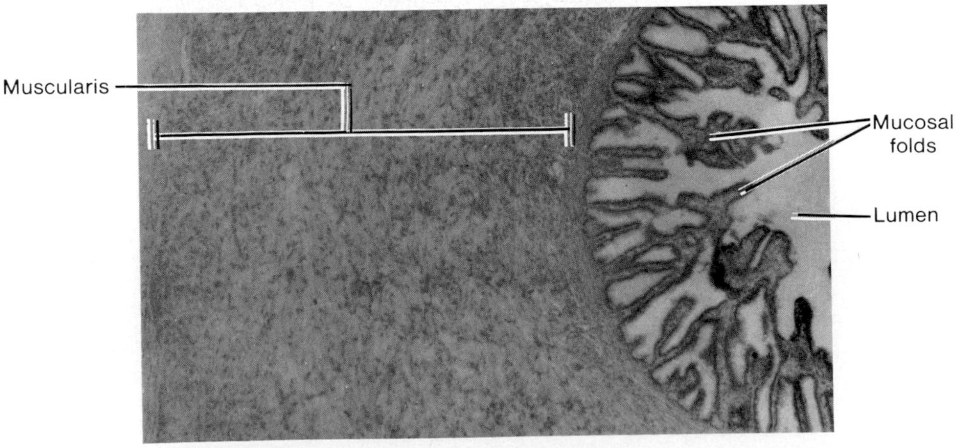

Figure 17-15. Ductus epididymidis. LM, ×250.
Figure 17-16. Ductus deferens. LM, ×150.
Figure 17-17. Ampulla of ductus deferens (human). LM, ×100.

17-18 Accessory Sex Glands

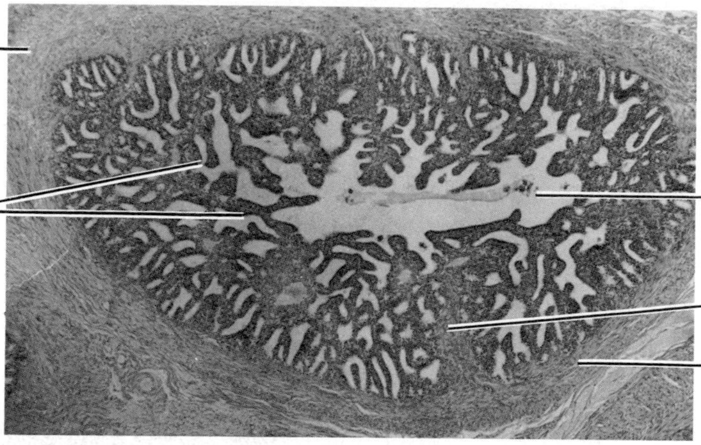

17-19

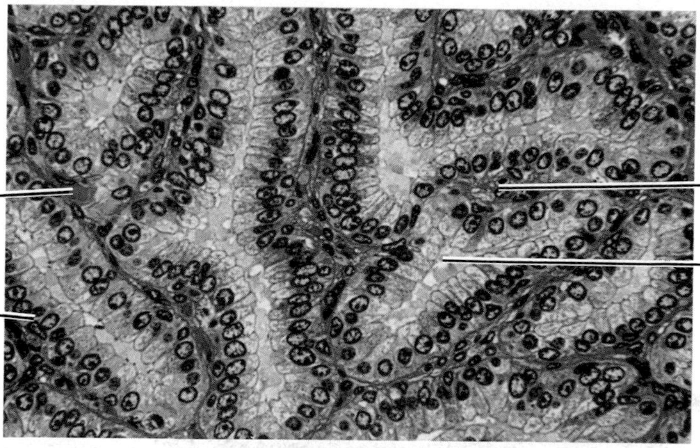

17-20

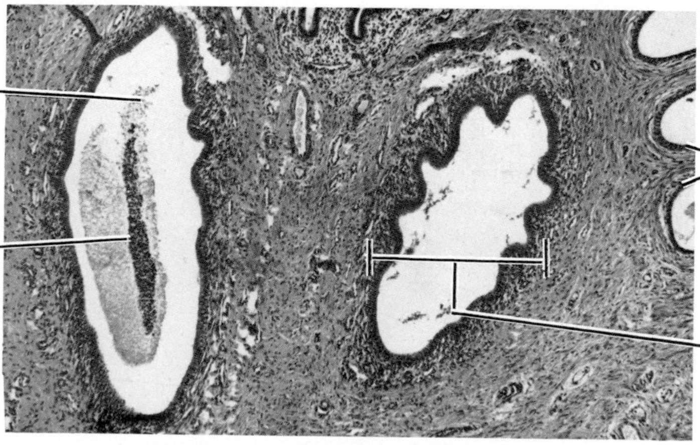

Figure 17-18. Seminal vesicle (human). LM, ×40.
Figure 17-19. Seminal vesicle. LM, ×250.
Figure 17-20. Ejaculatory ducts (human). LM, ×40.

17-21

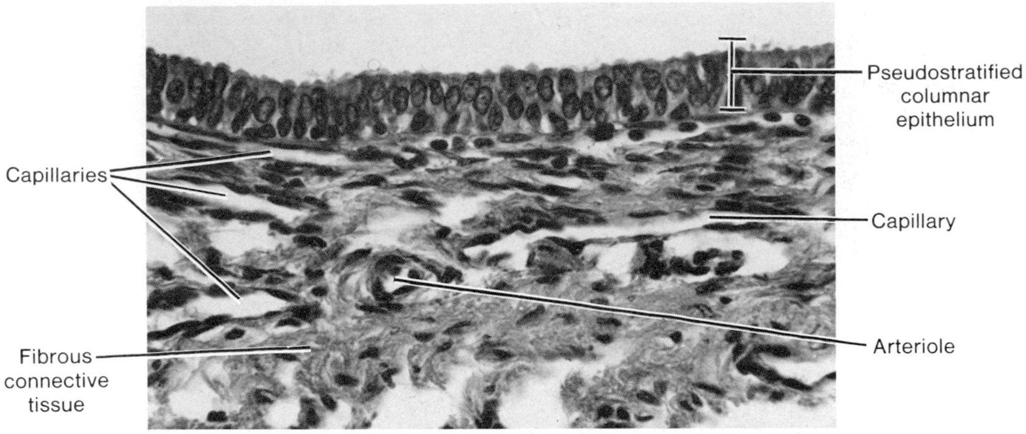

17-22

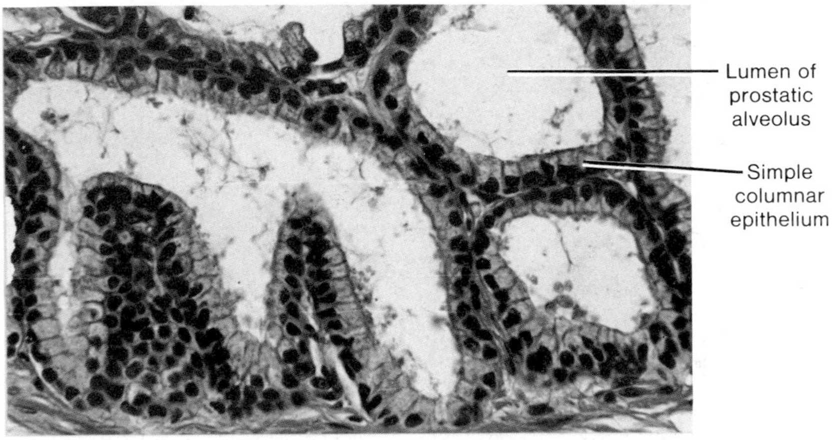

17-23

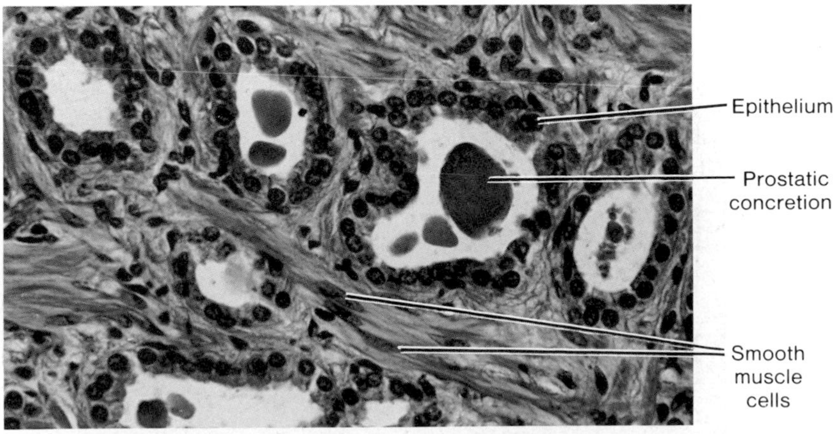

Figure 17-21. Ejaculatory ducts (human). LM, ×250.
Figure 17-22. Submucosal gland of prostate (human). LM, ×250.
Figure 17-23. Principal glands of prostate (human). LM, ×400.

17-24 Penis

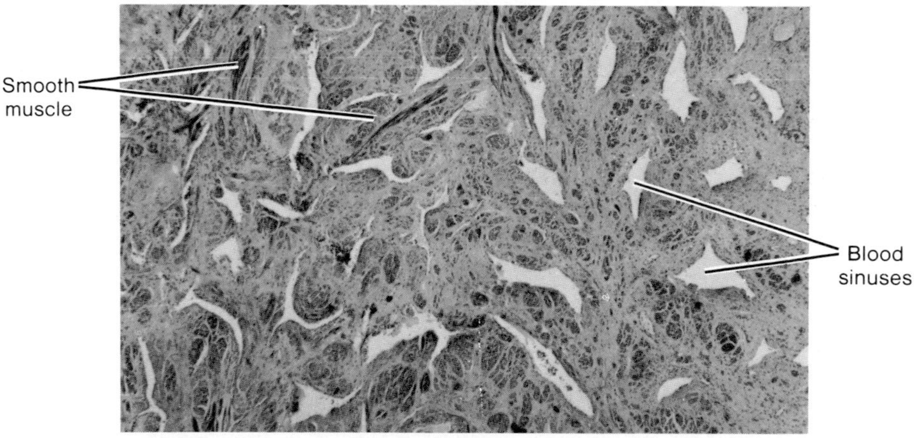

17-25 Spermatozoa

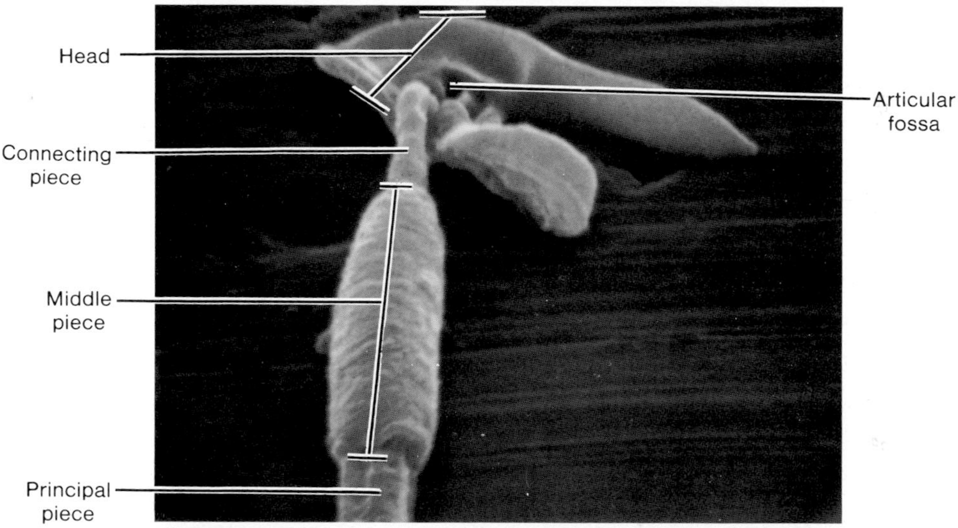

17-26

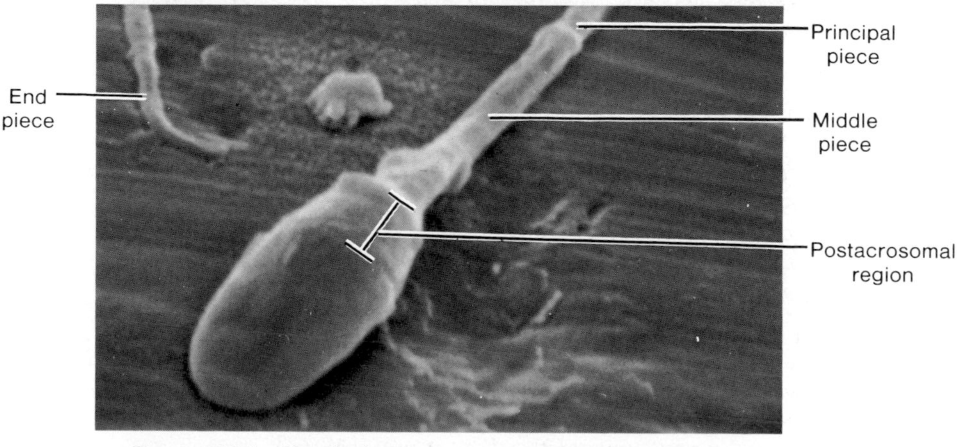

Figure 17-24. Erectile tissue-corpus spongiosum (human). LM, ×30.
Figure 17-25. Spermatozoon (opossum). SEM, ×5000.
Figure 17-26. Spermatozoon (human). SEM, ×10,000

17-27 Development

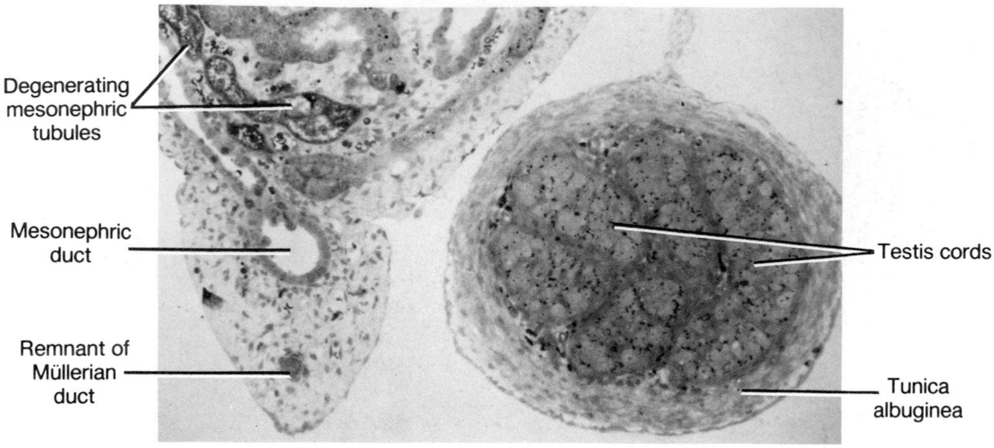

17-28

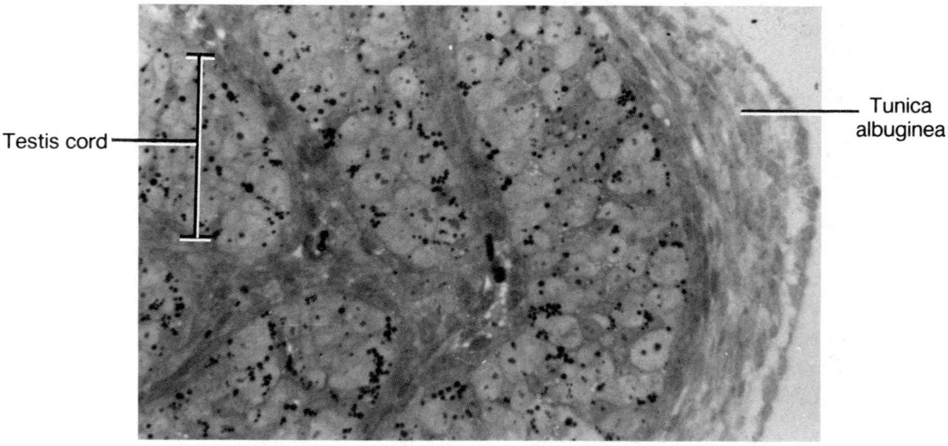

17-29

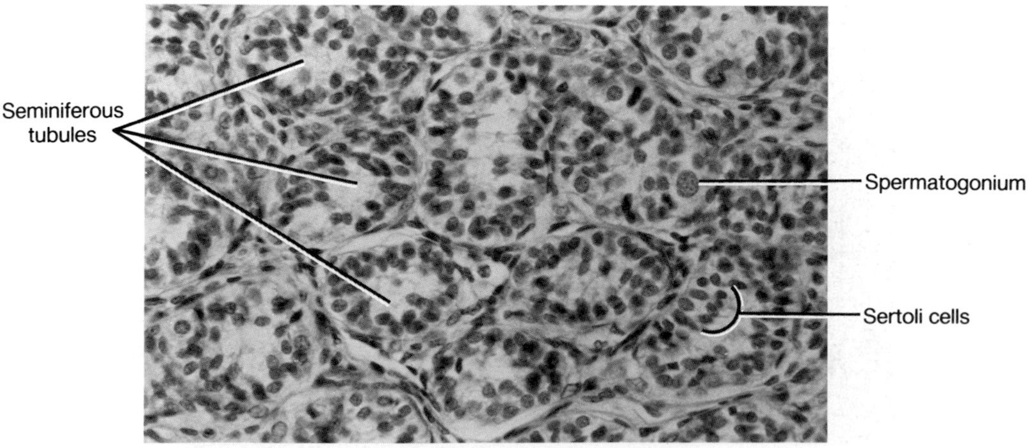

Figure 17-27. Developing testis. LM, ×100
Figure 17-28. Developing testis. LM, ×450
Figure 17-29. Prepubertal testis (human). LM, ×250

17-30

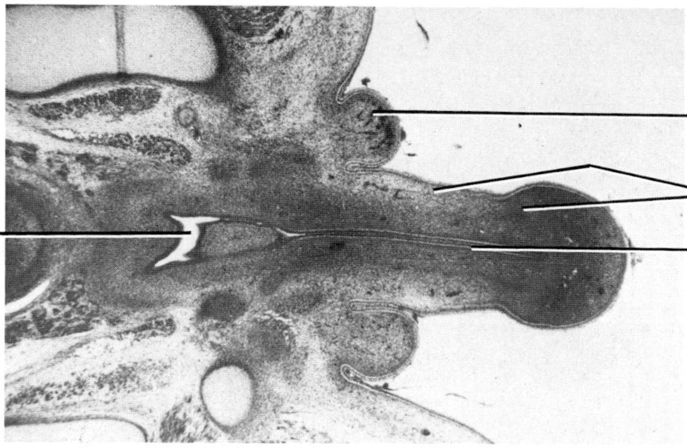

17-31

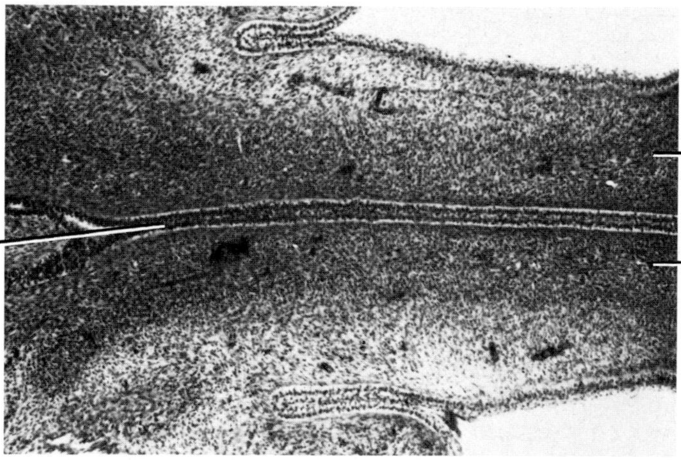

17-32

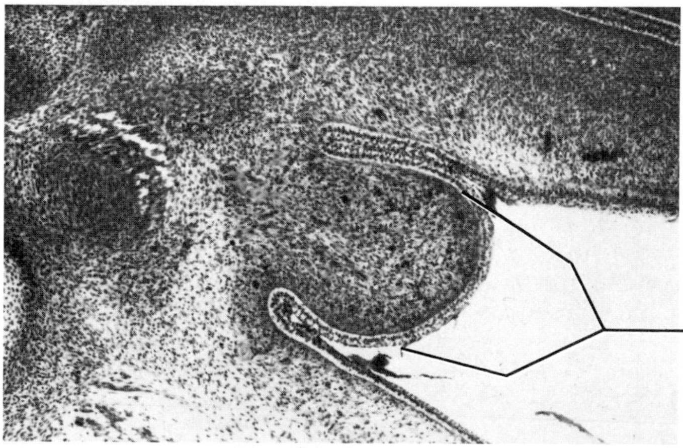

Figure 17-30. External genitalia (40 days, human). LM, ×15
Figure 17-31. Penis (40 days, human). LM, ×200
Figure 17-32. Scrotal swelling (40 days, human). LM, ×200

18

Female Reproductive System

The female reproductive system consists of a group of internal organs—the ovaries, oviducts, uterus and vagina—and external structures (the external genitalia) which include the labia majora, labia minora and the clitoris. Although not genital organs, the mammary glands are important accessory organs of the female reproductive system. Throughout the first 10 or 11 years of life, the reproductive organs remain immature and growth parallels that of the body generally. During the 2 or 3 years prior to the first menstrual period, the generative organs increase in size, the breasts enlarge and pubic and axillary hair appears. Following the first menses and thereafter throughout the reproductive period, the ovaries, oviducts, uterus, vagina and mammary glands undergo cyclic changes in function and structure associated with the menstrual cycle and with pregnancy. During menopause, the cycles become irregular and eventually cease; in the postmenopausal period the reproductive organs atrophy.

THE OVARIES

The ovaries are paired, oval bodies that lie one on either side of the uterus, where they are suspended from the broad ligament by a mesentery, the mesovarium. A fold of peritoneum extends from the upper pole of the ovary to the posterior abdominal wall and constitutes the suspensory ligament. It contains the ovarian blood vessels and nerves. The ovarian ligament proper is a short fibromuscular ligament that passes from the lower pole of the ovary to the lateral surface of the uterus, below the junction with the oviduct. The ovaries are homologous with the testes and like the latter are compound organs that have both exocrine and endocrine functions. The exocrine secretion consists of whole cells—the ova—and, thus, the ovary can be regarded as a holocrine or cytogenic gland. It also secretes, in cyclic fashion, female sex hormones directly into the blood stream and is, therefore, an endocrine gland.

Structure

KEY WORDS: surface epithelium cortex, tunica albuginea, ovarian follicles, medulla

Each ovary is covered by a mesothelium that is continuous with that of the mesovarium. As this membrane extends over the surface of the ovary, the squamous cells assume a cuboidal shape to become the **surface epithelium** of the ovary. Sections of the ovary show an outer cortex and an inner medulla but the boundary between these two regions is indistinct. The stroma of the **cortex** consists of a compact feltwork of fine collagenous fibers and numerous spindle-shaped cells. Elastic fibers are rare or absent in the cortex, except in conjunction with the walls of blood vessels. Immediately below the surface epithelium, the connective tissue of the cortex is less cellular and more compact, forming a more dense layer called the **tunica albuginea**. Scattered throughout the cortical tissue are the **ovarian follicles**, whose size varies with their stage of development. The stroma of the **medulla** consists of a loose connective tissue that is less cellular than that of the cortex and contains many elastic fibers and some scattered smooth muscle cells. Numerous large, tortuous blood vessels, lymphatics and nerves also are present in the medulla.

Ovarian Follicles

KEY WORDS: cortex, ovum, epithelial cells, primordial, primary, secondary, mature follicles

The follicles are located in the **cortex** of the ovary, deep to the tunica albuginea, and consist of an immature **ovum** enclosed by one or more layers of **epithelial cells**. At birth the human ovary contains some 300,000 to 400,000 ova embedded in the cortical stroma, but few reach maturity and become ovulated. During the menstrual cycle, several follicles begin to grow and develop, but only one attains full maturity; the rest degenerate. The size of the follicle and the thickness of the epithelial envelope varies with the stage of development. During their growth, the follicles undergo a sequence of changes in which **primordial, primary, secondary** and **mature follicles** can be distinguished.

Primordial Follicles

KEY WORDS: unilaminar, follicular cells, primary oocyte

In the mature ovary, follicles are present in all stages of development. The majority, especially in young females, are primordial, or **unilaminar** follicles, which are present in the periphery of the cortex just beneath the tunica albuginea. These follicles consist of an immature ovum surrounded by a single layer of flattened **follicular cells** which rest on a basement membrane. At this stage the ovum is a **primary oocyte**, suspended in the diplotene state of the meiotic prophase. The primary oocyte is a large cell situated in the center of the primordial follicle and contains a large vesicular nucleus with a prominent nucleolus. The Golgi apparatus is well developed and spherical mitochondria tend to be concentrated in the region of the centrosome.

As the primordial follicle develops into a primary follicle, changes occur in the ovum, follicular cells and adjacent connective tissue stroma of the cortex.

Primary Follicles

KEY WORDS: zona pellucida, granulosa cells, stratum granulosum, theca folliculi, theca interna, theca externa

During growth of a primary follicle, the oocyte increases in size, and the Golgi complex, which originally was a single organelle situated next to the nucleus, becomes a multiple structure scattered throughout the cytoplasm of the oocyte. Free ribosomes increase in number; the mitochondria become dispersed; and rough endoplasmic reticulum, although not prominent, becomes more extensive. A few lipid droplets and lipochrome pigments appear in the cytoplasm, and yolk granules accumulate; these, however, are smaller and less numerous than in nonprimate species. As the oocyte grows, a clear, refractile proteoglycan membrane, the **zona pellucida**, develops between the oocyte and adjacent follicular cells. The origin of this membrane generally is attributed to the follicular cells, but the oocyte also may contribute to its formation. Microvilli extend from the oocyte into the zona pellucida.

Concurrently with growth of the ovum, the flattened follicular cells of the primordial follicles become cuboidal or columnar in shape and proliferate to form several layers. These cells are now **granulosa cells** and the layer of stratified epithelium which they form is called the **stratum granulosum**. Mitochondria, free ribosomes and endoplasmic reticulum increase and the Golgi complex becomes prominent. Irregular, slender cytoplasmic processes extend from the granulosa cells and penetrate the zona pellucida to make contact with the processes from the oocyte. There is no cytoplasmic continuity between the oocyte and the cells of the stratum granulosum, but the processes of the granulosa cells may penetrate into the cytoplasm of the oocyte.

While these changes are occurring in the oocyte and follicular cells, the adjacent stroma becomes organized into a sheath, the **theca folliculi**, which surrounds the growing primary follicle. The theca folliculi is separated from the stratum granulosum by a distinct basement membrane. The cells differentiate into an inner secretory layer, the **theca interna**, and an outer fibrous layer, the **theca externa**. However, the boundary between the two layers is somewhat indistinct. The theca externa merges imperceptibly into the surrounding stroma. Many small blood vessels penetrate the theca externa to provide a rich vascular network to the theca interna. The stratum granulosum remains avascular until after ovulation.

Secondary Follicles

KEY WORDS: liquor folliculi, follicular antrum, antral follicle, cumulus oophorus, corona radiata

As the follicular cells continue to proliferate, the growing follicle assumes an ovoid shape and gradually comes to lie deeper in the cortex. When the stratum granulosum has become 8 to 12 layers thick, small, irregular, fluid-filled spaces appear between the granulosa cells. The fluid, the **liquor folliculi**, increases in amount and the spaces fuse to form a single cavity called the **follicular antrum**. The follicle is now a secondary or **antral follicle**. At this stage the oocyte has reached its full size and undergoes no additional growth. The follicle, however, continues to increase in size, due in part to the continued accumulation of the liquor folliculi. The ovum now occupies an eccentric position in the follicle, surrounded by a mass of granulosa cells that projects into the fluid filled-antrum as the **cumulus oophorus**. The cells of the cumulus oophorus are continuous with those that line the antral cavity. The granulosa cells that surround the oocyte form the **corona radiata** and are anchored to the zona pellucida by cytoplasmic processes.

Mature Follicles and Ovulation

KEY WORDS: endocrine gland, estrogen, secondary oocyte, ovulation, stigma (macula pellucida)

In the human female the follicles require 10 to 14 days to reach the stage of a mature follicle. At maximum size, the follicle occupies the thickness of the cortex and bulges from the surface of the ovary. Fluid spaces appear between the granulosa cells of the cumulus oophorus, and the connection between the ovum and stratum granulosum becomes weakened. The theca folliculi has attained its greatest development. The cells of the theca interna assume the cytological characteristics of a steroid-secreting **endocrine gland** and elaborate **estrogens**. Just prior to ovulation, the oocyte completes the first meiotic division and gives off the first polar body. Thus, at ovulation a **secondary oocyte** is liberated.

Rupture of the mature follicle and liberation of the ovum constitutes **ovulation**, which normally occurs at the middle of the menstrual cycle. Just prior to ovulation, a further expansion of the follicle occurs due to an increased secretion of liquor folliculi, and the follicle appears as though the contents were under pressure. However, direct measurements show no increase in pressure within the follicle. The wall of the follicle that bulges from the ovary becomes thinner and a small, avascular, translucent area appears. This is the **stigma**, or **macula pellucida**. The tunica albuginea thins out and the covering epithelium of the ovary becomes discontinuous in this area. A collagenase produced by granulosa cells adjacent to the tunica albuginea may be responsible for the breakdown of the collagen fibers at the site of the stigma. The stigma protrudes as a small vesicle or blister, ruptures and the ovum with its adherent corona radiata is extruded along with follicular fluid.

Corpus Luteum

KEY WORDS: estrogen, progesterone, granulosa lutein cells, theca lutein cells, corpus albicans

Following ovulation, the follicle is transformed into a temporary endocrine gland, the corpus luteum, which elaborates both

estrogens and **progesterone**. The walls of the follicle collapse and the stratum granulosum is thrown into folds. Bleeding from capillaries in the theca interna may result in a blood clot in the center of the corpus luteum. The granulosa cells increase greatly in size, assume a polyhedral shape and transform into pale-staining **granulosa lutein cells**. Lipid accumulates in the cytoplasm of the cells, and in electron micrographs, smooth endoplasmic reticulum is abundant and the mitochondria possess tubular cristae. Cells of the theca interna also enlarge and become epithelioid in character to form **theca lutein cells**. The lutein cells derived from the theca interna are somewhat smaller than the granulosa lutein cells.

The basement membrane separating the granulosa cells from the theca interna depolymerizes, and capillaries from the theca interna invade the lutein tissue to form a complex vascular network throughout the corpus luteum. Connective tissue from the theca interna also penetrates the mass of lutein cells and forms a delicate network about them. The fully formed corpus luteum secretes both estrogens and progesterone; secretion of progesterone increases rapidly during luteinization and is maintained at high levels until the corpus luteum involutes.

If the ovum is not fertilized, the corpus luteum persists for about 14 days, then undergoes involution. The cells decrease in size, accumulate much lipid and degenerate. Hyaline material accumulates between the lutein cells, the connective tissue cells become pyknotic, and the corpus luteum gradually is replaced by an irregular white scar, the **corpus albicans**. Over the following months the corpus albicans itself disappears. If fertilization occurs, the corpus luteum enlarges further and persists for about the first 6 months of pregnancy, then gradually declines. Following delivery, the involution of the corpus luteum is accelerated, resulting in the formation of a corpus albicans.

Atresia of Follicles

KEY WORDS: atresia, glassy membrane

During the early part of each menstrual cycle, several primordial follicles begin to grow, but usually only one attains full development and ovulates. The remainder undergo a degenerative process called **atresia**, which may occur at any stage in the development of a follicle. In an atretic primary follicle the ovum shrinks, degenerates and undergoes cytolysis; the follicular cells show similar degenerative changes. The follicle is resorbed and the small space left is rapidly filled by the connective tissue of the stroma. Similar degenerative changes occur in larger follicles, but the zona pellucida may persist for a time after dissolution of the oocyte and follicular cells. Macrophages invade the atretic follicle and engulf the degenerating material, including fragments of the zona pellucida.

The cells of the theca interna remain for a longer time than do those of the stratum granulosum, but they also show degenerative changes. The theca cells increase in size, lipid droplets appear in the cytoplasm, and the cells take on an epithelioid character resembling that of lutein cells. The theca cells assume a cord-like arrangement, the cords being separated by connective tissue fibers and capillaries. The basal lamina between the granulosa cells and theca interna frequently increases in thickness and forms a hyalinized, corrugated layer, the **glassy membrane**. This structure is characteristic of atretic growing follicles and aids in distinguishing a large follicle undergoing atresia from a corpus luteum. Other differences include degenerative changes in the granulosa cells and the presence of fragments of the zona pellucida at the center of the follicle without an associated oocyte. Ultimately the degenerated remains of the follicle are removed and a scar resembling a small corpus albicans results. This too eventually disappears into the stroma of the ovary.

Interstitial Cells

KEY WORDS: theca interna, hilus cells

In some mammals, especially rodents, clusters of epithelioid cells are scattered in the stroma of the cortex. These interstitial cells contain small lipid droplets and bear a marked resemblance to luteal cells. It is thought that these interstitial cells arise from the **theca interna** of follicles that are undergoing atresia. In the human, interstitial cells are most abundant during the first year of life, the period during which atretic follicles are most numerous. In the adult they are present only in widely scattered, small groups. Their role in ovarian physiology is unknown. In the human they elaborate estrogens, whereas in the rabbit, the interstitial cells produce progesterone.

Other large epithelioid cells, the **hilus cells**, are found in association with the vascular spaces and unmyelinated nerves in the hilus of the ovary. The cells appear to be similar to the interstitial cells of the testis and contain lipid, lipochrome pigments and cholesterol esters. Their function is unknown. Hilus cells are most commonly found during pregnancy and at menopause; tumors arising in these cells have a masculinizing effect.

The Ovarian Cycle

KEY WORDS: follicle-stimulating hormone, luteinizing hormone

Maturation of ovarian follicles, their endocrine functions and the phenomenon of ovulation are regulated by follicle stimulating hormone (FSH) and luteinizing hormone (LH). These are gonadotrophic hormones elaborated by the anterior pituitary. **Follicle-stimulating hormone** is responsible for the maturation of follicles and stimulates secretion of estrogens by cells of the theca interna. The initial development of the follicles is self-regulated and does not require FSH, but the hormone *is* essential for their maturation. In conjunction with FSH, **luteinizing hormone** induces ripening of the mature follicle and ovulation. Alone, LH converts the mature follicle to a corpus luteum and induces it to secrete estrogens and progesterone. The cyclic nature of follicle formation and ovulation is the result of a reciprocal interaction between pituitary gonadotrophins and ovarian hormones.

As production of estrogens by the theca interna increases, release of FSH from the pituitary is inhibited and the level of this hormone falls below that required for the maturation of new follicles. However, the rising level of estrogen also stimulates the release of LH from the pituitary, resulting in ovulation, formation of a corpus luteum and secretion of progesterone and estrogen by this body. The rising levels of progesterone in turn inhibit the release of LH from the pituitary, and as the level of LH declines, the corpus luteum no longer is maintained. With decline of the corpus luteum, estrogen levels decrease; inhibition of the pituitary is abolished; and the increased levels of FSH initiate a new cycle of follicle formation. The ovarian hormones do not affect the pituitary directly; their action is mediated through the hypothalamus.

OVIDUCTS

The oviducts (uterine tubes) are a pair of muscular tubes that extend from the ovary to the uterus along the upper margin of the broad ligament. One end of the tube is closely related to the ovary and, at this end, is open to the peritoneal cavity; the other end communicates with the lumen of the uterus. The oviduct delivers the ovum released at ovulation to the uterine cavity and provides an environment for fertilization and initial segmentation of the fertilized ovum.

Structure

KEY WORDS: infundibulum, fimbria, ampulla, isthmus, intramural (interstitial) portion, serosa, muscularis, mucosa

The oviduct is described as having several segments. The ovarian end, or **infundibulum**, is funnel-shaped and the margin is drawn out into numerous, tapering processes called the **fimbria**. The infundibulum opens into the **ampulla** of the tube, which is tortuous and thin-walled and makes up slightly more than half the length of the tube. The ampulla is continuous with the **isthmus**, a narrower, cord-like portion that constitutes about the medial one-third. The **intramural (interstitial) portion** is the continuation of the tube, where it passes through the uterine wall. Like other hollow viscera, the wall of the oviduct consists of several layers—an external **serosa**, an intermediate **muscularis**, and an internal **mucosa**.

Mucosa

KEY WORDS: plicae, columnar epithelium, lamina propria, ciliated cells, nonciliated cells, cyclic changes

The mucosa of the oviduct presents a series of longitudinal folds or **plicae**. In the ampulla these folds possess secondary and even tertiary folds to create a complex labyrinth of epithelial-lined spaces. In the isthmus, the folds are shorter with little branching, while in the intramural part the plicae form only low ridges. Throughout the tube, the plicae consist of a single layer of **columnar epithelial** cells and a **lamina propria** of richly cellular connective tissue that contains a network of reticular fibers and fusiform cells. Basally, the epithelial cells rest on an incomplete basement membrane. The epithelium decreases in height from ampulla to uterus and consists of ciliated and nonciliated cells. The **ciliated cells** are most numerous on the surface of the fimbria and progressively decrease in number through the ampulla, isthmus and intramural portion. The **nonciliated cells** appear to be secretory and may help to establish an environment that is suitable for the survival and fertilization of the ovum, and maintenance of the zygote. A third type of cell, an undifferentiated type with a darkly staining nucleus, may represent a precursor of the secretory cell or the exhausted secretory cell.

The epithelium shows **cyclic changes** associated with the ovarian cycle. During the follicular stage, ciliated cells increase in height, reaching their maximum at about the time of ovulation. There also is evidence of increased secretory preparations in the secretory cells during the follicular phase. In the luteal phase, the ciliated cells decrease in height and lose their cilia and there is an augmented secretory activity by the secretory cells. Loss of cilia is greatest in the fimbria and is less marked in the isthmus. The cilia are responsive to steroid hormones; estrogen appears to be responsible for the appearance and maintenance of the cilia while progesterone increases the rate at which they beat. Other ciliated cells of the body show no such hormone responsiveness.

Muscular Coat and Serosa

KEY WORDS: inner circular, outer longitudinal

The mucous membrane rests directly on the muscle coat and is not supported by a submucosa. The muscle coat consists of two layers of smooth muscle but there is no sharp boundary between the two coats. The **inner layer is circular** or closely spiralled; the **outer layer** of generally **longitudinally oriented** fibers is thinner. The muscularis increases in thickness toward the uterus due to the increased depth of the inner layer. Externally the oviduct is covered by a serosa which represents the peritoneal covering of the organ.

UTERUS

The human uterus is a single, hollow, pear-shaped organ with a thick muscular wall. It lies in the pelvic cavity between the bladder and rectum. The nonpregnant uterus varies in size from individual to individual but generally measures about 7 cm in length, 3 to 5 cm in its widest (upper) dimension and 2.5 to 3.0 cm in thickness. It is slightly flattened dorsoventrally and the cavity corresponds to the general overall shape. The uterus receives the fertilized ovum and nourishes the embryo throughout its development.

Structure

KEY WORDS: body, fundus, cervix, cervical canal, external os, fundus, endometrium, myometrium, perimetrium

Several regions of the uterus can be distinguished. The bulk of the organ consists of the **body**, which comprises the upper expanded portion. The dome-shaped part of the body between the junctions with the oviducts is referred to as the **fundus**. Below, the uterus narrows becoming more cylindrical in shape and this portion forms the **cervix** (neck), part of which protrudes into the vagina. The **cervical canal** passes through the cervix from the uterine cavity and communicates with the vagina at the **external os**.

The wall of the uterus is made up of several layers or coats to which special names have been applied. The internal lining or mucosa is called the **endometrium**; the middle muscular layer forms the **myometrium** and the external layer is referred to as the **perimetrium**. The perimetrium is the serosal or peritoneal layer, which covers the body and supravaginal part of the cervix posteriorly and the body of the uterus anteriorly.

Myometrium

KEY WORDS: smooth muscle, internal layer, middle layer, stratum vasculare, outer layer

The bulk of the uterine wall consists of the myometrium, which forms a thick coat about 15 to 20 mm in depth. The myometrium is composed of bundles of **smooth muscle** fibers separated by thin strands of connective tissue in which are collagenous fibers, fibroblasts, reticular fibers, mast cells and macrophages. Several layers of muscle are present but are not sharply defined because of the intermingling of fibers from one layer to another. Generally, however, the fibers form internal, middle and outer layers. The **internal layer** is thin and consists of longitudinal and circular fibers. The **middle layer** is the thickest and shows no regularity in the arrangement of the muscle fibers which run longitudinally, obliquely and transversely. This layer also contains many large blood vessels and has been called the **stratum vasculare**. The **outermost layer** of muscle consists mainly of longitudinally oriented fibers, some of which extend into the broad ligament, oviducts and ovarian ligaments proper. Elastic fibers are prominent in the outer layer but are not present in the inner layer of the myometrium, except around blood vessels.

In the nonpregnant uterus the smooth muscle cells are about 30 to 50 μm in length but during pregnancy they hypertrophy to reach lengths of 500 to 600 μm or greater. During pregnancy there is production of new muscle from undifferentiated cells and possibly from division of mature cells also. In spite of the total increase in the muscle mass, the muscle layers are thinned during pregnancy as the uterus becomes distended. The connective tissue of the myometrium also increases in amount. Following delivery, the muscle cells rapidly diminish in size but the uterus does not regain its original nonpregnant dimensions.

The myometrium normally undergoes intermittent contractions which, however, are usually not of sufficient intensity to be perceived. The intensity of the contractions may increase during menstruation to result in cramp-like pains. The contractions are diminished during pregnancy, possible as the result of the hormone relaxin. At parturition strong contractions of the uterine musculature occur, as a result of which the fetus is expelled. Uterine contractions are increased following administration of oxytocin, a hormone produced by the neurohypophysis. They also are increased in response to prostaglandins and a rise in the level of prostaglandins occurs just prior to delivery.

Endometrium

KEY WORDS: endometrial stroma, columnar epithelium, uterine glands, stratum basale (basal layer), stratum functionale (functional layer), arcuate arteries, radial branches, straight arteries, spiral arteries, lacunae

The endometrium is a complex mucous membrane that, in the human female, undergoes cyclic changes in structure and function in response to the ovarian cycle. The cyclic activity begins at puberty and continues until menopause. In the body of the uterus, the endometrium consists of a thick lamina propria, the **endometrial stroma**, and a covering epithelium. The stroma resembles mesenchymal tissue and consists of loosely arranged stellate cells with large round or ovoid nuclei, supported by a fine connective tissue network in which lymphocytes, granular leukocytes and macrophages are present. The endometrial stroma lies directly on the myometrium to which it is firmly attached and there is no intervening submucosa.

The stroma is covered by a simple **columnar epithelium** that contains ciliated cells and nonciliated secretory cells. The epithelium dips down into the stroma to form numerous **uterine glands** which extend deeply into the stroma and occasionally penetrate into the myometrium. Most are simple tubular glands but some branching may occur near the muscle. A basement membrane underlies both the glandular and surface epithelium.

The endometrium can be divided into the stratum basale (basal layer) and the stratum functionale (functional layer). These differ in their structure, function and blood supply. **Stratum basale (basal layer)** is narrower, more cellular and fibrous than the functional layer and lies directly on the myometrium. It undergoes few changes during the menstrual cycle and is not shed at menstruation, but rather serves as the source from which the **functional layer** is restored. The **stratum functionale** extends to the lumen of the uterus, and it is this portion of the endometrium in which cyclic changes occur and which is sloughed during menstruation. The stratum functionale is sometimes divided into the compacta, a narrow superficial zone, and the spongiosa, a broader zone that comprises the bulk of the functionalis.

The blood supply of the endometrium is unique and plays an important role in the events of menstruation. Branches of the uterine artery penetrate the myometrium to the middle layer, where they provide **arcuate arteries** which run circumferentially in the myometrium. One set of branches from these arteries supplies the superficial layers of the myometrium, while **radial branches** pass inward to supply the endometrium. At the junction of myometrium and endometrium the radial branches provide a dual circulation to the endometrium. **Straight arteries** supply the stratum basale, while the stratum functionale is supplied by highly contorted **spiral arteries**. As the latter pass through the functional layer, they provide terminal arterioles which then unite with a complex network of capillaries and thin walled dilated vascular structures, the **lacunae**. The venous system also forms an irregular network of venules and veins with irregular sinusoidal enlargements, then drains into a plexus at the junction of myometrium and endometrium. During the menstrual cycles the spiral arteries constrict periodically so that the functional layer is subjected to intermittent periods of blanching. The distal portion of the arterial supply in the functionalis undergoes degeneration and regeneration with each menstrual cycle, whereas the straight arteries of the basal layer show no such changes.

The arrangement of blood vessels in the endometrium is shown in Figure 18–1.

Cyclic Changes in the Endometrium

KEY WORDS: proliferative, maturation of follicle, secretory phase, corpus luteum, ischemic (premenstrual) and menstrual stages

During the normal menstrual cycle, the endometrium undergoes a continuous sequence of changes in which four stages can be described. The stages correlate with the functional activity of the ovaries and constitute the proliferative, secretory, ischemic (premenstrual) and menstrual stages.

The **proliferative** stage begins at the end of the menstrual flow and extends to about the middle of the cycle. This stage is characterized by the rapid regeneration and repair of the endometrium. The epithelial cells in the glandular remnants of the stratum basale proliferate and migrate over the raw surface of the mucosa. The stromal cells also proliferate and the endometrium increases in thickness. The endometrial glands increase in number and length and toward the end of the proliferative stage, glycogen accumulates in the basal region of the glandular epithelial cells. The spiral arteries lengthen but are lightly coiled and do not extend into the superficial third of the endometrium.

The proliferative phase corresponds to the **maturation of the ovarian follicle** up to the time of ovulation. Secretion of estrogens by the developing follicles stimulates growth of the endometrium. Some proliferative growth may continue for a day or two after ovulation.

During the **secretory phase**, the endometrium continues to increase in thickness as a result of hypertrophy of glandular cells, stromal edema and increased vascularity. The glands increase in length and become tortuous and convoluted with wide, irregular lumina. Glycogen and mucoid materials rapidly increase in the glandular cells, appearing basally at first, then moving to the apical portion of the cells and thence into the lumina of the glands. Elongation and coiling of the spiral arteries continues and the vessels extend into the superficial portion of the endometrium.

The secretory phase is associated with the development of the **corpus luteum** and is maintained as long as the corpus luteum remains functional. Progesterone secreted by the corpus luteum is responsible for the secretory changes in the endometrial lining.

The **premenstrual** or **ischemic** phase is characterized by changes in the spiral arteries which constrict intermittently, resulting in vascular stasis and reduced blood flow in the functional layer. The outer zone of the endometrium is subjected to anoxia for

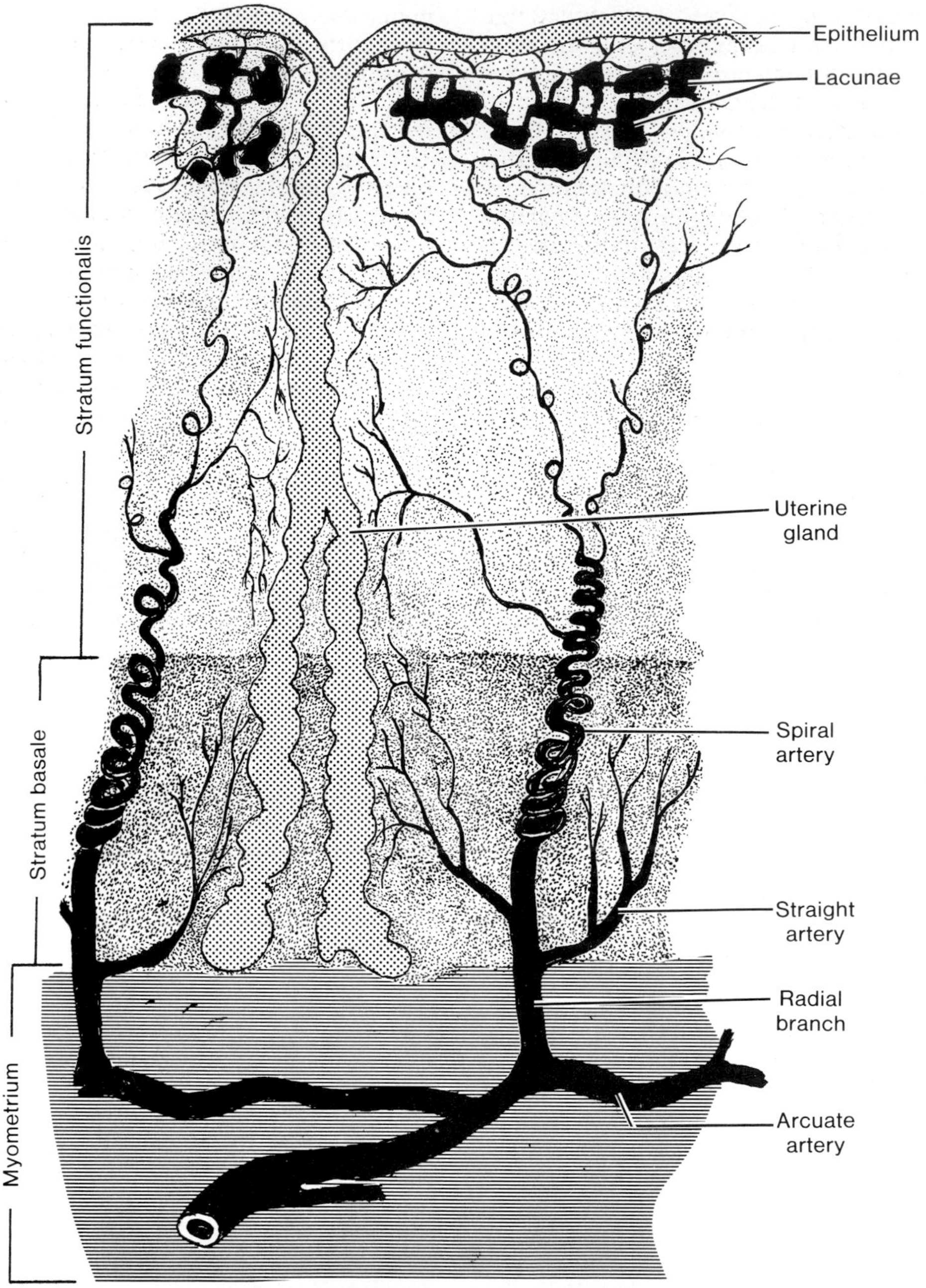

Figure 18.1. Arrangement of blood vessels in the endometrium.

hours at a time, resulting in the breakdown of the stratum functionale. The stroma becomes increasingly edematous and is infiltrated by leukocytes.

In the **menstrual stage**, the functional layer becomes necrotic and is shed. The spiral arteries also become necrotic and blood is lost from the arteries and veins. Small lakes of blood form and coalesce and patches of mucosa are detached, leaving a denuded stromal surface. Sloughing of endometrial tissue continues until the entire functional layer has been discarded. Blood oozes from the torn veins exposed by the shedding of endometrial tissue. The menstrual discharge consists of arterial and venous blood, autolyzed and degenerated epithelial and stromal cells and glandular secretions. The straight arteries of the stratum basale do not constrict during menstruation. The basal layer is preserved to provide for the restoration of the endometrium during the succeeding new proliferative stage.

The onset of the menstrual cycle coincides with the beginning involution of the corpus luteum.

The hormonal relationships of the ovary and uterine mucosa are shown in Figure 18–2.

Cervix

KEY WORDS: dense collagenous connective tissue, endocervix, nonkeratinized stratified squamous, secretory changes

The wall of the cervix differs considerably from that of the body of the uterus. Little smooth muscle is present and the cervical wall consists mainly of **dense collagenous connective tissue** and elastic fibers. In that portion which protrudes into the vaginal canal, smooth muscle is lacking. The cervical canal is lined by a mucosa, the **endocervix**, which forms complex, branching folds. The epithelial lining consists of tall columnar cells which secrete mucus and some ciliated columnar cells are present also. Numerous large, branched glands are present and are lined by mucus-secreting columnar cells similar to those of the lining epithelium. The cervical canal usually is filled with mucus. Occasionally the glands become occluded and filled with secretion and then form the Nabothian cysts.

The portion of the cervix that protrudes into the vaginal canal is covered by a **non keratinized stratified squamous** epithelium, the cells of which contain much glycogen. The transition from the columnar epithelium of the cervical canal is abrupt and

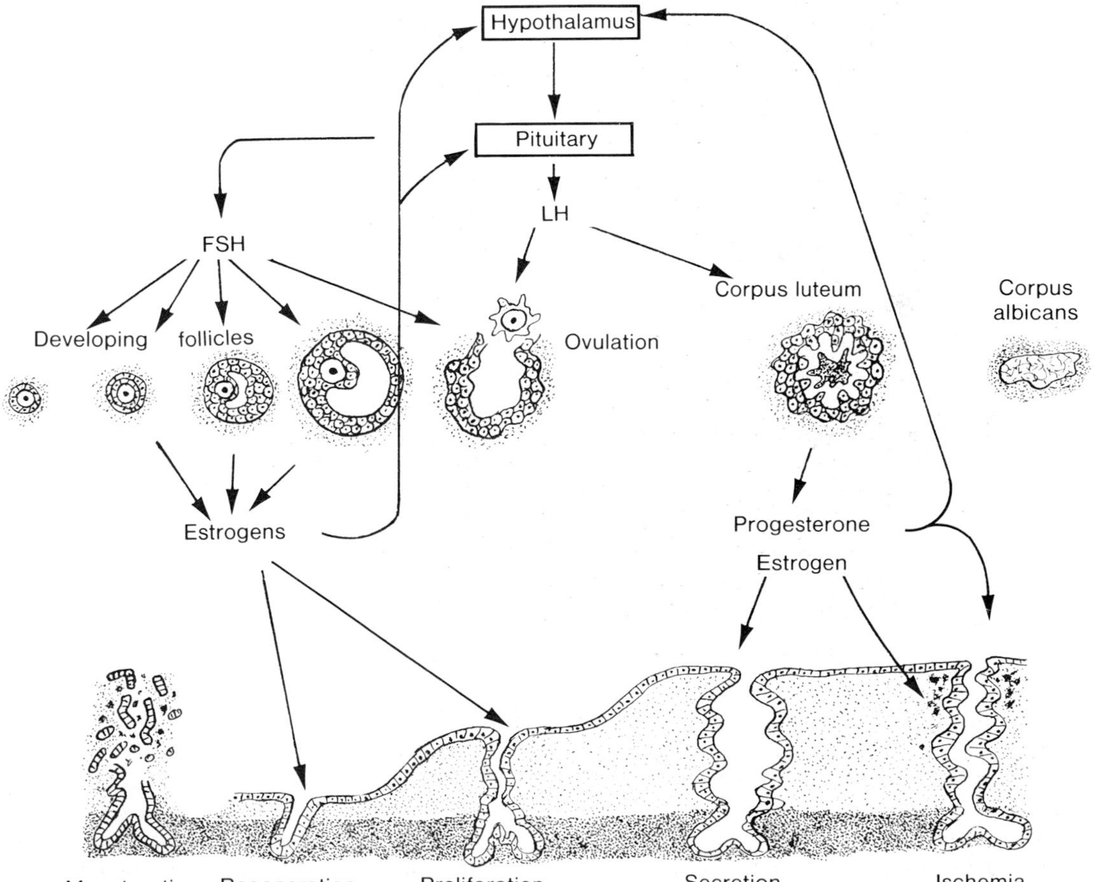

Figure 18.2. Hormonal relationships of the ovary and uterine mucosa.

usually occurs just inside the external os. The cervical mucosa does not take part in the cyclic changes of the body of the uterus and is not sloughed. The glandular elements of the cervical canal do show **changes in secretory activity**, however. At midcycle there is a copious secretion of a thin alkaline fluid, probably the result of increased stimulation by estrogens. Following ovulation and establishment of the corpus luteum, the amount of secretion diminishes and the mucus becomes thicker and more viscous.

VAGINA

The vagina is the lowermost portion of the female reproductive tract and is a muscular tube that joins the uterus to the exterior of the body. It represents the copulatory organ of the female. Ordinarily the lumen is collapsed and the anterior and posterior walls make contact.

Structure

KEY WORDS: mucosa, rugae, nonkeratinized stratified squamous, lamina propria, muscularis, adventitia

The wall of the vagina consists of a mucosa, a muscularis and an adventitial coat. The **mucosa** is thrown into folds, or **rugae**, and consists of a thick surface layer of **stratified squamous epithelium** of the **nonkeratinized** type overlying a lamina propria. The epithelial cells contain abundant glycogen, especially at midcycle. The **lamina propria** consists of a fairly dense connective tissue which becomes more loosely arranged near the muscle coat. Immediately below the epithelial lining, elastic fibers form a dense network. Diffuse and nodular lymphatic tissues are found occasionally and many lymphocytes invade the epithelium, along with granular leukocytes. The vagina has no glands and the epithelium is kept moist by the secretions from the cervix.

The **muscularis** consists of bundles of smooth muscle fibers that have a circular orientation in the inner layer and a longitudinal arrangement in the outer portion. The longitudinal fibers are continuous with similarly arranged fibers of the myometrium.

The **adventitia** is a thin outer layer of connective tissue and elastic fibers. It merges imperceptibly into the surrounding loose connective tissue about other organs.

EXTERNAL GENITALIA

The external genitalia of the female consist of the labia, the clitoris and the vestibular glands.

Labia

KEY WORDS: labia majora, homolog of the scrotum, labia minora

The **labia majora** are the **homolog of the scrotum** of the male and are folds of skin covering an abundant adipose tissue and a thin layer of muscle. In the adult, the outer surface is covered by coarse hair with many sweat and sebaceous glands; the inner surface, which is smooth and hairless, also contains sweat and sebaceous glands. The **labia minora** consist of a core of highly vascular, loose connective tissue covered by stratified squamous epithelium which is deeply indented by connective tissue papillae. The deeper layers of epithelium are pigmented. Both surfaces of the labia minora are devoid of hair, but large sebaceous glands are present.

Clitoris

KEY WORDS: erectile, corresponds to dorsal penis, corpora cavernosa, glans clitoridis

The clitoris is an **erectile** body which **corresponds to** the **dorsal part of the penis.** It consists of two **corpora cavernosa** enclosed in a layer of fibrous tissue and separated by an incomplete septum. The free end terminates in a small rounded tubercle, the **glans clitoridis** which consists of spongy erectile tissue. The clitoris is covered by a thin layer of stratified squamous epithelium with high papillae associated with many specialized sensory nerve endings.

Vestibular Glands

KEY WORDS: mucous, major vestibular glands, compound tubuloalveolar

The vestibule is the cleft between the labia minora and in it are the vaginal and urethral openings. It is lined by stratified squamous epithelium and contains numerous small vestibular glands concentrated about the openings of the vagina and urethra. The glands contain **mucous** cells and resemble the urethral glands of the male. A pair of larger glands, the greater or **major vestibular glands** are present in the lateral walls of the vestibule. These are **compound tubuloalveolar** glands which secrete a mucoid, lubricating fluid. The major glands correspond to the bulbourethral glands of the male.

THE FEMALE REPRODUCTIVE TRACT AND PREGNANCY

Pregnancy involves the implantation of a blastocyst into the prepared uterine endometrium, with the subsequent formation of a placenta for the nourishment and maintenance of the developing embryo. Prior to implantation, fertilization of the ovum and cleavage of the resulting zygote occur in the oviduct.

Fertilization

KEY WORDS: female pronucleus, male pronucleus

Before an ovum can be fertilized, it must undergo maturational changes, chief of which is the reduction of the chromosome complement to the haploid condition. The oocytes pass through the early stages of the first meiotic prophase during fetal life, and it is only just prior to ovulation that the division is completed and the first polar body given off. The resulting secondary oocyte immediately enters the second meiotic division which, however, proceeds just as far as metaphase and is completed only at fertilization.

At the time of ovulation, the oviduct shows active movement that brings the ampulla and the fimbria into close approximation with the ovary. Cilia on the surface of the fimbria sweep the ovum into the ampulla of the oviduct, where fertilization, if it is to occur, takes place. The human ovum probably remains fertilizable for about 1 day, after which it degenerates if fertilization does not occur.

Of the millions of sperm deposited in the female tract, only one penetrates the ovum. There is no evidence for a chemotactic attraction and random movements bring the ovum and spermatozoon together. The successful sperm pierces the corona radiata and zona pellucida, possibly by lysis of the membrane through enzymes in the sperm acrosome, and the entire spermatozoon is engulfed in the cytoplasm of the ovum. Electron micrographs suggest fusion of the plasma membranes of the ovum and spermatozoon, with that of the spermatozoon being left at the surface of the ovum. Penetration is followed by immediate changes in the permeability of the zona pellucida, which thereafter excludes entry by competing sperm.

The ovum now completes the second maturation division and extrudes the second polar body. The remaining chromosomes (23) reconstitute and form the **female pronucleus.** The nucleus of the head of the spermatozoon swells to form the **male pronucleus** and the body and tail disappear. The two pronuclei move to the center of the cell and two centrioles supplied by the anterior centriole of the spermatozoon appear. Nuclear membranes dissociate and the chromatin of each pronucleus resolves into a set of chromosomes which align themselves on the spindle to undergo a normal mitotic division of the first cleavage. Each cell resulting from this division will receive the full diploid set of chromosomes.

Cleavage

KEY WORDS: blastomeres, morula, blastocele, blastocyst, inner cell mass, trophoblast

The zygote undergoes a series of rapid divisions called cleavage that result in a large number of smaller cells, or **blastomeres.** The cells are located within the zona pellucida and a mulberry-like body, the **morula**, is formed. Cleavage is a fractionating process: no new cytoplasm is formed and at each division the cells become smaller until the normal cytoplasmic/nuclear ratios are achieved. Thus, the total size of the morula is not increased. Cleavage occurs as the morula is slowly moved along the oviduct by the waves of peristaltic contractions in the muscle coat. When the morula has reached the 12- to 16-cell stage, it is delivered to the uterine cavity. This occurs 3 to 5 days after fertilization.

At about the time the morula enters the uterine cavity, fluid penetrates the zona pellucida and diffuses between the cells of the morula. The fluid increases in amount, the intercellular spaces become confluent, a single cavity, the **blastocele**, forms, and the morula becomes a **blastocyst.** The zona pellucida disappears. The blastocyst remains free in the uterine cavity for about a day and then attaches to the secretory endometrium. At this time the blastocyst is a hollow sphere, containing at one pole a mass of cells called the **inner cell mass** that will form the embryo proper. The capsule-like wall of the blastocyst consists of a single layer of cells, the **trophoblast**, which establishes function relationships with the endometrium.

Implantation

KEY WORDS: secretory phase, syncytial trophoblast, cytotrophoblast, lacunae

At the time of implantation, the endometrium is in the **secretory phase** and, having been under the influence of progesterone from the corpus luteum for several days, has reached its greatest thickness and development. The trophoblast becomes fixed to the endometrial epithelium and at this point, the trophoblast proliferates to form a cellular mass between the blastocyst and maternal tissues. No cell boundaries can be made out in this mass of cells, which is called the **syncytial trophoblast.** The syncytium erodes the endometrium at the point of contact, creating a cavity into which the blastocyst sinks, gradually becoming more deeply embedded until the entire blastocyst lies within the endometrial stroma. The surface defect in the endometrium is closed temporarily by a fibrin plug. Later, proliferation of surrounding cells restores the surface continuity of the endometrial lining.

As the blastocyst sinks into the endometrium, the syncytial trophoblast rapidly increases in thickness at the original site of attachment and progressively extends to cover the remainder of the blastocyst. When completely embedded, the entire wall of the blastocyst consists of two layers—the thick outer syncytial trophoblast, and an inner layer, the **cytotrophoblast**, composed of a single layer of cells with well defined cell boundaries. The cytotrophoblast shows active mitosis and contributes cells to the syncytial trophoblast, where they fuse with, and become part of, that layer. The syncytial trophoblast continues to erode the uterine tissues, opening up the walls of maternal blood vessels. Spaces appear in the syncytial trophoblast and these **lacunae** expand, become confluent and form a labyrinth of intercommunicating spaces. Many of the spaces contain blood extravasated from the eroded maternal blood vessels; this blood supplies nourishment for the embryo and represents the first step in the development of uteroplacental circulation.

Placenta

KEY WORDS: primary villi, chorion, secondary villi, chorionic plate, chorion frondosum, chorion laeve, tertiary (definitive) placental villi, decidua, chorionic gonadotrophins

As the lacunae enlarge, the intervening strands of trophoblast form the **primary villi**, each villus consisting of a core of cytotrophoblast covered by a layer of syncytial trophoblast. The primary villi extend around the entire periphery of the blastocyst. The trophoblastic cells from the tips of the villi apply themselves to the endometrium and form a lining for the cavity in which the blastocyst lies. With establishment of the embryonic germ layers, mesoderm grows out from the embryo as the **chorion,** and forms a lining for the trophoblast that surrounds the blastocyst. The mesoderm extends into the primary villi to provide a core of connective tissue and convert the villi to **secondary villi.** The deeply embedded portion of the chorion constitutes the **chorionic plate**, from which numerous villi project to form the **chorion frondosum.** Villi on the chorion that faces the uterine cavity grow more slowly and are less numerous; ultimately these villi disappear. This surface of the chorion becomes smooth and forms the **chorion laeve.** Blood vessels develop within the mesenchymal cores of the secondary villi and soon establish connection with the fetal circulation. With vascularization, the secondary villi become the **tertiary** or **definitive placental villi.**

The endometrium also shows changes. At parturition all but the deepest layers will be shed and in consequence, the superficial part of the endometrium of pregnancy is called the **decidua.** A feature of the stroma is the alteration of its cells to form the enlarged decidual cells which contain abundant glycogen. According to the relationship with the implantation site, three regions of the decidua are recognized. The decidua capsularis is that part which lies over the surface of the blastocyst, while the decidua basalis underlies the implantation site and forms the maternal component of the placenta. The endometrium lining the remainder of the pregnant uterus is the decidua parietalis. As the embryo increases in size the decidua capsularis becomes increasingly attenuated and thinned. Eventually the decidua capsularis comes into contact with the decidua parietalis on the opposite surface of the uterus and the uterine cavity is obliterated.

The mature placenta thus consists of maternal and fetal components; the maternal part is the decidua basalis; the fetal portion consists of the chorionic plate and the villi arising from it. Maternal blood circulates through the intervillous spaces and bathes the surfaces of the villi, of which two types are identified. Some pass from the chorionic plate to the decidua basalis as the anchoring villi from which secondary and tertiary branches float in the intervillous spaces as free or floating villi. The structure of the two types of villi is identical and both consist of a core of loose connective tissue in which are fetal capillaries. Covering each villus is an inner layer of cytotrophoblast which have large nuclei and a lightly basophilic cytoplasm that contains considerable glycogen. External to the cytotrophoblast is a layer of syncytial trophoblast of variable thickness. The cells of the cytotrophoblast decrease in number in the latter half of pregnancy and only a few are present at term. The syncytial trophoblast also thins out to form a narrow layer.

A diagram of the structure of the placenta is shown in Figure 18-3.

The placenta serves to transfer oxygen and nutrients from the maternal to the fetal circulation and the waste products of fetal metabolism to the maternal circulation. Although the maternal and fetal circulations are in close proximity, they remain separated by the syncytial trophoblast (and early in pregnancy by the cytotrophoblast also), a basement membrane, the connective tissue of the villi and the wall of the fetal blood vessels. Transport of materials between fetal and maternal blood appears to be regulated by the syncytial trophoblast. Being without

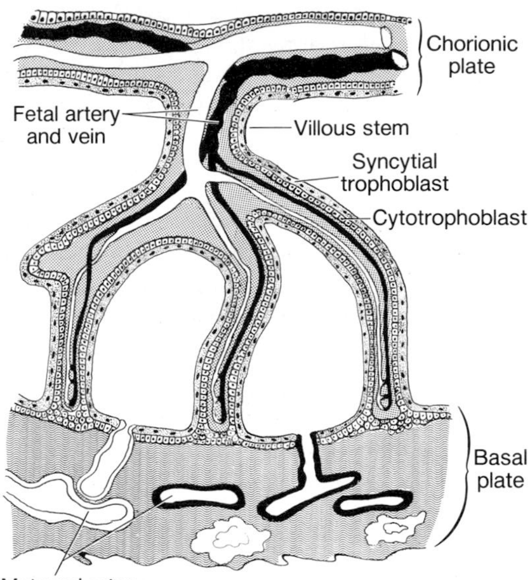

Figure 18.3. Diagram of the structure of the placenta.

cell boundaries and intercellular spaces, any materials passing into or leaving the fetal blood must pass through the cytoplasm of the syncytium. The cytotrophoblast appears to serve as the source of cells for the syncytial trophoblast. The placenta also is a multipotential endocrine organ, supplying estrogens, progesterone and **chorionic gonadotrophins.** The latter is produced by the syncytial trophoblast and stimulates secretion of estrogen and progesterone by the corpus luteum during early pregnancy.

MAMMARY GLANDS

Mammary glands are present in both sexes but in the male remain rudimentary throughout life. In the female, the size, shape and structure varies with age and with the functional status of the gland. Prior to puberty, the female breasts are undeveloped but enlarge rapidly at puberty due mainly to the accumulation of adipose tissue. They reach their greatest development during late pregnancy and lactation. In the adult female, the mammary glands are variably hemispherical and conical in shape and each is surmounted by a cylindrical projection, the nipple. Surrounding the nipple is a slightly raised, circular area of pigmented skin, the areola.

The mammary gland can be classed as a compound tubuloalveolar gland. It is considered to be of cutaneous origin and to represent a modified sweat gland.

Structure

KEY WORDS: lobes, septa, resting gland, lobules, lactiferous sinuses, alveoli, myoepithelial cells

Each mammary gland consists of 15 to 20 individual pyramidal-shaped **lobes** that radiate from the nipple. The lobes are separated by **septa** of dense connective tissue. Each lobe represents an individual gland and contains glandular tissue consisting of secretory and ductal components embedded in the intralobular connective tissue. The proportions of these components varies with the functional activity.

In the **resting gland** the principle glandular element consists of ducts which are grouped together to form the **lobules.** The smallest branches of the ductal system are lined by a simple cuboidal epithelium, but the lining increases in height as the ducts unite and pass toward the nipple. Just beneath the areola, the ducts expand to form the **lactiferous sinuses**, which are lined by a two-layered cuboidal epithelium. As the duct ascends through the nipple it becomes lined by stratified squamous epithelium.

The secretory units consist of a cluster of **alveoli** surrounding a small duct. The alveolar wall consists of a simple cuboidal epithelium resting on a basement membrane. Between the epithelial cells and the basement membrane are highly branched **myoepithelial cells.** The long, slender processes of the myoepithelial cells embrace the alveolus in a basket-like network. Alveoli are not prominent in the resting mammary gland and there is some question as to whether they are present at all. Generally, when present, they occur as small, bud-like extensions of the terminal ducts.

The connective tissue about the ductules and alveoli within the lobule is loosely arranged and cellular. That surrounding the ducts and lobules is variably dense and contains much adipose tissue.

Nipple and Areola

KEY WORDS: keratinized stratified squamous epithelium, lactiferous ducts, smooth muscle, areolar glands

The nipple is covered by **keratinizing stratified squamous epithelium**, continuous with that of the skin overlying the breast. The underlying dermis projects deeply into the epithelium to form unusually tall dermal papillae. The skin is pigmented and contains many sebaceous glands but is devoid of hair and sweat glands. The nipple is traversed by many **lactiferous ducts**, each of which drains a lobe and opens onto the tip of the nipple. The outer parts of these ducts also are lined by keratinizing stratified squamous epithelium. The dense collagenous connective tissue of the nipple contains bundles of elastic fibers, and much **smooth muscle** also is present. The smooth muscle fibers are arranged circularly and radially and on contraction produce erection of the nipple.

The areola is the pigmented area of skin that encircles the base of the nipple. During pregnancy the areola becomes larger and more deeply pigmented. It contains sweat glands, sebaceous glands and **areolar glands.** The latter appear to be intermediate in structure between sweat glands and true mammary glands.

The Mammary Glands during Pregnancy and Lactation

KEY WORDS: colostrum, apocrine secretion, oxytocin

During pregnancy, mammary glands undergo extensive development in preparation for their role in lactation. During the first half of pregnancy, the terminal portions of the ductal system grow rapidly, branch and develop terminal buds that expand to become alveoli. The increase of glandular tissue takes place at the expense of the fat and stromal connective tissue, which decrease in amount. The connective tissue becomes increasingly infiltrated with lymphocytes, plasma cells and granular leukocytes. During the late months of pregnancy, the proliferation of glandular tissue subsides, but the alveoli enlarge and there is some formation of secretory materials. The first secretion, **colostrum**, is thin and watery. It is poor in lipid but contains a considerable amount of antibodies which may give some degree of passive immunity to the newborn.

True milk secretion begins a few days after parturition, but not all of the breast tissue is functioning at the same time. In some areas the alveoli are distended with milk, the epithelial lining is flattened and the lumen distended; in other areas the alveoli are resting and have narrow lumina lined by tall epithelial cells. The secreting cells have abundant rough endoplasmic reticulum, a moderate number of relatively large mitochondria and a supranuclear Golgi complex. The milk proteins are elaborated on the rough endoplasmic reticulum and in association with the Golgi, form membrane-bound vesicles. These are carried to the apex of the cell, where the contents are released by exocytosis. The lipid arises as cytoplasmic droplets which coalesce to form large apical globules. The droplets and globules, apparently with portions of the plasmalemma and apical cytoplasm are cast off into the lumen. This method of release is a form of **apocrine secretion**, but only minute amounts of cytoplasm are lost.

Passage of milk from the alveoli into and along the ducts results from the contraction of the myoepithelial cells, stimulated by the hormone **oxytocin.** This hormone is released from the neurohypophysis as the result of neurostimulating responses to suckling.

With weaning, lactation soon ceases and the glandular tissue returns to its resting state. However, regression is never complete and not all alveoli completely disappear.

Hormonal Control

KEY WORDS: estrogen, progesterone, somatotrophin, prolactin, adrenal corticoids, neurohormonal reflex, oxytocin

Prior to puberty, growth of the mammary gland parallels general body growth, but as the ovaries become functional, the mammary tissue comes under the cyclic influence of estrogens and progesterone. While some structural changes can be observed, the cyclic response of the breast is minor. During pregnancy, the glands come under continuous stimulation by **estrogen** and **progesterone,** both from the corpus luteum and the placenta. Generally, growth of the ductal system depends upon estrogen, but for alveolar development both progesterone and estrogen are required. However, to attain the full development of late pregnancy, other hormones—**somatotrophin, prolactin** and **adrenal corticoids**—appear to be necessary.

At the end of pregnancy, the levels of circulating estrogen and progesterone fall abruptly and the increased output of prolactin by the hypophysis results in the secretion of milk. Maintenance of lactation requires continuous secretion of prolactin, which occurs as a result of a **neurohormonal reflex** estalished by suckling. The periodic suckling also causes release of **oxytocin** from the neurohypophysis and this hormone stimulates contraction of myoepithelial cells, resulting in the release of milk from the alveoli into and along the ducts.

DEVELOPMENT OF THE FEMALE REPRODUCTIVE TRACT

Early development of the female tract is related closely to that of the male tract and urinary system. All arise in the mesoderm of the urogenital ridges, within epithelial thickenings on each side of the midline. Initially the ovaries and testes are indistinguishable and form the primitive, indifferent gonad.

Ovary. The urogenital ridges give rise to the genital (gonadal) ridges which divide into lateral and medial parts: only the medial portion gives rise to the ovary. The epithelium of the gonadal ridge proliferates and a number of cellular gonadal cords penetrate the underlying mesenchyme. The cords at the periphery form a primary ovarian cortex while centrally, proliferation of mesenchyme establishes a primary medulla. The gonadal cords break up into irregular clusters separated by strands of mesenchyme, an extension of which cuts off the cell clusters from the surface epithelium, and forms the tunica albuginea. A second proliferation of surface epithelium gives rise to new cellular cords which invade the primary cortex, dissociate into isolated clusters and form the definitive cortex. The cell clusters surround one or more primitive germ cells and establish the first follicles. The ovary now has its full complement of germ cells (primary oocytes), which enter prophase of the first meiotic division. The primary medulla is replaced by a fibroelastic stroma to establish a permanent medulla.

Primordial germ cells, which give rise to the definitive oogonia and spermatogonia, are segregated early in development. They appear first in the yolk sac, then migrate to the dorsal mesentery and thence to the genital ridges. It is uncertain as to whether the primordial cells arise from particular blastomeres during cleavage or as clones of a single blastomere. Their early association with endoderm has suggested this as their tissue of origin.

Oviduct, Uterus, and Vagina. By 6 weeks in the human, male and female embryos have paired mesonephric and paramesonephric ducts. In the female embryo, paramesonephric ducts become predominant, giving rise to oviducts, uterus and, possibly, the vagina. Mesonephric ducts regress, except for a few remnants.

Each paramesonephric duct begins as an invagination of the celomic epithelium on the lateral side of the mesonephric ridge. Cranially, the duct opens into the celomic cavity as a funnel-shaped structure which gives rise to the fimbriated and ampullary parts of the oviduct. Caudally, the paramesonephric tubes lengthen and descend, then turn medially to meet each other and fuse into a single structure, the uterovaginal canal. The descending portions of the ducts give rise to the rest of the oviduct, the fused caudal portion forms the body and cervix of the uterus. Mesenchyme surrounding the uterovaginal canal supplies the endometrial stroma and myometrium.

The vagina arises from an epithelial proliferation, the sinuvaginal bulb, on the posterior wall of the urogenital sinus. It is not certain as to whether this epithelium is true sinus epithelium or epithelium of the mesonephric duct that descended into this region. The proliferating epithelium extends cranially as a solid bar, the vaginal plate. Beginning at the caudal end, cells in the center of the plate degenerate and a vaginal lumen is formed. In humans, canalization is complete by the 5th month. The fetal vaginal epithelium is under the influence of maternal hormones and in late fetal life becomes markedly hypertrophied. After birth, it regresses and assumes its inactive childhood form.

External Genitalia. Like the gonads, the external genitalia pass through an indifferent stage before they develop their definitive sexual characteristics.

The caudal end of the primitive hind gut is closed by a cloacal membrane, around which the urogenital folds develop. These folds unite at their cranial ends and form the genital tubercle which, in the female, elongates only slightly to give rise to the clitoris. A pair of genital swellings develops along each side of the genital folds: in the female, these remain separate and form the labia majora. Similarly, the urogenital folds do not fuse in the female but give rise to the labia minora.

Mammary Glands. Mammary glands represent modified apocrine sweat glands and are derived from ectodermal outgrowths. The primordia of the mammae develop as two ventral bands of ectoderm, the mammary ridges, that extend from axilla to inguinal region. In the human female, a single pair of glands develop in the pectoral region and the remainder of the mammary ridges usually disappears. As the glands develop, 15 to 20 solid buds of ectoderm invade the underlying mesenchyme. Each bud will form the branching lactiferous ducts of one mammary lobule. The ducts are lined by columnar epithelium and myoepithelial cells can be distinguished early. Alveoli do not develop until puberty, and even then alveoli are scarce and small. A further expansion of the ductal system occurs during pregnancy and some alveoli form, but they reach their greatest development during lactation. The surrounding mesenchyme forms the supporting connective tissue and at puberty becomes infiltrated with fat cells.

FUNCTIONAL SUMMARY

The ovary acts as a cytogenic gland, releasing ova, and also serves intermittently as an endocrine gland. During its growth in the follicles, the oocyte is nourished by the blood vessels of the ovary via the theca interna. When the corpus luteum is formed after ovulation, estrogens and progesterone are produced and are responsible for development of the uterine mucosa preparatory for reception of the blastocyst. The periodic nature of hormone production by the ovaries establishes the menstrual cycle during which, in the absence of pregnancy, the mucosa is shed. If pregnancy occurs, the corpus luteum persists and its hormonal activities maintain the endometrium in a prepared state.

The oviduct serves as the site of fertilization of the ovum and also transports the zygote to the uterus. Transportation along the oviduct is the result of muscular and ciliary activities. Conditions within the oviduct must be such as to maintain spermatozoa in a viable state prior to fertilization, and for survival of the zygote as it undergoes cleavage during tubular passage. The nutritional needs of the zygote are met from the materials stored in the cytoplasm of the ovum.

On entering the uterine cavity, the blastocyst lies in the secretions produced by the prepared endometrium. The secretion is rich in glycogen, polysaccharides and lipid, providing an excellent "culture" medium for the dividing cells of the blastocyst. The uterine endometrium, to which the blastocyst attaches, provides for the sustenance of the embryo throughout its development. A rich food source for the implanting blastocyst is provided by glandular secretions and cytolytic products from the breakdown of the uterine stroma. These products are absorbed by the syncytial trophoblast and diffuse to the developing embryo. Later, as the trophoblast continues to erode into the endometrium, blood-filled spaces form and the blastocyst becomes surrounded by pools of maternal blood which supply the nutritional needs of the embryo. When the placenta has been established, the nutritional, respiratory and excretory requirements of the developing embryo are met by this fetal-maternal organ. The placenta also has a protective function, preventing the passage of particulate matter such as bacteria to the embryo. It also has an endocrine function, elaborating the gonadotrophins, estrogen and progesterone. Gonadotrophins are produced very early and maintain the corpus luteum during early pregnancy. The basal layer of the endometrium is not shed either at parturition or at menstruation and provides for restoration of the uterine mucosa after these events have occurred. The myometrium, through its muscular contractions, is responsible for expulsion of the fetus at parturition.

Changes in the secretory activities of the cervical glands during the menstrual cycle may have significance in fertility. During most of the cycle, the glands produce a thick viscid mucus which appears inhibitory to the passage of sperm, whereas the thin, less viscid mucus elaborated at midcycle seems to favor the migration of sperm.

The mammary glands provide the nourishment for the newborn, which is delivered in an immature and dependent state. The colostrum contains a high complement of antibodies which may give some degree of passive immunity to the suckling young.

Atlas and Table of Key Features for Chapter 18

Table 18.1
Key Histological Features of Female Reproductive Tract

	Epithelial Lining	Support	Muscle
Oviduct	Simple columnar: ciliated and nonciliated cells	Lamina propria, cellular, thin collagen and reticular fibers	Well-defined inner circular smooth muscle; outer layer of scattered longitudinal fibers
Uterus	Simple columnar, with groups of ciliated cells: extends into lamina propria to form tubular glands	Lamina propria = endometrial stroma, similar to mesenchyme; richly cellular, fine reticular fibers, few collagen fibers. *Note:* The oviduct and uterus are the only hollow organs with this type of lamina propria	Myometrium. Thick coat of smooth muscle in 3 intermingling layers.
Cervix	(a) Tall columnar, some ciliated, some mucus-secreting cells (b) Vaginal part covered by nonkeratinized stratified squamous	Dense collagenous and elastic connective tissue	Smooth muscle much reduced in amount, lacking in vaginal part
Vagina	Stratified squamous nonkeratinized epithelium	Lamina propria of dense collagenous connective tissue. Dense elastic network below epithelial layer	Inner circular smooth muscle, outer longitudinal smooth muscle

18-4 Ovary

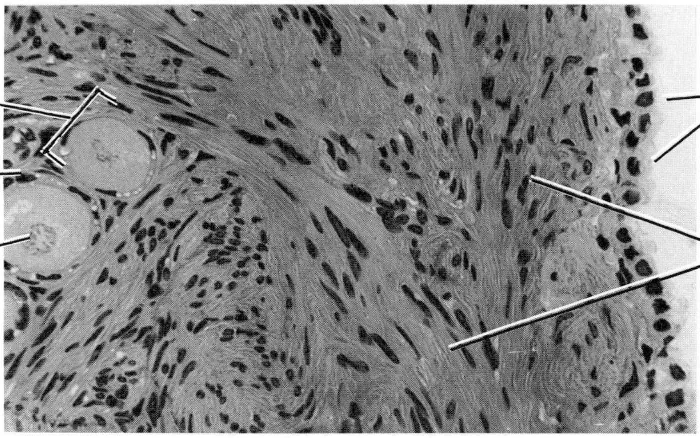

18-5

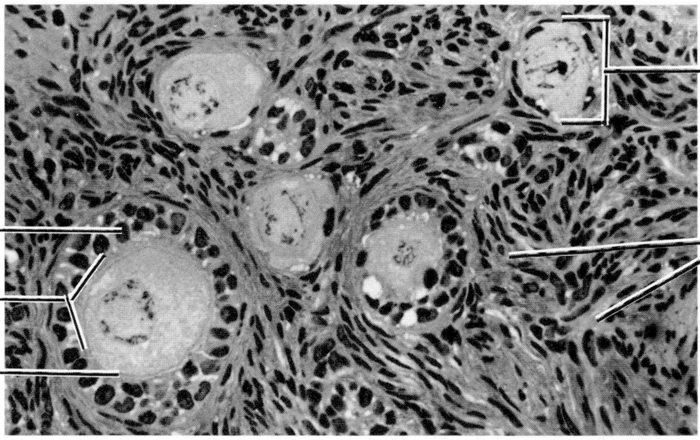

18-6

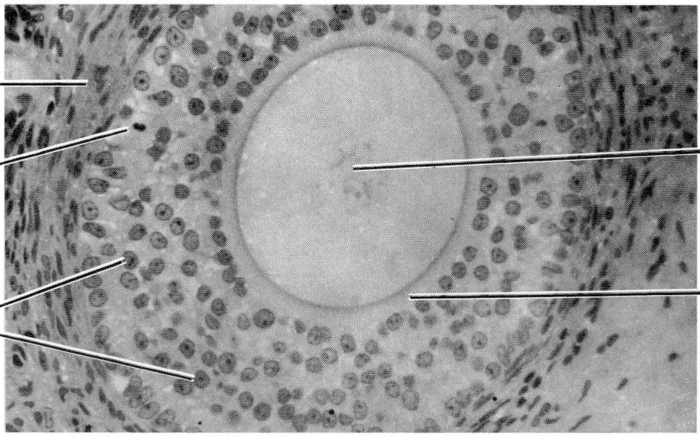

Figure 18.4. Cortex. LM, ×250.
Figure 18.5. Cortex. LM, ×250.
Figure 18.6. Primary follicle. LM, ×250.

18-7

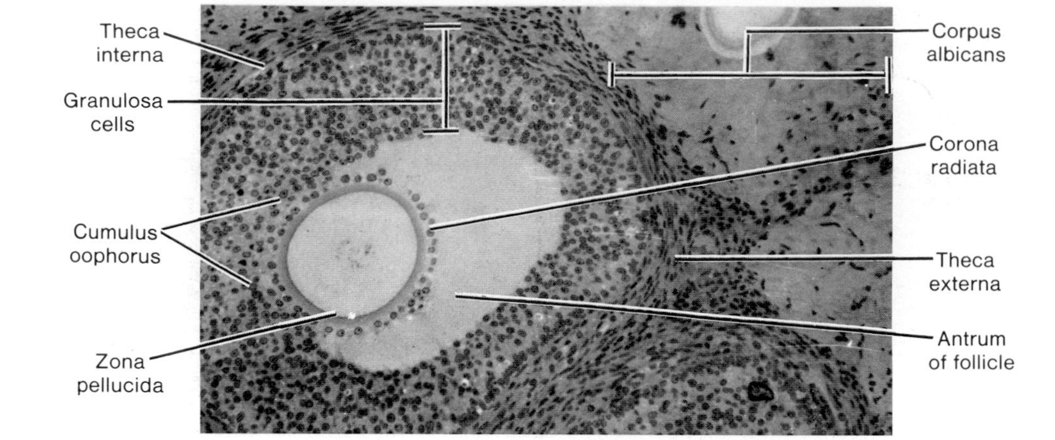

18-8

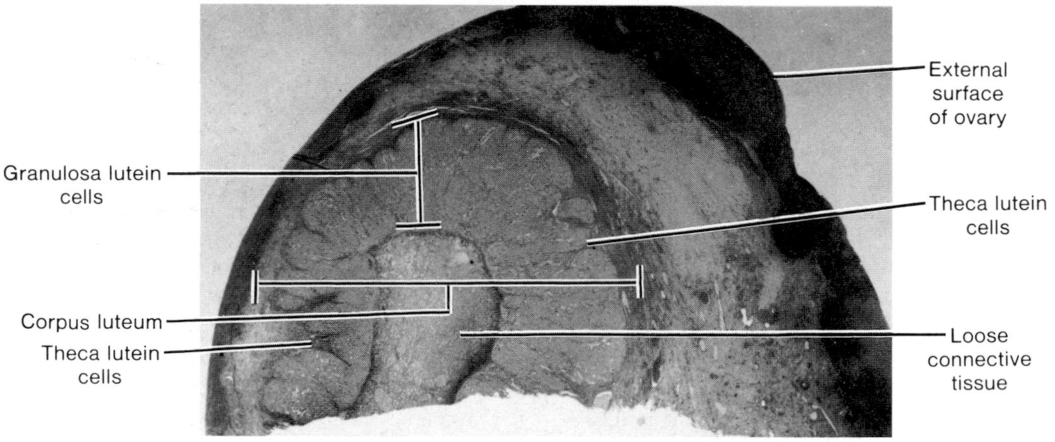

18-9

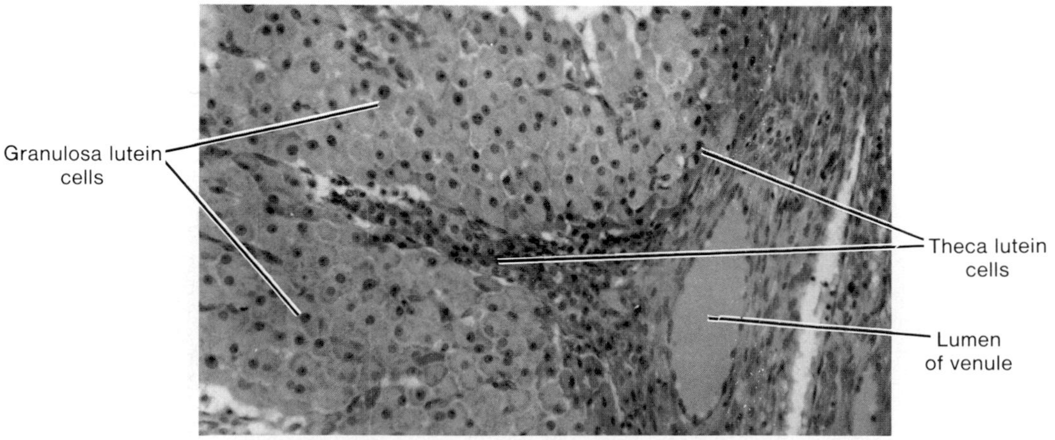

Figure 18.7. Secondary follicle. LM, ×100.
Figure 18.8. Corpus luteum (human). LM, ×25.
Figure 18.9. Corpus luteum (human). LM, ×100.

18-10

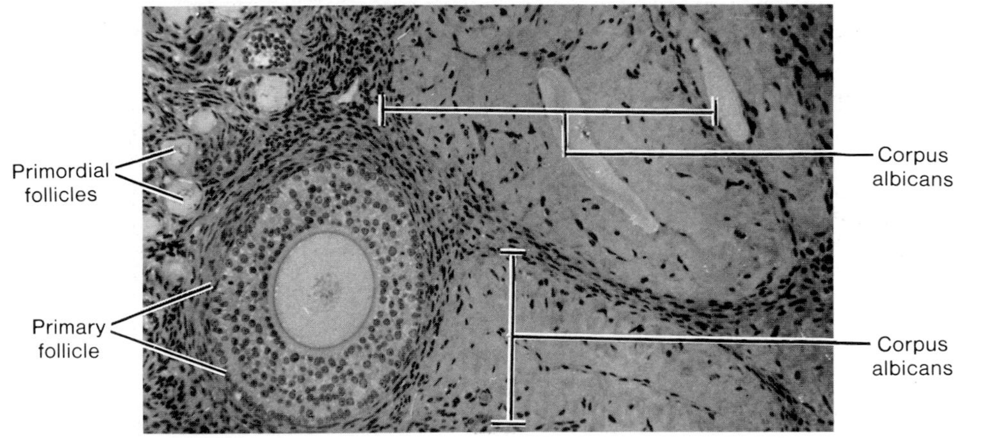

18-11

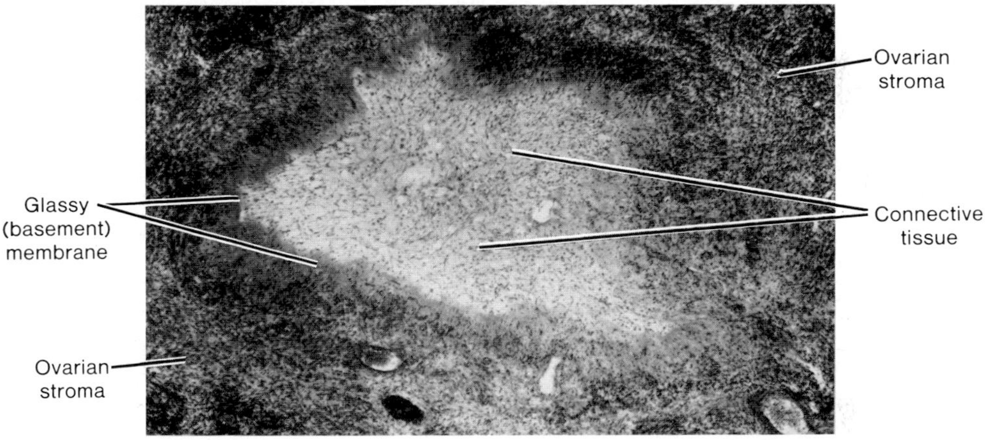

18-12 Oviduct

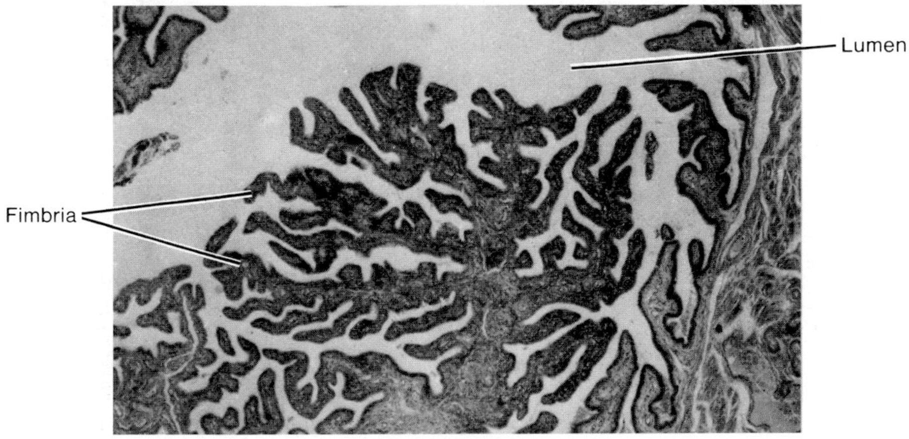

Figure 18.10. Cortex (ovary). LM, ×100.
Figure 18.11. Atretic follicle (human). LM, ×40.
Figure 18.12. Infundibulum of oviduct (human). LM, ×40.

18-13

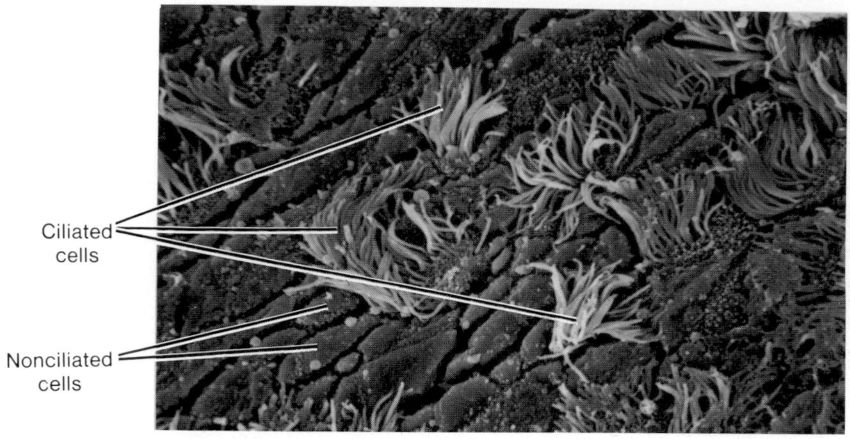

18-14

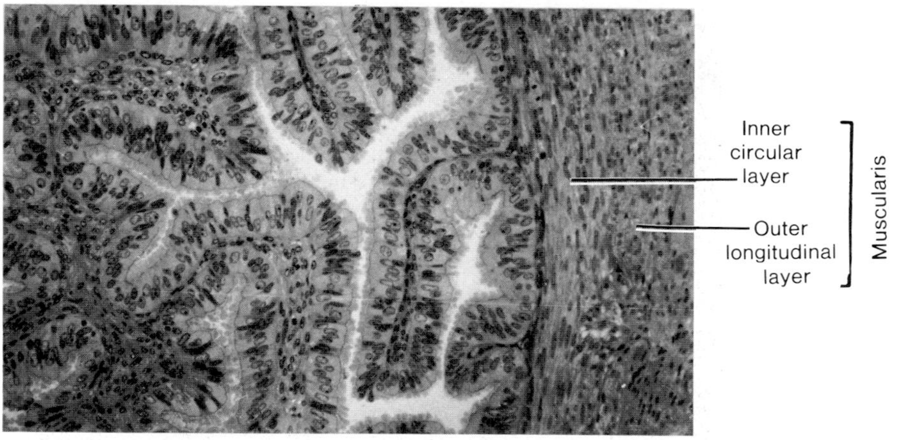

18-15

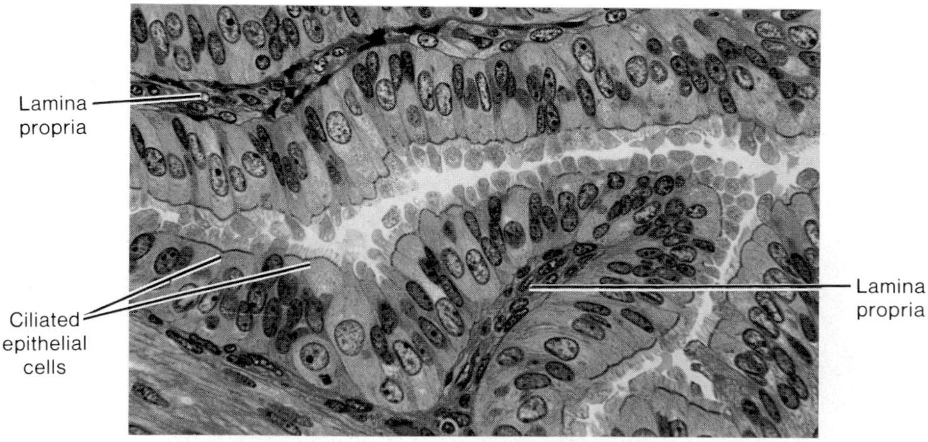

Figure 18.13. Mucosal surface of oviduct. SEM, ×2000.
Figure 18.14. Ampulla (oviduct). LM, ×100.
Figure 18.15. Ampulla (oviduct). LM, ×250.

18-16 Uterus

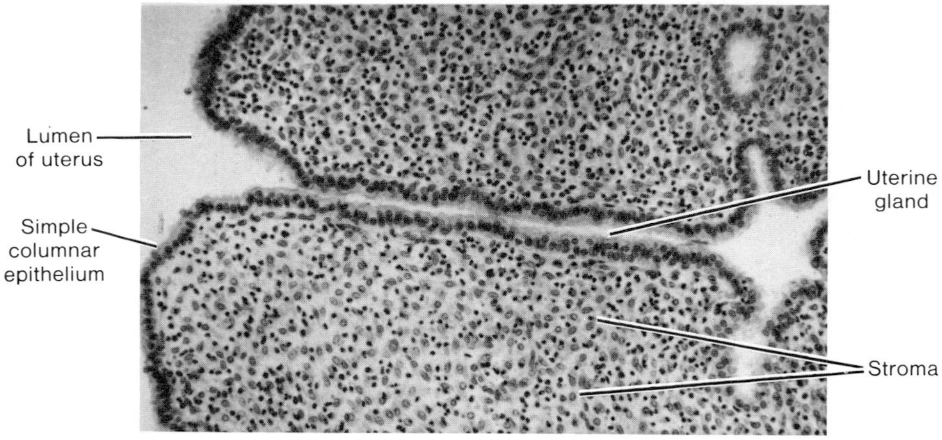

18-17

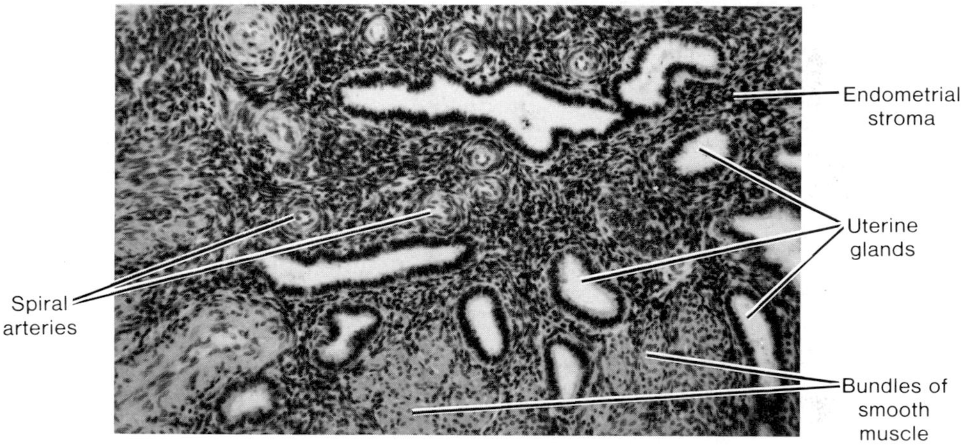

18-18

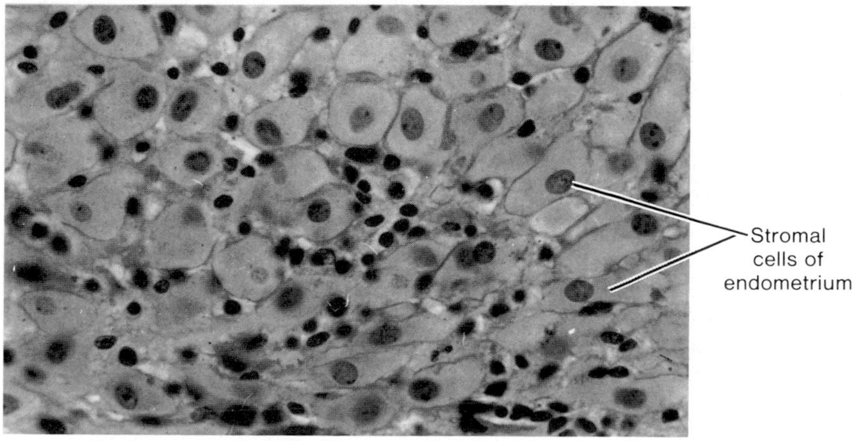

Figure 18.16. Endometrium (human). LM, ×100.
Figure 18.17. Stratum basale (human). LM, ×100.
Figure 18.18. Endometrium (pregnant human). LM, ×250.

18-19 Vagina

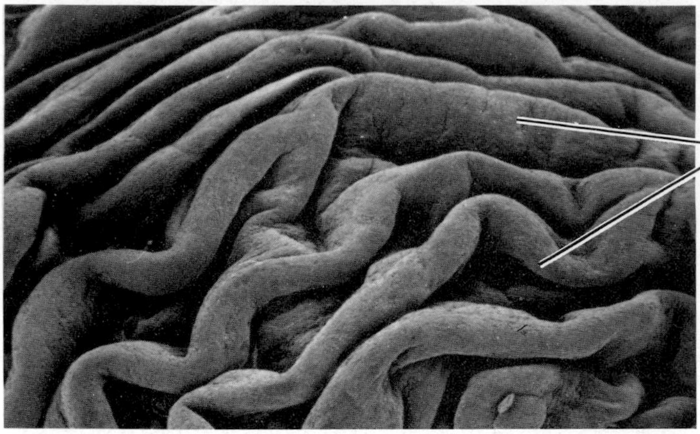

18-20

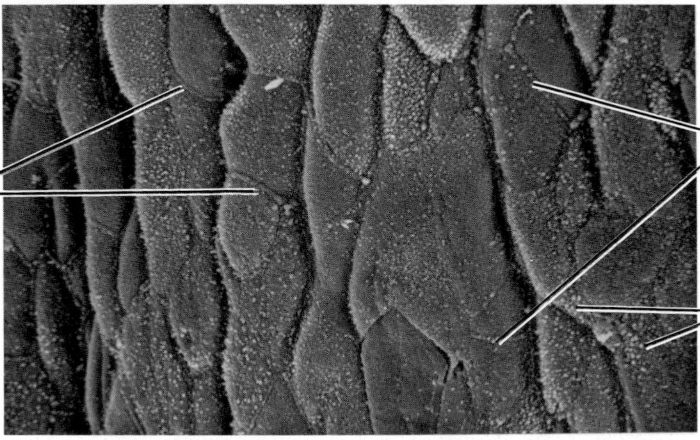

18-21

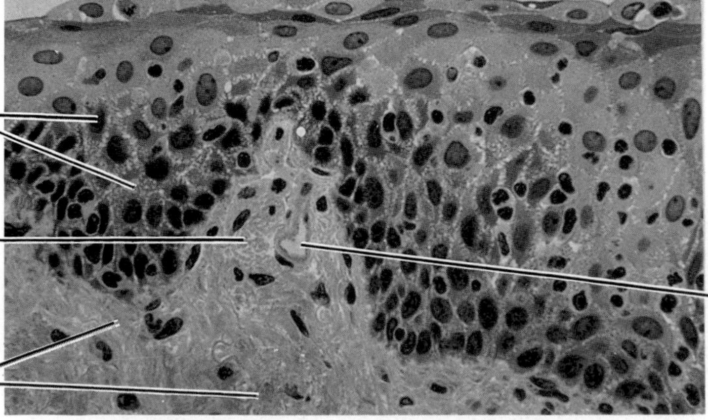

Figure 18.19. Vagina (mucosal surface). SEM, ×50.
Figure 18.20. Vagina (mucosal surface). SEM, ×1000.
Figure 18.21. Vagina. LM, ×250.

18-22 Zygote

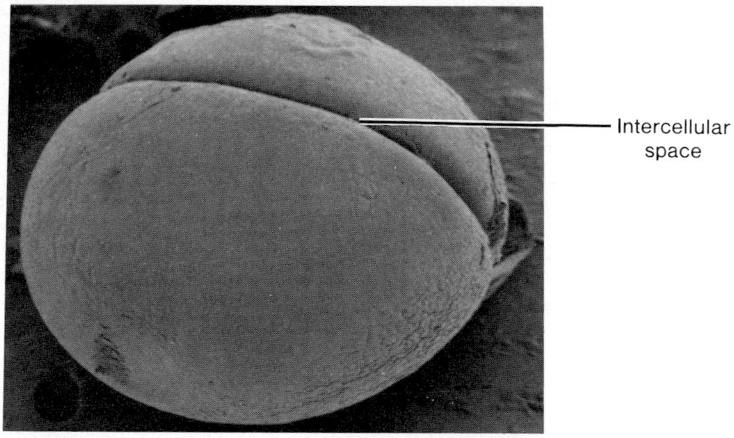

18-23

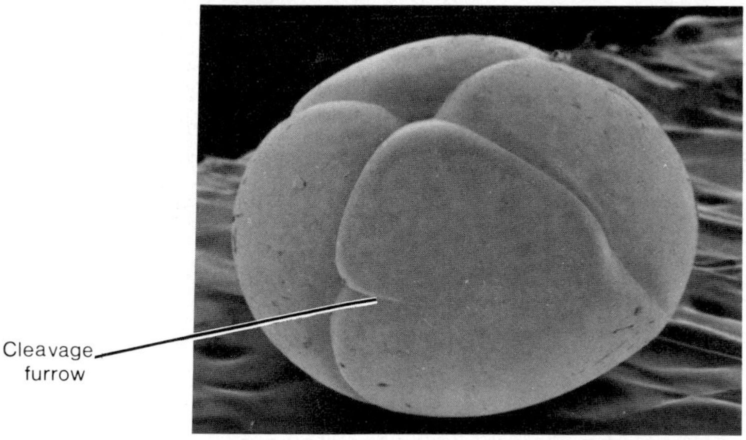

18-24

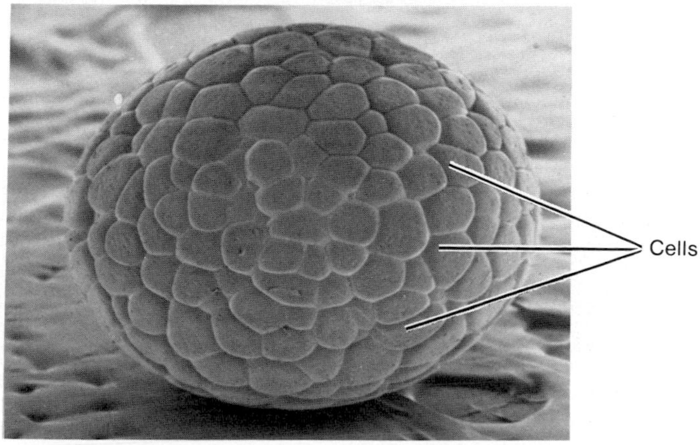

Figure 18.22. Zygote (two-cell stage). SEM, ×50.
Figure 18.23. Zygote (eight-cell stage). SEM, ×50.
Figure 18.24. Zygote. SEM, ×50.

Embryos

18-25

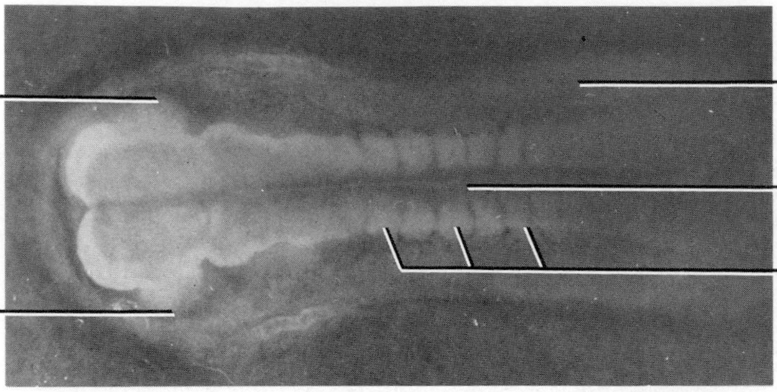

18-26

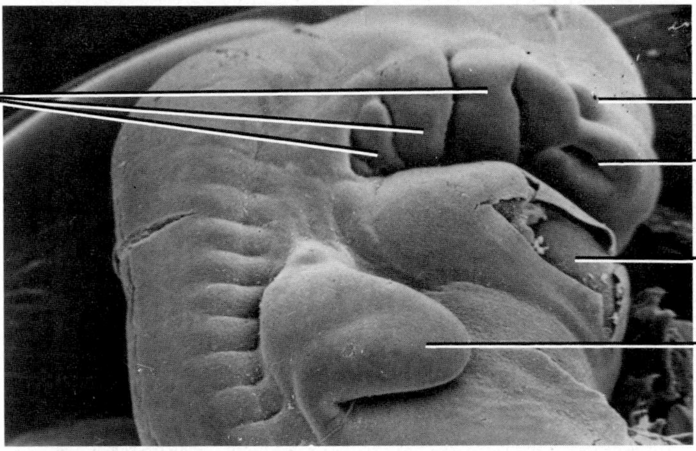

18-27

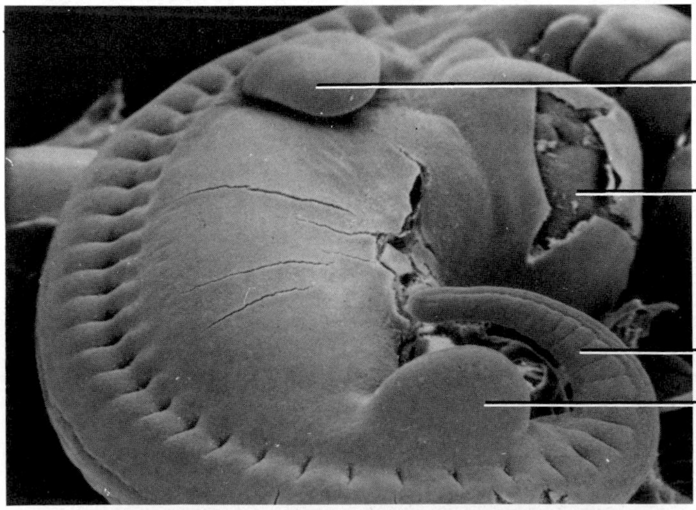

Figure 18.25. Opossum embryo (9 day). LM, ×100.
Figure 18.26. Pig embryo (9 mm). SEM, ×20.
Figure 18.27. Pig embryo (9 mm). SEM, ×20.

18-28 Placenta

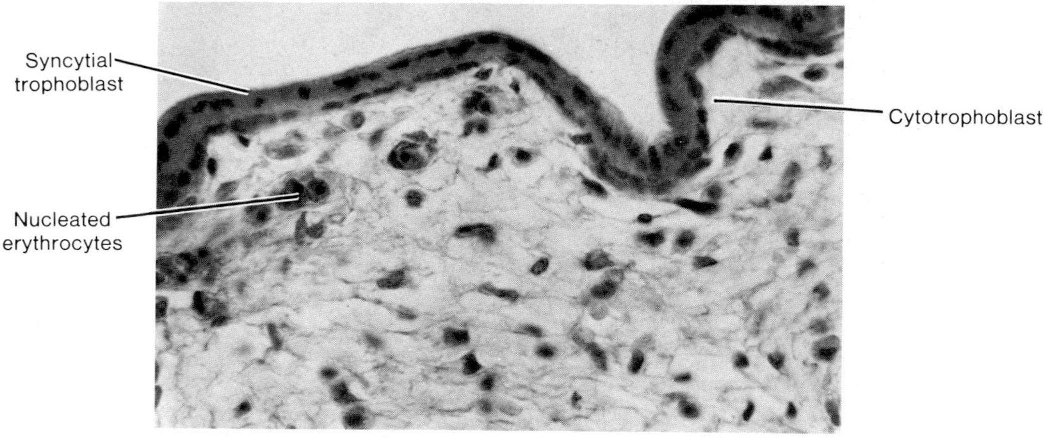

18-29

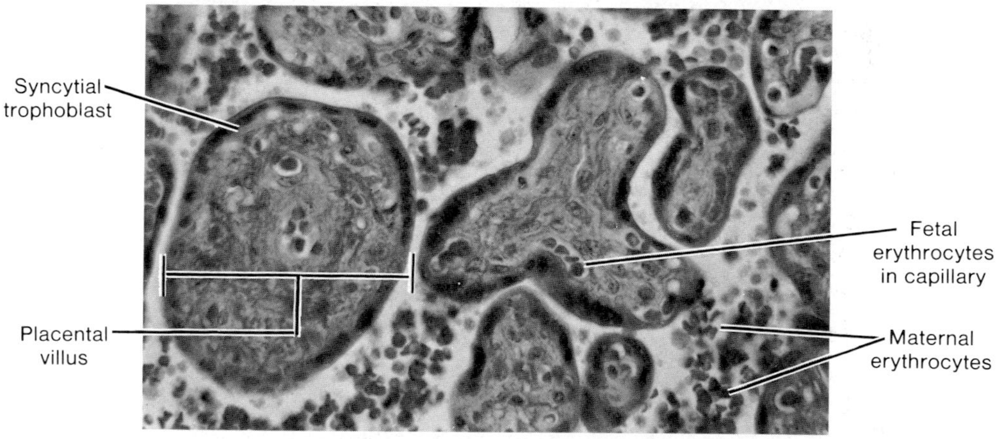

18-30 Mammary Gland

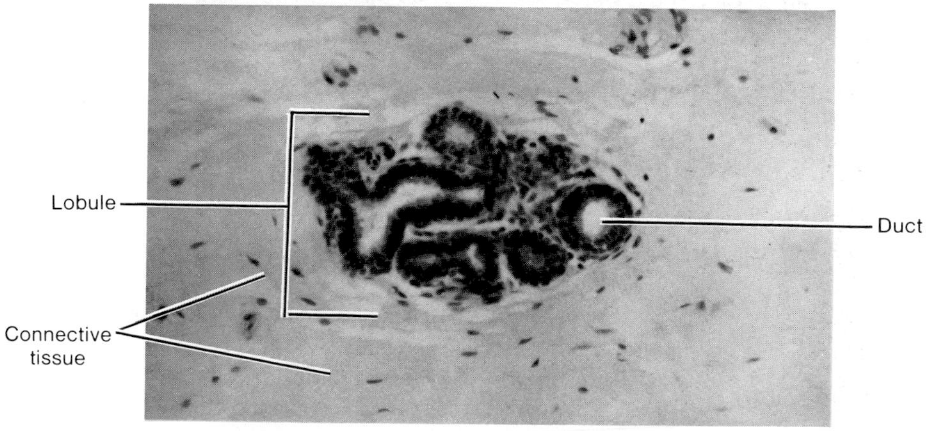

Figure 18.28. Human placenta (3rd week). LM, ×250.
Figure 18.29. Human placenta (6th month). LM, ×250.
Figure 18.30. Human mammary gland (inactive). LM, ×100.

18-31

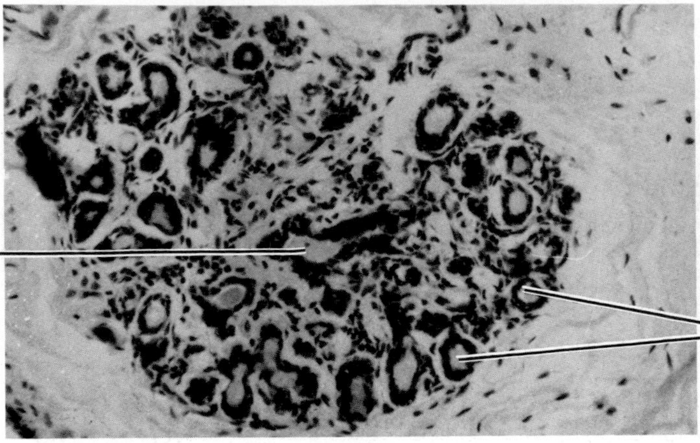

18-32

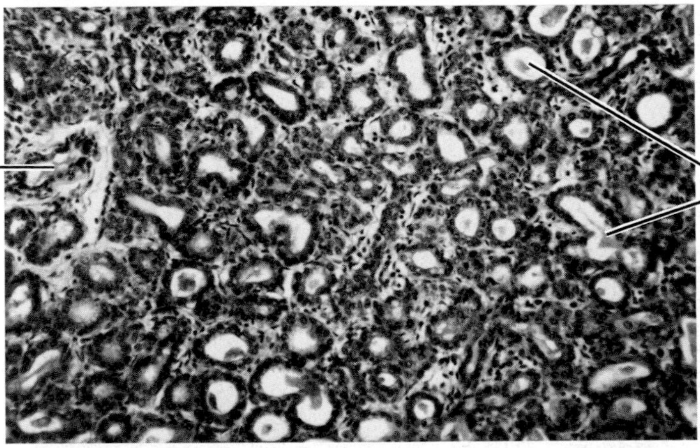

18-33

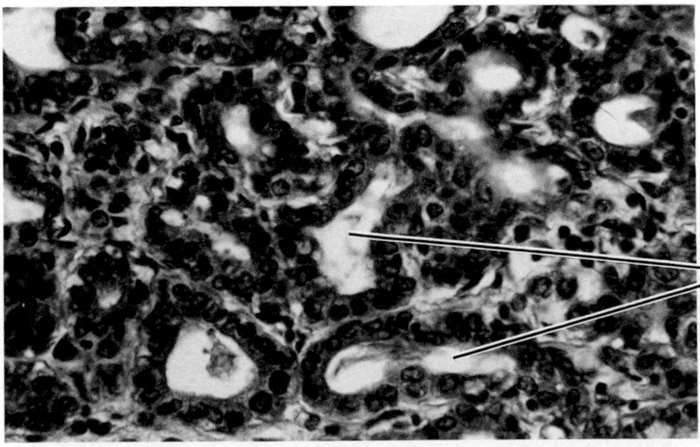

Figure 18.31. Human mammary gland (pregnancy). LM, ×40.
Figure 18.32. Lactating mammary gland (human). LM, ×100.
Figure 18.33. Lactating mammary gland (human). LM, ×250.

Development

18-34

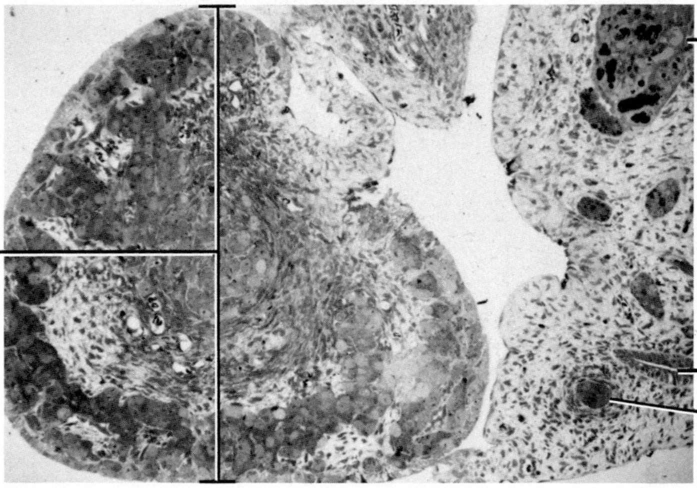

18-35

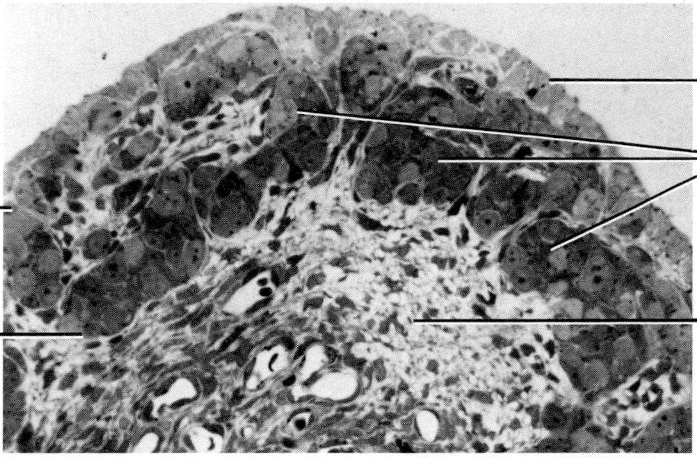

18-36

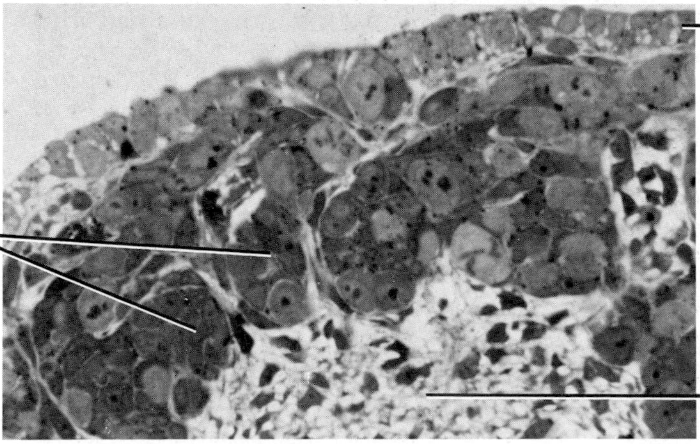

Figure 18.34. Ovary. LM, ×200.
Figure 18.35. Ovary. LM, ×250.
Figure 18.36. Ovary. LM, ×400.

19

Endocrine Glands

Endocrine glands lack ducts and their secretory products (hormones) generally pass into the blood or lymphatic circulation. In some instances, however, hormones are secreted directly into the intercellular space (paracrine secretion) to elicit a local effect on adjacent cells. Hormones that are secreted into the vascular system eventually enter the tissue fluids and, depending on the specificity of the hormone, can alter the activities of just one organ or influence several. The organs that respond to a specific hormone are the target organs of that hormone. Depending upon the endocrine gland of origin, hormones may be steroids, polypeptides, proteins or glycoproteins.

In some glands, such as the liver, the component epithelial cells have both exocrine and endocrine functions. Hepatocytes fulfill the definition of endocrine cells since they release glucose, proteins and other substances directly into the hepatic sinusoids, but the same hepatocytes also secrete bile into adjacent canaliculi (which represent the beginning of the liver duct system), thus satisfying the definition of exocrine cells.

Organs such as the pancreas, kidney, testis and ovary are a mixture of endocrine and exocrine components. In these particular glands, separate or isolated groups of cells secrete directly into the vasculature and form the endocrine portion. The remainder of the gland comprises the exocrine portion, which usually is drained by a duct system. The placenta is unique as an endocrine gland because of its transitory nature, lasting only about 9 months in man.

The classical endocrine glands consist of discrete masses of cells with a relatively simple organization into clumps, cords or plates supported by a delicate vascular connective tissue. Endocrine glands have a rich vascular supply and the component cells have direct access to nearby capillaries. The classical endocrine system consists of pineal, parathyroid, thyroid, adrenal and pituitary glands.

In contrast to these multicellular endocrine structures, a vast system of unicellular endocrine glands (cells) also exists, which collectively forms the diffuse endocrine system. It is represented by scattered, unicellar glands that often are at some distance from one another, separated by intervening cells of another type. This particular system occurs throughout the gastrointestinal tract, in the ducts of the major digestive glands and in the conducting airways of the lung. When the cells of this system are considered collectively, they form a mass that is larger than many of the individual organs of the classical endocrine glands.

PINEAL GLAND

The human pineal gland is a somewhat flattened body measuring 5 to 8 mm in length and 3 to 5 mm in width. It is attached to the brain (roof of the diencephalon) by a short stalk which contains some nerve fibers and their supportive elements.

Structure

KEY WORDS: pinealocytes (principal pineal cells), glial cells, corpora arenacea (brain sand), melatonin, serotonin

The pineal is covered by a thin connective tissue capsule that becomes continuous with the surrounding meningeal (pial) tissue. Richly vascularized and innervated septa extend into the parenchyma of the gland and subdivide it into poorly defined lobules. Two types of cell, pinealocytes and glial cells, are present and form clumps and cords.

Pinealocytes (principal pineal cells) have relatively large lobulated nuclei. Long cytoplasmic processes often radiate from the cell body and form club-shaped terminations near adjacent perivascular spaces or neighboring pinealocytes. Vesicles and membrane-bound dense granules are present in the swollen endings of the processes. Nearer the cell body the cytoplasm contains abundant, fairly large mitochondria, numerous free ribosomes, profiles of smooth endoplasmic reticulum, lipid droplets, lipochrome pigment, lysosomes and large numbers of microtubules. Although light and dark forms of pinealocytes have been described, it is not known whether each actually constitutes a distinct cell type or whether they represent differences in the activity of a single cell type.

Glial cells form an interwoven network within and around the parenchymal cords and clumps of the pineal gland. They are fewer in number than the pinealocytes and their nuclei are smaller and stain more deeply. Glial cells show elongated cytoplasmic processes and often are regarded as a form of astrocyte. The cytoplasm of the glial cell contains many fine filaments that measure 5 to 6 nm in diameter.

Corpora arenacea (**brain sand**) are concretions found in the pineal gland of man and some other mammals such as ungulates. These irregularly shaped structures occur in the capsule and substance of the gland and consist primarily of calcium carbonates and phosphates within an organic matrix. In man they increase in number with age, but their functional significance is unknown.

The mammalian pineal gland has an extensive vascular supply and is provided with numerous postganglionic sympathetic nerve fibers from neurons in the superior cervical ganglion.

Melatonin, an indolamine, is produced by the pineal gland and in amphibia causes blanching of melanophores. In mammals such as the rat, pinealocytes synthesize **serotonin**, a precursor of melatonin, which varies in amount according to diurnal and perhaps seasonal changes in the amount of light. Serotonin levels fall and melatonin levels rise during darkness. These circadian rythmns are controlled by the periodic release of norepinephrine from sympathetic fibers that enter the pineal from the superior cervical ganglion, which in turn is controlled by light perceived by the retina. In rodents and birds the pineal, through its secretion of melatonin, plays an active role in the reproductive cycles, which are influenced by the length of daylight. Hence, the pineal in these species acts as a neuroendocrine organ influencing the gonads in response to light. The functional significance of melatonin in man, however, is unknown. Pineal specific peptides are thought to influence or mediate hypophyseal function, but their exact role is uncertain.

PARATHYROID GLANDS

The parathyroid glands are small, brownish, oval-shaped bodies that measure 4 to 8 mm in length and 2 to 5 mm in width. In man, they are usually four in number, but as many as six or more may lie within the capsule of the thyroid gland or may be embedded within the substance of the middle third of this organ. In about 8% of the human population, additional parathyroid tissue may be found within the thymus. This particular association results from the common developmental origin of these structures from the third pharyngeal pouch. Parathyroid glands are present in all mammals and most vertebrates, with the exception of fishes and gill-bearing amphibia.

Structure

KEY WORDS: chief (principal) cells, oxyphil cells, parathyroid hormone

Each parathyroid gland is surrounded by a thin connective tissue capsule. The gland is subdivided by delicate trabeculae that extend from the capsule and contain the blood vessels, lymphatics and nerves which enter the substance of the parathyroid. In older individuals, fat cells often are abundant in the connective tissue stroma. The parenchyma consists of closely packed groups or cords of epithelial cells supported by a delicate framework of reticular fibers that support a rich capillary network and nerve fibers.

The parenchyma of the human parathyroid glands consists of chief or principal and oxyphil cells. **Chief cells** are the more numerous and measure between 8 and 10 μm in diameter. They have round, centrally-placed, vesicular nuclei and the clear cytoplasm contains, in addition to the usual organelles, large accumulations of glycogen, lipid droplets and small dense granules limited by a membrane. Lipofuscin granules also are often present.

Oxyphil cells form only a minor portion of the cell population and may be found singly or in small groups. This type of cell has been reported only in man, macaque monkeys and cattle, but even in these species, the oxyphils do not appear in significant numbers until puberty, becoming more abundant with age. Oxyphil cells are larger than chief cells and their cytoplasm stains intensely with eosin. Their small nuclei deeply stain and often appear pyknotic. The cytoplasm is packed with large, elongated mitochondria that show numerous cristae. Between the mitochondria are small accumulations of glycogen and occasional profiles of granular endoplasmic reticulum.

Numerous cells intermediate in appearance between the chief and oxyphil types also have been reported. The chief cell may represent the primary parenchymal element of the parathyroid gland and other cell types, such as the oxyphil and intermediate cells, represent only a modification or a state in the development of the chief cell.

The parathyroid gland secretes a polypeptide hormone, **parathyroid hormone** (PTH), which regulates the level of calcium in the blood plasma. Nearly half the blood calcium is in bound form, with the remainder present as free ions. The concentration of calcium ion governs the secretion of parathyroid hormone. If the concentration drops below normal levels, the hormone is secreted. Parathyroid hormone acts directly on osteoclasts and osteocytes to mobilize calcium ion from bone. It also acts directly on the renal tubules of the kidney to promote absorption of calcium ion and inhibit absorption of phosphate ion from the glomerular filtrate. With an increase in the concentration of calcium ion in the blood, there is a decrease in the amount of parathyroid hormone released. Blood levels of calcium are kept from exceeding the optimum by a second calcium-regulating hormone, calcitonin, which is produced by the parafollicular cells in the thyroid gland.

Parathyroid hormone is essential for life and complete removal of the parathyroid glands results in a precipitous drop in blood calcium, which ultimately leads to tetany and death.

THYROID GLAND

The thyroid gland normally weighs between 25 and 40 g in man and is located in the anterior region of the neck, inferior to the cricoid cartilage. It consists of two lateral lobes and an isthmus which forms a narrow connecting bridge across the trachea between the lateral lobes.

Structure

KEY WORDS: follicles, colloid, principal (follicular) cells, colloidal resorption droplets, thyroglobulin, triiodothyronine, tetraiodothyronine (thyroxine), binding protein, parafollicular cells (light cells, C cells), calcitonin (thyrocalcitonin), ultimobranchial body

The parenchyma of the thyroid gland is enclosed in a connective tissue capsule and is organized into spherical structures, the **follicles**. These vary considerably in diameter and contain a gelatinous material called **colloid**. The walls of the follicles consist of a simple epithelium which rests upon a thin basal lamina 50 nm thick. Each follicle is supported by a delicate reticular network that contains a vast capillary plexus, numerous nerve fibers and blindly ending lymphatic vessels.

The follicular epithelium consists mainly of the **principal** or **follicular cells**, which usually are squamous to cuboidal in shape. Depending on the functional state of the thyroid, the cells may assume a columnar appearance. The nuclei are spherical, contain one or more nucleoli and occupy a central position. The lateral cell membranes are united at the apex by junctional complexes and the luminal surfaces bear short microvilli. The basal plasmalemma is smooth and without infoldings. Mitochondria are evenly distributed throughout the cytoplasm and vary in number according to the activity of the cell. Active cells take on a cuboidal shape and show numerous profiles of rough endoplasmic reticulum, while the inactive cells are squamous and exhibit only a few elongated cisternae and profiles of rough endoplasmic reticulum. Golgi complexes usually occupy a supranuclear position in active cells and the apical cytoplasm shows numerous small vesicles, lysosomes and multivesicular bodies. **Colloidal resorption droplets** also are found in the apical cytoplasm.

The thyroid is unique among endocrine glands in that its secretory product, colloid, is stored extracellularly in the lumen of the follicle. Colloid consists chiefly of mucoproteins, proteolytic enzymes and a glycoprotein called **thyroglobulin**, the primary storage form of thyroid hormone. Synthesis of thyroglobulin occurs in the principal cells along the same basic intracellular pathway as does glycoprotein in cells elsewhere in the body. Amino acids are synthesized into polypeptides on the rough endoplasmic reticulum and then are carried in small transport vesicles to the Golgi complex, where the carbohydrate moiety is conjugated to the protein. From the Golgi complex the glycoprotein (noniodinated thyroglobulin) is transported to the apical surface in small vesicles, from which it is discharged by exocytosis into the follicular lumen where it remains as part of the colloid mass.

Simultaneous with the synthesis of thyroglobulin, thyroperoxidase is assembled in the granular endoplasmic reticulum, passes through the Golgi complex and is released by small vesicles at the apical surface of the follicular cells. Follicular cells have a unique capacity to take up iodide from the blood and concentrate it. The iodide subsequently is oxidized to iodine ion by intracellular peroxidase and used in the iodination of tyrosine groups in thyroglobulin. The formation of monoiodotyrosine and diiodotyrosine is thought to occur within the follicle immediately adjacent to the microvillus border of the follicular cells. When one molecule of monoiodotyrosine is linked to one of diiodotyrosine, a molecule of **triiodothyronine** is formed, whereas the coupling of two molecules of diiodotyrosine results in the formation of **tetraiodothyronine (thyroxin).** The thyronines make up only a small portion of the thyroglobulin complex but represent the only constituents that have hormonal activity. Both thyroglobulin and the thyronines are retained in the follicular lumen until needed.

When thyroid hormone is required, droplets of colloid are sequestered from the follicular lumen by endocytosis and enter the apical cytoplasm of the follicular cells. Lysosomes coalesce with the vacuoles and hydrolyze the contained thyroglobulin, liberating mono- and di-iodotyrosine as well as tri- and tetraiodothyronine (thyroxin) into the cytoplasmic matrix. The mono- and diiodotyrosine molecules are deiodinated and the iodine is reutilized by the cell. The thyroxin and triiodothyronine molecules diffuse through the cytoplasmic matrix and are released at the base of the cell to enter surrounding blood capillaries and lymphatic channels. Thyroxin is transported in the blood plasma complexed to a protein called **binding protein**. Triiodothyronine, which hormonally is the more potent of the two but not as abundant, is not as firmly bound to the protein as is thyroxin.

Synthesis of thyroid hormone is shown in Figure 19–1.

Binding protein plays an important role in regulating the amount of free hormone that circulates within the blood plasma. Both thyroxin and triiodothyronine are released from the binding proteins only in response to metabolic needs, thus preventing rapid

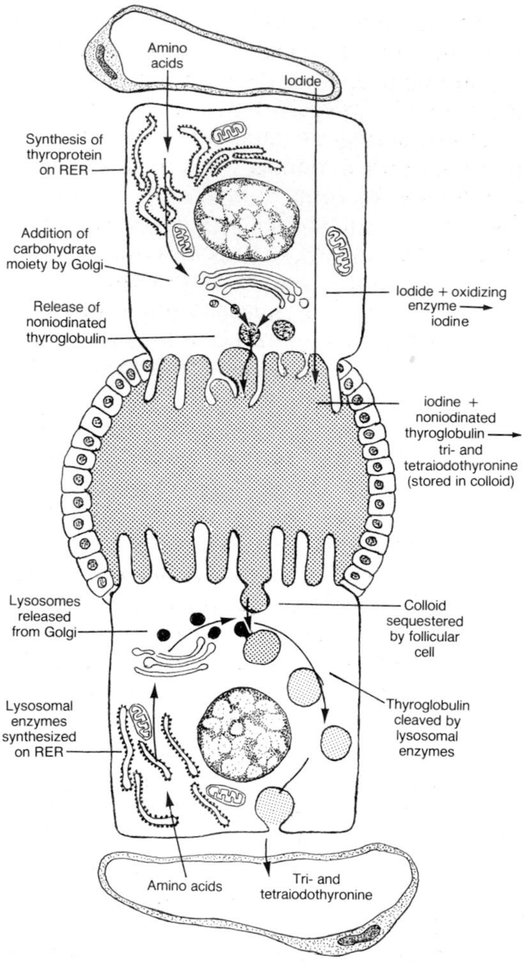

Figure 19-1. Synthesis of thyroid hormone.

fluctuations in the levels of these biologically active principals. As they are released and elicit their effects, both hormones are replaced by additional thyroxin and triiodothyronine molecules from the thyroid. The activity of the thyroid gland is regulated by a thyroid stimulating hormone (TSH) secreted by the anterior lobe of the pituitary.

Thyroid hormone has a general effect on the metabolic rate of most tissues of the body. It influences carbohydrate metabolism, the rate of intestinal absorption, heart rate, body growth, mental activities and has many other effects.

In addition to the follicular (principal) cells, the mammalian thyroid contains a smaller population of cells called **parafollicular cells (light cells, C cells)** which are present in the follicular epithelium and in the delicate connective tissue between follicles. The cells in the follicular epithelium usually appear to be sandwiched between two follicular cells and lie immediately adjacent to the basal lamina of the follicle; parafollicular cells never directly border the follicular lumen. Between follicles, they may occur singly or collect into small groups or nests. In electron micrographs, the parafollicular cells are characterized by numerous moderately dense, membrane-bound secretory granules that measure 10 to 50 nm in diameter. The cytoplasm also contains occasional profiles of rough endoplasmic reticulum, scattered mitochondria and poorly developed Golgi complexes.

The parafollicular cells secrete **calcitonin (thyrocalcitonin)**, a second polypeptide hormone that regulates blood calcium levels. Calcitonin lowers blood calcium by acting on the osteocytes and osteoclasts of bone to suppress bone resorption and the release of calcium into the blood. Thus, calcitonin has an effect opposite that of parathyroid hormone, serves to control the action of parathyroid hormone and helps to regulate the upper levels of calcium concentration in the blood plasma.

In lower vertebrates (fishes, amphibians, reptiles, and birds) the C cells form a separate epithelial mass called the **ultimobranchial body**. In these species, calcitonin is secreted from the ultimobranchial body and not the thyroid.

ADRENAL GLAND

The adrenal glands in man are a pair of flattened, triangular structures with a combined weight of 1 to 2 g. One adrenal is situated at the upper pole of each kidney. The adrenal glands of mammals are composite organs consisting of an outer surrounding cortex and an inner medulla, each of which differs markedly in structure, function and embryologic origin.

In lower vertebrates such as sharks and teleost fishes, the cortex (internal tissue) and medulla (chromaffin tissue) occur as separate entities. In amphibia the cortex and medulla may lie next to each other or, depending on the species, there may be some intermingling of the two tissues. In the adrenals of reptiles and birds, islets of chromaffin tissue generally are scattered throughout the cortical tissue. The distinct relationship of an outer surrounding cortex with a separate, centrally placed medulla is found only in the mammals.

Adrenal Cortex

KEY WORDS: zona glomerulosa, zona fasciculata, zona reticularis, mineralocorticoids (aldosterone, deoxycorticosterone), renin-angiotensin system, glucocorticoids (cortisol, cortisone, corticosterone), dehydroepiandosterone

The adrenal gland is surrounded by a thick connective tissue capsule composed primarily of collagen fibers and fibroblasts, together with scattered elastic fibers. In some species a few smooth muscle cells also may be present. The capsule contains a rich plexus of blood vessels (primarily small arteries) and numerous nerve fibers. Some blood vessels and nerves enter the substance of the cortex from the connective tissue trabeculae that penetrate the gland from the surrounding capsule.

The parenchyma of the adrenal cortex consists of continuous cords of secretory cells that extend from the capsule to the medulla, separated by blood sinusoids. The cortex is further organized into three strata or layers according to the arrangement of the cells within the cords and the strata comprise an outer zona glomerulosa, a middle zona fasciculata and an inner zona reticularis. The cytological changes from one zone to another are gradual.

The **zona glomerulosa** forms a narrow zone immediately beneath the capsule. The cells are arranged into ovoid groups or arcades and appear columnar in shape with centrally placed, spherical nuclei. In electron micrographs, the cells show a well developed complement of smooth endoplasmic reticulum and numerous mitochondria which are evenly distributed throughout the cytoplasm. Occasional lipid droplets and scattered profiles of rough endoplasmic reticulum also are observed.

The **zona fasciculata** constitutes the widest zone of the adrenal cortex and consists of long cords, generally one or two cells thick. The cords run roughly parallel to one another, separated by sinusoids that are lined by an attenuated endothelium. The cells of the zona fasciculata are larger than those of the other two zones, are polyhedral in shape and the lightly-stained, spherical nuclei are centrally located in the cell. The cells forming this zone often are binucleate. The cytoplasm shows numerous lipid droplets that contain neutral fat, fatty acids and fatty acyl esters of cholesterol. These forms of lipid represent stored precursor material for the synthesis of the steroid hormones that are secreted by the zona fasciculata. The cells of this zone also contain numerous, rounded mitochondria with tubular cristae and abundant smooth endoplasmic reticulum. The granular form of endoplasmic reticulum also is well developed and short microvilli often are present on the plasmalemma adjacent to sinusoids.

The **zona reticularis**, which forms the innermost zone of the cortex, is composed of a network of irregular, anastomosing cords that also are separated by sinusoids. The parenchymal cells are smaller than those of the zona fasciculata, the cytoplasm contains fewer lipid droplets, the nuclei stain more intensely, and lipofuscin granules are prominent. Except for these differences, the cells of the zona reticularis are similar to those of the zona fasciculata, both by light and electron microscopy. Light and dark forms of the parenchymal cells have been described in the zona reticularis but the significance of these forms is unknown.

The adrenal cortex synthesizes and secretes a variety of steroid hormones which generally can be placed into two broad categories: **mineralocorticoids**, which control water and electrolyte balance, and **glucocorticoids**, which effect carbohydrate metabolism. Both are derived from cholesterol.

The mineralocorticoids, **aldosterone** and **deoxycorticosterone**, are secreted primarily by the zona glomerulosa. Aldosterone acts on the distal tubules of the kidney to increase the rate of sodium absorption from the glomerular filtrate and, at the same time, to increase potassium excretion by the kidney. It also lowers the concentration of sodium in the secretions of the sweat glands, salivary glands and intestinal mucosa.

Aldosterone secretion is controlled primarily by the **renin-angiotensin** system, which is sensitive to changes in blood pressure and to the concentrations of sodium and potassium in the blood plasma. Although the exact mechanism is unknown, it has been suggested that the juxtaglomerular apparatus of the kidney receives signals created by decreased arterial renal blood pressure (which reduces the degree of stretch on the juxtaglomerular cells) or by a decrease in the amount of sodium detected by the macula densa. In response to the signal, the juxtaglomerular cells release renin, which converts circulating angiotensinogen to angiotensin I. A converting enzyme then acts on angiotensin I to transform it into angiotensin II which stimulates the zona glomerulosa of the adrenal cortex to secrete aldosterone. Angiotensin II also acts as a vasoconstrictor, thus directly increasing blood pressure. Aldosterone increases blood pressure due to increased sodium ion concentration. Both agents influence juxtaglomerular cells and renin release. The pituitary hormone, adrenocorticotropic hormone, may have a minor role in the activity of the zona glomerulosa.

The glucocorticoids (**cortisol, cortisone** and **corticosterone**) are secreted by the zona fasciculata and zona reticularis. They act primarily on the metabolism of fats, proteins and carbohydrates, resulting in an increase in blood glucose and amino acid levels, and in the movement of lipid into and out of fat cells. Cortisol also acts to suppress the inflammatory response and some allergic reactions. A weak androgen called **dehydroepiandosterone** also is secreted by cells of the zona fasciculata and zona reticularis, although cells of the reticularis are said to be the more active in androgen secretion.

The secretory activity of the zona fasciculata and zona reticularis is regulated by a polypeptide hormone, adrenocorticotropic hormone (ACTH), which is secreted by cells in the anterior lobe of the pituitary. Adrenocorticotropic hormone stimulates steroid synthesis and release, increases blood flow in the cortex, and promotes growth of the two inner zones of the adrenal cortex. The adrenal cortex is essential for life.

Adrenal Medulla

KEY WORDS: chromaffin cells, catecholamines, epinephrine, norepinephrine

The adrenal medulla is composed of large, round or polyhedral cells that are arranged in clumps or short cords. These parenchymal elements are the **chromaffin cells,** so named because they exhibit numerous brown granules when treated with chromium salts (the chromaffin reaction). The parenchyma of the medulla is supported by a framework of reticular fibers and the stroma contains numerous capillaries, veins and nerve fibers. Sympathetic ganglion cells also are present and may occur singly or in small groups. Chromaffin cells secrete **catecholamines**, and by special histochemical techniques, two types of chromaffin cells have been identified, one containing **epinephrine**, the other **norepinephrine**.

In electron micrographs, the chromaffin cells are characterized by numerous electron-dense granules that are limited by a membrane and measure 100 to 300 nm in diameter. The granules from norepinephrine secreting cells have intensely electron-dense cores, whereas cells that elaborate epinephrine possess a homogeneous, less dense form of secretory granules. Both cell types show profiles of granular endoplasmic reticulum, scattered mitochondria and well developed Golgi complexes that are localized close to the nucleus.

Although not essential for life, adrenal medullary hormones aid the organism in meeting stressful situations. Epinephrine increases cardiac output, elevates the level of blood glucose and increases the basal metabolic rate. Norepinephrine acts primarily to elevate and maintain blood pressure by causing vasoconstriction in the peripheral segments of the arterial system. Secretion of both hormones is under direct control of the sympathetic nervous system.

Blood Supply

Major arteries from several sources (inferior phrenic artery, renal artery and aorta) form a rich plexus of small arteries in the adrenal capsule. Cortical arteries arise from this plexus and enter the parenchyma of the adrenal to empty into a vast network of cortical sinusoids that surround the cords of epithelial cells. The attenuated endothelium of the sinusoids shows numerous fenestrations and is supported by a thin basal lamina and a delicate network of reticular fibers. After passing through all three layers of the adrenal cortex, the sinusoids begin to merge near the corticomedullary junction to form large collecting veins. These drain the medulla and ultimately empty into a single large suprarenal vein that drains the entire adrenal gland. The cortex has no separate venous drainage. Some arteries enter the cortex in the connective tissue trabeculae and provide a direct arterial supply to the medullary tissue. Hence, the medulla receives blood from cortical sinusoids and medullary arteries. The capillaries which surround the medullary cords also are lined by a thin fenestrated endothelium.

Adrenocorticosteroids (primarily glucocorticoids), in addition to their systemic effect, may influence cells in the adrenal medulla. Secretion of epinephrine or norepinephrine by the chromaffin cells of the medulla may be influenced by the steroid-rich blood entering from the cortex. Some experimental evidence does indicate that the glucocorticoids induce an enzyme which converts norepinephrine to epinephrine. In lower forms such as the shark, where the cortex and medulla exist as separate entities without an interconnecting blood supply, norepinephrine is the primary catecholamine secreted by the chromaffin tissue. In mammals where the adrenal is a composite gland, epinephrine is the major catecholamine secreted.

Paraganglia

KEY WORDS: chief cells, norepinephrine, supporting cells

Clusters of chromaffin cells located outside the adrenal medulla and normally associated with the sympathetic nervous system are referred to as paraganglia. They are invested by a thick connective tissue capsule that is composed mainly of collagen. Paraganglia are highly vascularized structures and consist of two cell types: chief cells and supporting cells. The **chief cells** contain numerous, membrane-bound, electron-dense granules similar to those observed in the chromaffin cells of the adrenal medulla and are thought to secrete **norepinephrine**. The chief cells are surrounded either in part or completely by elongate **supporting cells** that are devoid of secretory granules. Their function is unknown. Some paraganglia, such as the aortic chromaffin bodies, are paired and quite large. Paraganglia can be important clinically if they secrete abnormally high amounts of catecholamine.

HYPOPHYSIS

The hypophysis or pituitary is a complex endocrine gland located at the base of the brain, where it lies in the sella turcica, a small depression in the sphenoid bone. It is attached to the hypothalamic region of the brain by a narrow stalk and has both vascular and neural connections with the brain. The gland weighs about 0.5 g in the adult but is slightly heavier in females than in males. It may exceed 1 g in weight in the multiparous female. Despite the small size, the pituitary gland produces several hormones that directly influence other endocrine glands and tissues.

Organization

KEY WORDS: adenohypophysis, neurohypophysis, pars distalis (anterior lobe), pars intermedia, pars tuberalis, pars nervosa, infundibular stalk, median eminence

The hypophysis is composed of two major parts, an epithelial component called the **adenohypophysis** and a nervous component which constitutes the **neurohypophysis**. The adenohypophysis is further subdivided into the **pars distalis (anterior lobe)**, which lies anterior to the residual lumen of Rathke's pouch; the **pars intermedia**, which forms a thin partition behind the residual lumen; and the **pars tuberalis**, which is an extension of the pars distalis surrounding the neural stalk. The neurohypophysis also consists of three portions. The major portion is the **pars nervosa**, which lies just posterior to the pars intermedia and is continuous with the **infundibular stalk** and the **median eminence**. The pars intermedia of the adenohypophysis and the infundibular processes of the neurohypophysis are frequently regarded collectively as constituting the posterior lobe of the hypophysis. The infundibular stalk and the surrounding pars tuberalis constitute the hypophyseal stalk. The hypophysis is surrounded by a thick connective tissue capsule. The subdivisions of the hypophysis are shown in Figure 19–2.

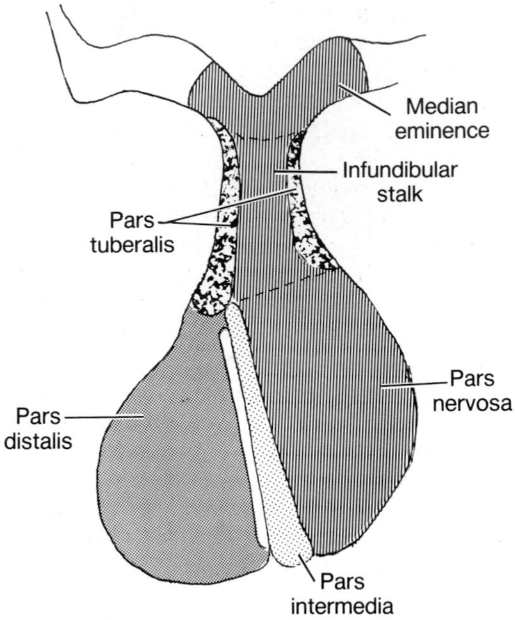

Figure 19-2. Subdivisions of the hypophysis and their relationships.

Vascular Supply

KEY WORDS: superior, middle and inferior hypophyseal arteries, common capillary bed

The pituitary is supplied by three pairs of arteries, namely, the **superior, middle and inferior hypophyseal arteries**, all of which supply directly to the neurohypophysis. The middle hypophyseal artery previously was believed to traverse the parenchyma of the adenohypophysis but recent evidence has shown that it, too, passes directly to the neurohypophysis. Thus, the adenohypophysis has no direct arterial blood supply but is linked to the neurohypophysis by a **common capillary bed** which extends throughout all three regions of the neurohypophysis and connects with the capillary bed of the hypothalamus. Contrary to previous belief, there is no system of pituitary portal veins separating the capillary bed of the median eminence and infundibular stalk from that of the adenohypophysis.

Venous drainage is accomplished by confluent pituitary veins that carry blood from the adenohypophysis, pars intermedia and neurohypophysis through a common trunk to the venous systemic circulation. Only a few lateral hypophyseal veins extend directly from the adenohypophysis to the cavernous sinus. The only direct drainage of the neurohypophysis is by the neurohypophyseal limbs of the confluent veins located at the lower end of the neurohypophysis. The pars intermedia is relatively avascular and few capillaries traverse it. The most prominent vessels of the pars intermedia are confluent pituitary veins.

Pars Distalis (Anterior Lobe)

KEY WORDS: chromophilic cells, acidophilic cells, somatotropes, somatotropin (growth hormone), mammatropes, prolactin, basophilic cells, corticotropes, adenocorticotrophic hormone, thyrotropes, thyrotropin (thyroid stimulating hormone), gonadotropes, follicle stimulating hormone, luteinizing hormone, interstitial cell stimulating hormone, chromophobes

The pars distalis, which makes up about 75% of the hypophysis, consists primarily of epithelial cells arranged in clumps or irregular cords. The parenchyma and surrounding sinusoidal capillaries are supported by a delicate network of reticular fibers. The parenchymal elements consist of chromophobic cells and chromophilic cells, distinguished by whether or not their secretory granules take up stain. **Chromophilic cells** are further subdivided into acidophilic and basophilic cells, terms which again refer to the staining properties of their secretory granules. All three cell types (chromophobes, acidophils and basophils) are present in the pars distalis.

Acidophilic cells are large, round or ovoid cells which measure 14 to 19 μm in diameter. They generally show a well-developed, juxtanuclear Golgi complex. Their secretory granules stain with eosin in routine preparations. Two types of acidophils are present in most mammalian species, the somatotropes and mammotropes. The cytoplasm of **somatotropes** contains well-developed profiles of granular endoplasmic reticulum and numerous electron-dense secretory granules that are spherical in shape and measure 350 to 400 nm in diameter. Somatotropes produce the protein hormone **somatotropin** (STH), or **growth hormone** (GH), which plays an important role in controlling body growth, acting primarily on the epiphyseal cartilages. The second type of acidophil, the **mammotrope**, tends to be more scattered within the parenchymal cords. Active cells show profiles of granular endoplasmic reticulum, Golgi complexes and scattered lysosomes. Their cytoplasm also contains irregular granules that measure 550 to 615 nm in diameter. Mammotropes secrete a protein hormone, **prolactin**, which promotes mammary gland development and lactation. In rodents, this hormone helps maintain the corpora lutea, hence its alternative name, luteotrophic hormone.

Basophilic cells of the pars distalis consist of three types of cells: corticotropes, thyrotropes and gonadotropes. **Corticotropes** generally are larger than most acidophilic cells and are round or ovoid in shape. They are most numerous in the central anterior portion of the pars distalis. In electron micrographs, the corticotropes in man show numerous secretory granules, 350 to 400 nm in diameter, that are similar in appearance to the granules observed in somatotropes. Their cytoplasm often contains lipid droplets and small filaments that measure 6 to 8 nm in diameter. Corticotropes secrete a polypeptide hormone called **adenocorticotrophic hormone** (ACTH) which stimulates the zona fasciculata and zona reticularis of the adrenal cortex to produce glucocorticoids.

The **thyrotrope** form of basophil often is angular in shape. The cells may form small groups deep in the parenchymal cords, at some distance from sinusoids. The secretory granules range from 130 to 150 nm in diameter and are the smallest of any granules found in the parenchymal cells of the hypophysis. Thyrotropes secrete the glycoprotein hormone, **thyrotropin** or **thyroid stimulating hormone** (TSH), which stimulates the thyroid gland to produce and release thyroid hormone.

Gonadotropes are the third type of basophil cells in the pars distalis. They generally are smaller than the corticotropic basophils, often show only scattered granules, usually are round in shape and frequently lie immediately adjacent to sinusoids. The cytoplasm contains profiles of granular endoplasmic reticulum, prominent Golgi complexes and scattered lysosomes. The sparse secretory granules are spherical in shape and measure about 150 nm in diameter. This type of basophil secretes two glycoproteins—follicle stimulating hormone and luteinizing hormone. **Follicle stimulating hormone** (FSH) stimulates growth of ovarian follicles in the female, and in the male stimulates the synthesis of androgen-binding protein (ABP) by the Sertoli cells of the seminiferous epithelium, thereby activating and promoting spermatogenesis. **Luteinizing hormone** (LH) is essential for ovulation, for simulating the secretion of estrogen by ovarian follicles and for promoting luteinization of follicles following the development induced by FSH. In the male, **interstitial cell stimulating hormone** (ICSH), the equivalent of LH in the female, also is secreted by this particular type of basophil. It stimulates production of testosterone by the interstitial cells of the testis. Testosterone is vital for sperm maturation and for development and maintenance of the secondary sex organs and characteristics.

The remaining general cell type, the **chromophobes**, usually are small and confined to the interior of the parenchymal cords. Lacking granules, they fail to stain with routine procedures, thus their name. Their existence as a distinct cell type has been questioned and they may represent a reservoir of cells from which chromophilic cells originate. This concept is in keeping with the hypothesis that cells of the pars distalis cycle, first accumulating secretory granules and then releasing them.

Pars Tuberalis

The pars tuberalis has been identified in all vertebrates studied and forms a sleeve, up to 60 μm thick, extending around the infundibular stalk. It is thickest anteriorly and may be incomplete posteriorly. The pars tuberalis is characterized by longitudinally arranged cords of parenchymal cells separated by sinusoids. The parenchyma of the pars tuberalis is continuous with that of the pars distalis and consists of acidophils, basophils and undifferentiated cells. The latter are usually columnar in shape and their cytoplasm shows numerous small granules and large amounts of glycogen. Nests of squamous cells also are observed. The pars tuberalis is not known to have a distinct hormonal function.

Pars Intermedia

KEY WORDS: chromophobes, basophils, melanocyte stimulating hormone

The pars intermedia is absent in some vertebrate species (whale, porpoise, manatee and some birds) and is rudimentary in man, where it forms only about 2% of the hypophysis. It consists of **chromophobe** and **basophil cells**, the latter often encroaching into the pars nervosa. Colloid-filled cysts lined by chromophobic or basophilic cells also may be present and remnants of Rathke's cleft may persist as fluid-filled cysts lined by a ciliated columnar epithelium. The pars intermedia of some species is responsible for the secretion of **melanocyte stimulating hormone** (MSH), a polypeptide hormone. In amphibia the hormone causes dispersion of melanin granules in the melanophores of the skin, resulting in increased pigmentation. In mammals its exact role is unknown. It may be involved in melanin production. In some species, MSH occurs in α and β forms, but only the precursor molecule for MSH occurs in man. Both forms of MSH contain amino acid sequences that are identical to portions of the ACTH molecule and the occurrence of these structurally similar regions is said to account for the melanocyte-stimulating effect of ACTH.

Control of the Adenohypophysis

KEY WORDS: releasing hormones, inhibitory hormones, somatostatin

Secretions from target endocrine glands that are under the control of the adenohypophysis influence cells in the adenohypophysis by acting through regulatory neurons located in the hypothalamus. Neurons in the hypothalamus produce **releasing hormones**, small peptides that enter the capillaries surrounding the infundibular stalk and then are transported to the capillaries of the pars distalis. The peptides are cell specific and stimulate the release of certain hormones by the pars distalis. Releasing hormones for somatotropin, thyrotropin, corticotropin and gonadotropin are known and their amino acid sequences have been determined. **Inhibitory hormones** such as **somatostatin** (a peptide consisting of 14 amino acids) also are secreted by hypothalamic neurons. Somatostatin inhibits secretion of growth hormone and thyrotropic hormone. Inhibitory hormones affecting the remaining cell types in the adenohypophysis are said to be produced by hypothalamic neurons but to date their biochemical nature is unknown.

Neurohypophysis

KEY WORDS: hypothalamohypophyseal tract, Herring bodies, pituicytes, neurophysin, oxytocin, antidiuretic hormone

Macroscopically, the neurohypophysis consists of the median eminence, the infundibular stalk and the infundibular process (pars nervosa). The greater part of the neurohypophysis consists of unmyelinated nerve fibers of the **hypothalamohypophyseal tract** which originates primarily from neurons in the supraoptic and paraventricular nuclei. The tract receives additional nerve fibers from other hypothalamic regions. The fibers end blindly in the pars nervosa close to a rich capillary plexus. The axons which comprise the hypothalamohypophyseal tract commonly contain spherical masses of secretory material which vary considerably in size. These are the **Herring bodies** which, by electron microscopy, are seen to consist of large accumulations of dense secretory granules that measure 120 to 200 nm in diameter. Hormone is thought to be synthesized in the perikarya of neurons in the supraoptic and paraventricular nuclei. The hormone is transported down the axons to be stored in the nerve terminals that comprise the pars nervosa. When released, the hormones traverse a thin, fenestrated endothelium to enter the capillaries in the pars nervosa from which they drain into hypophyseal veins and finally enter the systemic circulation.

Scattered among the nerve fibers are cells called **pituicytes** which vary in size and shape and may contain pigment granules. Pituicytes are considered to be the equivalent of neuroglial cells in the central nervous system, but whether they have a supportive function only or actively participate in the secretory process of adjacent nerve terminals is not known.

Two cyclic polypeptide hormones, oxytocin and antidiuretic hormone (vasopressin), are stored and released from the pars nervosa of the neurohypophysis. During axonal transport, each hormone is bound to a carrier protein called **neurophysin** and it is the neurophysin-hormone complex that constitutes the major part of the Herring bodies. **Oxytocin** is released in lactating mammals by means of a neuronal reflex that is initiated during suckling and transmitted to the hypothalamus through the cerebral cortex. Oxytocin causes contraction of myoepithelial cells surrounding alveoli in the mammary gland and aids in expressing milk into the ductal system, a phenomenon known as "milk letdown." Large exogenous doses of this hormone enhance contractions of uterine muscle during parturition, but whether or not this is a normal physiological function is unknown. **Antidiuretic hormone (ADH)** acts primarily on the collecting ducts and distal convoluted tubules of the kidney to increase their permeability to water, thus promoting its reabsorption from the glomerular filtrate. The perikarya of neurons in the supraoptic and paraventricular nuclei are thought to act as osmoceptors and to secrete in response to an increase in the osmolarity of the body fluids. Pharmacologic doses of ADH cause contraction of vascular smooth múscle and elevate blood pressure. Therefore, this hormone is sometimes referred to as vasopressin.

DEVELOPMENT OF ENDOCRINE GLANDS

Classical endocrine glands develop from invaginations of epithelium (ectoderm, endoderm, mesoderm) into underlying mesenchyme; connection with the epithelium of origin is lost.

Pineal Gland. The pineal arises from the roof of the developing brain by fusion of a solid anterior outgrowth near the habenular commissure, with a hollow saccular evagination from the roof the diencephalon. Cell proliferation first begins, and is more extensive in, the anterior portion. In this region, the differentiating pineal neuroepithelial cells form a network of anastomosing cords and follicles within the mesenchyme. Together with contributions from the neural crest, the mesenchyme forms the connective tissue capsule, trabeculae and stroma of the gland. Neuroepithelial cells differentiate into pinealocytes and neuroglial cells. As the gland matures, the lobules become more distinct and are composed mainly of pinealocytes.

Parathyroid Gland. The parathyroids develop in the endodermal epithelium of the third and fourth branchial pouches. Dorsolateral thickenings on each pouch form solid masses of cells, each of which represents a primordium of a parathyroid gland. As they invaginate, each cell mass forms a vesicle which loses its connection to the epithelium of the pharyngeal floor. The paired primordia from the third pouches migrate with the thymic rudiment to the caudal border of the thyroid to become the inferior parathyroids. The pair associated with the fourth pouches remains at the cranial border of the thyroid and forms the superior parathyroids.

The cells of the primordia mainly differentiate into chief cells which form anastomosing cords and sheets. Growth of the gland occurs as the cords of cells expand by addition of new cells derived by mitosis. The thin capsule and vascular stroma of each parathyroid originate from the surrounding mesenchyme. Initially, the stroma is relatively inconspicuous and free of fat, which accumulates with age. In man and the few other species where the cells are found, oxyphils do not appear in appreciable numbers until after puberty, and also increase with age.

Thyroid Gland. Generally, thyroid development can be divided into three major stages: formation and separation of the thyroid anlagen, early differentiation (prefollicular stage), and follicle formation.

Thyroid follicles are derived from ventral outpockets of the endodermal epithelium over the floor of the pharynx. These outgrowths form the median thyroid, which fuses with smaller caudal-lateral outpockets (the lateral thyroid) of the pharynx. The latter contribute to the ultimobranchial bodies of the thyroid. The median thyroid enlarges and an epithelial-lined vesicle forms which separates from the pharyngeal floor. As the vesicle migrates caudally, it expands laterally to form two lobes which fuse with the tissues of the developing ultimobranchial bodies. The lumen of the thyroid vesicle is lost, the epithelial cells of the vesicle wall proliferate, and numerous branching, anastomising cords expand into the surrounding mesenchyme. A minute lumen lies at the center of each cord. These features characterize the prefollicular stage. As a result of the secretory activities of the epithelial cells, the lumen expands and the epithelial cords segment to form primary follicles. Secondary follicles arise by budding and/or further subdivision and growth of the primary follicles. The capsule and stroma develop from the surrounding mesenchyme.

The origin of the parafollicular (C) cells is obscure. They may be derived from neural crest or from endoderm associated with the ultimobranchial bodies.

Adrenal Gland. The adrenal cortex is a derivative of mesoderm; the medulla arises from neural ectoderm.

A provisional fetal cortex first arises from the mesothelial cells over the dorsal mesentery. These rapidly proliferate and invade the adjacent vascular mesenchyme, which subsequently forms the capsule and stroma of the gland. Differentiation of the epithelial cells gives rise to a thick zone of large, acidophilic cells which constitute the provisional cortex. This soon is enveloped by an outer, compact layer of smaller, densely-staining cells that will form the permanent cortex. The provisional cortex continues to grow and at birth makes up almost 80% of the cortex. Immediately after birth, the provisional cortex involutes and disappears during the first few weeks of postnatal life. As the provisional cortex regresses, the cells of the definitive cortex differentiate and advance centrally. At birth, the zona glomerulosa is present and the zona fasciculata is in its initial stage of development. The zona fasciculata and reticularis become well-defined and assume adult form during the first few months of postnatal life.

The medulla arises during the 7th week in man by a migration of cells from developing ganglia in the region of the coeliac plexus. The cells invade the medial side of the cortical primordium, which subsequently envelops them. As a result, the presumptive chromaffin cells occupy a central position in the adrenal, late in fetal life. Ultimately, the chromaffin cells become arranged into cords and plates separated by sinusoids.

Hypophysis. The neurohypophysis develops as an outgrowth from the floor of the diencephalon, while the adenohypophysis arises from an (ectodermal) epithelial invagination of the developing oral cavity (Rathke's pouch). The vesicle loses its connection with the epithelium and comes to abut the rostral surface of the infundibulum. It differentiates into the three primary epithelial subdivisions of the adenhypophysis. The rostral wall thickens to become pars distalis; the caudal wall thins to form pars intermedia; and bilateral outgrowths of the dorsolateral wall wrap around the infundibular stem to become pars tuberalis.

As these events occur, the lumen of Rathke's pouch is obliterated, or may form a residual lumen which appears as cysts in the adult. Thickenings of the rostral wall occur at a time when the parenchyma of the developing pars distalis differentiates into cords or plates of cells that are separated by sinusoids. The latter arise from surrounding mesenchyme which is incorporated into the parenchyma as the two major subdivisions blend into one. The surrounding mesenchyme forms the capsule and septae of the gland. By the 10th week in man, the major cell types have differentiated.

FUNCTIONAL SUMMARY

The parenchymal cells of endocrine glands synthesize hormones which may regulate specific tissues of the body or which may have a more general systemic effect. Endocrine glands control and coordinate many of the physiological activities of the body and often act in concert with the nervous system. In many instances neurons perform endocrine functions through secretion of peptide hormones directly into the blood stream. Antidiuretic hormone and oxytocin are synthesized by neurons in the supraoptic and paraventricular nuclei of the hypothalamus, travel down their respective axons and are released into the vasculature of the pars nervosa. From here they enter the hypophyseal veins and make their way into the general systemic circulation. Antidiuretic hormone promotes the absorption of water from the glomerular filtrate, thus conserving body water and concentrating the urine. The stimulus for ADH secretion is an increase in the osmolality of the blood plasma. The cell bodies of neurons in the paraventricular and supraoptic nuclei are thought to act as osmoreceptors and to secrete ADH in response to this stimulus as well as to stimuli from other pressure-sensitive regions of the vascular system. Oxytocin, on the other hand, is released in response to the suckling reflex and stimulates the contraction of myoepithelial cells, which aids in expressing milk from the secretory units into the ductal system of the mammary gland.

Other hypothalamic neurons act on mediator cells, the gonadotrophes, of the adenohypophysis and through them control follicular growth, ovulation and hormone production in the female and spermatogenesis and hormone production in the male. Several hypothalamic neurons, acting through releasing hormones, influence somatotrophes and thyrotrophes of the pars distalis to control the levels of growth hormone and thyroid hormone. These specific hormones control general body growth and metabolism.

Adrenocorticotrophic hormone elaborated by the corticotrophes of the pars distalis, stimulates the zona fasciculata and zona reticularis of the adrenal gland to secrete and release glucocorticoids. Like other epithelial cells in the pars distalis, corticotrophes are controlled by releasing and inhibitory hormones secreted by hypothalamic neurons.

Unlike most of the classical endocrine glands, the chromaffin cells of the adrenal medulla are under the direct control of the sympathetic nervous system. When stimulated to secrete, the chromaffin cells release two biologically active catecholamines, epinephrine and norepinephrine which, although not essential for life, are important in meeting stressful and "flight or fight" situations by increasing cardiac output, metabolic rate and blood pressure.

Other classical endocrine glands are not under direct nervous stimulation or control by neural hormones. The activity of the parathyroid gland, for example, is influenced primarily by the concentration of calcium ion in the circulating blood plasma. If the concentration falls below a specific level, parathyroid hormone is secreted and acts on the osteocytes and osteoclasts of bone to promote resorption of calcium ion, and on kidney tubules to increase calcium absorption from the glomerular filtrate, thus restoring the calcium ion concentration in the blood. Blood calcium is kept from rising above optimal levels by calcitonin which is released from the parafollicular cells of the thyroid gland. Calcitonin counters the action of parathyroid hormone by suppressing the resorptive activities of osteocytes and osteoclasts. Thus, regulation of the calcium ion concentrations in the blood plasma is controlled by two endocrine glands that act in opposition to one another.

The hypothalamus is restricted by the blood-brain barrier, whereas the neurohypophysis is not. This may explain why oxytocin, ADH, and the hypophyseotropic releasing and inhibitory hormones (which are released by neurons in the hypothalamic region) must travel considerable distances along axons before being released into capillaries in the region of the median eminence, infundibular stalk and infundibular process to finally enter the hypophyseal or systemic circulations.

Atlas and Table of Key Features for Chapter 19

Table 19.1.
Key Historical Features of Classical Endocrine Glands

	Arrangement of Cells	Cell Types	Other Features
Neurohypophysis	Cells vary in size; arranged around unmyelinated nerve fibers	Pituicytes	Herring bodies
Adenohypophysis	Cells form irregular cords and plates	Basophils, acidophils, chromophobes	Numerous capillaries between cords
Parathyroids	Irregular cords and plates	Chief cells (majority) oxyphils, occur singly or in nests	Abundant fat in interlobular connective tissue
Thyroid	Follicles	Follicular cells, parafollicular cells; single (adjacent to follicles) or in small interfollicular nests	Colloid in follicular lumen
Adrenal Cortex			
(a) Zona glomerulosa	Ovoid groups or arcades	Columnar cells, occasional lipid droplets	Near capsule
(b) Zona fasciculata	Long cords	Polyhedral cells, numerous lipid droplets	Cords of cells separated by sinusoids
(c) Zona reticularis	Irregular, anastomosing cords	Polyhedral cells, few lipid droplets	Cords of cells separated by sinusoids
Adrenal medulla	Irregular clumps or short cords	Large, pale-staining chromaffin cells	Ganglion cells, "sympathetic neurons"; sinusoids
Pineal	Poorly defined lobules, clumps and cords	Pinealocytes; glial cells	Corpora arenacea

19-3 Hypophysis

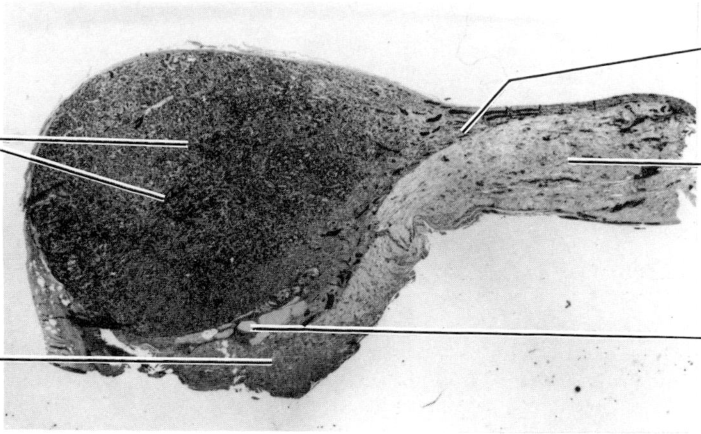

19-4

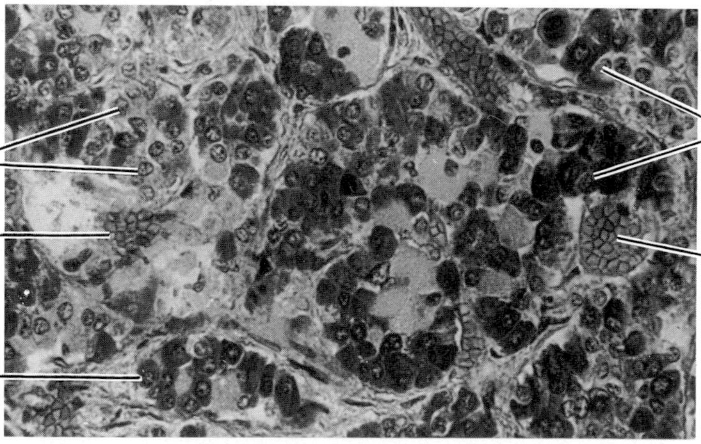

19-5

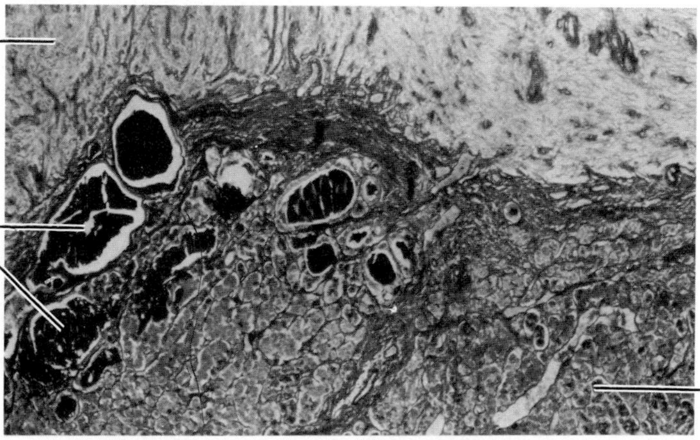

Figure 19-3. Hypophysis (human). LM, ×20.
Figure 19-4. Pars distalis (human). LM, ×250.
Figure 19-5. Pars intermedia (human). LM, ×100.

19-6

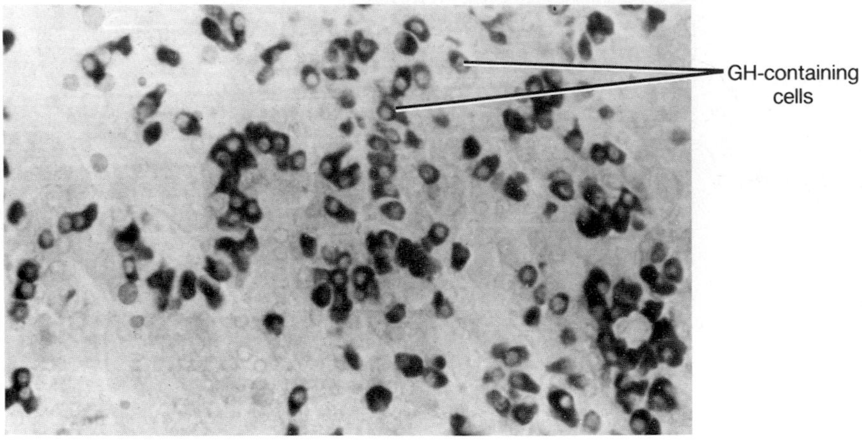

19-7

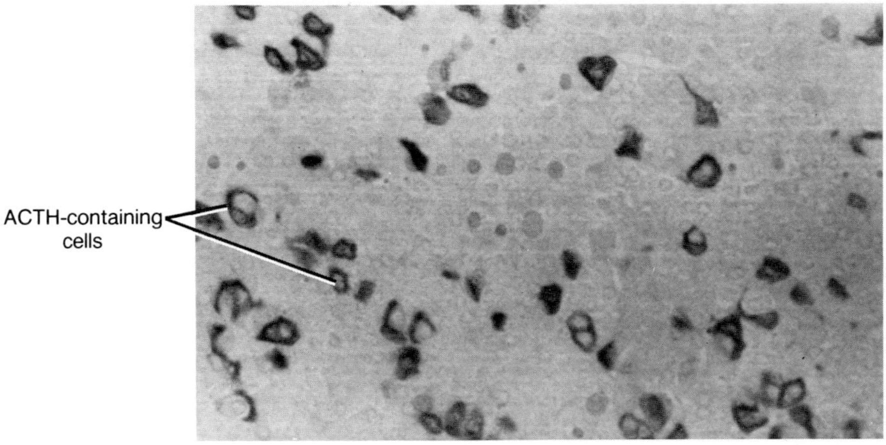

19-8

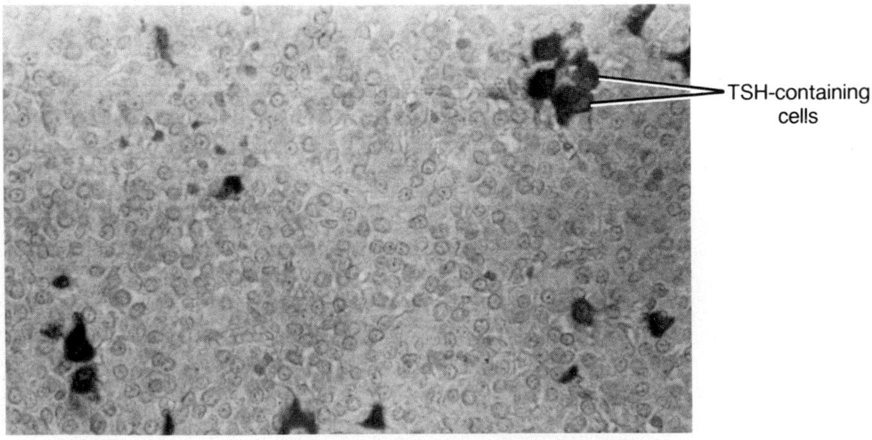

Figure 19-6. Growth hormone (PAP technique). LM, ×400.
Figure 19-7. ACTH (PAP technique). LM, ×400.
Figure 19-8. TSH (PAP technique). LM, ×400.

19-9

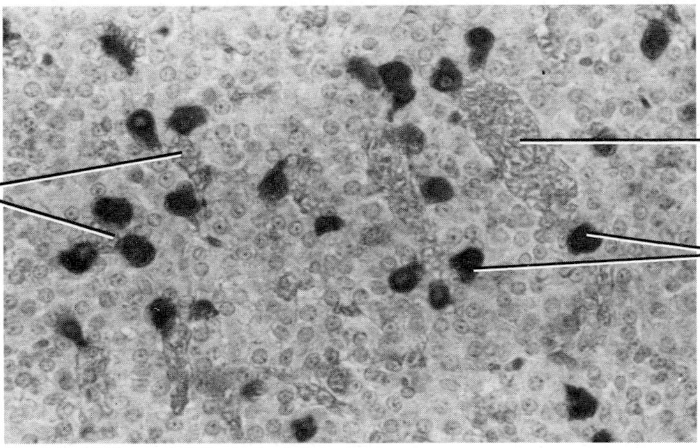

19-10

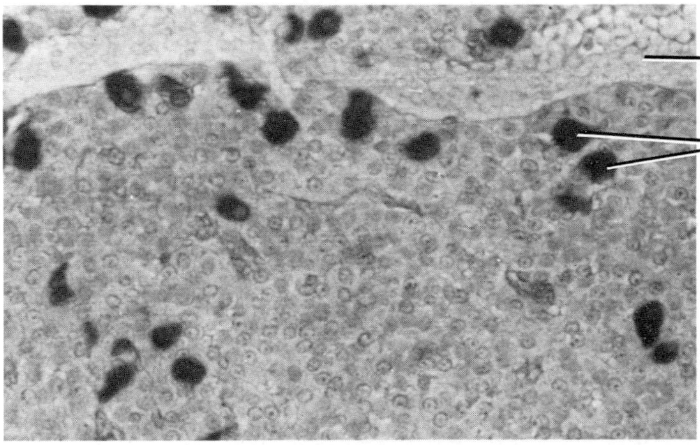

19-11 Median Eminence

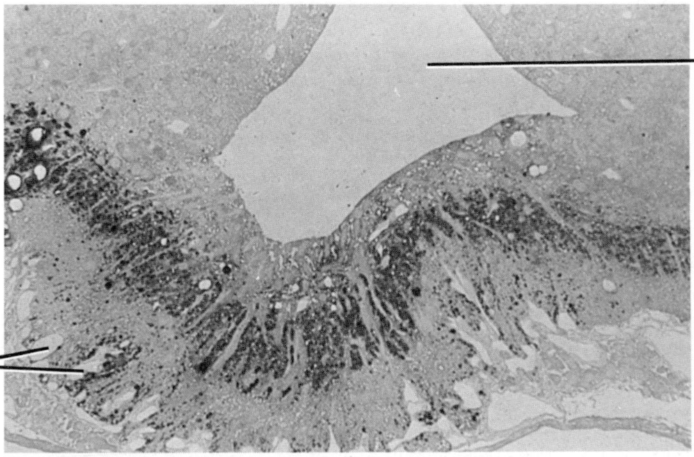

Figure 19-9. FSH (PAP technique). LM, ×400.
Figure 19-10. LH (PAP technique). LM, ×400.
Figure 19-11. Neurophysin (PAP technique). LM, ×100.

19-12 Infundibular Stem

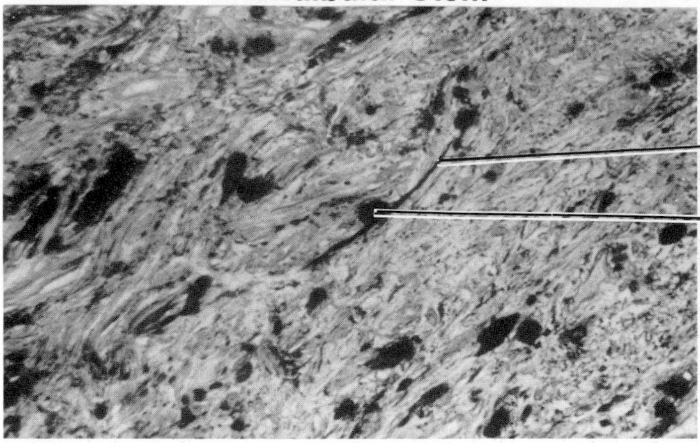

19-13 Pineal

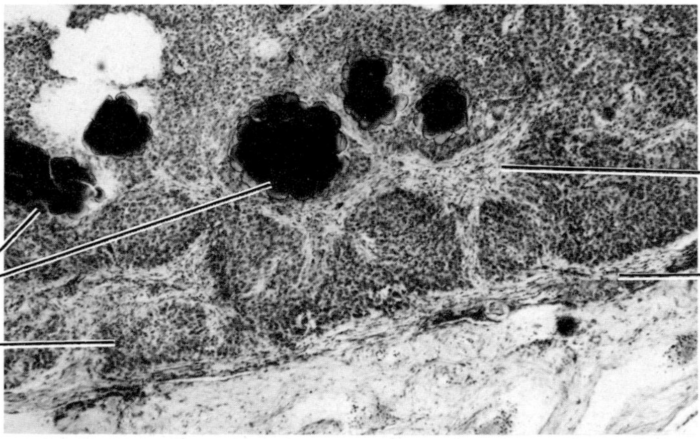

19-14 Thyroid

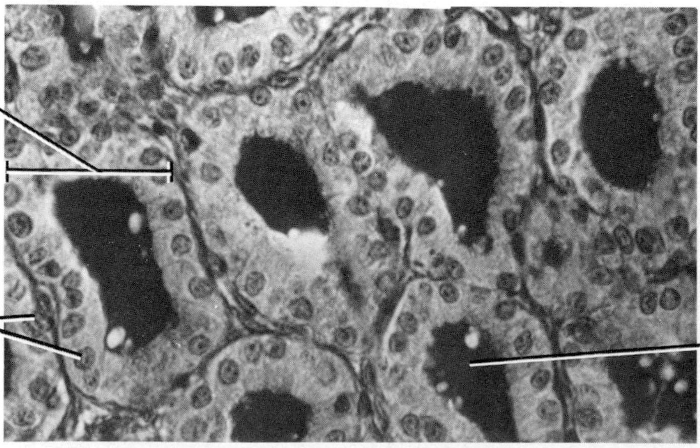

Figure 19-12. Infundibular stem (human). LM, ×250.
Figure 19-13. Pineal (human). LM, ×400.
Figure 19-14. Thyroid. LM, ×100.

19-15

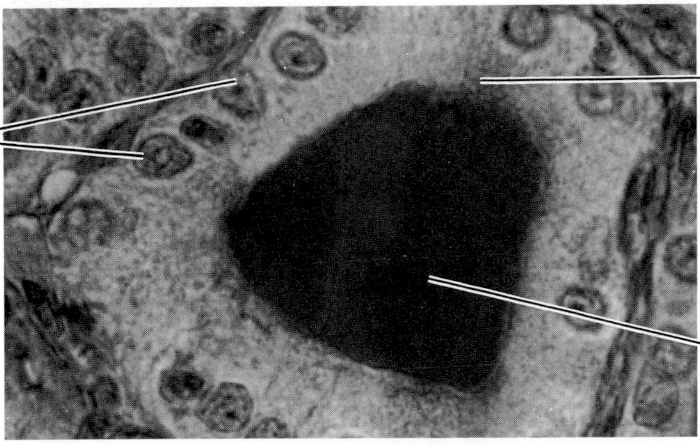

19-16

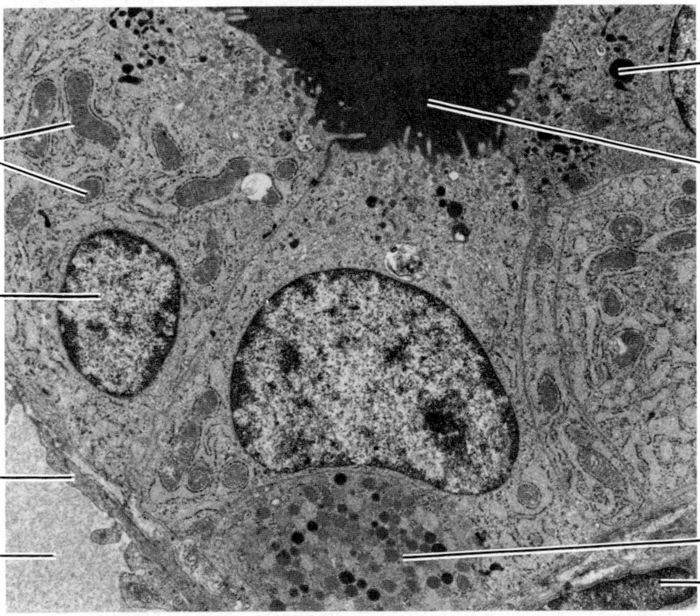

19-17

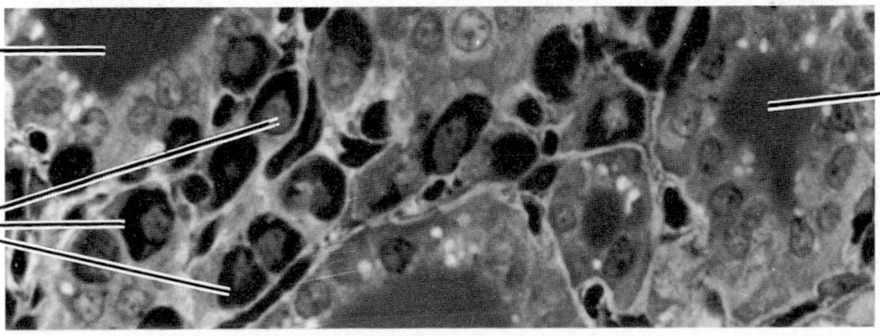

Figure 19-15. Thyroid follicle. LM, ×400.
Figure 19-16. Thyroid. TEM, ×3500.
Figure 19-17. Parafollicular cells (thyroid). LM, ×250.

19-18

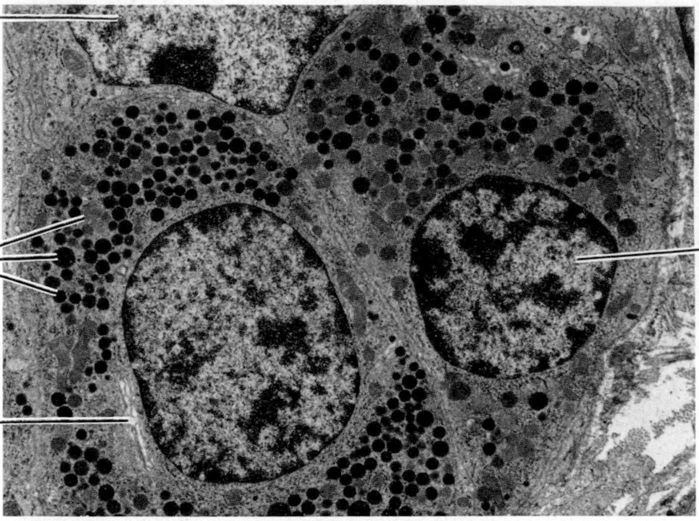

19-19 Parathyroid

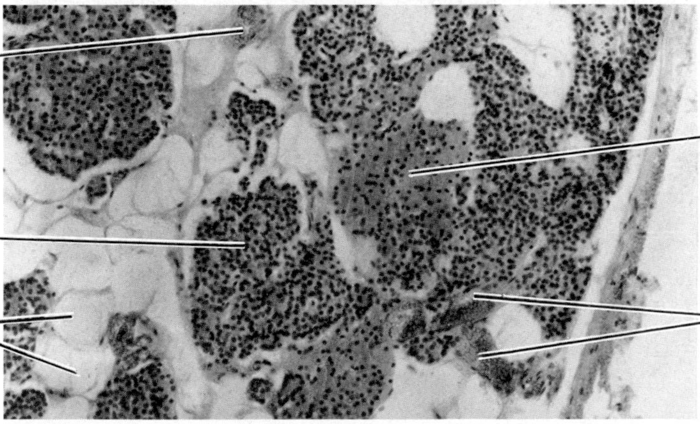

19-20 Adrenal

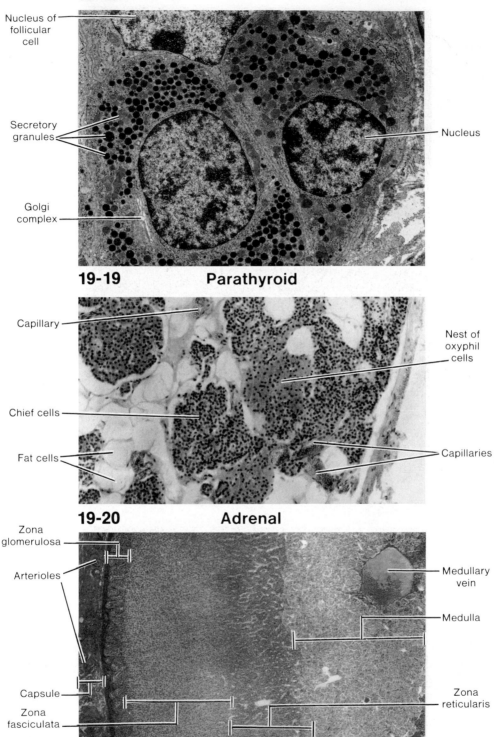

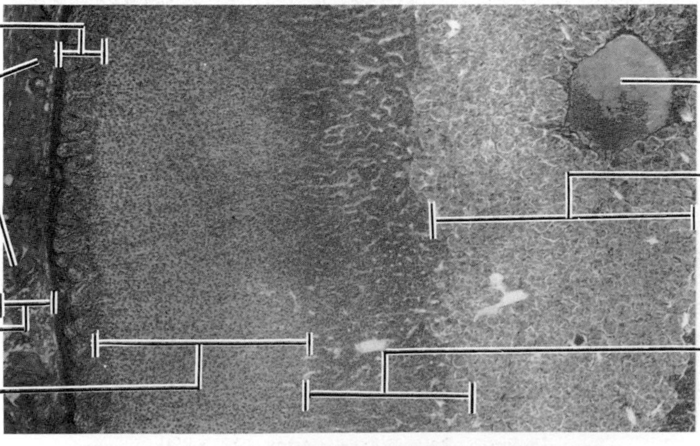

Figure 19-18. Parafollicular cells (thyroid). TEM, ×4000.
Figure 19-19. Parathyroid (human). LM, ×100.
Figure 19-20. Adrenal gland (human). LM, ×40.

19-21

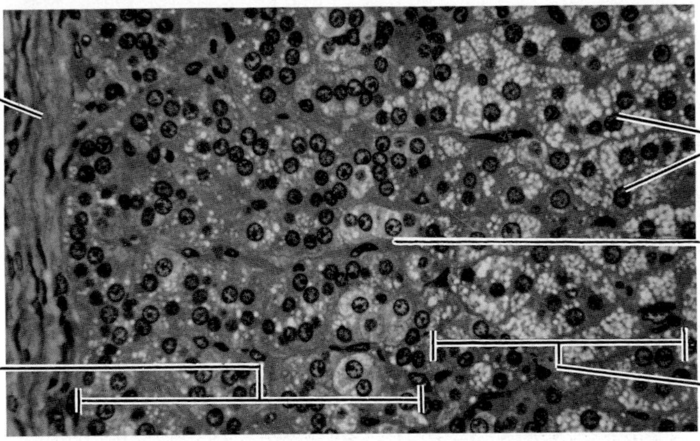

19-22

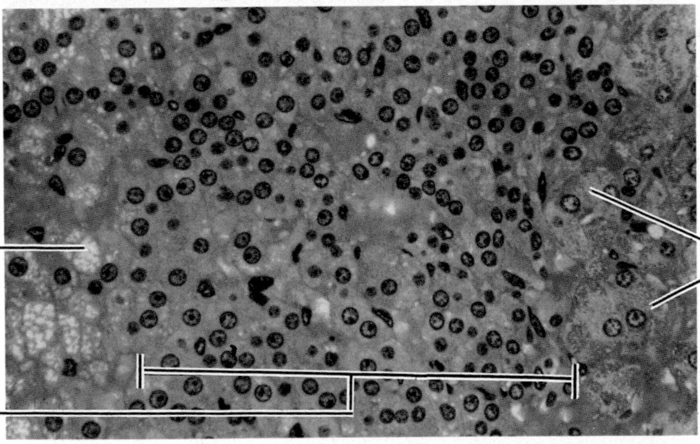

19-23

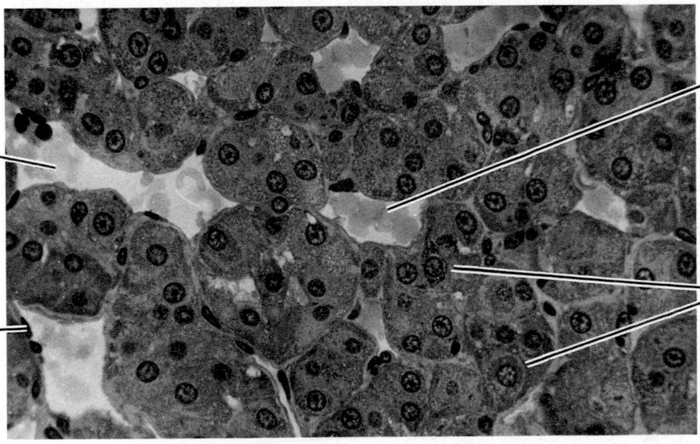

Figure 19-21. Adrenal cortex. LM, ×250.
Figure 19-22. Zona reticularis. LM, ×250.
Figure 19-23. Adrenal medulla. LM, ×325.

19-24 Development

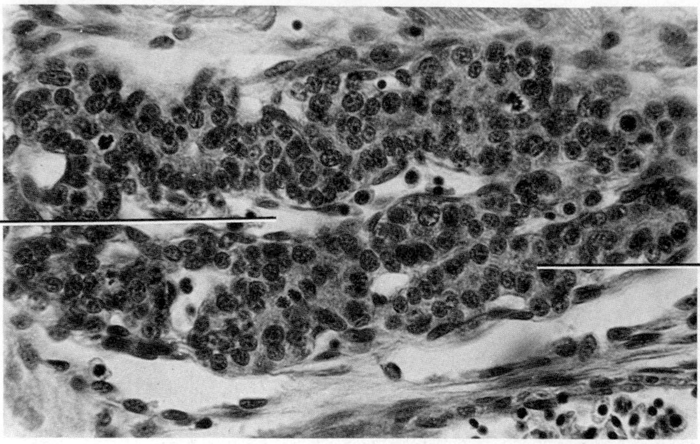

19-25

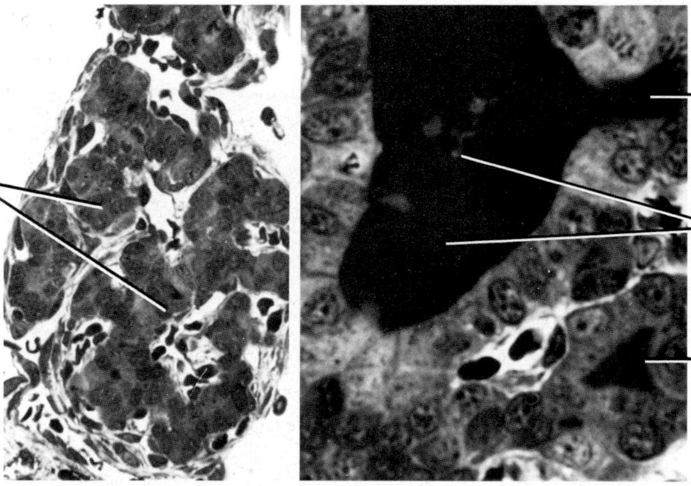

19-26

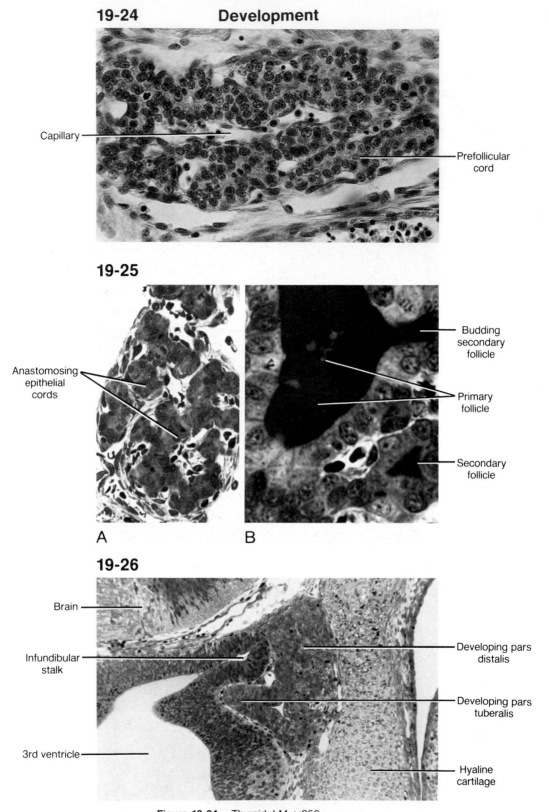

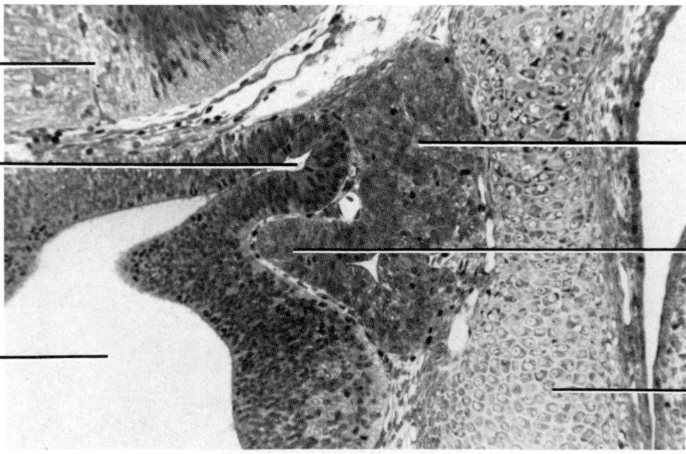

Figure 19-24. Thyroid. LM, ×250.
Figure 19-25. Thyroid. LM: *A*, ×200; *B*, ×400.
Figure 19-26. Hypophysis. LM, ×100.

19-27

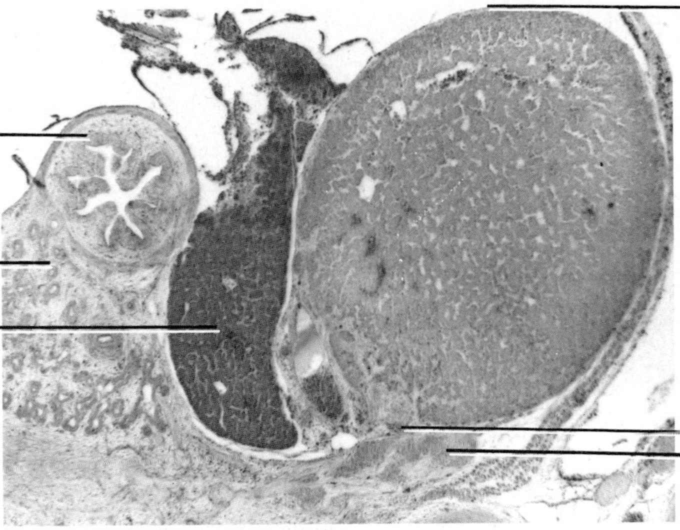

19-28

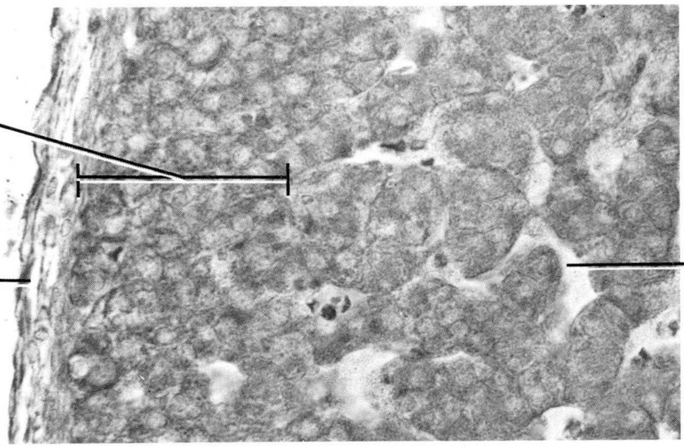

19-29

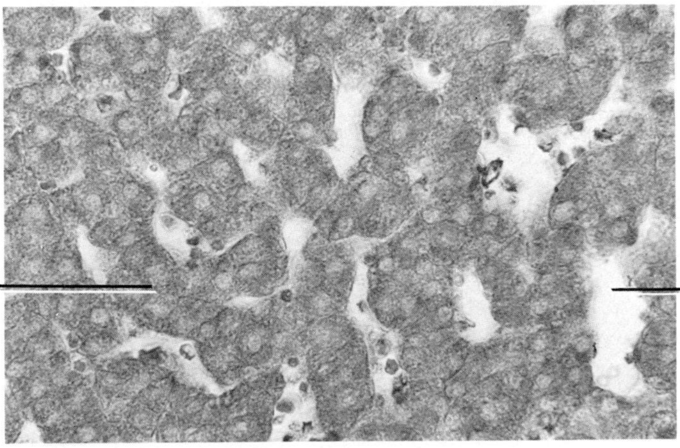

Figure 19-27. Adrenal (40-day human). LM, ×15.
Figure 19-28. Adrenal cortex (40-day human). LM, ×250.
Figure 19-29. Deep adrenal cortex (40-day human). LM, ×250.

Appendix

Key Features in the Recognition of Structures with Similar Morphology

Appendix Table 1.
Key Histological Features in Identifying Cartilage, Bone and Tendon

	Arrangement of Cells and Lacunae	Other Features
Hyaline cartilage	Glass-like matrix; lacunae randomly distributed, slit-like in appearance near perichondrium	Isogenous groups; territorial matrix
Elastic cartilage	Matrix more fibrous in appearance; elastic fibers (need to be stained selectively)	Large isogenous groups
Decalcified bone	Lacunae show organization within lamellae of osteons; Haversian canals	Tide marks; bone marrow
Ground bone	Haversian systems; interstitial and circumferential lamellae	Canaliculi between lacunae
Fibrocartilage	Dense fibrous connective tissue a dominant feature with a small amount of ground substance; lacunae few in number and scattered between fibers	Round-shaped chondrocytes
Tendon	Fibroblast nuclei are densely stained and elongate; lie in parallel rows between bundles and fibers of collagen	Lacunae absent

Appendix Table 2.
Key Histological Features in the Recognition of Connective Tissue, Muscle and Nerve

	Characteristics of Nuclei	Shape and Orientation of Cells and/or Fibers	Additional Features
Loose areolar connective tissue	Fibroblast nuclei stain either intensely or lightly, appear scattered within extracellular material	Fibroblasts and extracellular fibers are randomly oriented. Extracellular fibers stain intensely.	Scattered fat cells; adipose tissue
Peripheral nerve	Numerous Schwann cell nuclei, stain lightly, may be stippled in appearance	Schwann cells (nuclei) oriented parallel to nerve axons	Undulating or wavy appearance of discrete bundle; limited by perineurium; nodes of Ranvier and axons may be visible
Smooth muscle	Single, oval-shaped, light staining nucleus per cell	Small, spindle-shaped cells; single central nucleus; well-stained cytoplasm	Cells organized into sheets or layers; scant intervening connective tissue
Dense regular connective tissue	Dense-staining, elongate fibroblast nuclei organized in rows	Large, dense-staining fibers arranged in parallel; fibers and fibroblasts orderly arranged in same direction	
Skeletal muscle	Numerous light-staining peripheral nuclei within each cell	Cells arranged in same direction per fascicle; striations of cell visible in longitudinal section	Connective tissue visible around individual cells, organizes several cells into fascicles
Cardiac muscle	Usually a single, large, light-staining central nucleus; occasional cell (fiber) shows 2–3 nuclei	Large branching cells, orientated in same direction as others in a specific layer; cross striations as for skeletal muscle	Intercalated discs

Appendix Table 3.
Key Histological Features in Identifying Major Glandular Structures

	Secretory Units	Ductal System	Other Features
Parotid	All acini (alveoli) and tubules are serous	Prominent intercalated ducts; intralobular duct system prominent	Numerous fat cells in man
Pancreas	Acini and tubules are serous; cells pyramidal in shape	Centroacinar cells; prominent intralobular ducts	Islets of Langerhans
Lacrimal gland	All acini and tubules are serous; cells low columnar	Ductal system inconspicuous	Occasional fat cells, gland small in size
Submandibular gland	Most of acini and tubules are serous; some mucous tubules capped with serous demilunes	Very prominent intralobular duct system especially striated ducts—numerous profiles in each lobule	Occasional fat cells
Sublingual gland	Mucous and serous acini and tubules equal in abundance; mucous tubules capped by serous demilunes	Duct system not prominent	Occasional fat cells
Thyroid	Large follicles filled with gelatinous colloid	Absent	Nests of parafollicular cells between follicles
Lactating mammary gland	Large, expanded alveoli contain thin secretion	Ducts visible in interlobular connective tissue	Lobulated
Nonlactating mammary gland	Alveoli poorly developed	Intralobular and interlobular ducts visible	Lobulated, loose connective tissue and fat abundant
Parathyroid gland	Irregular cores of serous cells: individual or clumps of oxyphil cells	Absent	Abundant fat cells in gland and surrounding connective tissue
Adenohypophysis	Irregular cores or clumps of epithelial cells: basophils, acidophils, chromophobes	Absent	Abundant capillaries in surrounding connective tissue
Adrenal	Cortex: cells arranged into epithelial cords separated by sinusoids, three zones; Medulla: large, light staining cells	Absent	Cortex—dark staining Medulla—light staining
Ovary	Ovarian follicles in cortex	Absent	Surface covering mesothelium; cortex; medulla of connective tissue and blood vessels
Kidney	Parenchyma consists of tubules forming the nephrons; large scattered, renal corpuscles	Large, light staining collecting ducts in medulla and medullary rays	Cortex—dark staining tubules Medulla—light staining tubules running in parallel
Testis	Seminiferous tubules, spermatogenic cells	Rete testis Efferent ductules	Tunica albuginea, septae, interstitial cells

Appendix Table 4.
Key Histological Features of Major Tubular Structures

Organ	Epithelial Lining	Muscle Coats	Special Features
Esophagus	Nonkeratinized stratified squamous	Prominent muscularis mucosae, muscularis externa of inner circular and outer longitudinal skeletal (upper ¼), mixed smooth and skeletal (middle ¼), smooth (lower ½)	Glands present in submucosa; may occur in lamina propria at distal and proximal ends
Small intestine	Simple columnar, striated border; goblet cells	Muscularis mucosae and externa, inner circular, outer longitudinal smooth muscle	Villi; intestinal glands; glands in submucosa of duodenum, Peyer's patches in ileum
Colon	Simple columnar, striated border; more goblet cells	Outer longitudinal layer of muscularis externa thinner except for taenia coli	No villi, smooth luminal surface, intestinal glands
Appendix	Simple columnar, goblet cells	Muscularis mucosae obscured by lymphocytic infiltration	No villi; much nodular and diffuse lymphatic tissue
Trachea and main bronchi	Ciliated pseudostratified columnar; goblet cells	Thin muscularis mucosae	Cartilage rings
Aorta	Simple squamous (endothelium)	Tunica media dominant layer, smooth muscle and elastic laminae	Lumen usually circular in outline. Vasa vasorum
Muscular artery	Endothelium	Prominent muscular tunica media	Internal and external elastic laminae
Vena cava and large veins	Endothelium	Tunica, adventitia is main layer—collagen, elastic and smooth muscle fibers	Lumen often irregular
Vagina	Nonkeratinized stratified squamous	No muscularis mucosae. External coat of inner circular, and outer longitudinal smooth muscle	Prominent venous plexus in lamina propria; no glands
Oviduct	Simple ciliated columnar	External muscle—inner circular, outer longitudinal smooth muscle, cellular lamina propria	(a) Ampulla—mucosa elaborately branched, lumen narrow spaces (b) Isthmus—mucosa less branched, lumen a single space
Ureter	Transitional epithelium	Proximal ⅔, inner longitudinal, outer circular smooth muscle. Distal ⅓ inner longitudinal; middle circular, outer longitudinal	Stellate lumen
Vas deferens	Pseudostratified columnar	Inner longitudinal, middle circular, outer longitudinal smooth muscle	Irregular lumen bounded by a thick muscle coat

Appendix Table 5.
Key Histological Features in Identifying Major Abrupt Junctions

	Changes in Epithelium	Other Features
Olfactory—respiratory junction of nasal cavity	Olfactory to ciliated pseudostratified columnar with goblet cells	Thick lamina propria containing nerves, serous glands and venous sinuses *to* a thin, vascular lamina propria
Oropharynx—nasopharynx junction at edge of soft palate	Nonkeratinized stratified squamous *to* ciliated pseudostratified columnar with goblet cells	Central core of skeletal muscle, mucous/seromucous glands in connective tissue underlying epithelium
Integument—oral mucosal junction at vermillion border of lip	Typical thin skin with hair follicles, sebaceous glands and sweat glands *to* a thick, nonkeratinized stratified squamous	Typical dermis of thin skin *to* a thick submucosa with tall connective tissue papillae extending into the oral epithelium; labial salivary glands; skeletal muscle core between the skin and oral mucosa
Esophageal—gastric junction	Thick, nonkeratinized stratified squamous *to* simple columnar	Branched tubular glands of esophagus *to* gastric pits and simple branched tubular cardiac glands of stomach
Gastrointestinal junction	Simple columnar *to* simple columnar with striated (microvillus) border and goblet cells	Gastric pits, pyloric glands *to* villi, intestinal glands, Brunner's glands in submucosa
Rectoanal junction	Simple columnar with striated border and goblet cells *to* nonkeratinized stratified squamous epithelium	Intestinal glands and muscularis mucosae of rectum *lost* at rectoanal junction
Vaginal-cervical junction	Nonkeratinized stratified squamous *to* tall, light-staining simple columnar	Coarse, vascular lamina propria devoid of glands, muscularis of smooth muscle *to* dense connective tissue wall containing cervical glands, Nabothian cysts

Index

Page numbers in italics refer to Atlas illustrations.

James E. Rogers